Paediatric Intensive Care Nursing

For Churchill Livingstone:

Senior Commissioning Editor: Ninette Premdas
Project Development Manager: Dinah Thom
Design Direction: George Ajayi

Paediatric Intensive Care Nursing

Edited by

Carol Williams BA(Hons) MSc RGN RSCN
Clinical Nurse Specialist, PICU, Guy's and St Thomas' NHS Trust, London

Julie Asquith DipN DipMngt RGN RSCN
Senior Nurse Manager, Guy's and St Thomas' NHS Trust, London

Foreword by

Margaret Fletcher BSc(Hons) PhD RSCN MRCPCH
Professor of Children's Nursing, South Bank University, London

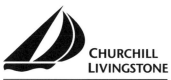

CHURCHILL LIVINGSTONE

EDINBURGH LONDON NEW YORK PHILADELPHIA ST LOUIS SYDNEY TORONTO 2000

Churchill Livingstone
An imprint of Harcourt Publishers Limited

© Harcourt Publishers Limited 2000

◢ is a registered trade mark of Harcourt Publishers
Limited 2000

First published 2000

ISBN 0 4430 5528 9

British Library Cataloguing in Publication Data
A catalogue record for this book is available from the British
Library.

Library of Congress Cataloging in Publication Data
A catalog record for this book is available from the Library of
Congress.

Note
Medical knowledge is constantly changing. As new
information becomes available, changes in treatment,
procedures, equipment and the use of drugs become
necessary. The editors, contributors and the publishers have,
as far as it is possible, taken care to ensure that the
information given in this text is accurate and up to date.
However, readers are strongly advised to confirm that the
information, especially with regard to drug usage, complies
with the latest legislation and standards of practice.

The
publisher's
policy is to use
**paper manufactured
from sustainable forests**

Printed in China

Contents

Contributors

Yvette Arendse AdvDipChildHealth RGN RSCN
Senior Staff Nurse, Paediatric Intensive Care
Unit, Great Ormond Street Hospital NHS Trust,
London, UK

Julie Asquith DipN DipMngt RGN RSCN
Senior Nurse Manager, Guy's and St Thomas'
NHS Trust, London, UK

S. Attard-Montalto MBChB FRCP FRCPCH DCH
Chairman, Department of Paediatrics, St Luke's
Hospital, Gwardamangia, Malta

Rebecca Brownlie RN RSCN
Formerly Senior Sister, Paediatric Intensive Care
Unit, St Mary's Hospital, London, UK

Mollie Cook BSc(Hons)Psychol DipCouns RGN RSCN
Ward Sister/Family Support Nurse-Counsellor,
Paediatric Intensive Care Unit, Guy's Hospital,
London, UK

Rebecca Dallmeyer DipPharmPrac MRPharmS
BPharm
Formerly Senior Paediatric Pharmacist, Guy's
and St Thomas' NHS Trust, London, UK

Karon Dyke RGN RSCN
Sister, The Birmingham Children's Hospital
NHS Trust, Birmingham, UK

Anne-Marie England BSc(Hons) RGN RSCN
Senior Lecturer in Intensive Care Nursing of
Children, Faculty of Health and Community
Care, University of Central England in
Birmingham, Birmingham, UK

Jayne Fisher DipICN RGN RSCN
Senior Sister, Paediatric Intensive Care Unit, The
General Infirmary at Leeds, Leeds, UK

Alison French BSc(Hons) SRD
Senior Dietitian, The National Centre for Brain
Injury Rehabilitation, St Andrew's Hospital,
Northampton

Alison Green RGN RSCN
Paediatric Community Nursing Sister,
Oldchurch Hospital, Romford, UK

Elizabeth Gibbons RGN RSCN
Sister, ITU, The Birmingham Children's Hospital
NHS Trust, Birmingham, UK

Caroline Haines PGDE BSc RGN RSCN
Lecturer/Practitioner, Paediatric Intensive Care
Unit, Bristol Royal Hospital for Sick Children;
Faculty of Health and Social Care, University of
the West of England, Bristol, UK

Kate Hall BSc RN RNT
Senior Lecturer, IHCS, Bournemouth University,
Bournemouth, UK

Judith Harris BSc(Hons) RGN RSCN
Lecturer-Practitioner, Paediatric Intensive Care
Unit, Guy's and St Thomas' NHS Trust, London,
UK

Dawn Harrison MA RGN RSCN
Lecturer in Child Health Studies, University of
York, York District Hospital, York, UK

Yvonne Hill RGN RN(Child) Diploma Child Health
Senior Staff Nurse, Paediatric Intensive Care
Unit, Great Ormond Street Hospital NHS Trust,
London, UK

Eiri Jones RGN RSCN
Cardiac Outreach Nurse, Guy's and St Thomas'
NHS Trust, London, UK

Jos Latour RN MScN
Nurse Manager, Paediatric Intensive Care Unit,
University Hospital 'Vrije Universiteit',
Amsterdam, The Netherlands

Karen Lockhart RSCN
Sister, Paediatric Haemodialysis Unit, Guy's and
St Thomas' NHS Trust, London, UK

Rachelle Lowe RGN RSCN
Sister, Paediatric Haemodialysis Unit, Guy's and
St Thomas' NHS Trust, London, UK

Alan G. Magee MRCP MRCPCH MB BCh
Consultant Paediatric Cardiologist, Royal
Brompton and Harefield NHS Trust, London,
UK

Michael Marsh FRCPCH MRCP MBBS
Consultant in Paediatric Intensive Care, Guy's
and St Thomas' NHS Trust, London, UK

Gavin Morrison MRCP DCH
Paediatric Intensive Care Unit, The Birmingham
Children's Hospital NHS Trust, Birmingham,
UK

Simon Nadel MRCP MB
Consultant in Paediatric Intensive Care, St
Mary's Hospital, London, UK

Tina Sajjanhar MRCPCH MRCP MBBS DRCOG DCH
Consultant Paediatrician, Lewisham Children's
Hospital, London, UK

Petra Shroff RGN RSCN Advanced Diploma Child
Health
Senior Staff Nurse, Paediatric Intensive Care
Unit, Great Ormond Street Hospital NHS Trust,
London, UK

Heather E. Steele DPSN RGN RSCN
Senior Sister, Paediatric Intensive Care Unit, The
Birmingham Children's Hospital NHS Trust,
Birmingham, UK

Bernie Steer DipM RSCN
Clinical Sister/ECMO Specialist, Cardiac
Intensive Care Unit, Great Ormond Street NHS
Trust, London, UK

Jenny Walker FRCPCH ChM FRCS MB ChB
Consultant Paediatric Surgeon, Children's
Hospital, Sheffield, UK

Trudy A. Ward BSc(Hons) RGN RSCN
Senior Clinical Nurse Manager, Chailey Heritage
Clinical Services, South Downs Health NHS
Trust, East Sussex, UK

Colin Way BSc(Hons) DipN(Lon) RGN RSCN
Lecturer Practitioner, Paediatric Intensive Care
Unit, Guy's and St Thomas' NHS Trust, London,
UK

Stephanie Wheeler BSc(Hons) RGN RM RHV PGCEA
Senior Lecturer, Institute of Health and
Community Studies, Bournemouth University,
Bournemouth, UK

Carol Williams BA(Hons) MSc RGN RSCN
Clinical Nurse Specialist, Paediatric Intensive
Care Unit, Guy's and St Thomas' NHS Trust,
London, UK

Michelle Wolstenholme DipAdvN RGN RSCN
Formerly Staff Nurse, Paediatric Intensive Care
Unit, Bristol Royal Hospital for Sick Children,
Bristol, UK

Foreword

Paediatric intensive care is more than simply a specialty. It requires more of the practitioner than technical skill, scientific knowledge and an ability to be caring. In a specialty noted for high levels of physical demands and emotional stress, all those involved in the care of the child and family must still provide knowledgeable, competent and caring professional support. Only with a secure understanding of the principles involved in the cycle of care can all members of the multi-disciplinary team contribute fully to managing these children with such very special needs.

As technology and science move the boundaries forward, so we need to consider the implications for, and of, our practice. Decisions become more complicated and families (and children) need ever more support and information to be able to participate in making these decisions.

The contents of this text provide a clear, concise, detailed resource to meet the theory needs of those giving care in what are becoming clearly distinct care settings. Paediatric intensive care is increasingly delivered through a hierarchical structure, demanding different skills of the practitioner. The skills and knowledge demanded at centres undertaking local stabilisation of the sick child will differ from those required for retrieval and subsequent care in a designated centre. In addition, we increasingly have the ability to maintain children with complex technological and monitoring needs in their own community and in transitional care facilities. Although this is seldom referred to as intensive care, the team supporting the child requires more than a passing understanding of the principles involved.

All these issues are addressed in the text, reinforcing the fact that this is a dynamic and changing field at the centre of which is the developing child and his or her family.

Margaret Fletcher

Preface

The purpose of this book is to provide all nurses working with critically ill children with information about current practice in this rapidly developing specialty. The layout of the book enables nurses to use it for quick reference information related to specific problems or as a text for study purposes. The use of professionals from multiple disciplines fulfils two aims:

- to provide expert knowledge in each aspect of management of critically ill children;
- to reflect the multidisciplinary framework outlined by the Department of Health in *Paediatric Intensive Care: A Framework for the Future* (1997).

The Departement of Health suggested that the most effective management of this group of children would be provided within the type of multidisciplinary team found in specialist centres. The key personnel constituting sucah a team include:

- paediatric intensivist (and medical team)
- specialist physician
- specialist surgeon
  paediatric intensive care nurses
- paediatric anaesthetist
- paediatric physiotherapist
- dietician
- specialist technicians.

In addition to the above, support services such as pathology, haematology, chemistry, portering, radiology and microbiology are essential.

This book is divided into three sections, each of which has a specific focus.

Section 1 addresses the issues of assessment, resuscitation and monitoring which are aspects of the management of all critically ill children. The chapter on retrieval amalgamates these concepts to provide an overview of the development and requirements of a retrieval service. Issues discussed in these chapters are not repeated elsewhere in the book.

Section 2 takes a systematic approach to the management of children with specific problems. The anatomy and physiology included in each chapter are those relating specifically to children. The book assumes the reader has an understanding of basic anatomy and physiology. The cardiac and respiratory systems have been divided into two chapters each, one dealing with the essential anatomy and physiology, and one with specific problems and their management. As editors, we believe that in-depth knowledge of these systems is essential for the management of all critically ill children. The contributors to these sections have considerable expertise in each specific area.

Section 3 addresses aspects of children's intensive care nursing that often are not immediately considered when faced with a critically ill child. The one exception to this is perhaps the pharmacological chapter. This chapter is placed here, despite having elements relevent to Section 1, as it deals mostly with the ongoing management of the critically ill child. The remaining chapters are essential when considering the holistic needs of the child and their family.

We hope that nurses reading this book find it easy to use and informative. Our aim was to provide a textbook that included all aspects of care relevant to the critically ill child. However, this rapidly developing specialty frequently provides us with new challenges and technology. This book will provide therefore the foundation on which nurses can develop their knowledge and expertise.

Carol Williams
London 1999   Julie Asquith

Acknowledgements

We would like to thank all contributors for their hard work.

Thanks to our family and friends, who supported us throughout this project.

1

Introduction

Julie Asquith

As a result of advances in technology, children with major illnesses now have greater chances of survival than previously. For example, children with congenital heart defects have benefited from advances in non-invasive techniques, aiding diagnosis and treatment. In addition surgical techniques and postoperative multiple organ support, such as extracorporeal membrane oxygenation, have enabled treatment in children who were previously considered inoperable. Organ transplantation has also had a major impact on the survival of infants and children with irreversible organ failure. Advances in ventilatory therapies in the last decade have included adapting ventilatory modes that are frequently used in adult intensive care, improving expertise in oscillation and, more recently, the developing area of liquid ventilation. Pharmacological advances have also played a major part in the intensive care revolution, with more effective pain relief and considerable advances in vasoactive drugs. The ability to treat major infections, for example pneumocystis in infants who are immunosuppressed, has largely been due to the development of antimicrobial therapy.

Paediatric Intensive Care (PIC) has developed in a piecemeal fashion alongside these advances in care, with little strategic planning. Critically ill children appear wherever there is an accident and emergency department. District General Hospitals have always been faced with a decision as to where to care for the child. A variety of solutions have been adopted, including caring for the critically ill child on a general children's ward, within Adult Intensive Care or Neonatal

Intensive Care Units or by transferring the child to another hospital with PIC facilities. The standard of care given therefore varies considerably depending on the skills and knowledge of the medical and nursing staff.

Those working within PIC have been aware of the shortfalls in provision for a significant period of time but have had little support to make changes. In 1987 the British Paediatric Association (BPA) produced the first report on PIC, followed in 1992 by a document produced by the Paediatric Intensive Care Society on *Standards for paediatric intensive care*. In December 1993 the BPA published a second report, *The care of critically ill children*, which highlighted the shortcomings of the current provision and made a number of key recommendations. However, it was only in 1996, after the public enquiry into the death of Nicholas Geldard, that the Department of Health set up a National Co-ordinating Group on Paediatric Intensive Care who produced the report *A framework for the future* in 1997. This document provided a strategic direction for PIC, applying a hub-and-spoke arrangement with a Lead Centre(s) within each region providing a PIC retrieval service. It is more likely that large Lead Centres will be able to meet the winter peaks in demand without wasting resources at other times in addition to effectively running the retrieval service. These arrangements should provide more equity of access to appropriate facilities for critically ill children.

In order to make this happen the training and education of medical and nursing staff is paramount. The availability of trained paediatric intensive care nurses was identified as one of the major issues in the BPA report (1993). A multidisciplinary task force led by the Chief Nursing Officer reviewed the nurse staffing of PIC and produced a report alongside that from the National Co-ordinating Group. This made some helpful recommendations regarding the recruitment and retention of these highly skilled nurses. Education and training was recognised as a key issue in the strategic development of this specialty. Larger units will be able to play an effective role in the training of nursing and medical staff in paediatric intensive care.

It should also be recognised that there is a great opportunity for multidisciplinary education. In this highly technical area the roles of the doctor and nurse are less clearly delineated. The advanced nurse practitioner has already been well defined in neonatal intensive care; whilst the requirements within paediatric intensive care may have a different emphasis, the concept is shared. As the education of junior doctors changes and their working hours become more restricted, it is likely that the nursing staff will provide the continuity in care and a high level of expertise. We must also recognise the significant contribution that professionals allied to medicine can provide.

It is clear from the survey for the BPA report (1993) and the Department of Health report (1997) that there are insufficient data on which to plan paediatric intensive care. There is also very little UK evidence of the benefits of PIC in terms of outcome. Some areas of the UK have now begun this work, to assess need and to map out provision. These data need to be qualitative and quantitative to demonstrate the real benefit of the service.

The internal market of the NHS did a great disservice to the development of this specialty, fostering a competitive culture that impaired strategic development; but, as we move into a more collaborative approach to healthcare, we should see health providers working together to provide the best service to the child and family. If we can keep the child and family as the central focus, we are more likely to get the model right. This is a high-cost service, and effective use of resources is essential.

The contributing authors of this book come from a variety of backgrounds, as befits a specialty which relies on multidisciplinary learning and collaboration to further develop the service provided to critically ill children.

REFERENCES

British Paediatric Association 1993 The care of critically ill children. British Paediatric Association, London

Department of Health 1997 Paediatric intensive care: a framework for the future. NHS Executive, Department of Health, London

Department of Health 1997 A bridge to the future. NHS Executive, Department of Health, London

Paediatric Intensive Care Society 1992 Standards for paediatric intensive care. Mosby-Year Book Europe Limited, St Louis

Resuscitation, Stabilisation and Monitoring

The section provides an overview of the issues surrounding resuscitation and stabilisation of all infants and children requiring intensive care. The cardiopulmonary resuscitation and transportation chapters will not relate to all children, but aim to provide an overview of the issues relevant to practice, including the current UK resuscitation guidelines. The monitoring and assessment chapters will underpin the management of all infants and children requiring intensive care treatment. These aim to provide practitioners with the knowledge to underpin and improve their practice in these areas.

2

Assessment of the critically ill child

Carol Williams

Assessment of the critically ill child is a complex process, which initially focuses on the physiological status of the child, but also includes information about development and psychosocial issues. This chapter addresses these areas and provides methods of ensuring a comprehensive assessment using a modification of Roy's Adaptation Model (Fraser 1996).

The purpose of assessment is to collect information about the critically ill child, identifying problems in order to plan the management required. This is essential at all stages of a child's treatment, but the most comprehensive assessment often takes place on or shortly after admission. The treatment and care that the child receives will be based on this information; therefore, thorough assessment is required.

Information is gathered by taking a history, undertaking a physical examination, collecting biochemical data and monitoring physiological signs. A variety of tools can be used to collect this information, including neurological and pain assessment tools. However, a formal structure or model for assessment enables practitioners to collect all relevant information. Nursing assessment can be structured around a nursing model, whereas medical assessment is often structured around biological systems.

The assessment tool described by Hazinski (1992) can be very useful for staff new to intensive care and can be adapted to provide a holistic approach (Box 2.1). This tool is particularly useful as it highlights areas that are important when assessing infants and children, including temperature, growth and development and the immune system. However, many experienced practitioners develop their own assessment structure. Whichever structure is used, it is important that practitioners remember to use their senses such as sight, hearing and touch. These are used during the processes of:

- observation
- palpation
- percussion
- auscultation.

Box 2.1 Adapted nine-point assessment tool

A: Airway/breathing
B: Brain
C: Circulation
· Creed and culture
D: Drips/drugs/drains
Discomfort
E: Electrolytes
Energy requirements
F: Fluids
Family
G: Gastrointestinal/genitourinary
Growth and development
H: Heat (thermoregulation)
I: Infection

Adapted from Hazinski (1992).

Observation. Observation should take place in a well-lit environment with the child at rest. Practitioners initially observe the child's body for position, activity, symmetry and colour. This enables immediate priorities to be established. Ongoing observation often includes monitoring of vital signs and physiological parameters.

Palpation. Palpation involves using the hands to determine the texture, temperature and abnormalities or painful areas over the surface of the body. It is important to observe the child's reaction to the examination to determine tender areas.

Percussion. Percussion involves determination of the type of sound produced when an area is percussed with the fingers. Hyperresonant sounds are indicative of air-filled cavities, whilst dull sounds suggest fluid or solid tissue. It is important to remember that the infant's lungs are often hyperresonant, making interpretation of sounds more difficult.

Auscultation. Auscultation involves assessing noises using a stethoscope and is particularly important in assessment of heart sounds, the respiratory system and gastrointestinal tract.

TAKING A HISTORY

When taking a history, all aspects of the child's life should be included. For inexperienced practitioners a rigid structure can be used to ensure that all relevant information is obtained which will provide a full picture of the child up to the time of his illness. This information should include:

- past medical history and details of the current illness
- a developmental history including education and language
- normal diet
- spiritual/cultural needs
- information about the child's 'community' including his major carer and family
- normal daily routine.

This information will be collected from the parents for the majority of critically ill children. However, in some situations, a teacher, childminder or other responsible adult may be the only person available to provide relevant details. Therefore, it may not be possible to take a full history on admission. This may have to be completed at a later time.

PHYSIOLOGICAL ASSESSMENT

Many treatments used in the management of critically ill children are based on weight. It is important for practitioners to be able to rapidly determine a child's weight when no accurate weight is available. The following formulae can be used to estimate weight in kilograms:

- infants: the average birth weight is 3.5 kg; infants double this by 5 to 6 months and treble it by 1 year
- 1 to 9 years: (age + 4) $\times$ 2
- 7 to 12 years: age $\times$ 3.

Oxygenation

During physiological assessment, the emphasis is on the cardiorespiratory system, which rapidly becomes compromised during primary and secondary illness. Both cardiac and respiratory systems are essential for effective oxygenation and removal of waste products of metabolism.

Initial assessment of the cardiorespiratory system includes:

- respiratory rate
- heart rate
- blood pressure
- peripheral pulses
- capillary refill time
- colour
- central and skin temperature (core–toe gap)
- level of consciousness.

It is important to know the normal parameters for age for respiratory and heart rates and blood pressure (Table 2.1). When assessing these, other factors should be considered including sleep, position and activity, pain, emotions, medications and fever, which all produce significant variation in vital signs for all age groups. Heart rate can double in infants from 90 beats per minute during sleep to 180 beats when crying. Respiratory rates should be assessed for a full minute, as it is normal for infants to have irregular breathing patterns.

Persistent bradycardia can significantly reduce cardiac output, as the infant's ventricle is unable to stretch to increase stroke volume and maintain cardiac output. Ventricular filling can be severely compromised by persistent tachycardias and dysrhythmias, such as nodal rhythm. This will result in a reduction in cardiac output and systemic arterial pressure.

Neonatal blood pressure will be lower than in older infants, as the left ventricle is small and thin-walled at birth. As the heart grows and the wall thickens, the force of contraction and stroke volume increase to provide effective circulation. Raised blood pressure (BP) is unusual in the resting child and is normally associated with renal disease, coarctation of the aorta or phaeochromocytoma. However, anxiety may increase BP, and failure to use equipment appropriately may produce abnormal readings. It must be remembered that a low blood pressure is a late sign of cardiovascular compromise.

When undertaking non-invasive BP recordings, the cuff should measure two thirds of the distance between the joints such as the shoulder and elbow. A wider cuff will produce low readings, and a narrow cuff high readings. The cuff should also encircle the whole of the limb to give an accurate recording. When invasive BP monitoring is available, it is important to calibrate the equipment prior to use.

Respiratory disease is the commonest cause of admission to intensive care during childhood. Therefore, when assessing respiratory function, it is important for practitioners to understand the anatomical differences in the airway and how this relates to assessment data.

The respiratory tract of the infant and young child is immature, with significant development occurring during early childhood (Engel 1997). The size and structure of the airways and lungs contribute to the signs observed in young children with respiratory difficulty.

Infants are obligatory nose breathers until the age of 6 months and will, therefore, exhibit signs of respiratory distress if the nostrils become blocked with mucus. The tongue is large in relation to the oral cavity in children below 2 years of age, increasing the risk of obstruction during alterations in consciousness level. The upper airway contains large amounts of lymph tissue, which can cause obstruction if local infection occurs.

Table 2.1 Normal vital signs in infants and children

Age	Heart rate	Blood pressure	Respiratory rate
1 month	100–180	85/50	30–80
6 months	120–160	90/53	30–60
1 year	90–140	91/54	20–40
2 years	80–140	91/56	20–30
6 years	75–100	96/57	20–25
10 years	60–90	102/62	17–22
12 years	55–90	107/64	17–22
16 years	50–90	117/67	15–20

Sources: Hazinski (1992), Engel (1997).

The larynx is situated anteriorly at the level of C2–3, making it difficult to visualise in infants and young children. Gentle cricoid pressure can facilitate intubation by aiding visualisation of the cords and preventing aspiration of stomach contents.

The epiglottis is a floppy, elongated structure, inserted at a 45° angle in the pharyngeal wall. This makes it less effective at occluding the airway, increasing the risk of aspiration of a foreign body. A straight laryngoscope blade is required to lift the epiglottis and visualise the vocal cords in infants.

The cricoid cartilage is the narrowest part of the airway in children under 8 years of age. This will limit the size of endotracheal tube used and provide a natural seal around the tube, making the use of cuffed tubes unnecessary. Cuffed tubes used in this age group cause pressure in the subglottic region, risking damage to the developing airway, causing long-term problems and, in severe cases, the need for ENT surgery.

The trachea is short, with compliant cartilage, which contributes to airway occlusion if the airway is flexed or hyperextended. The chest wall is also highly compliant in infants and toddlers, as the ribs are cartilagenous. In addition, the ribs are placed horizontally until the child is school age. With the poorly developed intercostal muscles, this makes it difficult for young children to lift the rib cage during inspiration. The child is reliant on its diaphragm to increase lung volumes. These factors contribute to recession and abdominal breathing patterns often seen in young children with respiratory illness. A full stomach or distended abdomen can further impede respiratory function.

The infant's chest wall is thin, making it difficult to assess air entry on auscultation. Therefore, it is important to assess pitch and symmetry of sounds. Crackles may indicate pulmonary oedema, which develops frequently in infants with respiratory distress. This is possibly due to the combination of high pulmonary capillary pressures and a limited amount of elastic tissue. This contributes to poor lung compliance during infancy.

When taking a history, it is important to determine whether the child:

- was intubated during the neonatal period
- has any neurological deficit
- could have inhaled a foreign body
- becomes worse when feeding or crying
- has a fever
- has experienced a change in vocal sounds
- has suffered trauma
- is able to swallow.

When assessing the respiratory system, practitioners are firstly observing for signs of respiratory distress. Early signs include:

- increased respiratory and heart rates
- recession above the sternum (cricoid tug), between the ribs (intercostal recession), below the rib cage (subcostal recession) and of the sternum
- nasal flaring
- respiratory noises such as stridor and wheezing
- altered level of consciousness
- altered skin colour
- decreased oxygen saturations, low PaO_2 and high $PaCO_2$.

Late signs include grunting, reduced air entry, cyanosis, apnoea and poor peripheral perfusion. These signs should be treated as an emergency, requiring endotracheal intubation, to prevent the child progressing to respiratory arrest.

When assessing respiratory noises, it is important to note at which point during the respiratory cycle they occur. Stridor is commonly found in children with respiratory problems and can indicate the associated pathology (Gilbert et al 1993). Stridor results from vibration, caused by disruption to airflow in the narrow airways. It can indicate a variety of problems from supraglottic and subglottic obstruction, aspiration of a foreign body and, more rarely, a vascular ring. Inspiratory stridor suggests obstruction above the glottis, whilst stridor associated with inspiration and expiration indicates a problem at or below the cords. Foreign body aspiration may produce noises with no fixed pattern, as the obstruction may move, whilst a constant pattern may be indicative of vascular ring. Epiglottitis is often associated with inspiratory stridor and expiratory snoring (Engel 1997).

Wheezing is another common noise heard in childhood and is often associated with bronchiolitis and asthma. Inspiratory wheeze suggests an obstruction high in the airway, whilst expiratory wheeze is indicative of lower airway obstruction. The loss of a wheeze, in a previously wheezy child, can indicate very little air movement and imminent respiratory arrest.

Respiratory crackles are indicative of pulmonary oedema and pneumonia. The site of the problem will be indicated by the intensity of the noise. Fine crackles suggest fluid in the alveoli, and loud or coarse sounds indicate fluid in the bronchioles and bronchi (Engel 1997).

Children with a history of spasmodic coughing followed by a 'whoop' will usually have whooping cough. However, infants do not whoop, but have periods of apnoea following coughing, often requiring assisted ventilation.

Radiographic assessment will provide information about pathophysiological processes, but should not be undertaken if it puts the child at risk of further deterioration. However, the following can be used to determine underlying pathology:

- neck/chest X-ray
- CT scan
- MRI scan
- barium swallow (to diagnose tracheo-eosophageal fistula or vascular ring).

Noninvasive monitoring can be used to assess oxygenation and CO_2 elimination. Pulse oximetry assesses the percentage of oxygen–haemoglobin saturation. It is important to consider this along side PaO_2, as small changes in PaO_2 below 8 kPa (60 mmHg) can result in a large reduction in saturation. This is explained by the oxygen–haemoglobin dissociation curve (McCance & Heuther 1994) which plots the relationship between PaO_2 and haemoglobin saturation. Several factors change this relationship by reducing or increasing the rate at which oxygen dissociates from haemoglobin (Table 2.2). These should be assessed when considering oxygenation. Initial

Table 2.2 Factors affecting oxygen–haemoglobin dissociation

Reduced O_2 dissociation	Increased O_2 dissociation
Alkalosis	Acidosis
Low $PaCO_2$	High $PaCO_2$
Reduced temperature	High temperature
Low 2,3-DPG	High 2,3-DPG
Carboxyhaemoglobin	Abnormal haemoglobin
Methaemoglobin	
Abnormal haemoglobin	

Source: McCance & Heuther (1994).

interventions to improve oxygenation include increasing FiO_2 and maintaining haematocrit at 35–45%.

Haemoglobin levels will be high at birth, due to the presence of foetal haemoglobin (HbF). HbF is replaced during the first month of life by HbA or adult haemoglobin. By the end of the first month Hb has fallen to around 11 or 12 and increases gradually during childhood to reach adult levels of 14 to 15 by adolescence. During periods of critical illness and infection, haemolysis occurs, causing significant falls in Hb, which may necessitate transfusion. Although blood transfusion carries risks, the oxygen-carrying capacity of the blood may need to be improved by increasing haemoglobin to normal levels. In children with severe haemolysis, red cell size and shape should be assessed, as disorders such as sickle cell disease may be present. Polycythaemia may be present in children with cyanotic heart lesions or dehydration.

End tidal CO_2 can be used with the intubated child to determine the concentration of exhaled CO_2 at the end of expiration. This represents the final portion of gas exhaled from the lungs and can, therefore, reflect the $PaCO_2$. Normal values are 5.1–5.3 kPa (38–40 mmHg). In neonates and young infants, transcutaneous CO_2 monitoring can offer an alternative estimation of $PaCO_2$.

In both cases the monitoring equipment should be calibrated against the arterial CO_2 to provide an accurate reflection of changes in $PaCO_2$.

In the ventilated child it is now possible to display ventilatory curves and loops on a screen either integral to or attached to the ventilator.

Changes in pressure, volume and flow can occur as a result of manipulation of the ventilator parameters or from changes in the child's lungs. When ventilatory settings remain constant, assessment of lung compliance, airway resistance and lung distension is possible (Rittner & Doring 1997).

All of the above can be used to assess respiratory function in the critically ill child, but the widely accepted method for assessment of respiratory gas exchange is evaluation of arterial blood gases. Respiratory failure is characterised by a reduction in CO_2 excretion and poor oxygenation due either to lung pathology or failure of the respiratory pump. Estimation of arterial blood gases enables assessment of management aimed at overcoming these problems. Arterial blood gases measure:

- hydrogen ion concentration (pH)
- CO_2 concentration ($PaCO_2$)
- O_2 concentration (PaO_2)
- bicarbonate levels ($SHCO_3$)
- base excess/deficit.

Bicarbonate and base are a reflection of the metabolic component of acid–base balance controlled by the kidneys. CO_2 and O_2 concentrations are a reflection of the respiratory component or respiratory function. Significant changes in respiratory and renal function will lead to changes in pH. Maintenance of pH within normal limits is essential for homeostasis. Cell membrane and enzyme functions are particularly affected by abnormal pH. Therefore, the buffer, respiratory and renal systems work to maintain pH within normal limits (Table 2.3) (Chapters 7 and 11). When interpreting blood gases, practitioners can quickly determine disturbances and the body's attempt to compensate for these (Table 2.4). Firstly, the pH should be observed to determine whether it is normal or reflects acidosis (< 7.35) or alkalosis (> 7.45). The practitioner then assesses the $PaCO_2$ and HCO_3 to determine whether the disturbance is metabolic or respiratory. For example:

pH	7.189
$PaCO_2$	10.18 kPa
$SHCO_3$	24.1
Base	−0.4

Table 2.3 Normal blood gas values during childhood

	Neonate	Infant/child
pH	7.3–7.4	7.35–7.45
$PaCO_2$	4.5–6.0	4.5–6.0
PaO_2	8–10	10–13
$SHCO_3$	20–24	22–26
Base excess/deficit	−2 to +2	−2 to +2

Table 2.4 Findings in acid–base disturbances with and without compensation

	Uncompensated			Compensated		
	pH	$PaCO_2$	HCO_3	pH	$PaCO_2$	HCO_3
Metabolic acidosis	L	N	L	H/N	L	L
Metabolic alkalosis	H	N	H	L/N	H	H
Respiratory acidosis	L	H	N	H/N	H	H
Respiratory alkalosis	H	L	N	L/N	L	L

L = low, N = normal, H = high.

suggests an acidotic child with an elevated CO_2, indicating a respiratory acidosis. The bicarbonate and base are normal, indicating an acute episode with no compensation. The body attempts to compensate by retaining bicarbonate in an attempt to return pH to normal:

pH	7.29
$PaCO_2$	7.5 kPa
$SHCO_3$	27.2
Base	+2.9

An elevated bicarbonate with abnormal pH would suggest partial compensation, whilst high HCO_3 with a normal pH would suggest full compensation:

pH	7.36
$PaCO_2$	7.3 kPa
$SHCO_3$	28.6
Base	+3.4

To determine which system is compensating for the other, practitioners should examine how the pH deviates from 7.4 (neutral) and which of the parameters reflects this. Therefore, the results above suggest a fully compensated respiratory acidosis, as pH is < 7.4. This tends towards acidosis, which is reflected in the high CO_2, whereas the high HCO_3 reflects alkalosis.

Practitioners can anticipate potential acid–base disturbances following assessment of history of the illness, vital signs and requirements for respiratory and cardiovascular support:

Respiratory alkalosis is seen in conditions where hyperventilation is a problem, including pulmonary disease, congestive cardiac failure and iatrogenic overventilation.

Respiratory acidosis is commonly seen in conditions interfering with normal ventilation, including CNS depression, conditions such as asthma which interfere with effective gas exchange, and problems which interfere with respiratory mechanics, such as chest trauma.

Metabolic alkalosis is commonly seen in infants and young children with a history of severe vomiting. However, iatrogenic causes include nasogastric aspiration and diuretic therapy.

Metabolic acidosis is commonly seen in conditions where the cardiovascular system cannot meet the body's requirements, such as sepsis. It is also seen in renal failure and diabetic ketoacidosis. The type of acidosis can be determined by calculating the anion gap:

$$(Na^+ + K^+) - (HCO_3^- + Cl^-) = 10–12 \text{ mEq (normal)}$$

An elevated anion gap indicates the presence of non-chloride ions such as lactic and keto acids, suggesting a non-renal cause of acidosis. Lactic acidosis (lactate > 2.2 mmol/L) is often seen in children with compromised cardiorespiratory function. This results in cellular hypoxia, anaerobic respiration and lactic acid production. Although not useful when measured in isolation, when recorded alongside other indices of cardiorespiratory function, lactate can be used to assess response to treatment and as an indicator of potential outcome (Nimmo & Nightingale 1996).

In addition to assessment of acid–base status, ongoing monitoring of the circulation includes measurement of:

- peripheral perfusion
- urinary output
- central venous or right atrial pressure (CVP/RAP)
- pulmonary artery wedge pressure (PAWP)
- cardiac output (CO) and cardiac index (CI)
- gastric pH.

Peripheral perfusion is assessed using a variety of methods. A well-perfused child will have warm, pink skin, with good peripheral pulses and a capillary refill of less than 2 s. In addition, the child will be alert, with normal vital signs and a urine output of > 1 mL/kg/h (>2 mL/kg/h in infants). Assessment of core–toe temperature gap and serum lactate (normal 0.5–2.2 mEq/L) provide information regarding circulation to the peripheral tissues. A core–toe gap of < 2°C indicates adequate perfusion. However, this should be assessed in relation to the environment, as extremes of temperature will affect perfusion. When assessing skin temperature, it is important to determine the severity of poor perfusion. This can be achieved by feeling the limbs to determine at which point the child's limb changes temperature.

Signs of poor perfusion occur as a result of inadequate circulating volume caused by hypovolaemia or failure of the cardiovascular system. Normal circulating volume is determined as 80 mL/kg. However, in infants this can increase to 85 mL/kg and fall to 75 mL/kg in older children. Assessment of the child's fluid status and cardiovascular function can be achieved both clinically, using the parameters above, and through invasive monitoring.

Assessment of CVP or RAP can be undertaken using a central venous catheter or a pulmonary artery flotation catheter. Measurement provides information about the circulating volume or preload on the heart. Normal pressure ranges between 1 and 5 mmHg in children. High pressures may be caused by hypervolaemia, necessitating the use of diuretics such as frusemide (1 mg/kg). If repeated doses are required, electrolytes should be monitored, as imbalances in Na^+ and K^+ will interfere with cardiac function. High pressures can also occur as a result of ineffective contractility of the heart and high afterload. Therefore, an inotrope such as dobutamine, which has beta 2 adrenergic effects, may improve ventricular function and dilate the systemic circulation, thus reducing afterload. Low CVP or RAP often occurs as a result of reduced circulating volume. Therefore, a fluid bolus of 10 mL/kg of colloid or 20 mL/kg of crystalloid may increase pressure. Repeated boluses should be given with care to prevent hypervolaemia and overdistension of the ventricles.

A pulmonary artery flotation catheter enables assessment of the function of left and right sides of the heart. The tip of the catheter sits in a pulmonary artery, but RAP is assessed from a port distal to the tip. PAWP is measured by inflating a balloon at the end of the catheter until a wedge pressure is achieved (normal 5–10 mmHg). Care should be taken not to inflate the balloon for longer than necessary, as pulmonary infarction can result. PAWP provides information about the preload or filling pressure on the left side of the heart, as it is a direct reflection of LAP (normal 5–10 mmHg) when the pulmonary vasculature is normal.

Measurement of right and left atrial pressures provides information about the ventricular end diastolic pressures (VEDP) in the absence of disease of the atrioventricular valves. This measurement enables assessment of ventricular filling, contraction and afterload or pulmonary and systemic vascular resistance. Although VEDP does not provide a direct reflection of ventricular end diastolic volume (VEDV), volume administration can increase VEDP. The relationship between VEDP and VEDV will depend on the contractility of the heart.

Contractility can be assessed using echocardiography, doppler or thermodilution. Pulmonary artery catheters have a thermistor at the tip, which can be used to determine the time taken for a known quantity of fluid at a known temperature to pass the catheter tip. This enables estimation of cardiac output. As CO changes with age, cardiac index can be calculated:

$$CI \ (L/min/m^2 \ BSA) = \frac{CO}{body \ surface \ area \ (BSA)}$$

(normal 3.5–4.5 L/min/m^2 BSA).

Assessment of the multiple parameters enables practitioners to titrate fluid boluses, inotropic therapy and vasodilators in order to maximise CO.

Fluid and electrolytes balance

Fluid requirements in infants and young children are higher per kilo of body weight than in older children and adults. This is due to a higher basal metabolic rate and evaporative losses, the inability of young infants to concentrate urine and a greater percentage of total body water in the very young. Infants have a greater percentage of extracellular fluid than older children and adults (Table 2.5). They exchange approximately 15% of the extracellular fluid each day, whereas adults exchange only 5%. Therefore, infants are at risk of developing fluid imbalances as a result of many illnesses, including:

- respiratory infection
- diarrhoea and vomiting
- sepsis
- burns and scalds.

As the percentage of body fat increases with age, total body water falls to adult values and fluid requirements are reduced. This makes older children less susceptible to severe fluid imbalances during minor illnesses. A simple formula for determining fluid requirements during infancy and childhood is widely used in practice:

- newborn infants: 60 mL/kg/24 h, increasing by 10 mL/kg/day for 4 days
- < 10 kg: 100 mL/kg/24 h

Table 2.5 Changes in fluid compartments in childhood

Age	Total body water (%)	Extracellular compartment (%)	Intracellular compartment (%)
Preterm infant	80–90	65	25
Term infant	70–80	35–44	33
6 month old	60	23	37
Adolescent	60 (male) 55 (female)	20	40

- 11–20 kg: 1000 mL + 50 mL for each kg over 10 kg
- 21–30 kg: 1500 mL + 25 mL for each kg over 20 kg.

Young children have a greater body surface area to weight ratio than older children and adults, making them capable of losing larger volumes of water from insensible losses through the skin. Insensible losses can be calculated using the formula:

$$300 \text{ mL/m}^2 \text{ BSA/24 h.}$$

These may be increased with raised respiratory rates and temperatures. For example a 1°C rise in temperature above normal can increase insensible losses by 12% and may necessitate an increase in fluid administration.

Assessment of fluid status includes:

- recording abnormal losses
- recording heart rate and strength of peripheral pulses
- assessing peripheral perfusion by measuring core–toe gap and capillary refill
- recording blood pressure
- assessment of renal perfusion by measuring urine output
- assessing cerebral perfusion by recording conscious level
- assessment of body surface to assess level of hydration
- measurement of blood and urinary electrolytes.

These parameters can be used to assess the severity of fluid loss by estimating the percentage of dehydration (Table 2.6). In addition, the weight of the child may assist this estimation, as rapid weight loss is often indicative of fluid loss.

It is important to assess the type of fluid lost, as this will influence the type of replacement fluid administered. It is important to understand the influence of electrolytes on fluid balance and to consider serum electrolyte levels when giving replacement fluids. The volume of extracellular fluid is maintained by sodium and plasma proteins. Intracellular fluid volume is maintained by proteins. The sodium–potassium

Table 2.6 Signs of dehydration in infants and young children

% Dehydration	Clinical signs
< 5% dehydrated	Moist skin and mucosa Thirst Normal anterior fontanelle and eyes
5–10% dehydrated	Dry mucosa Dry skin with tenting Soft anterior fontanelle and dark rings around eyes Loss of body weight Increased heart rate Oliguria (< 1 mL/kg/h)
10–15% dehydrated	Dry mucosa Poor skin turgor with clamminess Sunken anterior fontanelle and eyes Anuria Reduced blood pressure Reduced consciousness level

pump in the cell membrane works to maintain the balance between electrolytes across the two major fluid compartments. The osmotic pressure, created by the solutes within each compartment, is responsible for maintaining the fluid volume of that compartment. Serum osmolarity (normal 272–290 mOsm/L) can be estimated by totalling serum solute values. When serum sodium levels are reduced, water moves out of the circulation to produce oedema. High serum sodium levels will attract water into the circulation. This can produce signs of both congestive cardiac failure and cerebral problems, such as fitting, if fluid shifts are dramatic. Dehydration can be classified according to sodium levels:

- hypertonic: Na > 150 mmol/L
- isotonic: Na 130–150 mmol/L
- hypotonic: Na < 130 mmol/L.

The cause of fluid imbalance will determine the type of replacement fluid; for example:

- Increased temperature resulting from phototherapy, radiant heaters or sepsis may require a 12–30% increase in fluids. Electrolytes should be measured to determine additional requirements.
- Hypertonic dehydration will require administration of saline solution to prevent the sodium falling rapidly and fluid moving quickly

into the cells, as this can cause neurological deterioration.

• Gastrointestinal losses are associated with potassium loss. Replacement fluids will depend on serum potassium levels and renal function. Concentrated potassium infusions (up to 0.5 mmol/kg/h) can be given if the child is passing urine.

• Blood loss from trauma will require replacement with blood products.

In the infant or child who has cardiovascular compromise as a result of fluid loss, 4.5% human albumin solution or a synthetic colloid will be given initially to expand circulating volume and treat signs of shock. In infants and young children, it is important to assess the results of fluid replacement at regular intervals. Therefore, an initial bolus of 10 mL/kg of colloid will be given prior to reassessment. Further boluses of 5 mL/kg may be given to infants, especially those with congenital cardiac disorders, to prevent overstretching of the heart.

When administering replacement fluids, it is important to remember to meet the child's normal fluid requirements. Dextrose saline or 5–10% glucose should be given depending on the child's age and blood glucose level.

Alterations in antidiuretic hormone (ADH) and aldosterone secretion may occur, leading to sodium and fluid retention. This may necessitate administering 75% of normal fluid requirements with additional boluses, based on cardiovascular signs, to prevent fluid overload. Urinary electrolytes aid evaluation of renal and endocrine function, assisting in the diagnosis of diabetes insipidus and syndrome of inappropriate antidiuretic hormone (SIADH) secretion. Daily urinalysis, including osmolality, should be recorded.

Nutrition

Assessment of the child's nutrition involves assessment of:

• gastrointestinal function
• calorie requirements
• growth.

Enteral feeding is common in the critically ill child because it provides the best route for provision of calorie requirements. Energy requirements can increase significantly during severe illness, as infants and children have increased basal metabolic requirements and normal requirements for growth (Table 2.7). In addition sick children require additional calories to aid recovery. This can double normal requirements in children who have sustained large thermal injuries (Table 2.8).

For those infants and children requiring prolonged intensive care, appropriate calorie intake can be determined by plotting weight, length and head circumference on a growth chart at weekly intervals. Although fluid balance may affect the weight, growth should be observed when adequate calories are provided.

Gastric aspirate is assessed for volume and contents. Small amounts of old blood in the aspirate may be caused by tube placement. However, continued aspiration of fresh or old blood may indicate a stress ulcer. Partial digestion of feeds suggests some GI function; therefore, the presence of large aspirates alone should not lead practitioners to cease enteral feeds. If large, partially

Table 2.7 Normal calorie requirements of infants and children

Age	Calorie requirement
Premature neonate	Up to 150 cal/kg/day
Term neonate	Up to 120 cal/kg/day
1–2 years	Up to 100 cal/kg/day
2–6 years	Up to 90 cal/kg/day
7–9 years	Up to 80 cal/kg/day
10–12 years	Up to 60 cal/kg/day

Adapted from Hazinski (1992).

Table 2.8 Percentage calorie requirements during illness, compared with normal

Illness	Calorie requirements (%)
Pyrexia	10% increase for each 1°C temperature rise
Cardiac failure	125
Major surgery	130
Thermal injury	200
Severe sepsis	150

digested aspirates are obtained, replacement of the aspirate, with a break in feeds of 1–2 hours, may enhance absorption and allow for feeds to continue. Enteral feeding should be continued if possible, as it is thought to be protective against the translocation of Gram-negative organisms across the gut wall and into the circulation, thus preventing Gram-negative sepsis. Absent bowel sounds and abdominal distension indicate paralytic ileus. Parenteral nutrition is required to provide essential nutrients until GI function returns. Children with absent bowel sounds should be observed for passage of faeces, as both loose stools and constipation can occur. Administration of drugs known to reduce gastric motility, such as morphine, may be inadvisable in the child with no bowel sounds.

Gastric pH can be assessed each time the stomach is aspirated, using universal pH paper. A more accurate assessment in children with severe cardiovascular dysfunction may be achieved using a tonometer, although this has not been validated in practice (Nathan & Mythen 1997). Reduced circulation to the gut via the splanchnic circulation can lead to a similar picture of anaerobic respiration and lactic acid production to that seen in the peripheral circulation. It is thought that this causes reduced gut motility, mucosal oedema and translocation of bacteria.

Tonometry measures CO_2 production by the gastric mucosa. This is achieved by aspirating a sample of normal saline from the gas-permeable tonometer balloon. The measured CO_2 from this sample is used with arterial HCO_3 to calculate gastric intramural pH (Nathan & Mythen 1997). Changes in intramural pH are said to be an indicator of potential outcome, when used in conjunction with serum lactate and other indices of cardiorespiratory function. However, this is a time-consuming process, which necessitates interrupting enteral feeds. This needs refining and validating before being widely used in practice.

The neurological system

Assessment of the neurological system can be based on normal milestones for age. However, for an accurate assessment to take place, a full developmental history is required for individual children. This will enable practitioners assessing the child to determine the appropriateness of responses. Parents can assist with interpretation of responses, but it should be remembered that stressed parents of critically ill children may interpret information in the way that they wish it to be. This should not preclude involvement of parents, but an assessment of their stress levels may be useful.

Tools used to determine level of consciousness in children include:

- the Glasgow Coma Scale (GCS)
- the Modified GCS
- the Adelaide Scale
- the James Adaptation of the GCS
- the Pinderfield Scale.

These are discussed further in Chapter 10. Adaptations of the GCS have been made to account for the developmental age of infants and children. However, none of them is entirely accurate when assessing neurological status of the critically ill child, particularly when the child is paralysed and sedated. Additional investigations are required to determine neurological function, including:

- CT scan
- MRI scan
- daily or continuous EEG
- assessment of reflexes and brainstem responses
- assessment of posture
- assessment of the optic discs.

CT scan will provide information about structure of the brain, bleeds or space-occupying lesions, presence or absence of oedema, size of the ventricles, grey–white matter differentiation and infarction. Serial CT scans can be used to assess outcomes of management. MRI scans will provide greater detail about the structure of the brain, but may be difficult to arrange in children who are unstable, as the magnetic field does not allow use of metal objects such as monitoring devices during the procedure.

Electroencephalography (EEG) can be used to

assess brain activity and is particularly useful in the child who is paralysed or has been having seizure activity. In some instances, daily EEGs are recorded by trained staff who are able to assess the child's brain function in response to visual, auditory and somatic evoked responses. This is useful to assess a child's condition over a period of days. However, continuous EEG can be used to assess a child's response to interventions used on the PICU. The CFAM, or cerebral function analysing monitor, can be used to provide a continuous printout of cerebral activity. Interventions such as ET suction, physiotherapy and other nursing activities can be recorded on the printout to allow assessment of the child's responses. This is particularly useful in children in coma and those who are heavily sedated because of status epilepticus. It is important to remember that EEG is difficult to interpret in infants because of the immaturity of the brain.

Assessment of brainstem function, reflexes, posture and papilloedema may be carried out at intervals during the child's management. Paralysing agents will have to be discontinued for periods to assess all but papilloedema. Presence of papilloedema is indicative of raised intracranial pressure, as are decorticate and decerebrate posturing. It is important that all of these signs are detected early to attempt to prevent further deterioration in the child's condition. Therefore, the intervals between assessment will vary depending on changes in the child's condition.

Pain assessment is dealt with in Chapter 19. However, this should be based on knowledge of a child's experiences of and normal responses to pain. Children admitted to PICU for elective surgery can be prepared prior to admission. Older children can be involved in planning the methods used to relieve postoperative pain.

Protection

Assessment of surface of the child's body involves observation of the skin, hair, nails and limbs to detect abnormalities. The body should be observed for:

- posture
- symmetry
- bruising or signs of fracture
- evidence of infection or breaks in the skin surface
- colour
- temperature
- rashes or skin discoloration.

The child's posture can provide significant information about the child's condition. The child with a respiratory disorder may be most comfortable in an upright position with the neck extended to maximise oxygenation. This would indicate severe respiratory distress and the need for intubation. Posture and asymmetry may indicate a fracture; therefore, practitioners should assess limb alignment and position. Bruising over the surface of the body will indicate other sites of trauma. Bruising or fractures in infancy may lead practitioners to suspect nonaccidental injury, which should be reported to the appropriate professionals and investigated.

Catheter and drain sites should be assessed hourly for leakage, swelling and redness. Cannulae should be observed above the site for evidence of thrombophlebitis and extravasation. Either of these signs would require the cannula to be resited.

White cells, or leucocytes, are involved in fighting infection within the body. Therefore, the leucocyte count is often elevated in children with a variety of infections. The white cell differential can aid identification of the type of infection present (Table 2.9). Infants and young children are particularly susceptible to infection, because of their immature immune system. This matures during the preschool years, but the inability to produce antibodies in children under 2 years of age makes them particularly susceptible to viral infections.

Temperature control in neonates and infants is also immature. Neonates may not increase their temperature in response to infection, but may exhibit signs of hypothermia. However, it is important to protect infants and young children from extremes of temperature. Their high surface area to body weight ratio makes heat loss

Table 2.9   Functions of white blood cells

Type of white cell	Function
Lymphocyte	B lymphocytes produce antibodies to bacteria T lymphocytes attack nonbacterial organisms such as viruses; they are involved in rejection of foreign tissue, e.g. transplants
Neutrophil	Engulf and destroy invading bacteria
Monocyte	Phagocytosis of bacteria and debris Become macrophages outside the circulation
Basophil	Mediate inflammatory response
Eosinophil	Modulate inflammatory response Involved in antigen–antibody response

through evaporation, conduction and convection more rapid than in older children and adults. Young infants, in particular, can exhibit signs of stress if their temperature falls. Their inability to make heat from shivering increases oxygen consumption. This can progress to hypoxia, lactic acid production and hypoglycaemia if the infant's environment is not adjusted to increase body temperature. Measurement of skin and central temperature enables practitioners to maintain a core–toe gap of < 2°C and a central temperature around 37.5°C to reduce oxygen demand and consumption.

Disseminated intravascular coagulation

Thrombocytopenia is commonly seen in critically ill children as a result of disseminated intravascular coagulation (DIC). This is a clotting abnormality associated with multiple disorders, including:

- major sepsis
- trauma
- shock
- transfusion reactions
- malignancies
- hypoxia.

DIC is characterised by excessive activation of the clotting cascade (Fig. 2.1), causing concurrent clotting and bleeding. The exact cause is unclear, as pathophysiological processes vary between cases (Hambly 1995b). The intrinsic pathway appears to be activated by hypoxia, sepsis and compromised circulation where there is injury to the endothelial lining of the vascular system. Both intrinsic and extrinsic pathways are activated by endotoxins released in Gram-negative sepsis (McCance & Heuther 1994). The extrinsic pathway is activated by tissue thromboplastin released following tissue injury in disorders such as malignant disease, burns and major surgery. Whichever pathway is affected, the activation of the common pathway (Fig. 2.1) leads to high levels of circulating thrombin which stimulates fibrinogen to produce fibrin. This travels to the microcirculation, where it lodges to form clots. These block vessels, trapping platelets, consuming clotting factors and preventing oxygen and nutrients reaching the vital organs and peripheral tissues. Ischaemia and necrosis result if the process is not halted. Rapid clot formation leads to a fall in circulating clotting factors and uncontrolled bleeding. This is further exacerbated by fibrinolysis, which aims to dissolve the clots. The production of fibrin degradation products results in further bleeding, as these are powerful anticoagulants.

A further mechanism associated with the development of DIC is direct activation of Factor X, which appears to be associated with release of chemicals into the circulation. Poisons such as snake venom, pancreatic and liver enzymes act in this way. Blood transfusion causes DIC by one of two mechanisms. Firstly, dilution of clotting factors can occur as a result of administration of large volumes of blood. Secondly, adverse blood reactions, resulting in antigen–antibody reactions, cause increased levels of procoagulant which triggers severe haemorrhage and hypotension (McCance & Heuther 1994).

Clinical signs and symptoms

- bleeding from mucosa or catheter and cannula insertion sites
- extension of skin petechiae or haemorrhage
- poor peripheral perfusion, due to vascular obstruction
- evidence of clot formation in major organs such as the lungs, kidneys and brain.

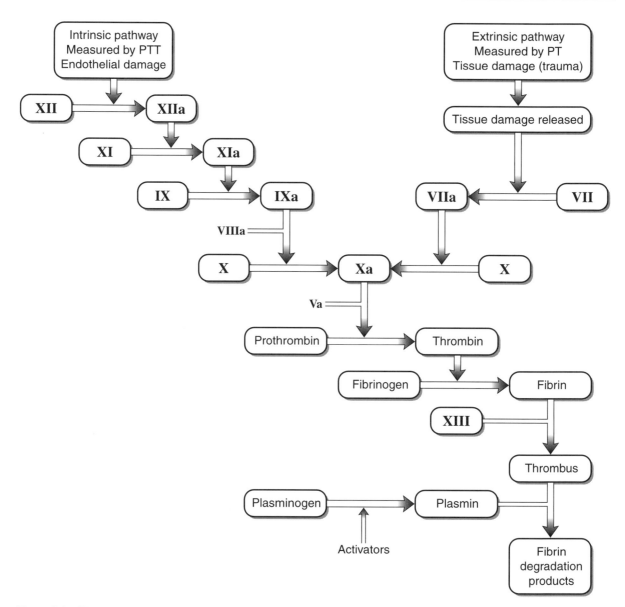

Figure 2.1 The clotting cascade. Adapted from Hazinski (1992), with permission, and Hambly (1995a).

Haematological findings

- low platelet count (< 150 000)
- increased prothrombin time/INR (ratio > 1.5)
- low plasma fibrinogen (< 175)
- increased partial thromboplastin time (ratio > 1.5)

- low Hb with fragmented red blood cells
- increased fibrin degradation products (> 10–40 or > 40).

In some cases, the only laboratory finding may be a low platelet count. It is important to interpret these findings in combination with clinical signs and symptoms and other treatments, as blood transfusion may dilute clotting factors with no other evidence of DIC.

Management of DIC

The most important aspect of management is to identify and treat the underlying problem. In addition, clotting factors and platelets should be replaced, with the aim of preventing further bleeding. Platelets are given when circulating levels are low and there is evidence of bleeding. Fresh frozen plasma (FFP) can be given to replace clotting factors, and cryoprecipitate will increase circulating factors VIII and V and fibrinogen levels.

Other treatments have been suggested, including heparin, oestrogens, DDAVP and antifibrinolytics. These products have been shown to work in specific situations and are, therefore, not effective in many cases (Hambly 1995b). Specific substances such as Protein C and Antithrombin III have been used in consultation with haematologists, but these products are not widely used in practice.

PSYCHOSOCIAL ISSUES

Roy's Adaptation Model aids assessment of psychosocial issues through assessment of:

- roles—who the child is
- self awareness—how the child sees him/herself
- interdependence—who is dependent on the child/on whom the child is dependent.

The roles the child fulfils can be further broken down into:

- primary roles—age and gender
- secondary roles—within a family
- tertiary roles—in relation to friends and hobbies.

Assessment of roles is closely linked to the assessment of interdependence, as this relates to individuals on whom the child is dependent, such as a child minder, and those that may be dependent on the child, such as pets. All of these issues can be illustrated using a diagram with the child as the focus (Fig. 2.2).

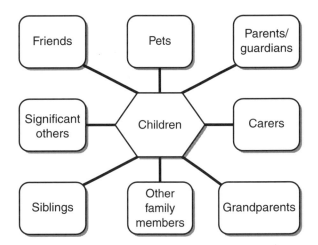

Figure 2.2 A child's roles and relationships. Reference: Evelina Children's Hospital Documentation Group (1998) Evelina Children's Hospital individual patient profile and assessment. Guy's and St Thomas' Hospital, London (unpublished).

Self awareness is assessed by asking the child (if appropriate) and family about the child's experiences of hospital, ill health and pain. Their knowledge of the child's current illness and expectations can be ascertained to enable information giving to be individualised. This is much easier to achieve for the child and family who are electively admitted to PICU. However, for families of children admitted as an emergency, the situation may make it less appropriate to ask about expectations. Other issues which may be assessed in relation to self awareness include:

- body image
- feelings
- response to family and significant others
- self esteem
- religion
- culture.

Assessment of psychosocial issues may not be essential during the early admission. However, this information is important when forming a relationship with the child and family. Knowledge of the child's normal routine, names of pets and past experiences can help practitioners reduce stress levels in both parents and the child.

Individualised discharge planning will be more effective when staff have knowledge of the child's normal routine and social contacts. Collection of this information may be made over a period of time, as the family builds relationships with the staff. However, practitioners should remember that it is important to ensure confidentiality and only collect information that is relevant to the child's current illness and ongoing health.

REFERENCES

Engel J 1997 Pediatric assessment, 3rd edn. Mosby Year Book, St Louis

Fraser M 1996 Conceptual nursing in practice: a research-based approach, 2nd edn. Chapman and Hall, London

Gilbert EG, Russell KE, Deskin RW 1993 Stridor in the infant and child. AORN Journal 58(1):23, 26–43

Hambly H 1995a Coagulation I — factors and pathways. Care of the Critically Ill 11(4):160–165

Hambly H 1995b Coagulation II — Clinical problems in coagulation disorders. Care of the Critically Ill 11(5):203–205

Hazinski MF 1992 Children are different. In: Hazinski MF Nursing care of the critically Ill child, 2nd edn. Mosby, St Louis

McCance KL, Heuther SE 1994 Pathophysiology: the biologic basis for disease in adults and children. Mosby Year Book, St Louis

Nathan AT, Mythen MG 1997 Gastric tonometry — its place in intensive care practice. British Journal of Intensive Care 223–229

Nimmo G, Nightingale P 1996 Tissue hypoxia and lactate — an update. Care of the Critically Ill 12(5):158, 160, 162–164

Rittner F, Doring M 1997 Curves and loops in mechanical ventilation. Drager, Germany

3

Monitoring physiological signs

Colin Way

Over the last ten years, physiological monitoring has grown in terms of its complexity and diversity; this can be attributed to advances in pharmacological management and the fact that children are surviving greater severity of illness requiring more intensive and varied monitoring. Paediatric intensive care practice has therefore become more aggressive in the use of invasive physiological monitoring. As a consequence, health care professionals working within the paediatric intensive care environment are faced with a wide variety of invasive and non-invasive monitoring (Rogers 1992).

In general terms, biomedical instrumentation may be used to monitor, measure or support the critically ill child. In essence, monitoring allows the health care professional to achieve four goals (Loach & Thomson 1987):

- evaluation of cardiac function, myocardial oxygen consumption, and physiological status of the critically ill child.
- assessment of oxygen uptake and delivery and the removal of carbon dioxide from the body
- evaluation of the results of pharmacological and physiological interventions in a number of responses: cardiac output, peripheral vascular resistance, pulmonary vascular resistance and stroke volume.
- monitoring of therapeutic and toxic levels of certain drugs such as nitric oxide.

This chapter will examine monitoring which allows assessment of respiratory and cardiac function (Box 3.1). It will include discussion of the principles of physiological monitoring, describe some of the equipment necessary for the care of critically ill children and discuss their uses and hazards. This equipment may be divided into two types:

- invasive — breaking the normal physiological barriers: for example, an arterial line
- non-invasive — not breaking the physiological barriers: for example, pulse oximetry.

Box 3.1 Common physiological monitoring

- invasive and non-invasive arterial blood pressure
- central venous and left atrial pressure
- pulmonary artery pressure
- cardiac output studies using thermodilution and mixed venous saturation
- co-oximetry
- capnography and end tidal CO_2
- pulse oximetry
- transcutaneous blood gas determination
- monitoring and delivery of nitric oxide

GENERAL SAFETY ISSUES — 'THE AT-RISK CHILD'

All critically ill children who are monitored using electrical equipment are at risk of injury or life-threatening events because of the close proximity of the equipment. Von der Mosel (1994) states that user error or careless handling of equipment causes some 64% of all accidental injury. To avoid accidents with monitoring equipment, healthcare professionals need to understand some of the basic principles pertaining to the physics of electricity and the dangers involved. The strength of electricity is measured in volts, but in order for it to be dangerous an electrical current must flow. Current is measured in amps, and the higher the amps the faster the flow of electricity. Lastly, electricity has to overcome a degree of resistance, which is measured in ohms. Using Ohm's law the following three equations become apparent:

1. voltage = current (amps) × resistance (ohms)
2. current (amps) = volts ÷ resistance (ohms)
3. resistance (ohms) = volts ÷ current (amps).

Von der Mosel (1994) states that there are three important factors for healthcare professionals to bear in mind, when considering the seriousness of an electrical accident. These are:

1. the amount of current that will flow through the child in the event of an electrical accident
2. the pathway the electricity takes through the child
3. the current density.

The electrical pathway is an important factor to consider because the current travelling through a limited area, for example one finger of a hand, may cause extensive burn damage to that area. However, if the same current were to enter one hand and leave through the other hand, vital organs may be damaged.

Macro and micro shock

Independent investigations have studied the effects of increasing levels of current on the human body when applied through normal intact skin (Box 3.2). This is sometimes referred to as macro shock and can be due to current leaking from monitoring equipment. However, if the electrical current is applied by bypassing the skin, for example through arterial monitoring or pacing wires, the effects can be far more devastating. It has been demonstrated that only 20–250 microamps (μA) are required to cause ventricular fibrillation (Von der Mosel 1994).

Effects of skin resistance

The skin provides resistance to the passage of electrical current. Normal human skin has a resistance of about 1000 ohms per cm^2 (Von der Mosel 1994). In the case of moist skin, resistance may be as low as 500 ohms. This is likely in the child who is, for example, pyrexial, has had electrode gel left on him or has skin that has not been properly dried following a wash. These factors can put the critically ill child at increased risk of having an electrical accident. For example in a child with normal skin integrity who is subjected to a current of 220 volts the resulting current would be 220 ÷ 1000 = 0.22 amps, which would be sufficient to cause fibrillation. However, in the critically ill child who is perhaps febrile and sweating, the resistance may be reduced to 250 ohms or 100 ohms where the skin is in contact with ECG electrode gel (Von der Mosel 1994). In this instance the resulting current would be 220 ÷ 100 = 2.2 amps.

disciplinary team has a vital role in reducing the incidence of electrical accidents, through regular checking of equipment and good practice when monitoring equipment is in use. Box 3.3 outlines some of the precautions health care professionals should take in order to reduce accidents (Von der Mosel 1994).

Box 3.2   How the body reacts to different levels of electrical current

1 mA (1 milliampere = 0.001 ampere)
The child will just be able to feel a slight tingling sensation

16 mA
Victim will not be able to remove her hand from the conductor
Strong muscular contractions can cause muscle damage
Although painful, the heart and lungs continue to function

50 mA
Death by suffocation due to contraction of the chest and respiratory muscles

100 mA
Ventricular fibrillation
Death if current is not stopped immediately

Source: Von der Mosel (1994).

Box 3.3   Suggested standards for avoiding accidents with electrical equipment

- Always disconnect equipment from the mains wall socket before disconnecting cable from the equipment.
- Never use multiple outlet extension leads.
- Extension leads should not be used. If a longer cable is required, install one.
- Be alert to potential electrical hazards and check equipment and cords daily.
- Damaged connectors, monitoring leads, socket outlets and cables should not be used but should be sent for repair.
- Ensure the cord sheathing is fully anchored to the plug and that wires are not showing.
- Ensure there is adequate instruction on the use of all equipment used on the PICU.
- If the equipment is used invasively, never touch the patient or invasive metal parts and the equipment at the same time.
- Hospital policies regarding the use of electrical devices should be clear and accessible.

Adapted from Von der Mosel (1994).

Although most medical equipment uses a low safety voltage of 25 volts, much of this is attached to devices which bypass the skin: for example, pacing wires. In this case, resistance can be as low as 10 ohms, producing a current of 2.5 amps. Current density has an important role in determining the severity of the injury. Devices that have a large surface area or low current density allow the current to be distributed over a larger area, which is not quite so hazardous. However, if electrical current is applied through a very small conductive area – for example, the tip of a temporary pacing wire – the current density is high and the danger is considerably greater. Therefore, extremely small amounts of current, which are undetectable to the health care professional, can be passed to the child and cause potentially fatal electrical accidents. The multi-

CARDIOVASCULAR MONITORING
General considerations

Monitoring is derived from the Latin word 'to warn', and therefore the proposed purpose for monitoring is to:

- measure, continuously or intermittently, key alterations in physiological data that aid diagnosis and guide treatment and nursing intervention
- provide alarms that inform the health care professional of important changes that have occurred in the child's condition
- record and evaluate trends that may help in the assessment of treatment, prognosis and nursing intervention.

Professionals involved in physiological monitoring should have a good working knowledge of each piece of equipment in order to understand its hazards and its usefulness to each individual child. Alarms may be turned off or malfunction, and so reliance on alarm systems can potentially be dangerous, allowing clinical deterioration to progress to a life-threatening state before detection. In light of the Allitt inquiry (Department of Health 1994), medical and nursing staff have a responsibility to ensure they have an up-to-date knowledge of all monitoring equipment used within their PICU and that alarm parameters are regularly reassessed and correctly set.

Lastly, if the data obtained from physiological monitoring is to be beneficial, health care professionals require knowledge to successfully interpret the accuracy and validity of the information being displayed and the factors which may affect its reliability (Campbell 1997). The following section will address these issues by focusing on the monitoring of arterial blood pressure and central venous pressure. However, in light of the potential for inaccuracy in invasive monitoring, the importance of combining this with good clinical assessment cannot be overstated.

Components of a monitoring system

Most instruments used to monitor critically ill children require a sensor, a transducer, an amplifier and a meter (Fig. 3.1). In haemodynamic monitoring systems, the sensor is the vascular catheter that provides access to the vascular pressure signal. The pulsatile vascular signal is converted to an electrical signal by a transducer. The amplifier in the monitor enhances the signal, to provide a digital display and waveform on the oscilloscope which functions as the meter (Blumer 1990).

Monitoring of arterial blood pressure

The pattern of the arterial waveform (Fig. 3.2) is the culmination of numerous events and reflects the function and pressure changes in the left ventricle and the resistance in the systemic arterial tree. After cannulation of an artery, the vessel

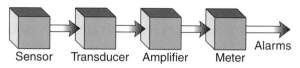

Figure 3.1 Components of a monitoring system. Adapted from Hazinski (1992).

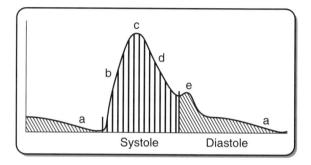

Figure 3.2 Components of the arterial waveform. Pulse wave a to c of the waveform occurs as blood is ejected into the aorta from the ventricle during systole. Volume displacement occurs at point c. Segment d occurs during late systole as the ventricles empty and forward movement slows. Closure of the aortic valve is reflected as the dichrotic notch, point e. At point e, the pulmonary valve is also closed and the atrioventricular valves are opening.

and catheter become part of a dynamic resonant monitoring system also consisting of a transducer and pressurised fluid-filled tubing. An electrical translation of intra-arterial pressure sensed at the end of the catheter results in a recognisable, high-pressure waveform on the monitor screen. The curved configuration of the arterial waveform is the result of a pressure wave preceding the ejection of blood from the left ventricle, followed by the actual forceful ejection of blood from the ventricle into the aorta. Pressure waves move to the periphery from the aorta and are reflected back from narrower vessels. The configuration of the waveform is the combination of the pressure wave and the reflected waves (Campbell 1997). Resistance is also seen as a reflection of pressure; for example, blood running against the closing aortic valve causes a pressure wave that is seen as the dichrotic notch in a normal waveform configuration (Campbell 1997). A properly functioning arterial line will have four distinguishing features (Loach & Thomson 1987):

1. Blood can be drawn from the catheter.
2. The system can be zeroed.
3. The system includes a mechanism to keep the catheter clear of obstruction between the transducer and the pressure source.
4. A dependable waveform is visible on the monitor.

Accuracy of arterial waveform

The accurate interpretation of haemodynamic information from invasive monitoring is dependent on a number of factors (Box 3.4). Today's technology has provided healthcare professionals with computerised monitors that provide very accurate interpretation of arterial waveforms in conjunction with monitoring lines that are better designed. Monitoring systems should have the following features to ensure accuracy (Gibbs & Gardner 1988):

Box 3.4   Factors affecting the accuracy of information obtained from the arterial waveform

- accuracy and design of the monitoring system
- air bubbles in the monitoring system
- length and compliance of tubing of monitoring system
- patency of tubing connections
- computer technology
- position of transducer relative to the child
- method of zeroing transducer
- position of the cannula in the vessel
- the child's underlying or changes in condition

---

1. Monitoring systems are simple with minimal non-compliant pressure tubing, flush devices and transducers.
2. Systems are air free when set up.
3. A continuous flush system minimises the potential for clot formation.
4. Long lengths or compliant interconnecting tube are eliminated.
5. Low-volume displacement transducers and flush devices are used.

There are other important factors that the professional needs to consider when ensuring accuracy of the information.

Zeroing of transducers

Zeroing the transducer is one of the most important aspects of obtaining accurate haemodynamic information. This is achieved by opening the transducer to atmospheric pressure. If the monitor does not read zero, the monitor's zero function is activated to offset any pressure on the transducer. This process references the vascular pressure to the atmospheric pressure, which is assumed to be zero. The transducer should be at the same level as the right atrium, and the limb in which the catheter is placed must be on the same plane as the right atrium during zeroing (Campbell 1997). The frequency with which transducers should be zeroed is unclear and is attributed to the lack of studies on newer, disposable transducers (Ahrens et al 1995). Research by Ahrens et al (1995) found that zero drift rates were only about 1%. Therefore, they suggest that transducers used for haemodynamic monitoring require zeroing only on initial set-up, following 20 minutes of warm-up time, and when disconnected from the monitor. Other literature suggests a compromise by zeroing every 24 hours (Loach & Thomson 1987). This is an important issue because unnecessary rezeroing takes up valuable nursing time and increases the risk of nosocomial infection by compromising the sterility of the system (Ahrens et al 1995).

Other considerations and safety issues

The arterial monitor may become over- or underdamped (Table 3.1) due to occlusion of the catheter, bleedback caused by the child's pressure exceeding the flush pressure, and change in position of the child in relation to the transducer. Bleeding can be a major problem and can occur either at the cannula site or at a loose connection within the monitoring system. Spasm within the cannulated artery can cause compromise in the circulation distal to the cannula (Rogers 1992). It is therefore considered good practice to regularly observe the monitoring system for secure connections and the child for signs of bleeding.

Table 3.1 Troubleshooting problems with arterial catheters

Problem	Cause	Treatment	Prevention
Dampened tracing	Occlusion of catheter tip	Try to aspirate clot but do not attempt to flush line	Adequate constant flushing
	Bleedback caused by patient's pressure exceeding the flush pressure	Regularly check all connections and that flush bag is at adequate pressure	Ensure connections and tubing are visible at all times
	Catheter tip against vessel wall		Ensure cannula is secured properly to prevent movement
	Clots or bubbles in pressure tubing or transducer	Flush system with three-way tap closed to child	Examine line regularly every 1–2 hours
Abnormally high or low readings	Change in position of transducer relative to patient	Check transducer level regularly	
	Bleeding at cannula site	Migration or dislodgement of catheter	Ensure cannula is taped securely and that entry site is visible
Compromise in circulation distal to insertion of cannula	Spasm of artery		Never flush line forcefully
No waveform visible or top of wave is flattened	Incorrect gain setting (scale)	Check monitor to see whether gain setting is inappropriately high or low (usually 60 or 120)	

Adapted from Hazinski (1992).

Significance of abnormal waveforms

Changes in the shape of the arterial waveform are often dismissed as artefact or system malfunction. However, predictable changes in waveform shape can occur in some disease processes (Loach & Thomson 1987). For example in hypertension the dichrotic notch disappears and is replaced by a 'shoulder' after the upward deflection. This can be attributed to the relatively non-compliant blood pressure, and such changes in compliance, resistance and pressure result in a compensatory wave reflected from the periphery to the aorta (Campbell 1997). Rapid upstroke of the arterial waveform is usually related to quick ventricular ejection, which may be seen in children with mitral regurgitation (Loach & Thomson 1987). Alternatively a slower than normal upstroke of the arterial waveform may be indicative of aortic stenosis. In any hypovolaemic state it is common for the arterial waveform to dip or become smaller in height, which may occur in conjunction with a numerical change. Arterial waveforms can therefore depict much more than just blood pressure. Like the ECG they can be used to help identify early changes in the child's condition.

Non-invasive blood pressure monitoring

Blood pressure measurement using the oscillometric method such as the Dinamap is common practice with children and is used where arterial access has proved very difficult or where invasive monitoring is felt unnecessary. Whereas arterial systems measure pressure, which is the amount of force exerted by circulating blood over a specific area, the oscillometric method measures the degree of oscillation produced by pulsatile blood flow through a vessel. It has been traditionally accepted as good practice to correlate the arterial blood pressure measurement to the manual blood pressure measurement. However, when properly functioning, invasive arterial monitoring is very reliable, and therefore this practice can be disregarded (Henneman & Henneman 1989). More importantly, because of the way in which each system measures blood pressure, the accuracy of an arterial catheter cannot be based on its comparison with a manual BP measurement in conditions marked by a disturbance in normal haemodynamics (Campbell 1997). For example, in a child with septic shock, where dilatation has occurred and is compensated by tachycardia and an increased cardiac output (flow), a manual reading may be higher than the arterial pressure because of the increased blood flow. This is because (Rogers 1992)

$$pressure = flow \times resistance.$$

Reliance on oscillometer readings may even be dangerous, because the literature suggests that these have only been validated as accurate in normotensive infants and children (Park & Menard 1987). In addition, poor correlation between oscillometric and arterial pressure has been documented in hypotensive neonates, whilst the oscillometric method overestimates low blood pressure in adults (Park & Menard 1987). Therefore, invasive blood pressure monitoring would appear most accurate when monitoring the critically ill child, with the key external factors influencing accuracy being the health care professional's ability to maintain and troubleshoot the system. In view of this, pressure values should not be considered in isolation when making clinical decisions but used in conjunction with physical assessment and other parameters such as urine output.

Central venous pressure lines

Central venous pressure (CVP) is the measurement of the pressure in the right atrium. Ideally, the tip of the central venous catheter should be positioned in the right atrium. However, because there are no valves between the superior vena cava (SVC), the inferior vena cava (IVC), and the right atrium, a catheter resting in the IVC or the SVC will reflect the pressure in the right atrium.

Indications for use

The CVP is used to measure right atrial pressure for the purpose of assessing blood volume, venous return, right ventricular function and determining fluid requirements (Loach & Thomson 1987).

A normal CVP waveform (Fig. 3.3) should be seen as a low-pressure waveform with no dichrotic notch. What is seen is a low-frequency curve characterised by 'a', 'c' and 'v' waves. The 'a' wave represents the forceful contraction of the right atrium, and the 'c' wave represents the closure of the tricuspid valve. The 'v' wave reflects a rise in right atrial pressure during right ventricular systole. This rise is caused by the bulging of the tricuspid valve into the right atrium as the right ventricle forcefully contracts.

Left atrial pressure line

The measurement of CVP provides valuable information about right heart function. In a child with a normally functioning heart, free of congenital malformation or haemodynamic problems,

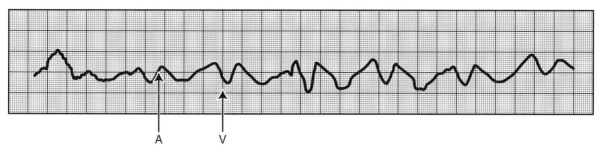

Figure 3.3 Normal CVP waveform.

the pressure in the right atrium can be used as an approximate measure of left ventricular function. In the critically ill child, however, or children with cardiovascular disease, the CVP may not be indicative of left heart function. This situation is problematic in children with mitral valve disease or left ventricular dysfunction because in both instances there will be some degree of back flow or regurgitation of blood. This would cause an elevation in left atrial pressure which would not be reflected by the pressures in the normally functioning left heart. In order to accurately measure left atrial pressure (LAP) in this group of children it may be necessary to insert a left atrial line. Because of the need for a thoracotomy, this type of monitoring is normally saved for children who have had cardiac surgery.

A normal LAP waveform should be a low-pressure waveform. As in a CVP waveform there is no dichrotic notch. The 'a' wave corresponds to the atrial kick, and the 'v' wave represents the bulging of the closed mitral valve into the left atrium, during left ventricular systole. The downward slope of the 'v' wave represents the decrease in pressure in the left atrium at the end of ventricular systole.

The consequences of air or particulate emboli are greater with left atrial lines than with right atrial lines, because of the direct route to the brain. These lines should be scrupulously monitored for clots and air bubbles and dedicated to monitoring only. Such lines should not be disconnected or used for sampling or administration of fluids except in extreme emergency (Rogers 1992). Left atrial pressure monitoring can be particularly useful in children with mitral valve dysfunction, as seen following repair of endocardial cushion defects.

A mean LAP of 4 to 12 mmHg is considered to be within normal limits. However, in some critically ill children, the optimum LAP will be that which provides maximum filling of the left ventricle and, in turn, maximum output. An increase or decrease in LAP may be due to interference, altered cardiac pathology or the effects of positive pressure ventilation. An elevated LAP may be due to a non-compliant left ventricle, left ven-

tricular failure or volume overload. The LAP may also fall below normal, with a decrease in volume intake, as in hypovolaemia.

For many critically ill children who require close, accurate cardiovascular monitoring, placement of an LA catheter may not be practical. In this situation a pulmonary artery flotation catheter may be a useful alternative.

Monitoring cardiac output

The clinician's ability to estimate cardiac function using indirect parameters such as urine output and capillary refill is too variable to be clinically useful (Tibby et al 1997). A tool is therefore required which objectively measures blood flow or cardiac output. Box 3.5 outlines both the common and newer methods available to measure cardiac output in the critically ill child. Ideally, haemodynamic monitoring techniques should be accurate, non-invasive, technically simple and cost effective (Tibby et al 1997). However, the literature suggests that this type of monitoring in children is still in its infancy and fraught with problems such as gaining access, technical constraints and the inability to compare new methods with a 'gold standard' (Tibby et al 1997).

Box 3.5 Methods of measuring cardiac function in the critically ill child

Invasive methods
- thermodilution (using pulmonary artery flotation catheter)
- dye dilution
- direct Fick method
- femoral artery thermodilution

Non-invasive
- doppler ultrasound (suprasternal, transtracheal, transosophageal)

Pulmonary artery catheter

The pulmonary artery catheter is a multi-lumen invasive device, which is able to measure right atrial pressure (RAP), pulmonary artery pressure (PAP), pulmonary artery wedge pressure

(PAWP) and mixed venous saturation. Using a thermodilution technique this device can also measure cardiac output, cardiac index, and many other haemodynamic parameters, including systemic vascular resistance and pulmonary vascular resistance (Bridges & Woods 1993).

Figure 3.4 details the position of the pulmonary artery catheter in the right side of the heart and the pressure waveforms generated. Pulmonary artery pressure reflects the systolic pressure generated by the right ventricle, and the waveform is comparable to a systemic arterial waveform. Pressure measurements displayed include the systolic, end diastolic and mean PAP, and all three should be routinely recorded (Stokes & Jowett 1985). The pulmonary artery wedge pressure is obtained by inflating the balloon at the tip of the pulmonary artery catheter. This causes occlusion of the vessel so that the pressure measurements obtained reflect the pressure distal to the balloon. If the balloon is placed appropriately (Fig. 3.4) and the transducer is zeroed and levelled correctly, this pressure should be interpreted as a close approximation of left ventricular end diastolic pressure (LVEDP). LVEDP and PAWP are usually within 2 to 3 mmHg of each other.

Blood taken from the pulmonary artery is termed mixed venous (SvO_2) because it represents the whole body's venous blood and not just part of it. Oxygen saturation of this blood can be measured continuously with some catheters and provides an acceptable reflection of cardiac output and oxygen uptake in the body as a whole. The mixed venous saturation will fall when oxygen delivery decreases. This occurs when cardiac output or arterial oxygen content fall. Mixed venous oxygen saturation will also fall if cell oxygen demand increases at a faster rate than oxygen delivery. If arterial oxygen content and oxygen demand are stable, the cardiac output will be directly related to the mixed venous oxygen saturation. Table 3.2 outlines normal childhood intracardiac pressures and mixed venous saturations.

The pulmonary artery catheter is used to:

1. measure right ventricular function by looking

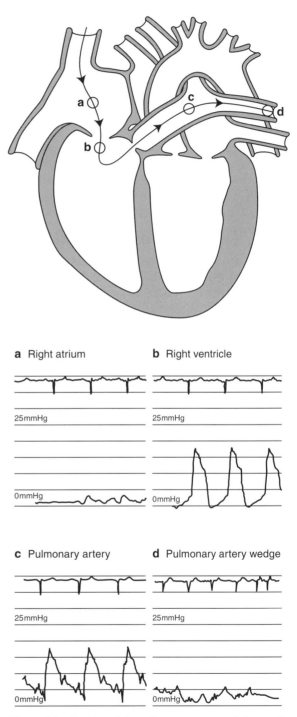

a Right atrium   **b** Right ventricle

c Pulmonary artery   **d** Pulmonary artery wedge

Figure 3.4 Position of the pulmonary artery catheter, and associated waveforms.

Table 3.2 Normal paediatric values in pulmonary catheter measurements

	Newborn	Child
RA	0–4 mmHg	0–4 mmHg
RV	50/3 mmHg	30/3 mmHg
PA	50/30 mmHg (M: 38)	30/12 mmHg (M: 18)
PAWP	4–8	4–8 mmHg
SvO$_2$	65–75%	65–75%

at pulmonary artery systolic pressure and CVP
2. assess flow and resistance in the pulmonary vascular bed
3. assess left ventricular function
4. measure cardiac output, from which systemic vascular resistance can be calculated
5. measure mixed venous oxygen saturation.

It is therefore useful in the following situations:

- evaluation of haemodynamic data in the child with myocardial dysfunction, particularly when vasoactive drugs are used
- evaluation of oxygen transport in a child with respiratory failure who requires manipulation of PEEP or other ventilatory support
- management of shock refractory to volume or use of inotropes
- management of septic shock.

Safety issues

The balloon should be inflated slowly to prevent rupture and should remain inflated for short periods only, to prevent trauma and infarction of the lung. Balloons are said to last 3–5 days or 70 inflations. If the child has a right to left shunt, there is an increased risk of myocardial or cerebral infarct. This is because of the potential for clots or air emboli travelling to the left side of the heart where there is direct access to the coronary and cerebral arteries (Merl & Pauly-O'Neil 1987). Therefore, it is advisable to flush the PA line before inflation, inflate briefly, look at the consistency of the trace and always close the port to air before removing the syringe. Potential complications (Box 3.6) necessitate the removal of the device as early as the child's condition indicates.

Box 3.6 Complications of pulmonary catheters

- infection and endocarditis
- thrombophlebitis
- balloon rupture
- pulmonary outflow tract obstruction
- arrhythmias
- knotting of catheter
- pulmonary infarct
- pulmonary artery trauma or rupture
- pulmonary embolism

Thermodilution and measurement of cardiac output

If a temperature-monitoring device is added, cardiac output can be studied using thermodilution techniques (Tibby et al 1997). A known volume of ice cold solution is injected into the right atrium. As it passes through the right ventricle, it mixes with blood at body temperature, cooling that volume of blood. When right ventricular blood and injectate are ejected into the pulmonary artery, the pulmonary artery thermistor measures the change in temperature of the blood and plots this change over time. This information is integrated into a time–temperature curve where the area under the curve reflects cardiac output, measured in litres per minute. The following formula describes this process:

$$CO = \frac{(T_b - T_i) \times V_i \times K}{\int \Delta T_b \, dt}$$

where T_b = blood temperature before injection, T_i = injectate temperature, V_i = injectate volume, K = correction constant, $\int \Delta T_b \, dt$ = area under the thermodilution curve.

Cardiac index can also be calculated if the child's body surface area is known; it can provide the clinician with a more reliable estimate of cardiac function.

The literature states that there are a number of errors relating to the method and to the patient (Tibby et al 1997). These include variation in injectate temperature and volume, loss of cold from the intracorporeal portion of the catheter, heart rate fluctuation with cold injectate and variation in cardiac output with mechanical ventilation. Tibby et al (1997) also state that, in paediatrics, low flow states and intracardiac shunting are two other sources of error. Despite this, thermodilution is the most commonly used method of measuring cardiac output, in children over 15 kg.

Because of the potential for error, particularly in relation to injectate volume and speed of injectate, one person should undertake these measurements and take the average of three consecutive readings. Because of all these technical problems, other methods for measuring cardiac output are being studied.

Dye dilution method

This technique requires the injection of a known quantity of dye rather than cold water. However, Tibby et al (1997) outline a number of limitations, including:

- time-consuming nature of calibration
- unreliability of readings with intra- and extracardiac defects
- toxic effect of dye accumulation.

Other methods for measuring cardiac output

Tibby et al (1997) are currently measuring cardiac output (CO) by measuring oxygen consumption-(VO_2), arterial and mixed venous oxygen content (C_aO_2 and C_vO_2) (direct Fick method). Cardiac output is calculated using the following equation:

$$CO = VO_2 \div (C_aO_2 - C_vO_2)$$

This requires a means of sampling blood from the systemic and pulmonary circulation and the ability to directly measure oxygen consumption from inspired and expired gases. The technology for this is new and cumbersome, e.g. Deltatract II Metabolic Monitor (Datex, Helsinki), and has limitations. For instance the child requires intubation with a cuffed tube.

A relatively recent feature involves modification of the traditional pulmonary artery thermodilution method. Tibby et al (1997) have used a 1.3 Fr thermistor placed in the femoral artery via a 22G cannula, and the temperature change is

sensed following an injection of cold 5% glucose. This is measured using the Cardiac Output and Lung Water Determination (COLD) machine. Although technically easier, this method appears to overestimate cardiac output when compared with pulmonary artery thermodilution.

Non-invasive methods of measuring cardiac output

Doppler ultrasound has been used to estimate cardiac output, based on the principle that the frequency shift (Δf) of reflected ultrasound will be proportional to the velocity (V) of the reflecting red blood cells (Tibby et al 1997):

$$V = \frac{\Delta f \times c}{2f_t \cos \theta}$$

where c = sound velocity in blood, f_t = transmitting frequency, θ = angle of insonation (i.e. between the beam and blood flow).

Suprasternal doppler measures velocity in the ascending aorta from a probe placed in the suprasternal notch. By combining the velocity versus time profile produced after spectral analysis, cardiac output can be estimated if the cross-sectional diameter of the aorta is known (Tibby et al 1997). Such problems as motion artefact and turbulent flow, as seen in aortic stenosis, can cause errors in readings. Transtracheal doppler is a relatively new technology which requires a probe attached to the distal end of an endotracheal tube. Tibby et al (1997) have used this technique on ten children and have found the major problem to be poor signal transmission due to the probe's requiring exact positioning.

With the oesophageal doppler method, a probe is placed in the mid oesophagus adjacent to the descending aorta. This technique does not measure absolute cardiac output but reflects changes with some accuracy.

Pulse oximetry

Pulse oximetry allows non-invasive, continuous measurement of oxygen saturation in arterial blood and has become very popular because of its simplicity of use (Von der Mosel 1994). Two light-emitting diodes emit red and infrared light through the tissue to a photo-detector. Red light absorption is inversely related to the amount of saturated haemoglobin passing through the tissue: well-saturated haemoglobin absorbs little red light, and poorly saturated haemoglobin absorbs a large amount of red light, so oxygen saturation is calculated from the degree of light absorption (Rogers 1992). In addition, the heart rate is also recorded, because blood flow is pulsatile.

Despite its simplicity, pulse oximetry has certain limitations. Most importantly, pulse oximetry can only estimate the percentage saturation of haemoglobin but cannot differentiate between different types of gas molecules. In a scenario where a child has carbon monoxide poisoning or methaemoglobinaemia, the pulse oximeter will incorrectly identify such molecules as oxyhaemoglobin (Rogers 1992). Also, pulse oximetry does not take into account the child's haemoglobin level, and cannot be relied upon to assess the oxygen-carrying capacity of the blood (Von der Mosel 1994). Therefore, paediatric intensive care units need the facility to measure blood gases using a co-oximeter. This machine measures the percentage saturation of arterial haemoglobin with oxygen, percentage of haemoglobin saturated with carbon monoxide, percentage of methaemoglobin and haemoglobin content. From this information the arterial oxygen content can be calculated (Martin 1992).

Inaccuracies are likely when the pulse oximeter is unable to measure the pulsatile changes in arterial blood. This becomes a problem in children with oedema or shock, when the peripheral circulation is poor. Bright external light sources can also affect readings, hence the recommendation that the probe be covered to keep light interference to a minimum (Von der Mosel 1994). Incorrect placement of the probe may allow light to hit the detector without first passing through the arteriolar bed, which will also cause inaccuracies (Rogers 1992).

Capnography and end tidal CO_2

The capnograph displays a respiratory wave-form and continuous reading of expired CO_2 during the respiratory cycle. An infrared detector is placed in between the child's endotracheal tube and ventilator tubing. This analyser determines expired CO_2 concentration, enabling evaluation of alveolar ventilation and CO_2 elimination (Rogers 1992). It is important to accept such readings as trends in pCO_2, because severe ventilation–perfusion mismatch, as with severe ARDS, can affect the relationship between end tidal CO_2 ($ETCO_2$) and pO_2 (Rogers 1992). Therefore, in children with severe respiratory disease, arterial blood gas monitoring is essential, whilst $ETCO_2$ can be used to monitor trends rather than absolute values.

Monitoring and delivery of inspired nitric oxide

Inhaled nitric oxide (NO) therapy has become increasingly popular in paediatric and neonatal intensive care units (Mupanemunda & Edwards 1997). Although it appears to have beneficial effects in certain disease processes, its safe delivery and effects on health professionals appears less straightforward (Woodrow 1997). Nitric oxide reacts readily with oxygen to produce nitrogen dioxide (NO_2), which is toxic to lungs in much smaller doses (Powroznyk & Latimer 1997). It also appears that NO_2 is formed much more quickly when NO is mixed in higher concentrations of inspired oxygen (Powroznyk & Latimer 1997). The 1988 Containment of Substances Hazardous to Health (COSHH) regulations limit employer exposure to 25 ppm of nitric oxide and 3 ppm of nitrogen dioxide (Grover 1993 cited in Woodrow 1997). There is less consensus on what constitutes a safe minimum and maximum dose range (Woodrow 1997). In a literature review by Mupanemunda & Edwards (1997) dose ranges varied depending on the condition being treated. However, most fell within the range 1–30 ppm. In view of this there should be:

1. facilities to safely monitor the levels of inspired NO and NO_2 and the levels expelled into the environment

2. a delivery system which accurately delivers between 0 and 60 ppm of NO (Powroznyk & Latimer 1997) with minimal production of NO_2
3. an integral scavenging system.

Monitoring of nitric oxide

Monitoring systems based on chemiluminescence and electrochemical cells are available. The chemiluminescence monitors remain the gold standard because of their accuracy (1%) and sensitivity (0.5 parts per billion) for measurement of constant or slowly changing concentrations of NO and NO_2 (Powroznyk & Latimer 1997). However, these machines are extremely expensive, cumbersome and have a slow response time (40 s) to increases in NO. Monitors using electrochemical cells are cheaper, more compact, with a minimal warm up time and acceptable accuracy (15%) and sensitivity (0.1 ppm) (Powroznyk & Latimer 1997). In older models the cells became quickly damaged from exposure to the NO and humidity. However, newer models have overcome these problems.

Nitric oxide delivery systems

To minimise NO_2 formation, NO must be injected into a stream of continuously flowing gas so that stasis is minimised and thorough mixing of the gases is ensured (Woodrow 1997). Once mixing with O_2 begins, the NO_2-forming reaction starts, and it is important to limit the time before the mixed gases are delivered to the lungs in order to reduce NO_2 production. In practice, this means reducing the dead space and avoiding reservoirs of static gas (Powroznyk & Latimer 1997). If the inspired NO concentration can be kept to below 20 ppm, then the formation of NO_2 is significantly reduced (Woodrow 1997).

Other considerations

Both NO and NO_2 are known to be toxic in high concentration, but the chronic effects of exposure to low concentrations are unknown. It is therefore important to scavenge the expiratory gases to prevent pollution (Woodrow 1997). In operating theatres, gases are removed using extractor systems; however, in PICU chemical scavenging appears popular using soda lime, activated charcoal or alumina. Soda lime appears variable in its ability to absorb NO and NO_2, whereas charcoal works better when dry.

Methaemoglobinaemia is a potential complication of NO therapy, as haemoglobin inactivates NO by binding to it and forming methaemoglobin (Powroznyk & Latimer 1997). Children receiving NO therapy should therefore have their methaemoglobin levels measured daily.

CONCLUSION

With the increase in the diversity and complexity of medical equipment, health care professionals are faced with the responsibility of collecting and synthesising a vast amount of technical knowledge and skills. This technology has the potential to help guide and perfect the management of the critically ill child. However, it is important for practitioners to understand the potential pitfalls and dangers of new and developing technology. As health care professionals, we are faced with the challenge of making this technology work in the best interests of the critically ill child.

REFERENCES

Ahrens T, Penick J C, Tucker M K 1995 Frequency requirements for zeroing transducers in hemodynamic monitoring. American Journal of Critical Care 4(6):466–471
Blumer J L 1990 A practical guide to pediatric intensive care, 3rd edn. Mosby, St Louis
Bridges E J, Woods S L 1993 Pulmonary artery pressure measurement: state of the art. Heart and Lung 22(2):99–111

Campbell B 1997 Arterial waveforms: monitoring changes in configuration. Heart and Lung 26(3):204–214
Department of Health 1994 The Allitt Inquiry. HMSO, London
Gibbs N C, Gardner R M 1988 Dynamics of invasive pressure monitoring systems: clinical and laboratory evaluation. Heart and Lung 17(1):43–51

Hazinski M F 1992 Nursing care of the critically ill child, 2nd edn. Mosby, St Louis

Henneman E H, Henneman P L 1989 Intracacies of blood pressure measurement: reexamining the rituals. Heart and Lung 18(2):263–271

Loach J, Thomson N B 1987 Hemodynamic monitoring. Lippincott, Philadelphia

Martin L 1992 All you really need to know to interpret arterial blood gases. Lea and Febiger, Philadelphia

Merl K E, Pauly-O'Neil S 1987 Nursing care of the child with a pulmonary artery catheter. Pediatric Nursing 13(2):114–119

Mupanemunda R H, Edwards A D 1997 Nitric oxide: physiology, pathophysiology and potential clinical applications. In: David TJ (ed) Recent advances in paediatrics – 15. Churchill Livingstone, New York, pp 119–136

Park M, Menard S 1987 Accuracy of blood pressure measurements by the Dinamap monitor in infants and children. Pediatrics 79(6):907

Powroznyk A V V, Latimer R D 1997 Progress in monitoring and delivery of inspired nitric oxide therapy. British Journal of Intensive Care (Jul/Aug):149–154

Rogers M C 1992 Textbook of pediatric intensive care. Williams and Wilkins, Baltimore

Stokes P, Jowett N 1985 Haemodynamic monitoring with the Swan-Ganz catheter. Intensive Care Nursing 1:3–12

Tibby S M, Brock G, Marsh M J, Murdoch I A 1997 Haemodynamic monitoring in critically ill children. Care of the Critically Ill 13(3):86–89

Von der Mosel H A 1994 Principles of biomedical engineering for nursing staff. Blackwell, Oxford

Woodrow P 1997 Nitric oxide: some nursing implications. Intensive and Critical Care Nursing 13(2):87–92

4

Cardiopulmonary resuscitation in infants and children

Jos Latour

A respiratory or cardiac arrest in infants and children is an acute, life-threatening event requiring immediate intervention. In spite of improved knowledge and advanced technology the mortality and morbidity rates among children following cardiopulmonary resuscitation are very high (Bos et al 1992, Zaritsky 1993).

Cardiopulmonary resuscitation (CPR) is the restoration of automatic and effective breathing and circulation. There are two stages to intervention in CPR:

1. Basic life support — the restoration of effective ventilation and circulation using non-invasive methods. That is, breathing expired air into the lungs without mechanical devices and using closed cardiac compression techniques.

2. Advanced life support — invasive procedures aimed at restoration of ventilation and circulation. These include bag–valve–mask ventilation, endotracheal intubation, intravenous, intraosseous and/or endotracheal drug administration and defibrillation.

HISTORICAL PERSPECTIVE

The history of cardiopulmonary resuscitation goes back to the Old Testament. This mentions the prophet Elijah bringing back to life an apparently dead child using mouth-to-mouth respiration and thoracic compression. In the 18th century, intubation techniques were used for the first time, but it was not until the 1950s that CPR techniques truly developed. Kouwenhoven and colleagues (1960) are credited with one of the first publications in this field, in which they described closed-chest cardiac massage. More recently, studies have assessed pharmacological agents and mechanical devices which improve vital organ perfusion and thus CPR outcome.

AETIOLOGY

The primary cause of a cardiopulmonary arrest in infants and children differs from that in adults. CPR in adults is often required following a primary cardiac arrest caused by arrhythmias, while a cardiopulmonary arrest in children is more often the consequence of respiratory failure. The initial hypoxia and acidosis result in bradycardia and subsequent asystole.

Common respiratory problems causing arrest in childhood include:

- asphyxia
- sudden infant death syndrome
- inhalation of a foreign body
- bronchiolitis
- pneumothorax.

A respiratory arrest can also occur secondary to neurological dysfunction such as convulsions, increased intracranial pressure, encephalopathy or intoxications.

Primary cardiac arrest in childhood is rare, observed mainly in children with congenital heart disease. Due to improved surgical techniques in the management of congenital heart defects, it may be that the number of children suffering from a primary cardiac arrest will increase in the future (Boisvert et al 1995).

Cardiac arrest also occurs secondary to circulatory failure with decompensated shock in children suffering from burns, trauma or meningococcal sepsis.

In paediatric intensive care (PIC), a cardiac arrest caused by progressive shock or arrhythmia will occur more frequently, as respiratory arrest is often prevented. Oxygen delivery and ventilatory support are sufficient to prevent deterioration in children with respiratory difficulties. The differing causes of cardiopulmonary arrest in children and adults are attributed to differences in anatomy and physiology, which influence the procedures used during resuscitation.

ANATOMICAL AND PHYSIOLOGICAL DIFFERENCES

The well-known statement 'Children are not small adults' implies that children need alternative treatments to adults. The most noticeable difference is the size and the variation with age. Rapid changes take place in the first year of life. An infant's weight increases from about 3.5 kg at birth to about 10 kg by 1 year. After the first year of life, weight gain is steady until the pubertal growth spurt. Medication is administered to children on the basis of a dose per kilogram, so it is important to know the child's weight in acute situations. A simple formula to calculate this is:

$$\text{weight (kg)} = 2 \times (\text{age} + 4)$$

This formula can be used for children between 1 and 10 years.

The anatomy of the respiratory tract changes as children grow older. Infants have a large head with a relatively short neck. The large tongue can easily obstruct the airway, particularly when the floor of the mouth is compressed.

The child's respiratory rate is considerably higher than in adults, because of the relatively high metabolic rate and oxygen consumption. The major developments in the cardiovascular system take place in the first months of life, the left ventricle becoming dominant by 6 months of age. The circulating blood volume of an infant is 70–80 mL/kg. This is a considerably larger volume per kilogram than in adults. However, the actual volume is small, leading to critical situations arising from relatively minor loss of circulating blood volume in infants and young children.

Knowledge of these differences in the respiratory and cardiovascular systems is important when performing CPR and is dealt with in the relevant sections below.

PAEDIATRIC BASIC LIFE SUPPORT

Basic life support should commence immediate-

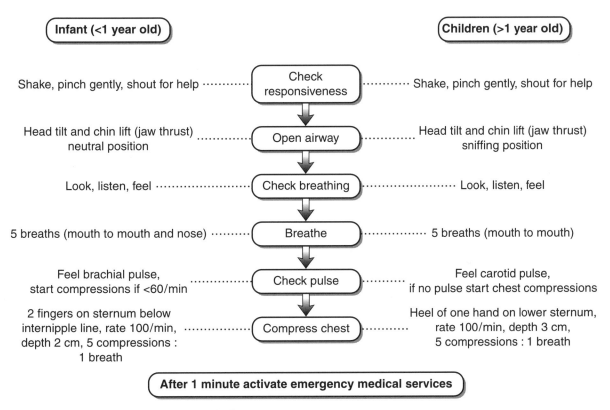

Figure 4.1 Primary steps in paediatric basic life support.

ly, once the rescuer has established a safe environment. The primary steps refer to the 'ABC of resuscitation' (Fig. 4.1):

- *Airway*
- *Breathing*
- *Circulation*.

Airway

A cardiopulmonary arrest in children is often caused by respiratory insufficiency. The anatomical and physiological differences in the airway between the child and adult often contribute to this. The airway of the child is much narrower than that of the adult. Obstruction from oedema or mucus can significantly reduce the airway diameter and increase resistance to airflow, consequently increasing the work of breathing (Chameides & Hazinski 1994). Infants under

6 months are obligatory nose breathers, which makes clearing of blocked nostrils essential in this age group. The tongue of the infant is large in proportion to the oral cavity. Posterior shifting of the tongue can cause severe airway obstruction. The epiglottis of young children is short and narrow, angling away from the axis of the trachea. This may cause some difficulties during endotracheal intubation, as visualization when passing the endotracheal tube may be difficult. In children under 10 years of age, the narrowest part of the airway is below the vocal cords at the level of the cricoid cartilage. In teenagers and adults, the narrowest area is at the glottic inlet.

Opening the airway is important in the unresponsive child. Unconscious infants and children often have airway obstruction because of displacement of the tongue. Establishing and maintaining airway patency is essential and can be

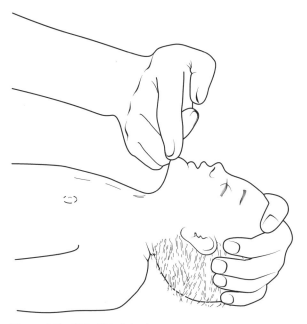

Figure 4.2   Chin lift in infants.

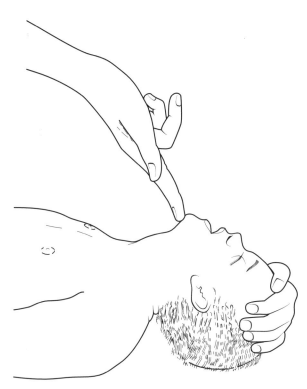

Figure 4.3   Head tilt / chin lift.

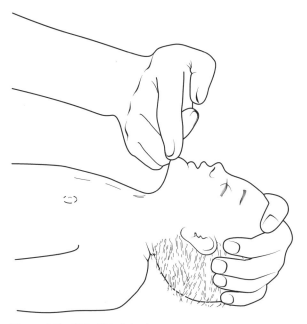

Figure 4.4   Jaw thrust.

achieved using one of two manoeuvres, as follows.

Head tilt / chin lift.   With one hand on the forehead, the head is tilted gently back into a slightly extended position. Overextension of the infant's head may result in airway obstruction due to the large tongue and collapsible trachea. The advisable degree of tilt is the neutral position for the infant and a sniffing position for the child (Figures 4.2 and 4.3). The lower jaw is lifted with the tip of a finger of the other hand. No pressure should be placed on the soft tissue under the chin, as the tongue can be pushed back into the airway.

Jaw thrust.   This manoeuvre is used where:

- cervical spine injury is suspected
- trauma has occurred
- head tilt / chin lift is ineffective.

Jaw thrust does not extend the neck. Three fingers are placed under the angles of the jaw, which is lifted upwards (Fig. 4.4). The mouth is opened by depressing the tip of the chin with the thumbs. Once the airway is opened the rescuer assesses breathing, for a maximum 10 s:

- *looking* for chest and abdominal movements
- *listening* for breath sounds via mouth and nose
- *feeling* for expired air movement on the cheek (ALSG 1997, Resuscitation Council 1997).

This is best achieved by putting the face above the child's head, the ear over the nose, the cheek over the mouth, and the eyes looking along the line of the chest and the abdomen.

Breathing

Children have a high oxygen demand per kilogram of body weight because their metabolic rate is high (ALSG 1997). Therefore inadequate ventilation rapidly leads to hypoxia in children. Hypoxia results from respiratory failure due to:

- decreased lung compliance
- increased airway resistance.

Both may increase the work of breathing and increase oxygen demand. Disease processes interfere with the exchange of oxygen and carbon dioxide. A mismatch of ventilation and perfusion may cause shunting of blood through the lungs, leading to hypoxia and hypercapnia. Hypothermia, intoxication, metabolic derangements, cervical spine injuries or dysfunction of the central nervous system may also compromise the ventilatory function of the child. Apnoea is relatively common in these cases, and the respiratory rate should be carefully observed.

If no spontaneous breathing is detected after airway opening manoeuvres, rescue breaths should be administered. While maintaining airway patency, expired air is blown into the infant's nose and mouth or into the child's mouth with the nose pinched. Up to five slow breaths, each lasting 1 to 1.5 s, should be delivered, whilst observing chest movement. Slow and steady inflation minimizes gastric distension. Initial inflation pressures may be high in infants in order to open the small airways. If the chest does not rise or if the movement is inadequate, airway opening manoeuvres and rescue breaths should be repeated. Foreign body obstruction should be excluded.

Circulation

Once the airway has been opened and the initial five breaths have been given, circulation should be assessed. The rescuer should feel for a pulse in a large artery for up to 10 s. This should assess rate and volume. Palpation of the carotid pulse is recommended in children, as it is easily accessible without removing clothing and is frequently palpable when the child is in shock. Palpating the brachial arteries is the easiest way to check the pulse in infants (Rogers & Helfaer 1995). The brachial pulse located on the inside of the middle of the upper arm can be palpated with two fingers over the abducted and externally rotated upper arm (Fig. 4.5). In all ages groups the femoral pulse is an alternative.

If there is an adequate rate but no effective breathing, ventilation should continue. If the pulse is less than 60/min in infants or absent for 10 s in older children, external chest compression is required. Chest compressions are serial, rhythmic compressions of the chest used to circulate blood to the vital organs until advanced life support can be provided. To achieve optimal compression the child must be supine on a hard surface.

In infants the area of compression is the lower half of the sternum, which can be located one finger breadth below the internipple line. Two fingers are used to compress the sternum about one-third the depth of the chest (Fig. 4.6). Another technique used in infants is the encircling method (Fig. 4.7). The thumbs are placed on the area of the sternum described above, and the fingers of both hands are placed behind the infant's back. The chest must re-expand between the compressions to enable optimal ventilation. In small children the compression area is two finger breadths above the xiphoid process. The heel of one hand is used to compress the sternum one-third the depth of the chest.

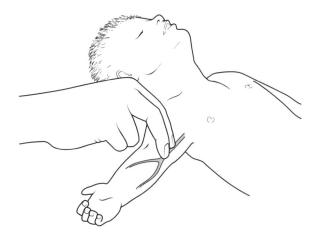

Figure 4.5   Feeling the brachial pulse.

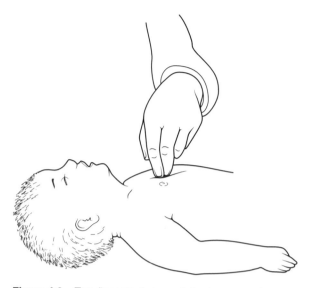

Figure 4.6 Two-finger technique of chest compression.

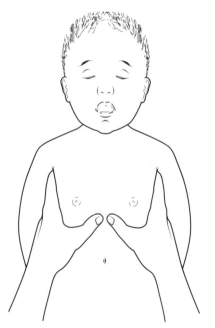

Figure 4.7 Hand-encircling technique.

During basic life support a compression rate of 100/min is maintained in infants and small children. The ratio of compression to ventilation is 5:1 for one or two rescuers. In older children the adult two-hand method of chest compression is used. The heels of the hands are placed on top of each other, two finger breadths above the xiphoid process. The depth of compression is one-third the depth of the chest at a rate of 100/min, with a compressions-to-ventilation ratio of 15:2 (Resuscitation Council 1997).

Basic life support should continue until medical intervention is available.

Foreign body obstruction

If airway obstruction by a foreign body is suspected, the airway must be cleared. If the object is clearly visible in the mouth, it can be removed by turning the head to one side and removing the object with one finger. Blind finger sweeps should not be used, as objects can be pushed further down the airway and mucous membranes can be damaged.

A common protocol for the management of choking in infants and children is seen in Fig. 4.8. Five back blows are delivered between the shoulder blades, while holding the infant or child in a prone position with the head lower than the chest. If the obstruction is not relieved, five chest thrusts are administered with the child in a supine position, the head again lower than the chest. The hand position for chest thrusts is the same as for chest compression, but the rate is slower, at 20 per minute, and the action is brisker.

The mouth is checked and visible foreign bodies removed before the airway is opened using the head tilt/chin lift or jaw thrust manoeuvre. If there is no effective spontaneous respiration, five rescue breaths are attempted. In children over 1 year of age abdominal thrusts (Heimlich manoeuvre) are substituted for chest thrusts after the second round of blows. This is not recommended in infants, as abdominal organs can be damaged. It is advisable to continue these procedures until the foreign body has been removed.

PAEDIATRIC ADVANCED LIFE SUPPORT

Paediatric advanced life support aims to perfuse the coronary and cerebral arteries with oxygenated blood to maintain vital cell function. This

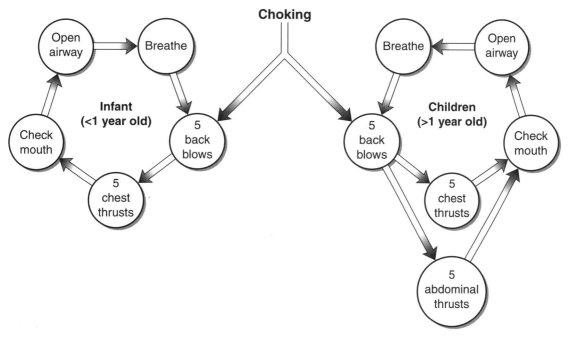

Figure 4.8 Choking protocol.

involves the use of airway adjuncts, drug therapy and defibrillation.

Airway adjuncts

A stable patent airway is necessary to ensure effective ventilation. To prevent the tongue obstructing the airway an oropharyngeal or Guedel airway can be used with bag–valve–mask ventilation. Guidance for the correct sizing of Guedel airways is that it should extend from the centre of the mouth to the angle of the jaw when laid against the child's cheek. Care should be taken when inserting this in infants and toddlers, as the soft palate can be damaged when inserted upside down. Adequate ventilation can be achieved using a bag–valve–mask system until personnel experienced in the intubation of infants and children are available.

During CPR, ventilation is best controlled with endotracheal intubation. Anatomical differences in infants and children dictate the type of laryngoscope blade used for intubation. A straight-blade laryngoscope is often preferred for infants, as it lifts the epiglottis to give a better view of the glottis. The curved-blade can be used in children over 1 year of age. The broader base and flange of the blade move the tongue to improve glottic visualization. During intubation, Magill's forceps may be used to guide the endotracheal tube through the vocal cords, and gentle cricoid pressure aids visualisation of the cords as well as reducing the risk of aspiration of stomach contents.

During resuscitation a plain sterile plastic endotracheal tube with a radiopaque marker is recommended. The use of cuffed tubes is not recommended in children below 8 years of age, as they can cause oedema at the cricoid ring. A 3 to 3.5 mm internal diameter endotracheal tube is required for full-term newborn infants, although premature neonates may need a 2.5 mm diameter. Rapid estimation of tube size in children can be achieved by choosing a tube with an outside diameter of about the same diameter as the child's little finger. Another useful guideline is the formula:

$$\text{internal diameter (mm)} = (\text{age}/4) + 4.$$

This formula is appropriate for children over 1 year of age. The correct length of the endotracheal tube is determined by assessing chest movement and breath sounds. Intubation must be achieved quickly; intervals in ventilation longer than 30 s may result in serious hypoxaemia. If intubation is not achieved within 30 s, bag–valve–mask ventilation should be recommenced. During CPR, orotracheal intubation is preferred because it can be performed more rapidly than nasotracheal intubation.

Ventilation adjuncts

A high concentration of oxygen is required during CPR. The face mask chosen must provide an airtight seal, which is achieved using a mask which extends from the bridge of the nose to the cleft of the chin. The face mask is used with a self-inflating bag–valve device with a reservoir bag to provide oxygen levels of up to 90%. A minimum oxygen flow of 10 L/min is required to maintain an adequate oxygen supply in the reservoir bag. Without this bag, maximal oxygen levels will be 60%.

The mask is held on the child's face with one hand performing the head tilt / chin lift manoeuvre, while the other hand is used for manual ventilation. There are three sizes of self-inflating bags available:

- 240 mL
- 500 mL
- 1600 mL.

Vascular access

Establishing reliable vascular access is essential during paediatric advanced life support. Evidence suggests that when vascular access is established within the first few minutes of resuscitation the outcome is improved (Rogers and Helfaer 1995). Peripheral venous access in children is difficult, but should be attempted unless the peripheral veins cannot be seen or palpated below the skin surface. In small children venous access should be established in the largest, most accessible veins without interruption of resusci-

tation. If venous access is not achieved within 90 s, intraosseous access should be attempted. Intraosseous needles provide a safe and reliable route for drug, fluid and blood administration in infants and children. It is a simple technique which in most cases can be applied within 60 s (Guy et al 1993). This route provides access to a non-collapsible venous plexus in the medulla of the bone. The proximal tibia is the site for intraosseous needle insertion in infants and children. A specially designed 16- or 18-gauge needle is inserted medial to the midline on the anterior surface of the tibia, 1–3 cm below the tibial tuberosity. The tibial tuberosity is identified by palpation. The needle is directed either at a 90° angle to the surface of the tibia or slightly inferior to avoid the epiphyseal plate.

If vascular or intraosseous access in an intubated child is not achieved within 3 min, adrenaline can be given via the endotracheal tube. In this case the dose should be 10 times the recommended intravenous dose (Quinton et al 1987). Atropine and lignocaine can also be given by this route but there is no scientific data regarding the dose. However, atropine 40–60 µg/kg and lignocaine 3 mg/kg diluted with saline have been recommended (ALSG 1997, Chameides and Hazinski 1994). The volume of endotracheal drug administration should not be too large:

- in small children, not more than 5 mL
- in older children, not more than 10 mL.

Dissolving the medication in normal saline decreases the possibility of damaging endothelial cells and destroying surfactant.

Intracardiac drug administration is no longer recommended, because complications such as damage to a coronary artery, cardiac tamponade or pneumothorax are common.

Drugs therapy

The most frequently used resuscitation drugs are epinephrine (adrenaline), atropine and sodium bicarbonate. Epinephrine has proven itself clinically in paediatric resuscitation, while atropine and sodium bicarbonate remain controversial (Goetting 1994). Epinephrine has alpha- and beta-adrenergic effects. The alpha-adrenergic actions increase peripheral vascular resistance, raising systolic and diastolic blood pressure. This increases coronary perfusion and cerebral blood flow during CPR. The beta-adrenergic activity increases myocardial contractility and heart rate. The initial intravenous or intraosseous dose of epinephrine recommended is 0.01 mg/kg (0.1 mL/kg of the 1:10 000 solution). The second and subsequent doses of epinephrine should be 0.1 mg/kg (1 mL/kg of the 1:10 000 solution or 0.1 mL/kg of the 1:1000 solution). After each dose of epinephrine a flush of at least 5 mL of normal saline should be given to move the drug to the central circulation. In non-VF/VT arrest, the dose is repeated at 3 min intervals during CPR.

Although atropine does not have proven benefits in paediatric CPR, it may be considered for the treatment of persistent bradycardia (Chameides & Hazinski 1994). Since cardiac output depends on the heart rate in young children, bradycardia must be treated even when the blood pressure is normal. A heart rate less than 60 beats/min in infants is associated with poor systemic perfusion. If hypoxia is the cause of bradycardia, adequate ventilation and oxygenation should be achieved before administering atropine. The recommended initial atropine dose for vagolytic effects is 0.02 mg/kg (20 µg/kg) with a minimum single dose of 0.1 mg and a maximum single dose of 0.5 mg. The maximum total dose is 1 mg in children and 2 mg in adolescents. Frequently, cardiopulmonary arrest in children is caused by hypoxia resulting from respiratory failure. Hypoxia leads to acidosis, which reduces the effectiveness of epinephrine (Chameides & Hazinski 1994). If epinephrine is not effective after two or three doses, sodium bicarbonate should be administered following assessment of the child's blood pH. The dose of sodium bicarbonate is 1 mmol/kg (1 ml/kg of 8.4%) given as a single bolus intravenously. A more accurate dose can be achieved using the following formula:

$$NaHCO_3 \text{ (mmol/kg)} = 0.3 \times \text{weight (kg)} \times \text{base deficit}$$

In infants, 4.2% solution should be used to reduce the hyperosmolar effects of sodium bicarbonate. Following sodium bicarbonate administration, the line should be flushed with normal saline, as catecholamines such as epinephrine are inactivated by bicarbonate. It should be remembered that the most effective method of correcting acidosis is by providing effective ventilation and chest compression during CPR. After any bolus of drugs used in CPR, a bolus of normal saline should be given whether the drug is given through an intravenous or an intraosseous line.

Fluid therapy

Fluid therapy is indicated for absolute or relative hypovolemia. The most common cause of circulatory failure in infants and children is hypovolemic shock, due to inadequate fluid intake or large volume losses. Distributive, septic and anaphylactic shock can also contribute to hypovolemia. When cardiac arrest occurs as a result of hypovolemia with poor or no response to the initial dose of epinenphrice, a bolus of fluid should be given. Fluid resuscitation therapy should consist of 20 mL/kg of a crystalloid such as Ringer's lactate, a colloid such as 5% human albumin or an artificial colloid solution. Caution is called for when administering glucose during CPR, especially in infants. Animal studies have shown that hyperglycaemia increases the possibility of ischaemic brain injury (Nakakimura et al 1990).

Cardiac arrest management

The Resuscitation Council of the United Kingdom (1997) has identified two cardiac arrest algorithms for use with infants and children (Figs 4.9 and 4.10).

Cardiac arrest is the absence of a palpable central pulse. In most cases, cardiac arrest is the final result of respiratory failure or shock in infants and children. Therefore attention must first be focused on the establishment of a patent airway, effective ventilation, adequate oxygenation and circulatory stabilisation. Where ventricular tachycardia (VT) or ventricular fibrillation (VF) occurs, the first intervention is defibrillation.

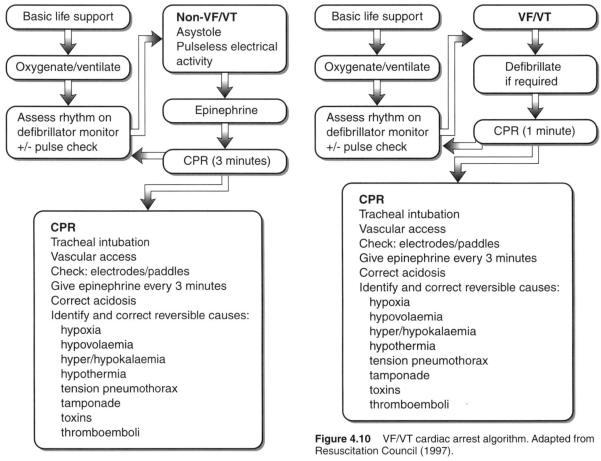

Figure 4.9 Non-VF/VT cardiac arrest algorithm. Adapted from Resuscitation Council (1997).

Figure 4.10 VF/VT cardiac arrest algorithm. Adapted from Resuscitation Council (1997).

The three commonest rhythms seen on electrocardiogram (ECG) of children suffering cardiac arrest are:

- asystole
- electromechanical dissociation or pulseless electrical activity
- ventricular fibrillation.

Asystole and pulseless electrical activity

These rhythms are incorporated into the algorithm for non-VF/VT arrest (Fig. 4.9). Asystole is a pulseless arrest with no cardiac electrical activity. In children, asystole is the most common arrest rhythm observed in respiratory and circulatory failure. The ECG shows a straight line along which occasional P waves can be observed. To determine asystole, clinical confirmation of the absence of pulse is obligatory since a straight line can also be caused by a loose lead or electrode.

Pulseless electrical activity or electromechanical dissociation is characterised by the absence of a palpable pulse but foresence of organised electrical activity on the ECG monitor. The most common cause of electromechanical dissociation (EMD) in children is hypovolaemic shock. Other common causes are:

- tension pneumothorax
- pericardial tamponade
- electrolyte disturbance
- intoxication
- hypothermia.

The cause of EMD should be detected and treated whilst CPR continues.

Ventricular fibrillation/tachycardia

Ventricular fibrillation is characteristically a disorganised series of ventricular depolarisations with absence of palpable pulses. No P, QRS, or T waves are identified on the ECG monitor. VF waves are chaotic and rough in structure, or fine when the waves are small.

VF is uncommon in children, but can be seen in children with

- hypothermia
- tricyclic antidepressant poisoning
- electrolyte abnormalities
- cardiac disease.

Ventricular tachycardia is rare in childhood, but is most often seen with cardiac disorder such as myocarditis or cardiomyopathy. Rates vary between 120 and 250 beats/min, but can increase to 400 (ALSG 1997, Chameides & Hazinski 1994).

Slow rates may be associated with an adequate cardiac output, but faster rates lead to poor perfusion, lack of palpable pulses and can deteriorate to VF. Causes of VT include:

- hypoxia
- acidosis
- electrolyte disturbances
- drug toxicity/poisons.

The ECG shows broad QRS complexes with absent or dissociated P waves and T waves of opposite polarity to the QRS. It is vitally important to identify VF or pulseless VT and treat immediately with defibrillation.

Defibrillation is asynchronous depolarisation of the myocardial cells to gain a spontaneously organised myocardial depolarisation (Chameides & Hazinski 1994). Paediatric paddles (4.5 cm) should be used when defibrillating infants under 10 kg of body weight, to optimise transthoracic impedance. In children, adult-sized paddles can be used if the entire surface of the paddles makes contact with the chest wall. One paddle is placed over the apex of the heart in the midaxillary line. The other is placed beneath the right clavicle

to the right of the sternum. Anterior–posterior placement of adult paddles can be used in infants if paediatric paddles are not available. In this position the paddles cover the total surface of the chest and back with the heart between them (Atkins et al 1988). The energy dose for the first two shocks is 2 J/kg, with subsequent shocks at 4 J/kg. The time between the three sets of shocks should be brief and limited to pulse checks using the appropriate artery for age. CPR should continue for 1 min prior to a second set of shocks at 4 J/kg. Consideration should be given to the cause of dysrhythmia, with correction of acid–base and electrolyte balance, which may enhance the effectiveness of defibrillation.

POST-RESUSCITATION MANAGEMENT

Following successful resuscitation, full intensive care facilities are required.

On admission to PIC, possible causes of the event should be explored. It is not uncommon for resuscitated children to die within the first 48 h of arrest, because of multisystem organ failure or cellular and homoeostatic abnormalities. Cellular damage may occur as a result of reperfusion injury. The post-resuscitation management in PIC aims to achieve and maintain homoeostasis in order to optimise the outcome of CPR.

Most children require ventilation to maintain oxygen saturation above 95% and blood gases within the normal range. Arterial and central venous pressure monitoring provide essential information about cardiovascular function. These parameters guide management in relation to circulatory expansion, inotropic support and vasodilatory agents. Kidney function is assessed clinically through observation of urine output and assessment of blood biochemistry. Acid–base and electrolyte balance have to be normalized in order to restore cellular homoeostasis.

Treatment aims to prevent secondary brain injury following hypoxic ischaemic insults. Therefore monitoring of neurological status is essential for 48 h following hypoxia, for early detection of signs of raised intracranial pressure. Temperature monitoring is essential; infants and children often become cold during resuscitation, because of their large surface area to weight ratio. Returning and maintaining temperature within normal parameters can help improve oxygenation and cardiovascular function.

Blood glucose monitoring is essential immediately after arrest, particularly in infants. Hypoglycaemia is not uncommon in critically ill infants. Symptoms similar to those seen in the hypoxic infant may occur, with a compromise in cardiovascular function. Correction of hypoglycaemia with 0.5 to 1 g/kg of 10% glucose solutions is recommended to prevent cerebral damage caused by hyperosmolar solutions. This equates to 5 to 10 mL/kg of the 10% solution, which should be given over 20–30 min on account of the volume.

TEAM APPROACH

Teamwork is essential during resuscitation. Ideally, the team consists of two doctors and two nurses. If possible, a third nurse can support parents and keep them informed. Team coordination is very important in this stressful situation. As medical decisions have to be taken, a doctor should lead the team, giving clear instructions to other team members. One nurse will be responsible for observing vital signs, informing doctors of changes, timing the resuscitation period and recording drugs given.

Protocols can be helpful to enhance efficiency and rapid decision-making. The Broselow paediatric resuscitation tape uses the child's length to calculate size of equipment and doses of drugs and fluid (Luten et al 1992). The Oakley chart provides a length–weight–age guide to drug and fluid dosage and ET tube sizes (Oakley 1988). It is important to know which system is used by the CPR team, to prevent unnecessary time delay.

Goetting (1994, p 1150) suggested that 'practice makes perfect, and poor CPR produces poor outcome'. It is essential for paediatric CPR teams to update their skills in order to maintain competence. It is recommended that people performing CPR update their skills through formal retraining programmes every 1–2 years, although frequency of recommended retraining is very

arbitrary. Study of CPR training shows a decline in competence between the training sessions (Berden et al 1993a). Practitioners must accept responsibility for maintaining their skills and undertaking retraining programmes (Berden et al 1993b, Maibach et al 1996).

Paediatric CPR training programmes should include both basic and advanced life support interventions. Emphasis in paediatric life support should rest with airway management, vascular access techniques and administration of cardiovascular drugs, since these techniques are the most common interventions in paediatric resuscitation (Schoenfeld & Baker 1993). Defibrillation techniques may only be relevant for practitioners working in PICU and accident and emergency departments. Therefore, they may not be included in all training programmes. Comprehensive evaluation of paediatric resuscitation is necessary to identify the content of future CPR courses.

ETHICAL AND MORAL ISSUES

When CPR is commenced, the child's parents should be informed immediately. Parents have often been anxiously kept away from their child during CPR. From the nursing and medical perspective this is considered to be a traumatic experience for parents to witness, and there are concerns that the parents' call for attention may be at a moment when the team has to concentrate on the resuscitation. Fortunately a change in this attitude has been observed in the past few years. More often parents are offered the opportunity to be present at the resuscitation of their child. Optimal support of the parents and explanation of this rather devastating event are essential. In this situation a nurse should stay with the parents constantly.

It is well known that the outcome of CPR in infants and children is very poor (Bos et al 1992, Zaritsky 1993). A child's death has a major impact on the lives of the parents and the other family members. It is the nurse's duty to support the parents in the grieving process.

By definition, resuscitation necessitates practitioners working under great stress. To prevent team members from developing psychological problems, it is important to evaluate everybody's actions after any CPR, whether successful or not. During this evaluation the team members should be allowed to express emotions. A social worker or counsellor can facilitate this process.

Ethical implications of treatments concerning withdrawal and limitation of life support are considered in many countries (Ryan et al 1993). When a 'do not resuscitate' order is considered, this will have to be discussed with the parents. Time is an effective variable in the parents' decision-making process. When the parents have to take a life support decision over their child in a very short time, they often authorise health care providers to do anything to offer their child a longer life. When life support has been discussed with the parents during the course of a child's illness, they are in a position to give careful consideration to this issue. In their considerations the main point is often the quality of the child's life (Kirschbaum 1996). Therefore it is the health care team's ethical and moral obligation to discuss the 'do not resuscitate' considerations with the parents at the earliest appropriate time.

THE FUTURE

Paediatric CPR techniques and guidelines have regularly been reviewed and updated over the past few decades. In spite of scientific evidence which has led to the update of these techniques and guidelines, the outcome of resuscitation in childhood is still poor. The question may be asked whether we have to wait for the findings of the next scientific contributions or if we can actively contribute to the improvement of paediatric resuscitation at unit or hospital level. Audit of paediatric cardiopulmonary resuscitation within the hospital may provide useful information about the standards of resuscitation in infants and children. It may result in change of equipment and drugs used for resuscitation (Innes et al 1993). Audit can also determine whether CPR training has to be intensified or adjusted. Periodic audit can determine whether the alterations made have influenced resuscitation. It has been documented that the competence of resuscitation skills of health care workers declines between CPR training sessions. Emphasis on training and audit of resuscitation skills for the purpose of maximising self-efficacy may benefit the commitment of staff performing CPR.

REFERENCES

Advanced Life Support Group (ALSG) 1997 Advanced paediatric life support, the practical approach. BMJ Publishing Group, London

Atkins D L, Sima S, Kieso R, Charbonnier F, Kerber R E 1988 Pediatric defibrillation: importance of paddle size in determining transthoracic impedance. Pediatrics 82(6):914–918

Berden H J J M, Williams F F, Hendrick J M A 1993a How frequently should basic CPR training be repeated to maintain adequate skills: retention of CPR skills in different training programmes. British Medical Journal 306:1576–1577

Berden H J J M, Williams F F, Hendrick J M A, et al 1993b Resuscitation skills of Dutch general nurses. Heart and Lung 22(6):509–515

Boisvert J T, Reidy S J, Lulu J 1995 Overview of pediatric arrhythmias. The Nursing Clinics of North America 30(2):365–379

Bos A P, Polman A, van der Voort E, Tibboel D 1992 Cardiopulmonary resuscitation in paediatric intensive care patients. Intensive Care Medicine 18(2):109–111

Chameides L, Hazinski M F 1994 Textbook of pediatric advanced life support. American Heart Association, Dallas

Goetting M G 1994 Mastering pediatric cardiopulmonary resuscitation. Pediatric Clinics of North America 41(6):1147–1182

Guy J, Haley K, Zuspan S J 1993 Use of intraosseous infusion in the pediatric trauma patient. Journal of Pediatric Surgery 28(2):158–161

Innes P A, Summers C A, Boyd I M, Molyneux E M 1993 Audit of paediatric cardiopulmonary resuscitation. Archives of Disease in Childhood 68(2):487–491

Kirschbaum M S 1996 Life support decisions for children: what do parents value? Advances in Nursing Science 19(1):51–71

Kouwenhoven W B, Jude J R, Knickerbocker G G 1960 Closed-chest cardiac massage. JAMA 173:1064–1067

Luten R C, Wears R L, Broselow J, et al 1992 Length-based endotracheal tube and emergency equipment selection in pediatrics. Annals of Emergency Medicine 21(8):900–904

Maibach E W, Schieber R A, Carroll M F B 1996 Self-efficacy in pediatric resuscitation: implication for education and performance. Pediatrics 97(1):94–99

Nakakimura K, Fleischer J E, Drummond J C, et al 1990 Glucose administration before cardiac arrest worsens neurologic outcome in cats. Anesthesiology 72(6):1005–1011

Oakley P A 1988 Inaccuracy and delay in decision making in paediatric resuscitation and a proposed reference chart to reduce error. British Medical Journal 297:817–819

Quinton D N, O'Byrne G, Aitkenhead A R 1987 Comparison of endotracheal and peripheral venous intravenous adrenaline in cardiac arrest: Is the endotracheal route reliable? Lancet i:828–829

Resuscitation Council (UK) 1997 The 1997 resuscitation guidelines for use in the United Kingdom. London, Resuscitation Council (UK)

Rogers M C, Helfaer M A 1995 Handbook of pediatric intensive care. Williams & Wilkins, Baltimore

Ryan C A, Byrne P, Kuhn S, Tyebkhan J 1993 No resuscitation and withdrawal of therapy in a neonatal and a pediatric intensive care unit in Canada. The Journal of Pediatrics 123(4):534–538

Schoenfeld P S, Baker M D 1993 Management of cardiopulmonary and trauma resuscitation in the pediatric emergency department. Pediatrics 91(4):726–729

Zaritsky A 1993 Outcome of pediatric cardiopulmonary resuscitation. Critical Care Medicine 21(9 suppl.):S325–S327

5

Transportation of the critically ill child

Gavin Morrison

Recent government interest in the development of paediatric intensive care (PIC) services has highlighted the need to rationalise and develop paediatric intensive care transport services. However, transport services can only function effectively if there is appropriate deployment of personnel and integration of transport teams into the network of paediatric services already established. This chapter will address issues to be considered when establishing an effective transport service.

Transport teams have formed an important component of adult and neonatal critical care services but have been relatively neglected in the provision of paediatric intensive care in the UK. In recent years an attempt has been made to produce guidelines for the establishment of a paediatric transport service within the UK. The Paediatric Intensive Care Society (1995) recommends that each PICU should provide a fully equipped, consultant-led transport team, available 24 hours per day, consisting of a doctor and senior nurse. These recommendations have been locally interpreted, which has resulted in over-provision and duplication of this service in some areas and inadequate provision in other areas of the country. The inadequacies of PIC transport services in the UK are highlighted in 'A framework for the future' (DoH 1997) and have been addressed through the recommendations for reorganisation and establishment of regional transport services from Lead Centres.

Review of the literature pertaining to interhospital transportation of critically ill children suggests recommendations can be made regarding the optimal configuration of this service. Indeed, to date, in the UK there has been a lack of consensus between physicians and health authorities regarding the ideal configuration of this service. There are lessons to be learned from North America and Australasia.

In the UK, PIC continues to be provided in units of widely variable bed capacity, often by staff with limited training in caring for critically ill children and in institutions lacking the full range of paediatric subspecialties. Many centres providing paediatric critical care do not have the ability to establish and maintain designated retrieval teams. Just as critically ill children benefit from being treated in large centres where care is managed by appropriately trained staff (Pollack et al 1991), evidence suggests that outcome is improved if transportation is undertaken by a specially trained transport team (Britto et al 1995, Edge et al 1994).

Why are specialised paediatric transport teams needed?

The transportation of critically ill children is not without risk to the child. Several studies have highlighted the morbidity associated with the interhospital transfer of the critically ill patient. Barry & Ralston (1994) conducted an observational study of the transfer of children to a tertiary critical care centre by transport teams originating from the referring hospital. The study was conducted over a period of 6 months and included 58 patients, 2 of whom were subsequently excluded due to failure to obtain full details of the transport episode. They identified one or more adverse events in 42 (75%) of these transfers, with potentially life-threatening events occurring in 13 (23%). Of the life-threatening events, 8 (61%) were related to failure to provide adequate airway support, a priority in the resuscitation and stabilisation of a critically ill child. Sharples et al (1996) recounted similar findings in a prospective audit of 143 children transferred to a tertiary critical care centre by teams from the referring hospitals. Nineteen (13%) children were transferred with no monitoring, whereas Barry & Ralston had documented 6 (11%) such cases in

their study. Failure to secure an adequate airway was again identified as a major failing, with 42 children transported without endotracheal intubation. Twenty-one (50%) of these 42 children required intubation on or shortly after arrival at the tertiary centre. In a further 10 children the endotracheal tube was occluded at the time of admission to PICU, necessitating immediate re-intubation. Other documented adverse events identified by these studies included:

- hypoxia
- failure to offer adequate fluid resuscitation
- infusion of inappropriate maintenance fluids
- absence of vascular access
- vital signs not recorded during the transfer.

The significance of the study by Barry & Ralston has been questioned on the grounds that many of their patients were infants with congenital abnormalities, but this does not detract from the relevance of the findings. A review of childhood deaths related to head injury in a single region over an 8 year period (Sharples et al 1990) again highlighted failure to provide adequate control of the airway as an avoidable factor contributing to death before and after hospital admission.

These studies suggest that standards of care during transport for critically ill children may be improved when performed by specialists. Edge et al (1994) compared the performance of transport systems involving two intensive care units. The participating units were similar in terms of the population served, rural/urban ratio and number of admissions per year. One centre received transported patients through a dedicated specialist transport team, whilst the second centre depended on the referring hospital to transfer the patient. The specialist team always consisted of:

- a physician with both neonatal and paediatric intensive care experience
- an intensive care nurse of 5 years experience and training in transportation
- a respiratory therapist with paediatric experience.

Both physician and nurse had completed an advanced life support course. The referring hospital team varied in seniority, training and paediatric experience, depending on the severity of illness of the child and the availability of staff. In some transport episodes undertaken by the referring team there was no physician present. The authors identified two categories of adverse event occurring during patient transport, based on criteria introduced by Kanter & Tompkins (1989), which can be grouped under one of the following:

(a) physiological deterioration, e.g.,
- respiratory arrest and/or desaturation
- circulatory arrest, hypotension, arrhythmia
- loss of consciousness, loss of brainstem reflexes and/or spinal cord function
- hypothermia $< 34°C$
- hypoglycaemia.

(b) intensive care/equipment related, e.g.,
- loss of intravenous access
- accidental extubation
- exhaustion of oxygen supply.

During the study period, 47 patients were transferred by the specialist team, while the referring hospital team were responsible for 92 transfers. The patients in each group were similar in terms of pre-transfer PRISM and Therapeutic Intervention on Severity Score (TISS) scores, duration of transfer and number of patients intubated. There was no difference between groups in terms of adverse physiological events, with deterioration occurring in 5 of the 47 and in 11 of 92 transfers (11% vs 12%), respectively. However in 19 of the transfers performed by the referring hospital team, an intensive care related adverse event occurred, whereas in only one transfer by the specialist team was such an event documented (20% vs 2%). This study suggests that specialist teams prevent avoidable secondary insults to the transferred patient. Drawing a conclusion from the failure of the specialist team to prevent physiological deterioration is hampered by the difference in age of the patients transported by the two teams and the incidence of trauma:

- 5 of 47 specialised transports
- 23 of 92 non-specialised transports.

Britto et al (1995) also used the criteria of Kanter & Tompkins (1989) as measures of morbidity in their study of 51 children transferred by a specialist team. Only 2 (4%) of these children experienced physiological deterioration, and no episodes of equipment failure were reported. In this study there were no patients transferred by non-specialist teams for comparison, therefore the data were compared with that provided by Barry & Ralston (1994). Drawing conclusions from such a comparison is difficult because of the difference in patient profile between the two groups (Logan 1995). Despite this, the findings reported by Britto reinforce the role of the specialist transport teams in the prevention of morbidity in the children that they retrieve.

Paediatric transport teams

Currently there is no consensus regarding the ideal composition of the paediatric transport team. However, the 'Framework for the future' document (DoH 1997) echoes the Paediatric Intensive Care Society (UK) (PICS) model of a consultant-led service, with each retrieval episode being undertaken by a clinician and a nurse. In the USA, guidelines have been issued on paediatric transportation, including the composition of the transport team (American Academy of Pediatrics Committee on Hospital Care 1986). Current practice is for teams to be led by a physician, who is at minimum a specialist registrar. This clinician will be an intensive care trainee, with an anaesthetic or paediatric medicine background. Each case is assessed by the Consultant Intensivist to determine the required experience of the medical personnel dispatched. The physician should be accompanied by at least one other person, usually an experienced nurse or an ITU technician. Solo transfers should never be undertaken. Inexperienced nurses should always be educated and supervised by senior nursing staff during critical care transfers until they have sufficient experience to undertake solo transport episodes safely. Nursing staff in North America undertaking paediatric transfer duties are required to undertake a comprehensive education programme (Beyer et al 1992, Edge et al 1994).

There has been extensive debate amongst providers of paediatric critical care in the USA as to the necessity of a physician-led team for every transfer. The knowledge and skills of the nurse combined with those of the respiratory therapist have challenged the need to have a doctor present. It has been demonstrated in both paediatric and neonatal transfers that suitably experienced and educated nursing staff are capable of performing patient transfers safely (Thompson 1980, Beyer et al 1992).

Edge et al (1994) documented a greater number of equipment-related but not physiological adverse events in transports performed by non-specialised teams. He speculated that the specialised team had performed better not because of the presence of a physician but because of the experience of nurse and respiratory therapist within the team. MacNab (1991) found that transfers led by physicians were associated with reduced morbidity compared with transport episodes led by a paramedic or emergency medical attendant (EMA) regardless of whether or not the EMA had received specialised paediatric training. (The EMA would be expected to be capable of basic life support skills, but would not be recognised as a specialist in the transport of the critically ill. The paramedic ambulance crews in the UK would have comparable skills.) He also found that specialist EMAs with paediatric training conducted safer transports than those undertaken by non-specialist EMAs even when accompanied by a referring physician. The combination of untrained physician and untrained EMA was associated with greater morbidity than transfers performed by untrained EMAs alone. Beyer et al (1992) reported on the transfer of 422 intubated patients by teams consisting of specialist nurses and respiratory therapists with paediatric critical care experience who had undergone an education programme in critical care transfer. Beyer correctly identified concerns for airway safety as a frequent argument for the presence of a physician. By studying only the intubated patients of a total 614 infants and children transferred, he sought to record the safety of non-physician transfers in terms of adverse physiological and equipment-related occurrences. An adverse event occurred in eleven out of the 422 transfer episodes. In only one case was the team unable to intubate/re-intubate a child deemed to require an endotracheal tube. This transfer was undertaken without the presence of a respiratory therapist but the child came to no lasting harm. The overall complication rate was only 2.6%. Unfortunately, drawing conclusions from this study is hampered by the disproportionate number of children aged less than 1 month who were included in the study group (295/422).

Smith & Hackel (1983) conducted a retrospective study of 115 patients transported between 1978 and 1979. Each transport was led by a physician. Each patient was assigned to one of four groups depending on the level of care required. Although not' addressed in their conclusion, the information provided suggests that over 50% of the patients could have been safely transported by experienced nursing staff alone. When Rubenstein et al (1992) interviewed transport physicians and nurses post-transport, these groups respectively identified 34% and 46% of transports as not requiring a physician. There is therefore sufficient evidence in the literature that non-physician-led transport teams are capable of safely retrieving many children for whom critical care has been requested and that the dispatch of such teams may be appropriate in 40–50% of transfers. However, a major difficulty lies in identifying a triage system capable of predicting the personnel required for each transport. In 1992, Rubinstein et al addressed this problem with a prospective evaluation of the three potential indicators of the requirement for a physician-led transport. The indicators utilised were:

- subjective evaluation of physician receiving the referral phone call
- PRISM score > 0 at time of referral
- presence of tachycardia (age adjusted).

The need to include a physician on the transport team was identified if a procedure or medical intervention normally undertaken by a physician was required during the transfer or on admission to the intensive care unit. By this criteria, only 50 (39%) transfers required a physician. However, pre-transfer physician assessment identified 114 (88%) transfers requiring a physician. This reflected a tendency to send physicians on transfers needlessly rather than mistakenly not send one. Likewise, use of PRISM score and presence of tachycardia failed to accurately predict transfers requiring a physician. This suggests that many paediatric critical care transfers can be safely performed without a physician, provided training in critical care procedures is undertaken and the members of the transport team are sufficiently experienced to make clinical judgements.

Regardless of the personnel profile of a transfer team, its establishment represents a significant commitment in terms of staff, especially if a unit seeks to be able to offer a 24 h retrieval service capable of undertaking concurrent transfers. Accurate data identifying the UK centres with a 24 h retrieval service is lacking. However, it appears that most UK centres are frequently unable to offer such a service, because of staff or resource limitations. Similarly, in the USA, 40% of paediatric centres with critical care or emergency medicine programmes included in a study were unable to offer regular patient transportation to their units, mainly because of staffing difficulties (McCloskey & Johnston 1990). All the literature cited originates in North America and at present may have little relevance to the situation in the UK. However, there are lessons to be learned from the experience of others, and a more multidisciplinary approach to transport of the critically ill in this country may result in more effective utilisation of human resources.

Whom should be transferred

Transfer is appropriate for those children whose condition may benefit from critical care intervention and where a reasonable quality of life can be expected upon recovery. The local paediatrician will often decide the appropriateness of referral to the tertiary critical care service for the continued therapy of the child. These decisions are relatively straightforward in the previously normal child with acute illness, but the value of critical care support to those children with advanced chronic disease or with a potentially fatal condition may be less clear and open to debate. Decisions regarding limitation of therapy are difficult but need to be addressed. The

child's best interests must be considered and decisions should not focus solely on sustaining existence. The local paediatricians may be best placed to make these decisions, particularly if the child and family are known to them. The request for critical care in situations in which the prognosis of a child is such that intervention is futile, is rare. Much more common is the request for critical care services for children who may require close monitoring or constant nursing attention but not intensive care. An audit of 145 consecutive retrieval episodes over a 4 month period, gave complete data on 135 children (McIntyre et al 1997). In this prospective audit, 32 (24%) of the children did not require intensive care therapy. Rubinstein (1992) identified 61% of the 129 transfers in his study as not requiring a physician or critical care intervention. Inappropriate referrals result in poor utilisation of the skills of critical care personnel and deskill other services. Inadequate provision of high-dependency care needs to be addressed to reduce the number of inappropriate referrals to intensive care. The role of intensive care units needs further clarification if transport services are to be used safely and appropriately. We must ensure that such transport services are not regarded as a paediatric-trained ambulance service.

Which centres should provide transfer of critically ill children?

To gain expertise in the transfer of critically ill children, transport teams must be regularly exposed to the challenges of providing effective critical care in multiple environments. No data exists to indicate the minimum number of retrievals required to ensure the skills of a transfer team are maintained. However, the reduction in adverse events associated with the deployment of specialist teams suggests that there is a negative correlation between the number of transfers undertaken and transfer-associated morbidity. This is recognised in the current strategy to establish regional transfer teams throughout the UK.

Provision of transport services also requires consideration of the local demographics and the distribution of specialised paediatric tertiary services. Critically ill children should have access to tertiary paediatric intensive care services which provide a transfer team with the ability to respond rapidly to requests. Specialist tertiary paediatric services are often required in the care of the critically ill child, therefore ready access to the expertise of subspecialists is essential to provide optimal care. Therefore, it would appear that transportation of the critically ill child should be conducted by teams arising from large PICUs in centres with a wide range of paediatric subspecialties, in order to provide for both the immediate and ongoing management of the child.

Rationalisation of PIC services in the UK is likely to result in the closure of small units, but the overall benefit of this strategy is that it provides equity in the quality of care and outcome for all critically ill children. Analysis of total admissions to paediatric intensive care units for 1987 indicated that, on the basis of admission rates of other developed countries, it was likely that a significant number of children were not given access to the care they required. Shann (1993) succinctly described the state of paediatric critical care in the UK, postulating that national paediatric intensive care requirements could be met by 12–14 units, each serving a population of approximately one million children. He highlighted the contribution to be made by specialised transport teams in improving the quality of critical care.

How should children be transported?

In the UK, patient transport is almost exclusively achieved by ambulance. This differs significantly from the experience in North America, where the use of aircraft occurs in approximately 70% of paediatric transports. Considerations when deciding the means of transport to be employed are well documented and include:

- nature of the illness
- distance from the tertiary centre
- weather conditions

- ease of access of the chosen mode of transport at both the referring and receiving centres.

The benefits of air evacuation have been demonstrated by the reduced mortality of adult trauma victims transported by helicopter compared with those transported by road. These studies originated in the USA, where large sections of the population live long distances from centres capable of providing expert tertiary care. The use of helicopter transport in such rural communities reduces the response time of the retrieval team and speeds up the transport of the patient to the tertiary centre. In Britain the population is more geographically concentrated and, with the exception of areas of low population density such as Scotland, it is unlikely that air transport offers any significant advantage over retrieval by road. Boyd et al (1989) suggested that trauma may be the exception. Outcome of rural trauma victims transported by air showed increased survival associated with a shorter arrival time at the tertiary care facility when compared with road transfer. Nicholl et al (1995) undertook a study comparing the performance of the London Helicopter Emergency Medical Service (HEMS) and land ambulance. There was evidence that patients with major trauma had improved survival if transported by HEMS. This advantage did not extend to non-trauma patients. Interestingly they found that, although medical attention was available at the scene an average of 25 min earlier if the team were delivered by helicopter, the land ambulance was capable of delivering the patients to the receiving units faster than the air service could. Given that helicopter air transfers are weather dependent and not undertaken at night within central urban areas, they do not constitute an efficient form of transport for the majority of episodes. Therefore, each region will have to consider local factors before deciding the merits of helicopter transportation.

Planning for retrieval of the critically ill child

Involvement of the critical care team in the management of a child begins at the time of referral.

To optimise the advice given and to allow for adequate planning on the part of the retrieval team, accurate clinical assessment of the child is required. Important clinical details may be omitted, making it difficult for the retrieval team to get a comprehensive view of the needs of the critically ill child. Britto et al (1995) utilise a transfer log to ensure the acquisition of all the relevant details at the time of referral, using a systematic approach. Difficulties in assessing the child prior to transfer are well documented. Scoring systems validated for intrahospital risk of mortality estimation perform poorly when utilised as triage tools. Recommendation of management strategies by the retrieval team have been shown to improve treatment in a significant number of children (McIntyre et al 1997). Appropriate advice was primarily related to securing the airway, fluid resuscitation and commencement of inotropes. The retrieval team can formulate a plan of management for the child whilst in transit to the referring hospital, including clarification of roles during the initial resuscitation and subsequent transfer. Relevant drug dosages are calculated prior to arrival at the referring hospital in order to save time.

Following assessment of the child, parents are informed of the interventions required and given the opportunity to ask questions. They should be given written information including directions to the retrieving hospital and contact telephone numbers. The referring hospital is asked to assist the parents in their travel arrangements, as only in exceptional circumstances is it possible for them to accompany their child in the ambulance.

The retrieval team maintains contact with their base unit, conveying information on the child's condition, expected time of arrival and any specific requirements. This facilitates a smoother handover of care from the retrieval team to the PICU team.

Responsibilities of the referring units

All staff in District General Hospitals caring for children will come into contact with those requiring resuscitation and intensive care. Many children referred to the transfer team will come from these hospitals. Therefore it is essential that staff have the skills to initiate resuscitation and level 2 critical care (DoH 1997). McIntyre et al (1997) identified 33 cases from 145 transport episodes in which specific management advice was ignored or not performed because it was deemed unnecessary. This represented 42% of all occasions when changes to management were recommended, with the commonest explanation given being the absence of a practitioner with the ability to undertake the intervention. Britto et al (1996) reported similar experiences, in a letter to the BMJ. In addition to this he found that failure to follow advice also occurred when personnel with the required skills were available. Raffles (1996) identified interventions undertaken by a specialised transport team which should or could have been performed by the referring centre. He recommended that local units be recognised for their contribution to critical care provision and that they themselves should recognise the contribution they have to make. Recognition of the importance of the concept of the golden hour or the platinum half hour is essential.

Legal issues in paediatric transport medicine

The respective responsibilities of the referring and accepting hospitals involved in the transfer of critically ill children has until now presented few problems, but potentially this presents a legal minefield. Currently, it is accepted that some responsibility rests with the receiving centre as soon as the child is accepted for retrieval. In the event that no bed is available, most centres recommend a second centre able to provide the appropriate level of care. Under the planned development of paediatric critical care services outlined in the document 'A framework for the future' (DoH 1997), the regional transport team will be responsible for ensuring that all referred children are found beds on units able to meet the child's needs.

The issue of legal responsibility arises at the time of the initial telephone referral when often advice is sought. If the advice offered is not followed, who bears the legal responsibility? A more complicated situation arises if the child experiences a significant complication secondary to undertaking the treatment recommended by the accepting hospital. Obviously the overall liability remains with the giver of care whether that care occurs within his/her own hospital environment or that of the referring hospital. All of these principles of responsibility have yet to be tested legally.

REFERENCES

American Academy of Pediatrics 1986 Guidelines for Air and Ground Transportation of Pediatric Patients. Pediatrics 78:943–950

Barry P W, Ralston C 1994 Adverse events occurring during interhospital transfer of the critically ill. Archives of Disease in Childhood 71:8–11

Beyer A J, Land G, Zaritsky A 1992 Nonphysician transport of intubated pediatric patients: a system evaluation. Critical Care Medicine 20:961–966

Boyd D R, Corse K M, Campbell R C 1989 Emergency interhospital transport of the major trauma patient: air versus ground. Journal of Trauma 29:789–791

Britto J, Nadel S, Maconochie I, Levin M, Habibi P 1995 Morbidity and severity of illness during interhospital transfer: impact of a specialised paediatric retrieval team. British Medical Journal 311:836–839

Britto J, Nadel S, Maconochie I, Levin M, Habibi P 1996 Impact of specialised paediatric retrieval teams (Author's reply to correspondence generated by their 1995 article). British Medical Journal 312:121

DoH 1997 Paediatric intensive care 'A framework for the future'. Department of Health, London

Edge W E, Kanter R K, Weigle C G M, Walsh R F 1994 Reduction in morbidity in interhospital transport by specialized pediatric staff. Critical Care Medicine 22:1186–1189

Kanter R K, Tomkins J M 1989 Adverse events during interhospital transport: physiologic deterioration associated with pretransport severity of illness. Pediatrics 84:43–48

Logan S 1995 Evaluation of specialist paediatric retrieval teams: commentary. British Medical Journal 311:839

MacNab A J 1991 Optimal escort for interhospital transport of pediatric emergencies. Journal of Trauma 31:205–209

McCloskey K A, Johnston C 1990 Critical care interhospital transports: predictability of the need for a pediatrician. Pediatric Emergency Care 6:89–92

McIntyre A, Nicoll S, Murdoch I 1997 Is the PICU retrieval team deskilling district general hospital staff. Abstract PICS conference, London

Nicoll J P, Brazier J E, Snooks H A, Lees-Mlanga S 1994 The costs and effectiveness of the London HEMS. Report to the DoH. Medical Care Research Unit, University of Sheffield

Paediatric Intensive Care Society 1995 Standards for paediatric intensive care

Pollack M M, Alexander S R, Clark N, Ruttiman U E, Tesselar H M, Bachulis A C 1991 Improved outcome from tertiary centre pediatric intensive care: a statewide comparison of tertiary and nontertiary care facilities. Critical Care Medicine 19:150–159

Raffles A 1996 Intensive care provided by local hospitals should be improved. British Medical Journal 312:120

Rubenstein J S, Gomez M, Rybicki L, Noah Z 1992 Can the need for a physician as part of the paediatric transport team be predicted? A prospective study. Critical Care Medicine 20:1657–1661

Shann F 1993 Australian view of paediatric intensive care in Britain. Lancet 342:68

Sharples P M, Storey A, Aynsley-Green A, Eyre J A 1990 Avoidable factors contributing to death in children with head injury. British Medical Journal 300:87–91

Sharples A, O'Neill M, Dearlove O 1996 Children are still transferred by non-specialist teams [letter]. British Medical Journal 312 (7023):120

Smith D F, Hackel A 1983. Selection criteria for pediatric critical care transport teams. Critical Care Medicine 11:10–12

Thompson T R 1980 Neonatal transport nurses: an analysis of their role in the transport of newborn infants. Pediatrics 65:887–892

Anatomical and Physiological Basis of Critical Illness in Infancy and Childhood

This section provides a systematic approach to the causes of critical illness in infancy and childhood and is written by medical and nursing experts from the UK. The common principles of management are addressed in relation to each physiological system. In addition, specific management of diseases and congenital problems is outlined where relevant. This approach has been taken to encourage a problem-solving rather than prescriptive approach to the management of specific disease processes.

6

Respiratory anatomy and physiology in infants and children

Michael Marsh

When considering paediatric respiratory disease it is useful to have a working knowledge of the developmental anatomy and physiology. This chapter describes the embryological development, adaptions at birth and major physiological functions of the respiratory system. In addition, basic principles of pulmonary mechanics, respiratory function tests and techniques available for respiratory support are included.

DEVELOPMENT OF THE RESPIRATORY TRACT

The respiratory system comprises:

- the nose
- nasopharynx
- larynx
- bronchi
- the lungs.

The development of the respiratory system is highly orchestrated with a clear pattern and rate of growth. Airway multiplication is complete at birth, although many alveoli and blood vessels have still to form. Differentiation of the respiratory system can be divided into four phases:

- The embryonic phase occurs between conception and 5 weeks and leads to initiation of airways formation.
- The pseudoglandular phase occurs between 5 and 16 weeks of gestation when the lower airways are formed.
- The canalicular phase, occurring from 17 to 24 weeks, sees the development of the acinus.

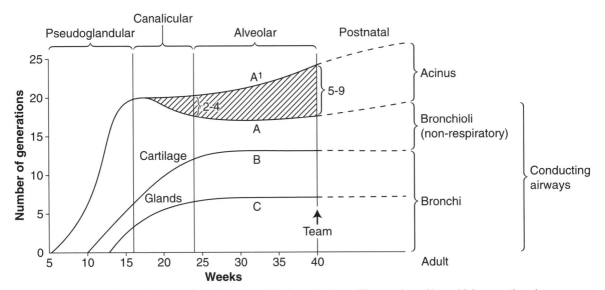

Figure 6.1 Intrauterine and postnatal development of the bronchial tree. The number of bronchial generations is represented by line A, respiratory bronchioles and terminal sacs by the shaded area A–A¹. B represents the extension of cartilage along the bronchial tree, and C the extension of mucous glands. Adapted from Bucher & Reid (1961), with permission.

• The alveolar phase, when the first respiratory units are formed (traditionally said to start in the perinatal period) (Thurlbeck 1981), has been shown to commence at about 27 weeks gestation (Langston et al 1984, Hislop et al 1986) and continue until term (Figs 6.1 and 6.2).

The upper airways

The endoderm appears about the 8th day. After the separation of the primitive endoderm from the blastodisc at about day 14, the cells of this layer form the primitive yolk sac. Around the 20th day the yolk sac becomes tucked under the head fold forming the foregut. The endodermal part of the mouth and much of the pharynx arises from the cranial portion of the foregut. At the end of the 4th week two ectodermal thickenings, called the nasal placodes, appear on the frontal prominence, which give rise to the nasal pits (Fig. 6.3a). When the embryo measures about 10 mm the nasal pits are seen and bounded by the medial and lateral nasal folds, the mandibular and maxillary processes (Fig. 6.3b). The maxillary process grows forward and meets the medial

nasal fold, which has formed the frontonasal process, hence forming the anterior and posterior nares. The lower deep aspect of the frontonasal process forms the primitive palate. Mesodermal tissue from the maxillary process grows medially, forming the palatal processes, towards the developing nasal septum. The palatal processes fuse with the posterior aspect of the primitive palate and subsequently with each other and the lower edge of the nasal septum.

Between the 3rd and 4th week a ventral diverticulum, the respiratory primordia, which gives rise to the larynx, trachea and lungs, appears caudal to the hypobronchial eminence. The caudal part of the foregut lengthens rapidly, forming the primitive oesophagus, with a longitudinal ridge developing on each side which subsequently fuses and separates the oesophagus from the respiratory diverticulum. At the end of the 4th week the epithelial component of the larynx develops rapidly, producing the hypopharyngeal eminences on either side, later to become the right and left arytenoid swellings, which form the primitive laryngeal aditus.

During the 5th and 6th week the epiglottis

Age	Length from TB to pleura (mm)	
(a) 16 week gestation	0.1	
(b) 19 week gestation	0.2	
(c) 28 week gestation	0.6	
(d) Birth	1.1	
(e) 2 months	1.75	
(f) 7 years	4.0	

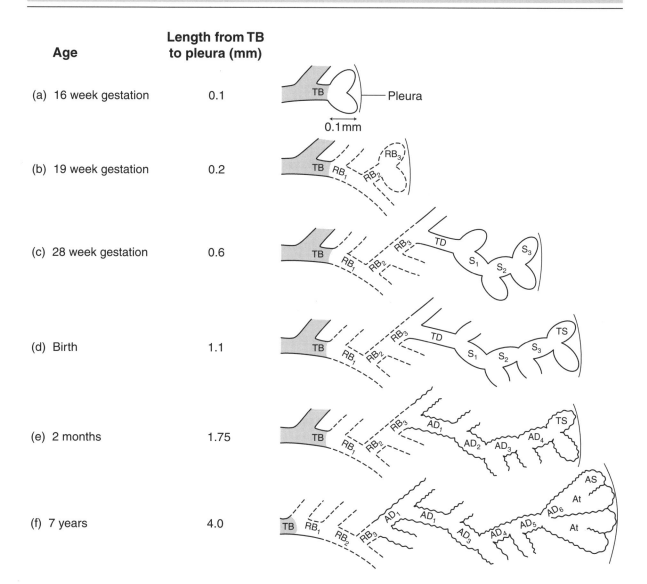

Figure 6.2 Diagrammatic representation of the acinus at six stages of development. At all ages, airway generations are drawn the same length, so that increase in length represents an increase in generations. A given generation may be traced down the same vertical line, permitting remodelling of its structure to be followed. Actual increase in size is shown by the length from terminal bronchiolus (TB) to pleura. RB, respiratory bronchiolus; TD, transitional duct; S, saccule; TS, terminal saccule; AD, alveolar duct; At, atrium; AS, alveolar sac. From Reid (1979), with permission.

appears as a midventral prominence at the base of the 3rd and 4th arch, cephalic to the glottis. The arytenoid swellings grow towards the base of the tongue, enfolding the epiglottis. At this stage epithelium temporarily obliterates the entrance to the larynx. In the following weeks the larynx grows rapidly and the lumen is re-established. By the 10th week the larynx is almost completely formed and the vocal cords appear on either side of the laryngeal lumen. The subsequent growth is slower, with the definitive form attained during the last trimester.

The bronchial tree

The tracheobronchial groove, part of the respira-

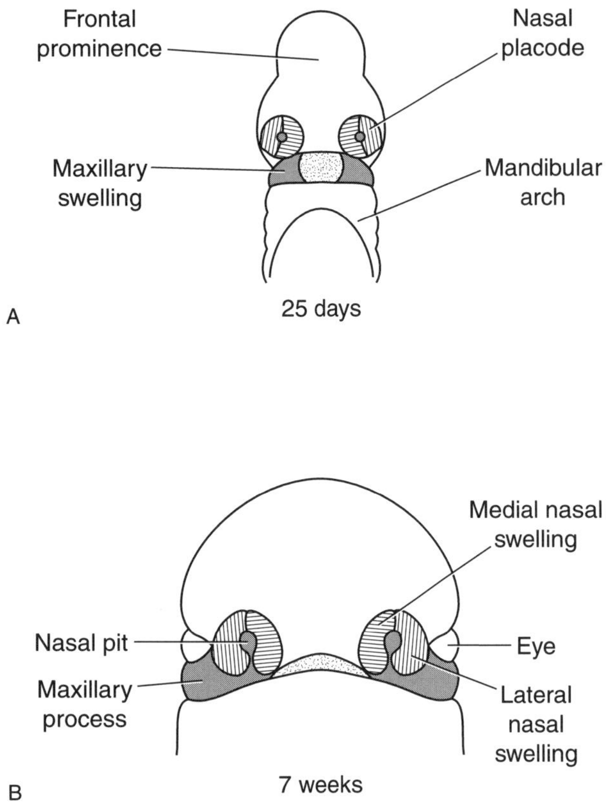

Figure 6.3 Frontal view of developing nasal placodes, maxillary swelling and the nasal swellings: (a) 25 days; (b) 7 weeks. Adapted from Larsen (1993), with permission.

tory primordia (lung bud), appears between the 3rd and 4th week as a ventral diverticulum, giving rise to the trachea and lungs. The distal portion of the groove, which gives rise to the trachea, lies ventral to and parallel with the oesophagus. The blunted end forms the primary bronchial buds. Endodermal tissue arises from the pharynx and gives rise to the epithelial lining and glands of the trachea, whilst surrounding mesenchyme gives rise to cartilage, muscle and connective tissue investing the developing trachea. Cartilage rings are identifiable by 10 weeks and epithelial glands by 16 to 18 weeks. By 20 to 24 weeks the main anatomical features of the trachea are established (Fig. 6.1).

The bronchial buds are usually asymmetrical and made up of two lobes: a large right and small left lobe separated by a shallow sulcus. From the

4th to 7th weeks, a series of monopodial and irregular dichotomous branchings occur, giving the principal bronchi with 10 principal branches on the right and 8 on the left (Fig. 6.4).

Between 10 and 14 weeks there is active division and ramification of the bronchi, resulting in 70% of the bronchial tree being complete. By the 16th week it is fully developed, with the lungs having a glandular appearance. Capillaries rapidly penetrate the epithelium, giving this a canalicular appearance. The number of bronchial generations is now complete and later decreases when alveolarisation of some non-respiratory bronchioles occurs, leaving about 27 generations.

Hence the bronchial tree consists of the trachea and the two main bronchi, which divide into lobar bronchi, segmental bronchi, lobular bronchi and alveolar ducts. The first 19 divisions do not take part in gas exchange and form the conducting zone. The first 7 divisions are cartilaginous in type, with the remaining 12 being membranous non-respiratory bronchioles and terminal bronchioles. The last 8 divisions take part in gas exchange, 4 divisions forming the respiratory bronchioles and the last 4 the alveolar ducts (Figs 6.1 and 6.2).

The terminal airways and alveoli

The terminal respiratory unit consists of those structures distal to the terminal bronchiole. At 16 weeks the terminal bronchiole opens directly into the terminal saccule, and the distance between the terminal bronchiole and pleura is 0.1 mm (Fig. 6.2). By 20 weeks the lung is midway through the canalicular stage. There is continued branching of the respiratory bronchioles, vascularisation of the terminal tubules and thinning of the epithelium. Each terminal bronchiole gives rise to between 2 and 5 orders of respiratory bronchioles between 19 and 28 weeks (Fig. 6.2c). The last respiratory bronchiole leads into the first alveolar ducts (for a period this exists as a transitional duct; Fig. 6.2d) which can vary in number between 2 and 6. At birth the final division opens into a terminal saccule, and the distance between the terminal bronchiole and the pleura is now 1.1 mm. Each alveolar duct opens into between

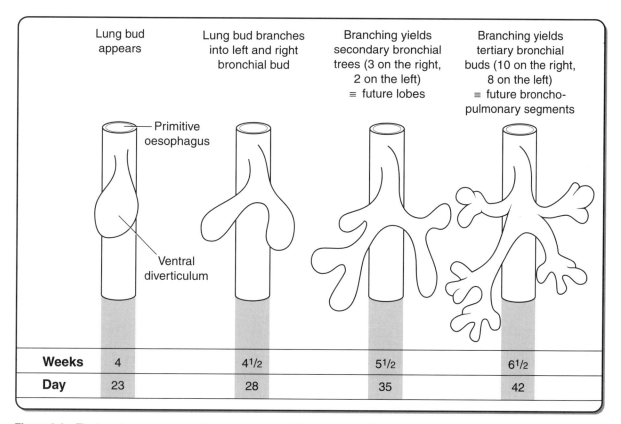

Figure 6.4   The lung bud giving rise to the principal bronchi between 4 and 7 weeks. Adapted from Larsen (1993), with permission.

10 and 16 alveoli. The alveoli begin to appear as shallow indentations between 32 weeks gestation and term. Most true alveolar development occurs after birth, increasing in number from 20–50 million in the newborn (Langston et al 1984) to about 300 million between 7 and 8 years of age. The alveoli are separated by an interalveolar septum made up of the alveolar epithelium, capillary and interstitial tissue (Fig. 6.5). Collateral ventilation between adjacent terminal airways is limited at birth, since the pores of Kohn have not yet developed.

The alveolar epithelium consists of two cell types both attached to a continuous basement membrane. Type I pneumocytes have a broad, thin cytoplasm and cover 90% of the alveolar surface, whilst Type II pneumocytes, which are more numerous because of their shape, only cover 5% of the alveolar surface. Type II cells develop cytoplasmic osmiophilic lamellar bodies at about 25 weeks and are responsible for the production and excretion of surfactant and epithelial cell regeneration.

The alveolar septa have a single capillary network. The capillaries have a basement membrane and a single layer of endothelial cells. The interstitial tissue consists of collagen and elastic fibres and some contractile myofibroblasts with a variable number of macrophages. The connective tissue is important in determining the elastic properties of the lungs and the relationship between lung units to try and ensure even expansion.

The lungs develop significantly after birth, with marked expansion of the acinus over the first 2 months of life. The distance from the terminal bronchiole to pleura now measures 1.75 mm. Alveolar proliferation occurs first on the saccules and the alveolar ducts, then the respiratory bronchioles and in later childhood on the terminal

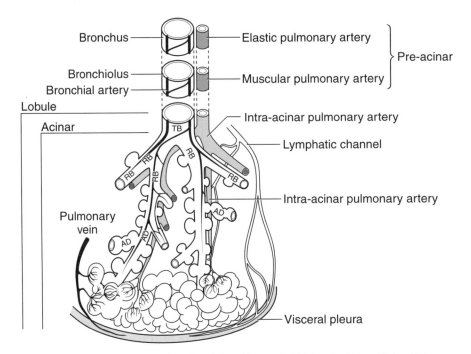

Figure 6.5 Schematic illustration of peripheral lung unit. TB, terminal bronchiolus; RB, respiratory bronchiolus; AD, alveolar duct. From Haworth (1987).

bronchioles, reaching 300 million by 7–8 years. The alveoli continue to grow in size until the chest wall growth ceases during early adulthood.

Adaptation of the respiratory system at birth

Effective adaptation takes place when structural, biochemical and neurophysiological maturation occurs in utero. Adaptation of the cardiorespiratory system at birth relies on the smooth transition from placental gas exchange to alveolar gas exchange.

After birth the lungs have to perform effective exchange of oxygen and carbon dioxide and play a vital role in acid–base balance. The fluid-filled lungs must empty and become aerated with adequate perfusion. These processes are centrally controlled by the brainstem.

Lung expansion

In utero the lungs are filled with fluid secreted by

the pulmonary epithelium. This has similar osmolality to fetal plasma, with a higher chloride content. The volume of this fluid is 20–30 mL/kg, which approximates to the functional residual capacity (FRC) established shortly after birth. During labour some of this lung fluid is cleared from the lungs by absorption. This process is affected by secretion of catecholamines (Brown et al 1981). As the infant passes through the birth canal, it is compressed. Intrathoracic pressures frequently reach above 50 cmH$_2$O and sometimes up to 200 cmH$_2$O (Saunders & Milner 1978). Lung fluid is expressed from the nose and mouth at about 10 mL/kg of body weight during labour.

As the chest emerges from the birth canal the elastic recoil of the chest wall contributes only a small part to initial aeration. On theoretical grounds and observations from stillborn and some healthy term infants, an opening pressure of 25–40 cmH$_2$O was thought to be necessary to expand the lungs. More recent studies on first breaths show that few require an opening pressure of greater than 10 cmH$_2$O. The onset of respiration usually occurs within 10 s of birth. A first breath of about 38 mL is taken with a mean inspiratory effort of between 30 and 35 cmH$_2$O. Of this breath about 16 mL is retained. A large intrathoracic pressure of up to 70 cmH$_2$O is almost always generated on the first expiration, because of closure of the pharynx and larynx (Saunders & Milner 1978). The remaining lung fluid is absorbed via the pulmonary lymphatics and across the pulmonary capillary membranes. Positive pressures during expiration in these early breaths and adequate surfactant are important in the maintenance of the established FRC.

Lung perfusion

In utero only 10–20% of the cardiac output flows through the lungs. Prior to delivery, the fetal pulmonary vascular resistance is higher than systemic vascular resistance, causing the remaining 80–90% of cardiac output to shunt through the foramen ovale and the ductus arteriosus. At birth, increased oxygenation and, to a lesser extent, the mechanical expansion of the lungs relieves pulmonary vasoconstriction. With the resulting fall in pulmonary vascular resistance the pulmonary artery pressure falls from around 60 mmHg at birth to around 30 mmHg at 24 h of age. Increased pulmonary blood flow causes a rise in the partial pressure of oxygen (PaO$_2$) and an accompanied rise in pH stimulating further pulmonary vasodilation. When the umbilical cord is clamped there is no longer any blood flow through the ductus venosus, causing a fall in right atrial pressure. Together with a rise in left atrial pressure, caused by increased pulmonary blood flow, functional closure of the foramen ovale is achieved. The ductus arteriosus closes under the influences of increased PaO$_2$ and inhibition of locally acting prostaglandins derived from the endothelial cells. The majority of measurable changes in the cardiopulmonary haemodynamics occur within 8 h of age (Berger et al 1977).

Control of respiration

The control of breathing after birth is a complex process which is unlikely to be fully mature at birth (Berger et al 1977). Components include:

- controllers—cerebrum, reticular activating system, brainstem and spinal cord
- effectors—spinal cord, diaphragm, intercostal muscles, upper airways and lungs
- sensors—peripheral and central chemoreceptors, proprioceptors, upper airway and lung receptors (Fig. 6.6).

Fetal breathing movements have been observed from 11 weeks gestation, the frequency and percentage of time performing these movements increases with gestational age, though even at term they occur less than 50% of the time. The chemoreceptors appear to be relatively insensitive in utero since the fetal PaO$_2$ is less than 4 kPa, a level that would cause intense respiratory drive after birth.

The levels of PaO$_2$ and PaCO$_2$ required to initiate breathing are PaO$_2$ 0.6 kPa in presence of PaCO$_2$ 5.5 kPa, rising to PaO$_2$ 2.5–3.0 kPa in the presence of PaCO$_2$>13.3 kPa. These blood gas changes occur rapidly after birth and, following the first breath, regular respiratory efforts are soon established.

The brainstem respiratory neurons do not appear to have inherent rhythmicity, but it occurs when the overall level of excitability is high. Non-specific factors (arousal, pain, temperature, touch) leading to reticular activation are likely to stimulate the respiratory neurons. The output of respiratory neurons is also modulated by afferents from mechano- and chemoreceptors.

Chemoreceptors have an important role in controlling respiration. The central receptors are affected mainly by changes in carbon dioxide detected by changes in brain tissue pH. Term infants seem to have the equivalent respiratory response to changes in PaCO$_2$ as adults, which is more marked during REM sleep. The response to changes in PaO$_2$ occurs mainly via the carotid body, and the newborn term infant responds to relative hypoxia by initial hyperventilation with increases in tidal volume and respiratory rate. The response to 100% oxygen is hypoventilation, suggesting a resting hypoxic drive in the newborn. The PaO$_2$ level is relatively low and unstable

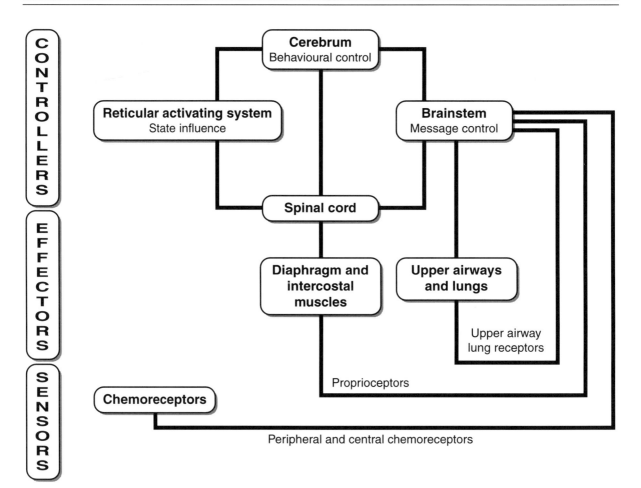

Figure 6.6 Schematic view of how respiration is controlled.

due to small lung oxygen stores and high metabolic consumption. This is therefore likely to generate powerful intermittent stimuli to breathe, contributing to the irregular periodic pattern observed in the newborn. In healthy infants this does not interfere with the normal response to raised CO_2 and low O_2 but may affect the infant with respiratory compromise. In light of this, care should be taken with infants who are at risk of respiratory depression from:

- major head trauma
- CNS infection
- narcotic administration
- raised intracranial pressure.

Vagal afferents from the lung, and receptors in the respiratory muscles and ribs, send information about lung mechanics. If less inflation occurs with a breath there is decreased afferent inhibition and hence increased inspiration signalled via efferents. The Hering–Breuer inflationary reflex probably has a protective role, preventing overinflation of the lungs by inhibiting inspiration. Similarly the Hering–Breuer deflationary reflex probably protects lung volume by initiating an inspiration if the lung volume falls below functional residual capacity (Marsh et al 1994).

Growth and development of the respiratory tract

The child's respiratory tract continues to grow

and develop throughout the first 8 years of life. It is important to appreciate the anatomical differences and the relevance of these during respiratory illness.

Structural differences in the upper airway relative to size can impede respiration. These include the following.

- Infants under 6 months of age are obligatory nasal breathers, therefore blockage of the nasal passages can lead to respiratory distress.
- Large amounts of lymphoid tissue can obstruct the airway during periods of infection.
- Size of tongue relative to the oral cavity.
- Size of airway predisposes increased airway resistance with any reduction in diameter, e.g. increased mucous production.
- Epiglottis is longer and floppier in infants and is positioned at a more acute angle, making it less effective at occluding the airway.
- The anterior position of the larynx is at the level of C2–3. Therefore cricoid pressure aids intubation by moving the larynx posteriorly, assisting the clinician to visualise the cords.
- The cricoid is the narrowest part of the airway in infants and children under 8 years, limiting the size of endotracheal tube used.
- Trachea is shorter, with more compliant cartilage, contributing to airway occlusion if the neck is hyperextended or flexed. When intubated, it is possible to dislodge the tube with excessive extension or flexion of the neck.
- More rapid growth of large airway produces a higher peripheral airway resistance in childhood. Inadequate exhalation can lead to air trapping, alveolar distension and possible pneumothorax. Therefore an appropriate ventilation regime would include:
  — small tidal volumes
  — short inspiratory times
  — low peak airway pressures.

The chest wall is cartilagenous in infants, giving a higher compliance than in older children and adults. Respiratory distress leads to retractions, reducing functional residual capacity and tidal volume, and thus increasing the work of breathing. The intercostal muscles do not assist the infant in elevating the rib cage but act only as a stabiliser. As the chest wall is thin, referred sounds are often heard. Therefore, when listening for air entry, the pitch is more important than the intensity of the sounds. In addition, the diaphragm of a newborn infant is higher in the thorax and contracts less efficiently than in the older child. It is positioned horizontally rather than obliquely into the chest wall, increasing the tendency to draw the lower edge of the rib cage inwards when distressed, especially when the infant is supine. Abdominal distension can severely impede the diaphragm. If present, infants should be nursed with a head-up tilt to reduce the pressure from abdominal contents.

BASIC RESPIRATORY PHYSIOLOGY

The primary function of the respiratory system is to facilitate oxygen delivery and uptake by the alveolar capillaries and allow alveolar carbon dioxide elimination. The lungs are responsible for exchange of oxygen and carbon dioxide, which contributes to the maintenance of acid–base balance. Both gases move between the air and blood by simple diffusion, and, according to Fick's law of diffusion, the amount of gas that moves is proportional to the area of the blood–gas barrier but inversely proportional to the thickness. In human lungs, these conditions are met by the enormous number of alveoli producing a large surface area for gas exchange. The alveoli are in direct contact with the pulmonary capillaries that are wrapped around them, providing a blood–gas barrier in the order of 0.5–1.0 μm.

Respiration consists of:

- *external respiration* or the exchange of gases between the blood and the lungs
- *internal respiration* or the exchange of gases in body tissues. More specifically, this involves the transfer of CO_2 from cells into the bloodstream and transfer of O_2 from the bloodstream into the cells.

Ventilation relates to the mechanical processes that move air in and out of the lungs during inspiration and expiration.

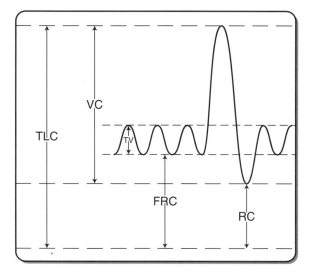

Figure 6.7 Lung volumes: TLC, total lung capacity; VC, vital capacity; TV, tidal volume; FRC, functional residual capacity; RV, residual volume. After Tortora & Anagnostakos (1990).

Inspiration

Negative pressure created within the thoracic cavity facilitates the movement of air into the lungs along a pressure gradient. Gas flows between the alveoli and capillaries according to the laws of diffusion, from areas of high concentration to areas of low concentration.

When considering the movement of gas into the lung, knowledge of static lung volumes is important (Fig. 6.7). Significant parameters are:

- tidal volume (TV) — normal breathing
- vital capacity (VC) — the volume exhaled following maximal inspiration followed by a maximal expiration
- residual volume (RV) — remaining volume of gas in the lungs after maximal expiration
- functional residual capacity (FRC) — volume of gas in the lungs after normal expiration
- minute ventilation (MV) — $MV = TV \times RR$
- alveolar ventilation (V_A) — $V_A = (TV - DS) \times RR$; this takes into account the anatomical dead space (DS).

In order for this process to occur successfully, gas must be brought to the blood–gas interface in the alveoli via the airways and blood to the pulmonary capillaries. The conducting airways carry inspired air to the gas-exchanging zone (Fig. 6.1). Since the conducting zones take no part in gas exchange, they constitute the anatomic dead space. The gas-exchanging zone is called the acinus or lobule (Fig. 6.5). During inspiration the volume of the thoracic cavity increases and air is drawn by bulk flow to about the level of the terminal bronchioles. Contraction of the diaphragm and intercostal muscles changes the thoracic volume as the diaphragm descends and the ribs are raised, increasing the cross-sectional area of the thorax. In the respiratory zone the massive increase in the cross-sectional area of the lungs results in a marked fall in the forward velocity of the gas. The mechanism of ventilation beyond this point is hence predominantly achieved by diffusion of the gas molecules. Return to the pre-inspiration volume is achieved through expiration caused by the elastic recoil of the lungs.

Perfusion (Q) and ventilation (V) are equally important. For perfect gas exchange, ventilation must equal perfusion of the lungs:

$$V/Q = 1$$

If either ventilation or perfusion alter, gas exchange will be affected. Physiologically a $V{:}Q$ ratio of 1 is never seen throughout the lungs of the normal child. When the child is upright the upper portions of the lungs are well ventilated but less well perfused. Therefore, Q is less than 1. The bases of the lungs are well perfused but less well ventilated, therefore V is less than 1. During respiratory illness or compromise the $V{:}Q$ ratio can be greatly affected, preventing adequate gas exchange.

Approximately 2% cardiac output fails to reach the right ventricle, as the bronchial circulation arises directly from the aorta. This supplies the intrapulmonary airways and drains into the pulmonary veins. In addition, the coronary circulation arises from the aorta, feeds the myocardium and drains via the Thebesian veins into the left ventricle. This small volume of deoxygenated blood leaving the left side of the heart forms the physiological shunt.

Diffusion — how gas crosses the alveolar wall

Diffusion is the process by which gas is transferred across the blood–gas barrier. Both oxygen and carbon dioxide move across the alveolar wall by passive diffusion. Diffusion through tissue is described by Fick's Law:

$$V_{gas} = \frac{area \times diffusion\ constant \times (P_1 - P_2)}{thickness}$$

The rate of diffusion of a gas (V_{gas}) through a barrier is proportional to the area and the difference in the partial pressure ($P_1 - P_2$) between the two sides, and inversely proportional to the thickness of the barrier. In the human lung the area of the blood–gas barrier is enormous and the barrier is less than 0.5 μm thick, making it ideal for diffusion. The diffusion constant is proportional to the solubility of the gas and inversely proportional to the square root of the molecular weight:

$$diffusion\ constant\ \alpha \frac{solubility}{\sqrt{molecular\ weight}}$$

Since carbon dioxide has a much higher solubility than oxygen despite a slightly higher molecular weight, it diffuses about twenty times more rapidly. Under normal conditions the transfer of oxygen across the blood–gas barrier is perfusion limited. The rise in the partial pressure of oxygen in the capillary virtually reaches the partial pressure of oxygen in alveolar gas when a red blood cell is about one-third of the way along the capillary.

In order to appreciate the effects of disease on diffusion it is useful to look at this in more detail. Normally the partial pressure of oxygen (PaO_2) in the red blood cell entering the capillaries of the lung is about 40 mmHg (5.4 kPa). In the alveoli on the other side of the blood–gas barrier the PaO_2 is about 100 mmHg (13.5 kPa). Oxygen therefore passes down this pressure gradient, and the PaO_2 in the red cell rises rapidly. This means that the difference between the PaO_2 in the alveolar gas and end-capillary blood is neglible.

Where cardiac ouput is high the pulmonary blood flow will be greatly increased and the time spent by a red blood cell in the capillary may be about a third of the normal time. Despite the reduced time available for oxygenation, there is still no measurable fall in the end-capillary PaO_2. However, if the blood–gas barrier is increased, as occurs in pulmonary oedema, oxygen diffusion may be impeded. The rate of rise in the PaO_2 is slowed and thus PaO_2 may not reach that of alveolar gas before the red blood cell has passed through the capillary. In this situation a significant fall between the alveolar gas and end-capillary blood PaO_2 may occur.

Oxygen transport

Oxygen is transported both bound to haemoglobin and in solution. Oxygen has extremely low solubility in solution, and therefore the majority is transported bound to haemoglobin. Each haemoglobin molecule has four binding sites for oxygen. The binding of each oxygen molecule alters the shape of the haemoglobin molecule such that loading and unloading for each subsequent molecule becomes easier. The relationship between the partial pressure of oxygen and the saturation of haemoglobin is referred to as the oxygen dissociation curve. Haemoglobin is fully saturated at approximately 100 mmHg (13.5 kPa). Alterations in pH, temperature and $PaCO_2$ can all affect the oxygen dissociation curve. Increases in $PaCO_2$, temperature and reducing pH all have the affect of shifting the oxygen dissociation curve to the right. This renders the unloading of oxygen much easier in the tissues. Reductions in temperature, $PaCO_2$ and increased pH shift the curve to the left, which has the effect of making the release of oxygen more difficult. In the fetus the main form of haemoglobin is fetal haemoglobin (HbF) rather than adult haemoglobin (HbA). HbF has a stronger affinity for oxygen than does HbA, and the oxygen dissociation curve in the fetus is shifted to the left of normal. This shift in the curve would appear to facilitate the transfer of oxygen across the placenta to the fetus. HbA starts to be produced by the fetus close to forty weeks' gestation.

Carbon dioxide transport

Removal of CO_2 from the blood by the lungs is a vital part of maintaining acid–base balance in the body. Respiring cells produce CO_2, and, unless this is removed from the body, life-threatening acidosis occurs. The kidneys also play an essential part in the removal of CO_2 from the body and maintaining acid–base balance.

Approximately 10% of CO_2 is carried away from the cells dissolved in plasma. This relates to the $PaCO_2$ and reflects the solubility of CO_2. Approximately 70% of CO_2 is carried as bicarbonate:

$$CO_2 + H_2O \rightarrow H_2CO_3 \rightarrow HCO_3^- + H^+$$

This reaction occurs mainly in the erythrocytes, which contain large quantities of carbonic anhydrase. This enzyme acts as a catalyst in the formation of carbonic acid from carbon dioxide and water. In the lungs the equation is reversed and CO_2 is removed. The remaining CO_2 (approximately 20%) combines with haemoglobin to form carbaminohaemoglobin. Whilst Hb can carry O_2 and CO_2 at the same time on different binding sites, the presence of one reduces the bonding ability of the other. The presence of dissolved CO_2 is also influenced by the PaO_2. If this decreases, the amount of dissolved CO_2 increases.

MEASUREMENT OF RESPIRATORY FUNCTION IN CHILDREN

Measurement of respiratory function can aid diagnosis and management of pulmonary pathology in adults and children. This has not been the case for the neonate and infant until relatively recently. The newborn infant presents special problems to the investigator, but information can be obtained about basal breathing patterns, mechanical properties, lung volumes and respiratory control using a range of techniques whilst the infant is in quiet sleep after a milk feed. The measurement of, for example, tidal volume may bring about changes in its baseline value, and investigators must be aware of this potential source of error. The more invasive the techniques the more likely this is to happen. Although these measurements still have a limited role in the management of individual children, they can increase our understanding of respiratory function and lung development.

Basal breathing patterns recording tidal volume, respiratory rate and minute ventilation are easy to perform in the sleeping newborn infant, using a face mask and pneumotachograph. The pneumotachograph ensures laminar flow across a small resistance, and under these conditions the flow is directly proportional to the pressure drop across the resistance. Measurements are affected by temperature, constituent gas and water vapour, but during tidal breathing the errors introduced are cancelled out. Volume is obtained by electronically integrating the flow signal against time.

Tidal breathing patterns give limited information. By simultaneously measuring intrathoracic pressure changes, it is possible to obtain a large amount of information about lung mechanics. This involves the passage of an oesophageal balloon (Beardsmore et al 1980), water-filled catheter or micropressure transducer (Vyas et al 1986) into the lower third of the oesophagus. With simultaneous measurements of flow, volume and oesophageal pressure, one can calculate dynamic compliance, a measure of lung stiffness, obtained by dividing a change in volume brought about by a change in pressure. Dynamic compliance is a reliable measure of lung stiffness when the infant's lungs are relatively healthy, the respiratory rate is less than 60 per minute (Milner 1990) and the oesophageal balloon is correctly positioned. Further information can be obtained by selecting the mid-inspiratory and mid-expiratory points on the volume trace and dividing the change in oesophageal pressure by the change in flow between these points. This gives the total pulmonary resistance, which provides a measure of airways obstruction.

More recently, techniques have been developed that allow non-invasive measurements of compliance and resistance. There are several variations of the technique, but all involve brief occlusion of the infant's airway at a lung volume above end-expiratory volume. The Hering–Breuer inflationary reflex produces respiratory muscle relaxation, and, on release of the occlusion, passive expiration occurs. This requires a face mask with an attached pneumotachograph, with a side port to measure mouth pressure at airway opening. Respiratory system compliance can then be calculated by dividing the volume expired on release of the occlusion by the pressure at airways opening (Mortola & Saetta 1987, England 1988).

Lung volume measurements can be useful for providing indirect information about lung growth and airways obstruction. Whole-body plethysmography enables you to measure resting lung volume. The infant is nursed in an airtight chamber with a face-mask–pneumotachograph–shutter system placed over the infant's face. By closing the shutter for 3 to 4 breaths the infant's continued respiratory efforts produce a pressure change within the face mask, which equals alveolar pressure in the absence of airways obstruction. The small changes in lung volume with these respiratory efforts can be calculated by calibrating the pressure changes within the chamber produced by the child's respiratory effort against a syringe. Using Boyle's Law the lung volume can easily be calculated.

RESPIRATORY SUPPORT

The goals of respiratory support in infants and children are similar to those of any critically ill patient. However, growth and development are important to consider as these often influence the type of support provided.

Goals for respiratory support

- Establish airway patency.
- Assess respiratory function to determine the respiratory support required. This could range from supplemental oxygen to full mechanical ventilation or even extracorporeal membrane oxygenation (ECMO).
- Preserve normal lung function.
- Reduce the metabolic expenditure on the work of breathing.
- Manipulate ventilation: for example, deliver abnormally high rates or large tidal volumes to control raised intracranial pressure.

Oxygen therapy

The infant with bronchiolitis may require no more than supplemental oxygen therapy, for the duration of the illness. Conversely, oxygen may be required for short or long periods following extubation after ventilation. Oxygen therapy can be delivered in a number of ways:

- headbox
- face mask
- nasal cannulae
- directly into the incubator.

Humidification is most easily provided through head box circuits or via a face mask using a heated wet humidity system. Heat–moisture exchange units are available for use with endotracheal tubes or tracheostomy tubes, and supplemental oxygen can be provided via an adaptor on the heat–moisture exchange unit.

There are two main difficulties associated with delivering oxygen therapy to infants and children: accuracy of the amount delivered and patient compliance may both influence the choice of delivery system. Hypoxic children become agitated, making them unlikely to tolerate oxygen therapy.

Oxygen delivery through a headbox can be measured directly using an oxygen analyser. Oxygen delivery via face mask is not easy to measure accurately. Different types of mask deliver different maximal percentages, but generally the nurse/doctor has to refer solely to the oxygen flow rate. However, masks utilising the venturi system are particularly accurate at low flow rates, but maximum O_2 is around 55% for most masks. It is impossible to measure accurately the oxygen amount received through nasal cannulae, but they nevertheless provide a useful method of delivery to infants requiring long-term therapy.

Whilst undergoing supplemental oxygen therapy, the infant or child requires monitoring of:

- oxygen saturations

- respiratory rate and pattern
- presence of respiratory distress
- heart rate.

Airway intubation and protection

Indications for artificial airways are:

- respiratory failure
- airway protection secondary to seizure control
- airway protection secondary to facial/neck swelling due to thermal injuries
- respiratory support for cardiac failure
- respiratory support for airway obstruction.

The narrowest part of a child's airway is at the level of the cricoid cartilage, whilst in adults it is near the glottis. For this reason, children are easily ventilated using uncuffed endotracheal tubes with minimal air leak. The diameter of the endotracheal tube is extremely important: too small and a large air leak will render ventilation difficult due to small inspiratory tidal volumes; too large a tube increases the risk of pressure on the airway and cricoid cartilage resulting in subglottic oedema and stenosis. A formula for calculating tube sizes in children over 1 year can be seen below:

$$\text{internal diameter (mm)} = \frac{\text{age} + 4}{4}$$

$$\frac{\text{length}}{\text{(cm)}} = \frac{\text{age} + 12}{2} \text{ (oral tube) or } \frac{\text{age} + 15}{2} \text{ (nasal tube)}$$

However, a quick estimation of tube diameter can be gained by looking at the diameter of the child's little finger.

Coles shouldered endotracheal tubes are still occasionally used. However, there is a substantial risk of the shoulder passing through the vocal cords and causing oedema, trauma and stenosis. Endotracheal intubation is a skilled procedure and where possible should be performed by appropriately trained personnel. In an emergency, airway maintenance with a pharyngeal airway or oropharyngeal airway and manual inflation with bag and mask, or bag and laryngeal mask is effective in trained hands. However, aspiration of stomach contents cannot be excluded unless a full length endotracheal tube is placed.

Once the oral or nasal tube is in position with its tip just above the carina, air entry at the mid axilla level should be bilateral and equal, with the presence of a small airleak around the uncuffed endotracheal tube.

Complications of intubation and mechanical ventilation

Complications include the following.

- Damage to the nasal and oral mucosa and the teeth may occur during intubation.
- In infants, damage to the gums and palate can occur.
- Damage to the vocal cords and subglottic region is more common with multiple attempts at intubation.
- Damage to the upper airway may result from prolonged intubation.
- Repeated episodes of intubation may result in subglottic oedema and stenosis. On extubation, the child may experience hoarseness and stridor. Marked stridor that results in re-intubation may later require the advice of ENT specialists. Infants can develop significant subglottic stenosis after short periods of intubation and ventilation.
- Barotrauma may present as pneumothorax, pneuomomediastinum, pneumopericardium or surgical emphysema. This may result from tears in the pleura, leaks around tracheostomy tubes, or high levels of positive pressure ventilation with high levels of PEEP. In extreme forms, barotrauma can result in the development of acute respiratory distress syndrome.
- Impaired cardiac output as a result of high levels of PEEP or CPAP (see below) is a well-recognised complication. Venous return is restricted by the high intrathoracic pressure, which also affects filling time.
- Arrhythmias may result from hypercapnia, hypoxia or vagal stimulation by the endotracheal tube.
- Stomach distention may result from the use of CPAP or high PEEP in children and infants with uncuffed endotracheal tubes, causing discomfort and possible splinting of the diaphragm, restricting ventilation.

- Alterations in the levels of antidiuretic hormone secretion have been associated with respiratory illnesses and mechanical ventilation. This results in fluid retention and may cause pulmonary oedema, pleural effusions or abdominal ascites.

Methods of fixing endotracheal tubes

There are a variety of methods used to secure endotracheal tubes in infants and children. All methods aim to secure the tube and minimise the risk of accidental extubation.

In small children it is thought that prolonged intubation using nasal tubes avoids injury to the hard palate, but it may cause nasal septum deviation and ulceration. The final choice for position of tube and preferred method of fixation will lie with individual practitioners.

Children who present with croup or subglottic stenosis may only require intubation for airway protection, and therefore not require any additional form of respiratory support once sedation, anaesthetic and muscle relaxants have worn off. These children may be allowed to breathe spontaneously without CPAP, and with supplemental oxygen and humidification provided through a heat–moisture exchange unit and oxygen adaptor. With developmentally appropriate reassurance and minimal sedation, the majority of children will tolerate the endotracheal tube well. Arm splints can be used to prevent the risk of accidental extubation.

Should the child who is breathing spontaneously through an ET tube require high amounts of oxygen or more humidification than is possible with a heat–moisture exchange device, a standard humidified T-piece circuit can be used effectively.

In addition to standard cardiorespiratory monitoring of the child requiring oxygen therapy, it should be remembered that these parameters do not necessarily reflect the arterial carbon dioxide content. The child developing increasing respiratory distress may be quite hypercapnic before hypoxia is noted. Arterial blood gas measurements are invaluable, but if the child has no arterial access, end-tidal CO_2 measurement can be a reliable guide to the CO_2 levels. Airway suction must be performed to ensure airway patency, and the frequency required will depend upon the quantity and consistency of secretions present. Chest physiotherapy may also be required to prevent collapse of airways or to treat lung disease.

Continuous positive airway pressure (CPAP)

CPAP prevents alveolar collapse by maintaining a pressure above atmospheric pressure in the alveoli during expiration. CPAP can be delivered through a tight-fitting mask, via nasal prongs, shortened ET tubes or via a full-length ET tube. CPAP is used for patients who are spontaneously breathing. When used in conjunction with artificial ventilation it is referred to as positive end expiratory pressure (PEEP).

Mechanical ventilators can provide CPAP for small children. For larger children and adolescents who might find it difficult to breathe on CPAP mode on adult ventilators, a T-piece circuit with a PEEP valve can be used.

The level of CPAP delivered may vary from 1 to 10 cmH_2O. Increasing the CPAP pressure may temporarily increase oxygenation, but at higher levels CO_2 removal may be compromised. CPAP via an uncuffed ET tube or face mask may cause abdominal distention and predispose to pneumothorax and pneumomediastinum. Increasing levels of CPAP may also compromise cardiac output by increasing the intrathoracic pressure and reducing venous return. CPAP may be used as a weaning mode from full ventilation or may be used as a means of avoiding ventilation in children with chronic lung disease.

Humidification is essential and is best provided by a wet humidity system for the infant and small child. Older children may tolerate heat–moisture exchange units. There is still much controversy as to which method provides the better form of humidification.

Ventilatory modes

Once the child is intubated, there are many varied forms of ventilation that can be used to achieve full respiratory support and facilitate adequate gas exchange.

Continuous mandatory ventilation (CMV)

CMV is also known as intermittent positive pressure ventilation. This mode of ventilation provides complete respiratory support for the child. Generally, ventilators providing this mode are time cycled and pressure or volume controlled, although some models may be pressure limited. Using CMV it should be possible to control $PaCO_2$ and PaO_2 levels by manipulating the following:

- inspiration times (I time)
- expiration times (E time)
- inspiration:expiration ratio (I:E ratio)
- frequency (f)/rate (r)
- peak inspiratory pressure (PIP)
- positive end expiratory pressures (PEEP)
- gas flow
- FiO_2.

Increasing breath frequency or inspiratory pressures reduces $PaCO_2$; increasing breath frequency and FiO_2 may increase PaO_2. Increasing peak inspiratory pressures (PIP) leads to increased oxygenation and removal of CO_2 but adds to the risk of both acute and chronic barotrauma. Increasing PEEP may improve alveolar recruitment but can decrease cardiac output and increase the risk of air trapping. Inspiration times of 0.7 s would be a starting point for infants, increasing to 1 s in older infants and toddlers. When increasing the rate it may be necessary to reduce the inspiration time to prevent the reversal of I:E ratio. In the presence of severely reduced lung compliance, for example, in infants with chronic lung disease, it may be necessary to deliberately invert the I:E ratio, but this should be closely monitored to prevent severe air trapping once compliance begins to improve.

In children with severe respiratory disease it may, however, prove impossible to achieve the levels of CO_2 and O_2 desired and alternative or additional therapies may be required such as nitric oxide therapy with ventilation or in extreme situations the use of extracorporeal membrane oxygenation (ECMO).

Infant ventilators generally function in time-cycled pressure-controlled modes. Although some of the more recent ventilators offer pressure-limiting facilities, the older forms of infant ventilator deliver a constant flow which is manually adjustable and intermittent positive pressure breaths. More recent ventilators used in adult units have pressure ventilation modes suitable for children and infants, although these function in a slightly different manner to infant ventilators. They also allow manipulation of PIP, PEEP, Rate, I:E ratio and FiO_2.

CMV may also be delivered in volume-controlled modes. Most commonly used for adults or older children with cuffed endotracheal tubes, this system is time cycled and delivers a preset volume to the patient. Variables include frequency, tidal and/or minute volumes, I:E ratio and FiO_2. In addition some ventilators offer a pressure-limiting facility. In the older child, tidal volumes of 10–15 mL/kg/breath can be used as a guideline before adjusting according to arterial blood gases, auscultation and chest movement. Infant tidal volumes are less predictable, hence the difficulty in using volume-controlled ventilation for them, but a rough guideline would be 5–10 mL/kg/breath. However, this will depend on the air leak around the endotracheal tube and the effectiveness of ventilation assessed on arterial blood gas analysis.

Patient trigger ventilation (PTV) and pressure support (PS)

PTV and PS offer support to the spontaneously breathing infant or child. The child is required to trigger the ventilator before receiving a preset pressure. The sensitivity level of the trigger can be adjusted to determine the level of respiratory effort required by the child before receiving the breath.

Infant ventilators offering PTV deliver a preset back-up breath if the infant fails to trigger the ventilator. If pressure support is utilised on some adult ventilators, no back-up breath is available should the patient fail to trigger the ventilator.

Therefore, this mode is often used in combination with synchronised intermittent mandatory ventilation (SIMV). PTV and PS are useful for weaning ventilation, as it is possible to decrease the pressure delivered during triggered breaths whilst increasing the work of breathing. In both modes the pressure support delivered is above the level of PEEP.

Oscillation

High-frequency oscillation ventilation (HFOV) is increasingly being used for infants and children who fail to respond to conventional ventilation. It can be used successfully in the following situations:

- decreased lung compliance caused by neonatal respiratory distress syndrome
- acute lung injury/acute respiratory distress syndrome caused by:
  — meconium aspiration
  — aspiration syndrome
  — severe sepsis
  — near drowning
  — pneumonia.

HFOV may be considered as an alternative to ECMO for infants and children with respiratory distress syndrome who meet the criteria for ECMO treatment. More recently, HFOV has been shown to result in significant improvements in oxygenation compared with conventional ventilation strategies. A reduction in the incidence of barotrauma has been shown in infants and children with respiratory failure (Arnold et al 1994). By having a constant distending pressure (MAP) during HFOV, recruitment of previously unventilated alveoli becomes possible. Small tidal volumes are delivered to the infant at very high frequencies. Tidal volumes as small as 3 mL may be delivered at frequencies of 5–15 Hz (300–900 times per minute) at a selected constant mean airway pressure (MAP). Both inspiration and expiration are active because of the oscillatory action of the ventilator, and therefore air trapping is reduced. The constant MAP reduces the risk of increasing the lung damage, and CO_2 removal is possible.

HFOV involves recruitment of maximal lung expansion by increasing MAP in small increments until arterial oxygen saturations of 90% are achieved with an FiO_2 less than or equal to 0.6. Lung hyperinflation is identified by chest X-ray. Variables include frequency in herz, FiO_2, amplitude (pressure) and MAP. Some ventilators offering HFOV provide an additional facility of delivering concurrent superimposed CMV.

Weaning from this mode is achieved by initially reducing the FiO_2 and MAP and increasing the frequency to reduce tidal volume. Limitations of HFOV include:

- using infant ventilators for larger children because it is impossible to generate the MAP required
- difficulties above 50 kg on the standard oscillator for the same reason
- impacted secretions and inability to perform airway suction without losing airway pressure.

Removal of secretions can be facilitated using closed suction systems available for infants and children.

Negative pressure therapy

Negative pressure ventilation is physiologically normal and has existed in the form of 'Iron Lungs' since the early 1900s. It can be applied as continuous negative extrathoracic pressure (CNEP), allowing the child or infant to breathe spontaneously but with added continuous negative pressure. Alternatively, it can be applied as intermittent negative extrathoracic pressure (INEP) delivering complete negative pressure respiratory support.

Today negative pressure can be delivered using:

- a rigid box system encompassing the child's body up to the neck
- a cuirass or jacket fitting tightly over the child's chest.

Both of these techniques are non-invasive, allowing the child's face to be free from tubes and tapes. This allows for better communication with the child and enables him/her to feed orally. Disadvantages of the system are:

- reduced access to the child, as disruption of jacket or box seal results in pressure loss
- heat loss in the fixed box system
- noise.

Supplemental oxygen therapy may be given via face mask, nasal specs or head box. CPAP or full positive pressure ventilation via ETT have been administered concurrently in some centres.

Extracorporeal membrane oxygenation (ECMO)

ECMO should be mentioned here as a form of total cardiovascular and respiratory support when attempts to improve oxygenation by all other methods have failed. As the use of HFOV continues to develop, respiratory ECMO is less likely to be used in practice. The invasive nature of this therapy presents increased risks for the child, which are not associated with less invasive techniques.

Liquid ventilation

Liquid ventilation has been shown to be effective in animal models of acute respiratory failure and in neonates with hyaline membrane disease, by improving gas exchange and reducing ventilator-induced lung damage. The effectiveness of this treatment is dependent on the perfluoro-chemical liquid decreasing alveolar surface tension, allowing homogenous alveolar expansion at low distending pressures and reducing the need for high peak inspiratory pressures. Bubble formation is facilitated by the low surface tension of the medium, and the high solubility of oxygen provides a gas exchange reservoir.

Perfluorocarbons (PFC) are well suited to this purpose, with excellent respiratory gas solubility (50 mL of O_2 and 210 mL CO_2/decilitre), low surface tension and only moderate viscosity. PFCs are not soluble in water, not metabolised, and only small amounts are absorbed systemically. In addition, they may act as antiinflammatory agents, provide pulmonary lavage, removing debris, and effectively deliver drugs such as nitric oxide.

There are two modes of liquid ventilation: total and partial. Total liquid ventilation (TLV), where PFC is instilled to equal the functional residual capacity, requires specialised bulky equipment and therefore may not be the treatment of choice. Partial liquid ventilation or perfluorocarbon associated gas exchange (PAGE) involves similar volumes of PFC, but utilises conventional gas ventilation techniques. Although this technique is not currently widely used, it shows promise in the treatment of conditions involving an abnormal pulmonary surfactant system or where multiple atelectasis contributes to V/Q mismatch. Further trials and evaluation of this treatment are required (Hatherill et al 1996).

REFERENCES

Arnold J H, Hanson J H, Toro-Figuero L O, Gutierrez J, Berens R J, Anglin D L 1994 Prospective, randomized comparison of high-frequency oscillatory ventilation and conventional mechanical ventilation in pediatric respiratory failure. Critical Care Medicine 22(10):1530–1539

Beardsmore C S, Helms P, Stocks J, Hatch D J, Silverman M 1980 Improved oesophageal balloon technique for use in infants. Journal of Applied Physiology 49:735–742

Berger A J, Mitchell R A, Severinghaus J W 1977 Regulation of respiration. New England Journal of Medicine 297:92–97, 138–143, 194–201

Brown M K, Olver R E, Ramsden C A, Strang L B, Walters D V 1981 Effects of adrenaline infusion and spontaneous labour on lung liquid secretion and absorption in fetal lamb. J Physiol 313:13

Bucher U, Reid L 1961 Development of the intrasegmental bronchial tree: the pattern of branching and development of cartilage at various stages of intrauterine life. Thorax 16:207–218

England S J 1988 Current techniques for assessing pulmonary function in the newborn and infant: advantages and limitations. Pediatric Pulmonology 4:48–53

Hatherill M, Murdoch I A, Marsh M J 1996 Paediatric ventilation. Current Anaesthesia and Critical Care 7:248–253

Haworth S G 1987 Paediatric cardiology. Churchill Livingstone, Edinburgh, p. 124

Hislop A A, Wigglesworth J S, Desai R 1986 Alveolar development in the human fetus and infant. Early Human Development 13:1–11

Langston C, Kida K, Reed M, Thurlbeck W M 1984 Human lung growth in late gestation and in the neonate. American Review of Respiratory Diseases 129:607–613

Larson W J 1993 Human embryology. Churchill Livingstone, Edinburgh

Marsh M J, Fox G F, Hoskyns E W, Milner A D 1994 The Hering–Breuer deflationary reflex in the newborn infant. Pediatric Pulmonology 18(3):163–169

Milner A D 1990 Lung function testing in infancy. Arch Dis Child 65:548–552

Mortola J P, Saetta M 1987 Measurements of respiratory mechanics in the newborn: a simple approach. Pediatric Pulmonology 3:123–130

Reid L M 1979 American Review of Respiratory Diseases 119:531–546

Saunders R A, Milner A D 1978 Pulmonary pressure/volume relationship during the last phase of delivery and the first postnatal breaths in the human subjects. Journal of Pediatrics 93:667–673

Thurlbeck W M 1981 Growth, development and ageing of the lung. In: Scadding J G, Cumming G, Thurlbeck W M (eds) Scientific foundations of paediatrics. Heinemann Medical, London

Tortora G T, Anagnostakos N P 1990 Principles of anatomy and physiology, 6th edn. HarperCollins, New York

Vyas H, Field D, Hopkin I E, Milner A D 1986 Determinants of the first inspiratory volume and functional residual capacity at birth. Pediatric Pulmonology 2:189–193

7

Management of the child with respiratory disease

Judith Harris   Michael Marsh

This chapter outlines the basic principles of managing the child with respiratory disease and some of the more common disorders of the respiratory tract. Causes of respiratory failure in children are:

- upper airway obstruction
- lower airway obstruction
- pnuemonias
- bronchopulmonary dysplasia
- respiratory distress syndrome
- near drowning
- respiratory muscle failure
- physical restrictions of respiratory function such as pneumothoraces.

PRINCIPLES OF MANAGEMENT OF THE CHILD WITH RESPIRATORY DISEASE

Respiratory failure may result from a variety of different causes but is characterised by inability of the child's respiratory system to meet metabolic demand by removing carbon dioxide and oxygenating adequately. Singh (1997) suggests that a $PaCO_2$ greater than 50 mmHg (6.6 kPa) with a pH less than 7.30 is characteristic of hypercarbic respiratory failure, while a PaO_2 less than 50 mmHg (6.6 kPa) with an FiO_2 above 0.5 is characteristic of hypoxaemic respiratory failure. A child presenting with respiratory failure requires investigations into the cause once initial resuscitation has been achieved. The aims of management are to ensure airway patency and facilitate adequate gas exchange. Therefore, the

ABC of resuscitation is as appropriate here as in all resuscitation events. Assessment of respiratory function is essential and includes:

- examination of respiratory rate and pattern
- observation of the child's colour
- O_2 saturations
- arterial blood gas measurement
- heart rate
- blood pressure
- use of accessory muscles
- presence of wheeze, stridor or other respiratory noises.

In intensive care the child may initially require only supplemental oxygen and/or CPAP (continuous positive airway pressure). However, intubation and ventilation is often essential when the child has respiratory failure. Skilled personnel are essential when rapid sequence induction is required in an emergency to prevent aspiration of stomach contents. This is achieved by applying cricoid pressure as the endotracheal tube is inserted.

The anaesthetic agents and muscle relaxants used during intubation will vary but those commonly used include:

- ketamine (1–2 µg/kg)
- morphine sulphate (0.1–0.2 mg/kg)
- fentanyl (1–2 µg/kg)
- midazolam (0.05–0.15 mg/kg)
- thiopentone (2–7 mg/kg)
- suxemethonium (1–2 mg/kg)
- atracurium (0.3–0.6 mg/kg) (Guy's et al 1997)
- vecuronium (0.8–0.1 mg/kg)
- pancuronium (0.03–0.10 mg/kg)
- propofol (2.5 mg/kg).

Propofol, whilst useful, is not recommended for use in children under 3 years of age, and has been associated with convulsions following anaesthesia in children. Anaesthetic gases which may be used for induction of anaesthesia include isofluorane, halothane and sevoflurane.

During either nasal or oral intubation, the presence of upper airway obstruction can be assessed by direct vision and ease of intubation (Fig. 7.1).

- Advantages of oral route:
  — Nasal intubation is difficult for all but skilled personnel
  — Oral intubation avoids damage to the nasal passages and nares

- Disadvantages of oral intubation:
  — The distressed child may bite through the tube
  — Damage to the hard and soft palate may occur in infants
  — Saliva production renders strapping with sticking plaster difficult

- Advantages of nasal route:
  — Avoidance of damage to the soft and hard palate
  — Easier to secure, therefore more stability of the tube
  — Infant or child may use an oral comforter

- Disadvantages of the nasal route:
  — Technically a more difficult and lengthy procedure
  — In the bigger child the size of the nasal cavity may restrict the size of endotracheal tube.

Once the airway is secure, the child will require full ventilatory support until muscle relaxants have been metabolised. Ventilatory support can then be adjusted to aid CO_2 removal and provide adequate oxygenation. Endotracheal and nasopharyngeal secretions should be obtained and sent for microbiological and virological examination. Once intubated and ventilated, a further respiratory assessment is made.

Respiratory assessment

- Chest X-ray is assessed for the placement of endotracheal tube, appearance of lung fields and exclusion of pneumothorax, effusions or a foreign body.
- Auscultation will determine the quality of air entry and aid assessment of respiratory sounds.
- Observation of colour and consistency of secretions will provide evidence of the presence of infection.

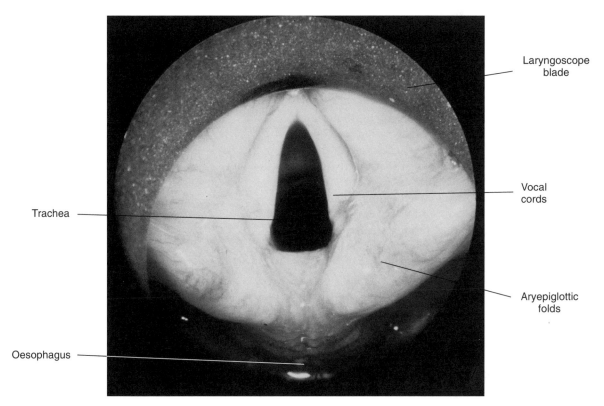

Laryngoscope
blade

Vocal
cords

Trachea

Aryepiglottic
folds

Oesophagus

Figure 7.1 Endoscopic view of normal larynx.

• Observation for signs of respiratory distress will provide information related to the amount of work the child has to do to breathe.

• Analysis of blood gases provides information about the amount of respiratory support required.

Supportive measures may include:

• physiotherapy
• administration of nebulised bronchodilators
• administration of inhaled nitric oxide when oxygenation is impaired with conventional ventilation alone.

Ongoing care of the ventilated child involves:

• continuous observation of ventilatory parameters
• assessment of breath sounds
• endotracheal suction to remove secretions and maintain tube patency

• humidification to reduce viscosity of secretions
• change of position to promote lung expansion, lung perfusion and postural drainage
• administration of sedation, analgesia and muscle relaxants if necessary to enable ventilatory therapy to achieve satisfactory gas exchange.

Weaning artificial ventilation

Weaning from mechanical ventilation can be considered either when the underlying disease process is resolving or when an improvement in gas exchange is noted. The support given by the ventilator is reduced as the child's respiratory effort increases. Assessment of the patient includes monitoring respiratory effort as characterised by chest movement, strength of effort, presence or absence of intercostal, subcostal or sternal recessions, and respiratory pattern. Abnormal blood gas results are usually a late sign that the child is struggling to achieve the increased respiratory effort required for the weaning process.

When considering weaning from ventilation the increased work that the infant or child will be required to undertake must be considered. In order to facilitate weaning of ventilation, drugs that inhibit breathing and movement are reduced. It may be difficult to achieve a balance between weaning sedation, to allow the child to breathe spontaneously, and having a distressed child who is endangering the safety of his airway. In addition the increased effort required to breathe may place additional demands for energy upon a child who is stressed and undernourished and potentially catabolic. Therefore, calorific requirements should be considered to facilitate weaning of ventilation.

The use of pressure support or CPAP modes may cause a degree of air swallowing in the infant or child with an uncuffed endotracheal tube. Marked abdominal distention can result from air swallowing and if allowed to continue may ultimately cause diaphragmatic splinting and hinder chest expansion.

Ventilation allows manipulation of both oxygenation and carbon dioxide removal and may be necessary for treatment of conditions other than primary respiratory disease:

- to support the cardiovascular system following major surgery
- to allow wound healing following complex tracheal or laryngeal surgery
- to manipulate $PaCO_2$ when intracranial pressure is raised
- to maintain respiratory function when pharmacological therapy interferes with effective respiration, for example in the management of status epilepticus
- where airway obstruction may be anticipated following facial or airway thermal injury.

In these instances the duration of ventilation will depend entirely upon the primary problem.

MANAGEMENT OF UPPER AIRWAY DISORDERS

Upper airway problems in children are commonly associated with inspiratory stridor. Problems can either be infectious, structural or mechanical by nature but all have the potential to cause complete airway obstruction (Box 7.1).

Box 7.1 Causes of stridor in childhood
- croup - epiglottitis - inhaled foreign body - vascular ring

Croup

Croup, or acute laryngo-tracheobronchitis, is most commonly seen in infants and toddlers between the ages of 3 months and 3 years. Spread is by droplet infection, with 85% of cases occurring as a result of viral infection. These include:

- parainfluenza
- respiratory syncitial virus
- rhinovirus.

Croup results from narrowing of the upper airway caused by mucosal oedema and secretions. It is distinguished by inspiratory stridor, caused by obstruction in the larynx, in association with pyrexia, hoarseness, a barking cough and signs of respiratory distress. The risk of increasing the child's distress and exacerbating airway obstruction makes it inadvisable to attempt arterial blood sampling. In this case the decision to intubate is based upon clinical assessment and pulse oximetry readings.

Croup scoring can be used to assess the severity of illness. An example of the scoring system is shown in Table 7.1.

Management includes careful assessment of cardiovascular parameters, respiratory rate, pattern, oxygen saturations, level of consciousness, level of hydration, urine output. The child with severe stridor and tachypnoea should receive adequate intravenous hydration but no oral fluids.

Table 7.1 Croup scoring system

Symptoms	0	1	2
Stridor	None	Inspiratory	Inspiratory/expiratory
Cough	None	Hoarse	Bark
Air entry	Normal	Reduced	Significantly reduced
Flaring/recessions	None	Flaring sternal	Sternal, subcostal, intercostal
Colour	Normal	Cyanosis in 21%	Cyanosis in 40%

Adapted from Rogers (1992).

This will help prevent gastric distention and also reduce the work of breathing. Antipyretics should be given as required. Humidity may have a role in loosening secretions, but there is no other conclusive evidence regarding its benefits in croup.

Indications for intubation include drowsiness, restlessness due to hypoxia, tachypnoea and tachycardia. Children are often able to breathe spontaneously through the endotracheal tube, without assisted ventilation, once the effects of muscle relaxants have been metabolised. Humidification and oxygen can be provided through a heat–moisture exchange device, or 'Swedish Nose', with oxygen adaptors. The majority of children tolerate the ET tube with only moderate sedation and arm splints to prevent accidental extubation. Occasionally, children may become very distressed, requiring large doses of sedation and assisted ventilation.

Children with croup usually remain intubated for 4 days, receiving enteral prednisolone at a dose of 1 mg/kg 12-hourly from intubation to 24 h post-extubation. The timing of intubation with concurrent enteral steroid administration in the authors' institution is based upon the Kaplan–Meier survivor distribution curve for length of intubation for children with croup (Altman 1991, Tibbals et al 1992). After this period, extubation is then attempted. The decision to extubate does not depend on the presence or absence of an air leak, although this is an encouraging indicator of reduced swelling.

If re-intubation is required the child will rapidly show signs of acute respiratory distress. A further period of 72 h intubation is usually required with a further course of antiinflammatory drugs. If the child is not successfully extubated at the second attempt, microlaryngobronchoscopy is indicated to exclude any structural abnormality which may be contributing to the stridor.

Children with croup often have copious endotracheal and oropharyngeal secretions requiring regular suction. Support and distraction is vital, particularly during suction which can cause great distress.

Acute epiglottitis

This is a severe bacterial infection of the epiglottis seen in children between 2 and 6 years and most commonly caused by *Haemophilus influenzae*. Incidence of this illness has decreased significantly following introduction of the HIB vaccine. The inflamed and swollen epiglottis can completely occlude the airway if a gag reflex is stimulated by examination or suctioning of the upper airway. Therefore, it is essential not to attempt to upset the child or visualise the epiglottis unless full resuscitative facilities are available, including emergency tracheostomy equipment. Presenting features include:

- barking cough
- pyrexia
- tachycardia
- stridor
- sternal recession with or without subcostal recession
- drooling caused by inability to swallow
- impaired level of consciousness due to increasing hypoxia.

Intubation should only be undertaken by skilled staff who are able to perform an emergency tracheostomy if necessary. It is common practice to arrange transfer of the child to theatre where an ENT surgeon is available and intubation can be undertaken in a controlled environment. Although it takes longer to achieve, gas induction of anaesthesia is preferable, as insertion of an intravenous cannula for IV sedation and anaesthesia could increase the child's distress and precipitate complete airway occlusion. Once intubated, the child is allowed to wake and breathe spontaneously. Heat–moisture exchange units provide humidification, and supplemental oxygen can be delivered if required. With appropriate sedation and distraction, these children may tolerate the ET tube well. The child is usually intubated for a period of 24–48 h during which time appropriate intravenous antibiotic therapy must be given. Extubation is usually undertaken once the child is apyrexial.

Inhaled foreign body

Foreign body inhalation should be considered in the child presenting with acute stridor and little history of previous upper respiratory tract infection. This can constitute a life-threatening emergency, as occlusion of the main bronchus can result from something as small as a sausage fragment or peanut (Fig. 7.2).

Presentation is usually acute with coughing, gasping and choking followed by wheeze, chest recession and cyanosis. Chest X-ray (lateral and AP) should identify the foreign body, but failure to identify it does not preclude its presence. Direct visualisation should only be attempted under general anaesthesia in the operating theatre. If the child is unconscious, laryngoscopy may allow visualisation and removal of the foreign body. If laryngoscopy fails to identify the foreign body, a tracheostomy may be necessary to achieve airway patency and ventilation before attempting to remove the object.

Following removal of the foreign body, the child will require careful monitoring of respiratory and cardiovascular status. Chest physiotherapy may be helpful when there is associated consolidation and/or collapse. Complications of inhaled foreign bodies can include erosion of the bronchial or tracheal wall from infection, pneumonitis, perforation and haemorrhage, and death from asphyxia.

Vascular ring

Although a rare cause of stridor, external compression of the trachea can be caused by vascular

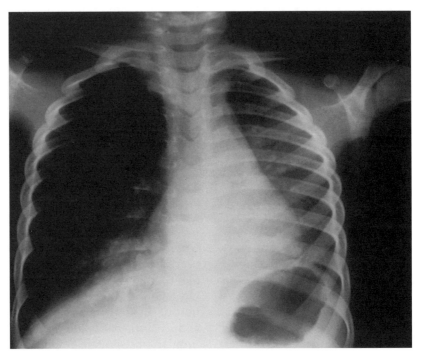

Figure 7.2 Inhaled foreign body — ball valve effect with foreign body in right main bronchus, causing hyperinflated right lung.

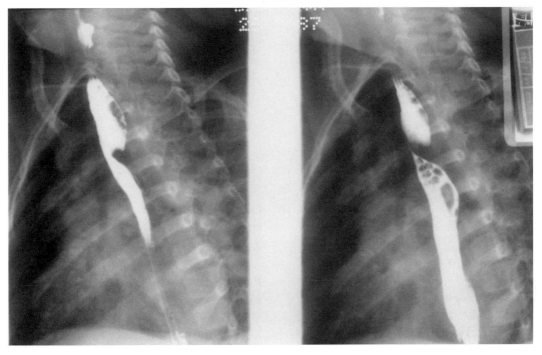

Figure 7.3   Contrast swallow — vascular ring (aberrant right subclavian artery) — defect in oesophagus as a result of compression; presenting symptom, stridor.

anomalies. Persistent stridor, with or without difficulty in swallowing, is often a feature of this defect. The commonly associated anomalies include a double sided aortic arch, where the right sided arch encloses the trachea, or anomalous origin of the left subclavian artery. Diagnosis, suggested by barium swallow, is confirmed by cardiac angiography (Fig. 7.3). Treatment is by surgery on cardiopulmonary bypass to release the trachea from the ring. Following removal of the obstruction the tracheobronchial tree may remain distorted and tracheomalacia may persist (Thompson et al 1990). Vascular rings may also be associated with other congenital facial and laryngeal anomalies which may still persist after removal of the ring.

SUBGLOTTIC STENOSIS

Subglottic stenosis is usually associated with episodes of repeated intubation during the neonatal period. It can, however, be associated with intubation with an endotracheal tube that is too large. The stenosis arises from thickening of soft tissue in the trachea wall, which can extend from the vocal cords to the cricoid cartilage. Infants and children with subglottic stenosis present with stridor, which usually occurs with upper respiratory infections. It may be difficult to differentiate between the infant with croup and the infant with subglottic stenosis. Both present with stridor but the infant with croup is not as likely to present with severe respiratory distress. Laryngoscopy following the acute episode will confirm the diagnosis. The child that presents with severe airway obstruction with every respiratory tract infection may require surgical intervention to relieve the obstruction. A cricoid split procedure may be performed or a single or two stage laryngotracheal reconstruction.

RESPIRATORY INFECTIONS
Pneumonia

Pneumonia is one of the most common infections

in the critically ill child and may be bacterial or viral in origin (Box 7.2). Treatment and prognosis vary according to the cause. Pneumonia may be classified as:

- lobar (Fig. 7.4)
- broncho
- interstitial (Fig. 7.5)

Box 7.2

The most common bacterial causes of pneumonia are:

- *Diplococcus pneumoniae*
- *Streptococcus pneumoniae*
- *Staphylococcus aureus*
- *Haemophilus influenzae*
- *Mycobacterium tuberculosis*
- *Escherichia coli*
- *Klebsiella pneumoniae*
- *Salmonella* species

The most common viral causes are:
- Syncytial virus RSV
- Parainfluenzae and influenza viruses
- Adenovirus
- (*Mycoplasma* species)
- Other causes may be fungal:
  — *Histoplasma capsulatum*
  — *Aspergillus* species
  — *Candida albicans*

Bacterial pneumonia

In general this occurs in children under 3 years of age. However, the critically ill child of any age is at risk of developing pneumonia secondary to endotracheal intubation. Bacterial infection may also occur in association with viral pneumonia. Most lobar pneumoniae are caused by *Streptococcus pneumoniae*. Chest X-ray demonstrates areas of consolidation rather than infiltrates.

Viral pneumonia

Viral infection is far more common than bacterial, most commonly causing interstitial pneumonia. Common findings are interstitial pneumonitis, mucosal inflammation of the bronchi and bronchioles and, occasionally, secondary bacterial infection.

Presenting features include:

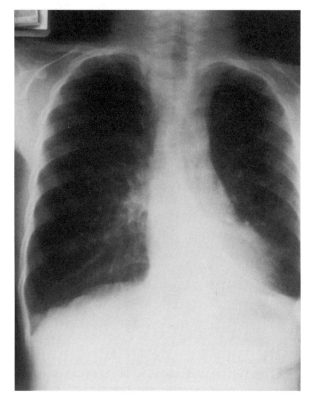

Figure 7.4 Left lower lobe collapse — pneumonia; shadow behind heart with clear lung.

- fever
- tachycardia
- tachypnoea
- respiratory distress
- wheezing
- haemoptysis may or may not be present.

Chest X-ray will confirm the diagnosis of pneumonia, demonstrating areas of consolidation and/or collapse. The chest X-ray will often demonstrate a hyperinflated lung with patchy infiltrates. Sputum from the endotracheal tube or nasopharyngeal aspirates should be obtained prior to commencing antibiotic therapy, to check sensitivity.

Management of the child includes careful assessment of both respiratory and cardiovascular status:

- patient's colour
- respiratory rate and pattern

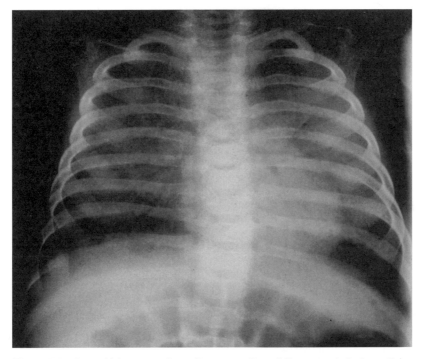

Figure 7.5 Interstitial pneumonia — *Pneumocystis carinii* pneumonia in 4-month-old child with severe combined immune deficiency (SCID).

- presence or absence of sternal or subcostal recession
- presence and appearance of secretions
- oxygen saturations and blood gases
- cardiovascular observations.

The child should be given intravenous hydration, usually restricted to 75% of normal requirements, because of the incidence of increased ADH secretion causing water retention. Physiotherapy will aid lung expansion and removal of secretions.

The child presenting with a primary pneumonia may not require intubation and ventilation and may be adequately supported with oxygen therapy via headbox or face mask. Alternatively, nasopharyngeal airway with CPAP may provide adequate respiratory support, reducing the need for intubation.

The decision to intubate must be based on the degree of respiratory failure, hypercapnia and acidosis. The child with a raised $PaCO_2$ alone may not necessarily need to be intubated if the pH is greater than 7.30. If, however, the $PaCO_2$ is rising with an associated fall in pH below 7.30, intubation and respiratory support should be initiated.

The ventilated child who develops pneumonia may require increased oxygen and ventilation, with increased inspiratory pressures or tidal volumes to achieve adequate gas exchange. Infants who develop lobar pneumonia may not tolerate lying with the affected side uppermost, although this would be preferable for postural drainage.

Whilst adults with unilateral lung disease can tolerate lying with their normal lung in the dependent position, infants find this difficult. When infants are placed with their good lung in the dependent position, their oxygenation worsens. This may be due to differences in lung mechanics and diaphragm function or merely because the gravitational effects on regional pulmonary blood flow are reduced relative to those of adults (Heaf et al 1983, Davies et al 1985).

Perhaps the best guideline for positioning the child or infant with lobar pneumonia is to alter her position according to her tolerance.

Complications of pneumonia include:

- development of emphysema
- pleural effusion
- tension pneumothorax
- acute respiratory distress syndrome.

Atypical pneumonias

These are usually found only in severely immunosuppressed children and include:

- *Candida albicans*
- *Aspergillus*
- *Pneumocystis carinii*.

Mortality rates in this group of children are high. These children require aggressive ventilatory support with or without the addition of high-frequency oscillation and nitric oxide therapy. Those infants and children who present with atypical pneumonia require investigation into immune status. This may be the first presentation of a child with a severe immunodeficiency disorder, such as HIV, AIDS or SCIDs.

Bronchiolitis

This is an acute inflammatory disease of the lower respiratory tract, leading to obstruction of the small airways. Bronchiolitis generally affects infants in the first year of life, but can be seen in children up to 3 years of age (Beck Koff et al 1993, Singh 1997). Children with underlying chronic lung disease, infants born prematurely and those with congenital heart disease are particularly at risk from bronchiolitis.

The majority of children with bronchiolitis are found to have respiratory syncytial virus (RSV), but other causes include rhinovirus, para-influenza virus, influenza virus and adenovirus. It has been suggested that there may be an immunological component to RSV bronchiolitis, and that an IgE-mediated hypersensitivity response may account for the severe symptoms of RSV bronchiolitis (Welliver et al 1981). In the 1970s it was suggested that a protective factor may be found in secretory IgA and it appeared that breast-fed babies were relatively protected from bronchiolitis, possibly from the IgA in colostrum and breast milk (Downham et al 1976).

Initially the infant presents with a cough, sneezes and rhinorrhea and subsequently develops respiratory distress characterised by tachypnoea, wheeze, sternal and intercostal recession and nasal flaring. On chest X-ray the lungs appear hyperinflated, and, on auscultation, diffuse wheezes and prolonged expiration are heard.

The infant requires careful assessment and observation of respiratory rate and pattern, heart rate, colour, oxygen saturations and levels of hydration. Arterial blood gas analysis will determine pH, $PaCO_2$ and PaO_2, assisting in the decision-making process regarding the level of respiratory support required. Naspharyngeal secretions should be obtained and sent for viral studies and immunofluorescence, to determine the cause of the infection. Treatment commonly involves oxygen therapy to correct hypoxia. Infants suffering with bronchiolitis are at risk from apnoeas. The risk is increased in premature infants and in situations of increasing respiratory failure. Apnoeas may be due to fatigue or airway obstruction resulting from increased secretions and swelling.

Nasal CPAP may produce an improvement in both respiratory effort and blood gases in those infants with persistent apnoeas who appear tired by the effort of breathing. Many infants can be managed successfully in this manner, avoiding the need for intubation and mechanical ventilation. $PaCO_2$ levels in premature infants with chronic lung disease are often higher than normal term infants, as damage to the lung tissue impairs gas exchange. Permissive hypercapnia refers to the process of accepting a higher than normal $PaCO_2$ provided that the child or infant is not acidotic. Therefore, levels of permissive hypercapnia have to be based on the presence or absence of acidosis in these infants. The infant who becomes acidotic, or continues to have apnoeas despite nasal CPAP, will require intubation and mechanical ventilation. Once ventilated, a degree of permissive hypercapnia is desirable. In the authors' institution infants with bronchiolitis have tolerated $PaCO_2$ levels of 12 kPa at times without developing acidosis. Where possible, arterial oxygen saturation should be maintained in the low 90s. However, if excessively high inspiratory pressures and high FiO_2 are required to achieve this, the risks of barotrauma outweigh the need for saturations at this level. Therefore, levels in the mid to high 80s may be accepted. The infant who remains hypoxic despite full mechanical ventilatory support with high inspiratory pressures and 100% O_2 may benefit from inhaled nitric oxide therapy.

Moderate hypoxia in these infants is generally a reflection of a basic gas exchange problem. Severe hypoxia despite high levels of ventilatory support reflects a severe mismatch between ventilation and perfusion. This is most likely to occur in the infant with pre-existing lung disease. Nitric oxide (endothelial derived relaxing factor) administered in gaseous form enhances smooth muscle relaxation, leading to vasodilation, and is presumed to improve V/Q mismatching by improving perfusion to ventilated lungs. This will improve oxygenation which will in turn improve pulmonary capillary pressure through further vasodilation. Physiotherapy would appear to have no beneficial effects in these infants and children unless they have an accompanying pneumonia. The infant with bronchiolitis has difficulties with air trapping and wheezing. Physiotherapy may exacerbate the wheeze and compound the air trapping. If the infant will tolerate postural drainage, drainage of secretions into the larger airways from where they can be expectorated or removed by endotracheal suction may be of benefit. However, large quantities of secretions draining into the large airways may block the endotracheal tube. Therefore the need for suction should be regularly assessed.

Ribavirin is a synthetic nucleotide analogue of guanosine with a specific anti-RSV action. It may be inhaled via a head box and has been administered to ventilated infants via the ventilator circuit but with the inherent risks of crystallisation in the circuit and ventilator. Early studies in the USA suggested that it played a significant role in the treatment of infants with RSV. It is no longer used universally for all children with RSV, but may have a place for those children with congenital heart defects, chronic lung disease or severe immunocompromise. There is little evidence that Ribavirin shortens the course of intubation; it is thought, however, to shorten the time of viral shedding.

It has been demonstrated that infants suffering from respiratory syncitial virus bronchiolitis have increased levels of secretion of antidiuretic hormone (ADH) (Gozal et al 1990, van Steensel-Moll et al 1990). Although some studies have shown that this elevated secretion is inappropriate, others have shown that it does appear appropriate (Gozal et al 1990). Decreased renal water excretion results, and the increased accumulation of fluid may cause increased respiratory and ventilatory difficulties. It has been suggested that the increased secretion of ADH in children and infants with RSV bronchiolitis may be compounded by interactions between osmotic control of ADH and a misleading picture of fluid depletion (van Steensel-Moll et al 1990). Large quantities of fluid replacement with hypotonic fluid should be avoided, and fluid restriction is therefore recommended. Diuretics may also prove useful in ventilatory management to reduce the amount of free lung water.

SEVERE ACUTE ASTHMA

Asthma is defined as lung disease with reversible obstruction of both large and small airways. Airway inflammation and airway responsiveness to varying stimuli result in wheezing and dyspnoea. In severe acute asthma, there is minimal air exchange with presence of CO_2 retention and increasing hypoxia. Despite advances in treatment over recent years, children and adults still die from asthma, and the seriousness of the disease should not be underestimated.

The exact cause of asthma is unknown, but there is an increased risk of asthma in children with family histories of atopic disorders. Asthma attacks which start with an antigen/antibody reaction are explained by the allergy theory. In children prone to allergic asthma, IgE is present in the body in abnormally large amounts. This appears to be associated with large quantities of the allergen-specific antibody. IgE binds to the high-affinity Fc receptors on mast cells and results in degranulation. Preformed mediators released from the granules include histamines, heparin, eosinophil and neutrophil chemotactic agents. Leukotrienes (slow-releasing substances of anaphylaxis [SRS-A]) and thromboxanes are released as a result of the metabolism of arachidonic acid. It would appear that interleukins IL-3, -4, -5 and -6 are also released (Roitt 1994). Ordinarily these mediators contribute to the acute inflammatory reaction but in the setting of release through atopic, allergic illness, they cause bronchoconstriction and vasodilation.

Dilation of the blood vessels, mucus production, airway oedema and contraction of the small airways result. The lungs become rapidly hyperinflated with air trapping (Fig. 7.6). Severe hypoxia and respiratory acidosis induce marked pulmonary vasoconstriction and a right-to-left shunt.

Signs and symptoms of severe acute asthma include:

- respiratory distress
- fever
- audible wheeze
- decreased air entry with air trapping
- decreased oxygen saturations
- tachycardia
- severe sternal and intercostal recession
- nasal flaring.

Peak expiratory flow rates will be significantly reduced, although to attempt measurement in the child with respiratory failure would be unwise, as it may exacerbate the condition. A chest X-ray should be carried out to exclude the presence of a foreign body, as presentation is similar. It should be noted that the degree of wheezing is not necessarily indicative of the severity of the attack. However, the absence of wheeze in the presence of respiratory distress and poor air entry is an indicator of severe airway obstruction. Presence of pulsus paradoxus (over 10 mmHg change in systolic pressure between inspiration

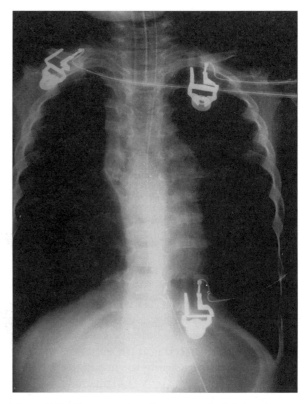

Figure 7.6 Severe acute asthma — marked air trapping, narrow mediastinum, black lung fields, pneumothorax.

and expiration) is also a good indicator of the severity of the disease.

Following initial assessment of respiratory rate, pattern, air entry, presence of recession, colour, cardiovascular status and level of consciousness, oxygen therapy should be administered via a face mask. Intravenous fluids should be given to correct or prevent dehydration, but only in restricted quantities. Usually half to three quarters of normal maintenance allowance will minimise or reduce the effects of raised levels of antidiuretic hormone which are associated with various forms of respiratory failure and mechanical ventilation.

Relief of bronchospasm is attempted through nebulised sympathomimetic agents (Table 7.2). Intravenous aminophylline may be considered if there is little or no improvement from the nebulisers. Aminophylline has a relatively narrow therapeutic range, however, and toxic side effects

Table 7.2   Drug treatments for asthma

Group	Name	Action	Side effects
Beta 2 antagonists	Salbutamol Terbutaline	Bronchodilator	Tachycardia, tremor
Acetylcholine antagonist	Ipratropium bromide	Reduces vagal tone to airways. Blocks bronchoconstriction caused by antigen/antibody response	Tachycardia
Xanthine	Aminophylline Theophylline	? Causes antagonism of adenosine receptors. ? Causes inhibition of intracellular calcium release	Nausea, vomiting, tachycardia, arrhythmias
Antiinflammatory	Corticosteroids	Inhibits eosinophil infiltration into tissue.	
	Beclomethasone Budesonide	Inhibits release of cytokines and mediators from macrophages and eosinophils	
Mast cell stabiliser	Di-sodium cromoglycate	Non-steroidal antiinflammatory	

include tachycardia, nausea, vomiting and tremors. Levels must be carefully monitored, particularly if children are also receiving phenytoin or phenobarbitone, which affect the drug clearance of aminophylline. Steroids are commenced to reduce the inflammatory response, but their effects are not immediate in this setting.

If these treatments fail to halt respiratory failure, intubation and ventilation are required. Ventilation is altered according to arterial blood gas results, chest movements and the presence of air trapping on chest X-ray. A lower PaO_2 than normal may be tolerated to reduce the risk of increased air trapping and barotrauma. Volume-controlled ventilation may be more effective at reducing and preventing further air trapping in these children. Manipulation of the I:E ratio to prolong expiratory time may also contribute to a reduction in air trapping. The use of PEEP in this group of children is controversial. Early works demonstrated beneficial effects of PEEP from 10 cmH$_2$O (Martin et al 1982) to 25 cmH$_2$O (Qvist et al 1982) but, more recently, high PEEP is

thought to be detrimental to the management of the child with asthma.

After the initial stages, physiotherapy will be essential to assist removal of secretions and prevention of consolidation. Secretions should be collected and sent for microscopy, preferably before the commencement of antibiotic therapy.

Complications of asthma include:

- hypotension
- pneumothorax
- pneumonia
- sepsis
- pulmonary embolus
- pneumomediastinum
- arrhythmias and ventricular failure.

ASPIRATION PNEUMONIA

Aspiration pneumonia is a major cause of nosomial infection in the child in intensive care. Children in intensive care are particularly at risk from aspiration pneumonia because of the following factors:

- intubated patients, mainly with uncuffed endotracheal tubes
- poor nutritional status due to illness
- sedation or reduced level of consciousness
- increased risk of aspirating due to reflux, reduced cough and gag responses.

Suspicion of an aspiration pneumonia may be raised by a history of severe coughing and choking or an episode of vomiting. The child may then develop a more frequent cough with increased sputum production. Sputum may or may not be purulent. Fever, increased oxygen requirements and increased ventilatory requirements are often seen with aspiration. Aspiration matter is most likely to cause problems to the right middle and lower lobes in view of the more vertical arrangment of the right main bronchus. It is possible that the initial chest X-ray after the vomiting or choking episode may be normal. This does not necessarily mean that the child will not subsequently develop a pneumonitis.

The aim of treatment is to continue to manage the child's underlying reason for admission. Ventilation should be adjusted according to patient requirements based upon clinical assessment and laboratory investigations. Physiotherapy may be of benefit to this child. Antibiotics should only be prescribed for the confirmed presence of a specific bacterial organism.

CHRONIC LUNG DISEASE

Chronic lung disease is difficult to define but is perhaps best characterised by significant respiratory and medical problems which warrant frequent hospitalisation. The spectrum of illness is inevitably wide. An infant who is slow to wean from headbox oxygen in the neonatal period may be classified as having chronic lung disease, as is the infant who has been ventilated for weeks in a neonatal unit following an episode of meconium aspiration. Chronic lung disease may affect the very preterm infant following respiratory distress syndrome or the term infant following meconium aspiration or with congenital malformations of the chest or heart.

Chronic lung disease in infancy is no longer solely the remit of neonatal units. Because of the aggressive management of preterm infants in neonatal units, more and more preterm infants are surviving the neonatal period and requiring subsequent admissions to PICUs with primarily respiratory problems.

The physiology of chronic lung disease is complex and is covered only briefly here. Specific neonatal texts will give a more comprehensive discussion. It generally occurs following an acute injury. Infant lungs are more susceptible to injury because of their prematurity and either deficient or dysfunctional surfactant. The insult leads to increased alveolar capillary permeability, and pulmonary oedema results. This further inhibits the formation of surfactant and reduces the compliance of the lungs. This causes more oedema and ultimately will cause atelectasis. Infection may also play a part in the lung disease process by causing the accumulation of neutrophils and macrophages which will in turn cause endothelial damage. Secondary lung injury may result from mechanical injury in the premature infant. Damage to the immature airways and lungs can result from positive pressure ventilation and from oxygen therapy. Oxygen may react with macrophages and neutrophils to produce oxygen free radicals which will compound any injury already present.

Management of chronic lung disease within the neonatal unit involves:

- early use of surfactant therapy in those infants at risk of respiratory distress syndrome
- careful management of ventilation to avoid oxygen toxicity and barotrauma.
- considering the use of HFOV
- ensuring adequate haemoglobin to facilitate good oxygen delivery
- regulation of fluid therapy to avoid fluid overload
- good nutritional provision
- avoidance of infection.

The infant or child with chronic lung disease admitted to the paediatric intensive care unit may have complex problems. The presenting illness or disease must be considered in conjunction with the chronic respiratory picture. It is particularly important to remember that the infant with chronic lung disease will not necessarily have the typical normal blood gas values for carbon dioxide. Over a period of time the infant will have developed compensatory mechanisms for a higher than normal $PaCO_2$. This may be seen as a high $PaCO_2$ with normal pH but high base excess and bicarbonate. Should this infant need to be ventilated it is vital to consider the picture that is normal for that particular child. It would not be appropriate to aim to keep the $PaCO_2$ as low as 6 kPa in an infant who usually runs his $PaCO_2$ at 8 kPa. The point at which the infant starts to show a respiratory acidosis is the point at which the $PaCO_2$ is too high for that infant. With careful management in PICU most of these infants and children can be successfully weaned from mechanical ventilation despite their underlying chronic disease.

SMOKE INHALATION INJURY

Smoke inhalation is one of the major causes of mortality and morbidity in children involved in house fires (Thompson et al 1986). Smoke inhalation injuries result from the combined effects of direct thermal injury to the respiratory tract and the effects of inhalation of the byproducts of combustion. These include:

- carbon monoxide
- cyanide
- hydrocyanic acid
- sulphur dioxide
- hydrochloric acid
- phosgene
- chlorine
- ammonia.

Carbon monoxide (CO) and cyanide are highly toxic and both are rapidly absorbed into the bloodstream, causing tissue damage. CO has a two hundred fold greater affinity for haemoglobin than oxygen. CO binds with Hb, forming carboxyhaemoglobin. This results in a shift of the oxygen dissociation curve to the left, reducing the rate at which O_2 is released to the cells. Thus already-hypoxic tissues are further damaged.

Levels of carboxyhaemoglobin in excess of 60% are usually fatal.

Carbon monoxide also has a direct effect on cytochrome oxidase (Prien & Traber 1988). Cytochrome oxidase is an enzyme involved in the electron transport system in which the potential energy stored in chemical bonds in fats, carbohydrates and proteins is released to create adenosine triphosphate (ATP). The ATP manufactured by this mitochondrial process through a series of oxidation and reduction reactions is used in every active cell and tissue in the body.

In lungs damaged by smoke, increased permeability of pulmonary capillaries and alveolar epithelium directly results in a leak of proteins into the alveolar space. Pulmonary oedema results from destruction of surfactant and the decrease in alveolar surface tension. Ventilation perfusion mismatch results in further hypoxia. Acute respiratory distress syndrome is commonly precipitated by smoke inhalation injury and requires aggressive management if the child is to survive. Initial assessment should follow the ABC of resuscitation. Children often present with respiratory failure, but cardiopulmonary arrest is not uncommon.

In the child who is cardiovascularly stable following a house fire, intubation and ventilation are indicated if there is any suspicion of smoke inhalation. This may be indicated by the presence of soot around the mouth and nostrils, burns to the head and neck or damage to the oral mucosa. Presence of soot below the vocal cords during intubation indicates the severity of the injury and may warrant bronchoalveolar lavage. Although pulse oximetry and arterial blood gas sampling are vital following smoke inhalation, it should be remembered that pulse oximetry and PaO_2 measurements are not accurate in situations of carbon monoxide poisoning. The only method for directly measuring arterial PaO_2 is by using a direct co-oximetry technique, which gives a breakdown of percentages of different types of haemoglobin.

Once intubation and ventilation has commenced, the child will need aggressive management with endotracheal suctioning and toilet, frequent monitoring of arterial blood gases, and close observation for onset of pulmonary oedema. Carboxyhaemoglobin levels should be measured, and concentrations greater than 5% should be treated with an FiO_2 of 1.0 despite arterial PaO_2 results. Manipulation of ventilation may include high PEEP to reduce pulmonary oedema, high PIP or tidal volumes to allow oxygenation despite stiff non-compliant lungs and potentially a reversed I:E ratio. Treatment with prophylactic steroids is not considered beneficial.

The child with severe hypoxia who fails to respond to conventional ventilation may benefit from trials with high-frequency oscillation ventilation or perhaps even ECMO. Hyperbaric oxygen treatment can be used for carbon monoxide poisoning, but facilities for this treatment only tend to exist in specialist centres.

NEAR DROWNING

Drowning is defined as submersion resulting in asphyxia and death within 24 h. The definition of near-drowning is less clear. Singh (1997), however, defines near drowning as submersion of sufficient gravity to require hospitalisation but not severe enough to result in death within 24 h.

Drowning in childhood may occur in baths, swimming pools, fishponds, rivers or the sea. Lack of supervision, for even brief periods, can result in submersion. Fresh or sea water may be involved and, in the past it was thought that the problems faced by the child may vary depending on the type of water involved (Swann & Spafford 1951). Swann thought that in freshwater drowning, hypotonic fluid enters the alveolar space and is then quickly absorbed into the capillaries. This leads to haemodilution and therefore a low haemoglobin and low serum electrolytes. Atelectasis may result from the dilution of surfactant. Salt water submersion fills the alveolar space with hypertonic fluid and fluid then shifts from the capillaries into the alveoli, causing pulmonary oedema and haemoconcentration. More recent opinion holds that the type of water holds little significance.

In practice, very few children aspirate any water at all, because of laryngospasm. Loss of

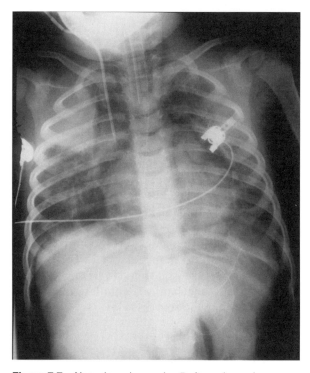

Figure 7.7 Near drowning — day 5 after submersion episode. ARDS with severe air leak (pneumomediastinum, pneumopericardium and pneumoperitoneum.

consciousness then results from anoxia, and at this point water may enter the airways, causing inflammation, airway obstruction, and destruction of alveolar and capillary membranes. Hypoxia, hypercapnia and acidosis develop quickly. Victims of submersion injury swallow vast quantities of water, however. This swallowed water contributes to the development of pulmonary oedema and predisposes to a more significant risk of aspiration during resuscitation. Additional problems may be pneumonia, ARDS, seizures and disseminated intravascular coagulation (Fig. 7.7). Neurological outcome is often better in victims of cold-water drowning due to the degree of cerebral protection afforded by the diving reflex. Hypothermia in children reduces the cerebral metabolic rate such that the demands for oxygen are reduced and the child will better tolerate relative hypoxia.

Initial assessment of the child admitted following a submersion episode entails airway protection, assessment of respiratory rate and pattern if any, assessment of cardiovascular status and, if possible, neurological assessment. The child with fluctuating or decreased level of consciousness and respiratory failure or apnoea will require intubation and ventilation.

High peak inspiratory pressures are often required because of reduced compliance, and high PEEP improves oxygenation. Pneumothorax is a risk of high inspiratory pressures. Analysis of arterial blood gases will determine ventilatory requirements.

Cardiac output may be compromised, and the cardiovascular system should be assessed and continually monitored. Control of electrolyte imbalance is a vital part of the management of these children. It may be particularly difficult to warm the child with severe hypothermia following submersion injury. If heating mattresses and warmers fail, other options include peritoneal lavage with warm isotonic fluid or warming through extracorporeal membrane oxygenation.

It may be desirable to keep the child ventilated, paralysed and sedated for 48–72 h to reduce the risk of secondary injury due to cerebral oedema. Once it is felt that the child's neurological condition is stable and respiratory status allows, the child could be woken and weaned. Seizures may occur because of initial hypoxia or cerebral oedema and should be treated to prevent raised ICP and increased cerebral O_2 consumption. There is controversy surrounding the usefulness of prophylactic anticonvulsants in these children. However, children having multiple seizures may benefit from a period of treatment, to reduce damage that may result from seizure activity.

Hypothermic children following submersion injury are at great risk from infection, due to impaired immune response. Neutrophil release may be effected by hypothermia. Particular care should be taken when obtaining central venous and arterial access. Maintaining adequate nutritional input is vital to provide sufficient energy for cell growth and repair. However, this is difficult in the initial stages following the injury.

ACUTE RESPIRATORY DISTRESS SYNDROME

Acute respiratory distress syndrome (ARDS) is characterised by:

- dyspnoea
- severe hypoxia
- bilateral pulmonary infiltrates
- reduced pulmonary compliance.

ARDS was first described by Ashbaugh and colleagues in 1967. It is clinically similar to respiratory distress syndrome in neonates but can appear in children and adults. Many disorders can lead to ARDS in children, including near drowning, sepsis, trauma and aspiration, but cardiopulmonary bypass, major burns, disseminated intravascular coagulopathies and aspiration pneumonia have been associated with ARDS. The diagnosis of ARDS is a clinical one with varying features. However, common factors are:

- a life-threatening event, pulmonary or other, in a child without left ventricular failure or congestive heart failure and with previously normal lungs
- severe respiratory distress: tachypnoea and dyspnoea, severe sternal and intercostal recession, hypoxia, reduced lung compliance and increased intrapulmonary right-to-left shunting
- radiological evidence of bilateral, diffuse pulmonary interstitial or alveolar infiltrates (Fig. 7.8).

The hypoxia, reduced compliance and reduced lung volumes seen in ARDS result from several features:

- protein leaking into the interstitial space because of alveolar capillary membrane damage
- decreased compliance, with V/Q mismatching, because of increased interstitial fluid and narrowing of the small airways
- intrapulmonary shunting from right to left, caused by alveolar flooding due to overloaded lymphatic drainage
- closure of alveoli and terminal airways.

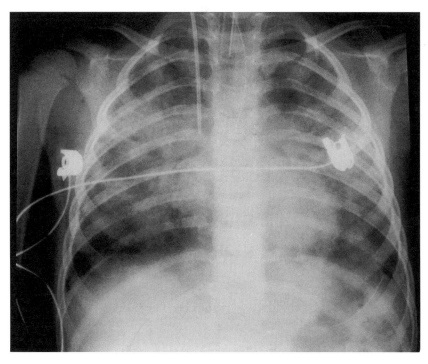

Figure 7.8 ARDS — 2 days after near-drowning episode, ARDS developed with bilateral pulmonary infiltrates.

The activated neutrophil has been suggested as one of the main agents of tissue damage within the lungs in ARDS. However, ARDS is seen in neutropenic patients, indicating the involvement of other agents in the process causing lung damage.

When ARDS occurs secondary to a non-pulmonary injury, the damage to the vascular endothelium occurs in the presence of circulating activated macrophages, neutrophils and lymphocytes. Chemotaxis attracts activated molecules, which adhere to the vascular endothelium. Cytokines such as tumour necrosis factor (TNF), interleukin (IL) 1, 6, and 8, leukotrienes and endotoxins have all been linked to the process of damage to the endothelium, which results in increased vascular permeability (Mulnier & Evans 1995). Additional current evidence points to the activated granulocytes as the mediator of microvascular damage in ARDS (Beck Koff et al 1993). It is suggested that the C5a part of the alternative complement pathway may be the major stimulant for activation and sequestration of granulocytes within the lungs. Activated granulocytes are involved in two potential mechanisms for lung damage: firstly the release of liposomal proteins, and secondly the release of free radicals. Proteolytic enzyme levels increase and both damage the lung microvasculature and form a positive feedback loop generating activated complement. Substances such as histamine and fibrinogen degradation products may also be involved in the lung injury process (Fig. 7.9).

Surfactant production appears inadequate, possibly due to damage to type II alveolar cells, causing reduced functional residual capacity. Alveolar collapse results from increasing alveolar surface tension and reduced surfactant production.

The aim of management of the child with ARDS is to support the cardiorespiratory system in order to maximise oxygen delivery. Adequate hydration, nutrition and prevention of infection are also vital components of the management.

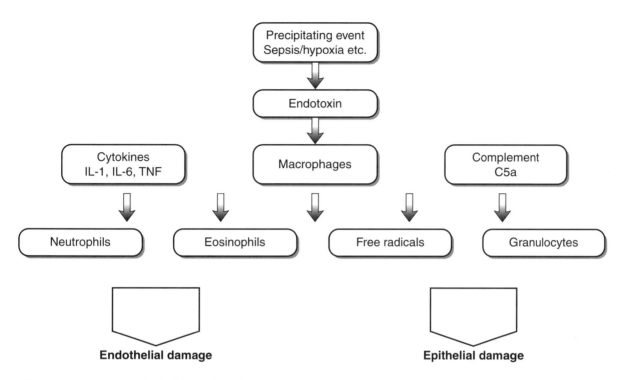

Figure 7.9 Mediators of acute respiratory distress syndrome.

Oxygen delivery is dependent upon haemoglobin, arterial O_2 saturations, heart rate and stroke volume:

$$\text{oxygen delivery } (DO_2) \text{ (mL/min)} = O_2 \text{ content} \times \text{cardiac output, CO}$$

where $CO = HR \times \text{stroke volume (SV)}$ and

$$O_2 \text{ content} = (SaO_2 \times Hb \times 1.34) + (0.003 \times PaO_2)$$

Manipulations of any or all of these parameters may increase O_2 delivery to the tissues. Much controversy exists, however, regarding the relationship between oxygen delivery and oxygen uptake.

Children suffering from ARDS frequently have compromised cardiac output usually resulting from decreased stroke volume rather than reduced heart rate. Increasing preload by ensuring central venous pressure is within desirable limits aims to improve cardiac output. If this remains low, inotropic and vasoactive agents are required to raise cardiac output. Cardiovascular management includes monitoring heart rate, blood pressure, central venous pressure, pulmonary artery wedge pressure and adjusting fluid administration, inotropic and vasoactive drugs to maximise stroke volume.

Respiratory support involves intubation and ventilation with sedation and muscle relaxation in the acute phase. High peak inspiratory pressures and PEEP are needed to combat decreased lung volumes and compliance. High PEEP must be carefully introduced, as reduction in cardiac output may result from reduced venous return.

Volume or pressure control modes of ventilation may be used and will be dictated by the child's clinical condition and physician preference. Recent advances in ventilator performance allow use of a pressure-limited volume control mode that may be of benefit in these children. Frequent blood gas analysis allows appropriate manipulation of ventilatory parameters to maximise oxygenation and CO_2 removal. Potential problems for these children include pneumothoraces from high peak inspiratory pressure and reduced cardiac output from high PEEP. It may not be possible to achieve adequate oxygenation and CO_2 removal, due to the difficulties faced when ventilating these children. Therefore, it may be necessary to accept a raised $PaCO_2$ and a degree of acidosis rather than increasing the risk of barotrauma. Reversing the inspiration:expiration ratio is one strategy used to improve oxygenation but this may be poorly tolerated.

The child with ARDS who continues to be unstable and have poor O_2 delivery despite full ventilatory support may benefit from inhaled nitric oxide (NO) therapy.

NO, or endothelial derived relaxing factor (EDRF), was discovered by Furchgott and Ingarro separately in 1986. Endogenous NO is synthesised from L-arganine present in endothelial cells. NO diffuses from the endothelial cell into the smooth muscle cell and activates guanylate cyclase, which by converting GTP (guanosine triphosphate) to cGMP (cyclic guanosine monophosphate) causes relaxation of the muscle cell and vasodilatation (Fig. 7.10). Research over the last 15 years has demonstrated that when additional NO is inhaled, selective pulmonary vasodilatation occurs without the systemic vasodilatation caused by conventional nitrovasodilators. It has been suggested that inhaled NO may improve V/Q mismatching by being delivered directly to ventilated areas of lung. In contrast, intravenous vasodilators may increase perfusion to unventilated lung areas (Tibbals 1993). NO is now considered to have an established role in the control of pulmonary vascular resistance.

Pulmonary hypertension generated by hypoxia responds to inhaled NO therapy. When pulmonary hypertension develops it appears that EDRF activity is lost in the pulmonary vessels and this is restored by inhalation of NO. It has been demonstrated that administration of low doses of NO improves oxygenation by reducing pulmonary vascular resistance in children, in adults with severe respiratory failure (Abman et al 1994) and ARDS and in children with pulmonary hypertension following cardiac surgery.

The systemic uptake of NO by haemoglobin to form methaemoglobin would appear to eliminate its systemic effect. Concerns regarding NO therapy relate to a lack of knowledge of tolerable levels of methaemoglobinaemia, levels of nitrogen dioxide (NO_2), and long-term effects of using inhaled NO. Careful monitoring of NO levels, NO_2 levels and metHb levels are essential when using NO therapy, and a scavenging system should be in place to prevent the risk of inhalation by PIC personnel.

Other methods of treatment include the use of ECMO, surfactant therapy and the use of liquid

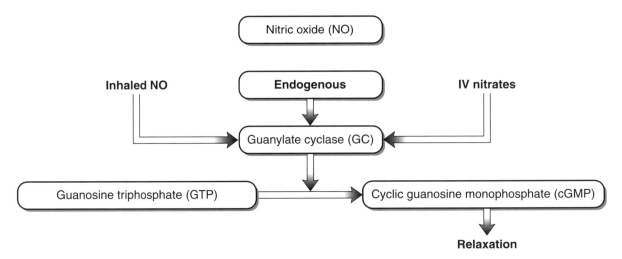

Figure 7.10 Schematic drawing of the action of nitric oxide in the smooth muscle cell. Adapted from Tibbals (1993).

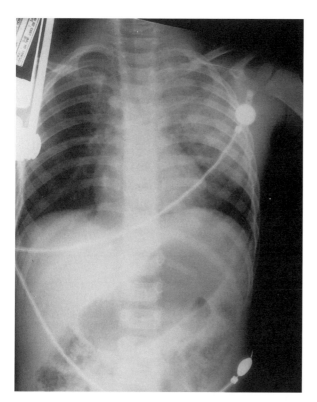

Figure 7.11   Left lung contusion following road traffic accident. Note associated acute gastric dilatation requiring nasogastric tube.

ventilation, which currently remains experimental. At present there is little evidence that surfactant therapy is of use in other than the neonatal population with respiratory distress syndrome. Partial liquid ventilation is thought to improve oxygenation in patients with severe lung disease and has had some success in studies with animal models.

CHEST TRAUMA

Chest trauma results from penetrating or non-penetrating injury. The most common injuries seen in children are non-penetrating, those resulting from contact with blunt objects through non-accidental injury, falls, and road traffic accidents (Fig. 7.11).

Types of injury include:

- rib fractures
- pneumothoraces
- haemothoraces
- sternal fracture
- rupture of the larynx
- tracheal and bronchial lacerations
- cardiac tamponade.

Rib fractures and flail chest are amongst the most common injuries seen in children. Assessment of the child with suspected rib fractures includes full assessment of respiratory rate and pattern. Painful shallow respirations and uneven chest expansion may give an indication of the presence of fractures. The condition of flail chest results in chest wall retraction during inspiration. The presence of pneumothorax and rib fractures can easily be identified with auscultation and chest X-ray.

Tension pneumothorax occurs when air becomes trapped in the pleural space, increasing in volume with each breath. This results in mediastinal shift and tamponade from compression of the heart. This condition constitutes a life-threatening emergency and must be diagnosed and resolved swiftly. Immediate decompression of the air collection is required and is performed by inserting a large-gauge needle into the pleural space. Chest drain insertion following decompression then facilitates complete lung re-expansion.

Children suffering from an acute flail chest require intubation and ventilation to provide adequate ventilation and gas exchange. Once stabilised, the child may benefit from continued ventilation for a week or more until adequate healing has occurred to prevent paradoxical chest movement.

The child in the PICU can suffer chest trauma as a direct result of intravenous cannulation of the internal jugular or subclavian veins. Pneumothorax or haemothorax can result from these procedures. To reduce the risks of complications, skilled personnel should carry out this procedure. The child should be monitored throughout the procedure and immediately following it. Careful monitoring of heart rate, blood pressure, oxygen saturations and chest movement will identify early problems and a routine post-insertion chest X-ray will identify pneuomthoraces.

CONGENITAL LOBAR EMPHYSEMA

This is a clinical syndrome in which compression of the lung and mediastinum results from progressive hyperinflation of the affected lobe. The infant presents at or shortly after birth with respiratory distress. A few infants progress undiagnosed until later in the first year and present with repeated upper respiratory tract infections.

Upper lobes are more commonly involved than lower lobes, although the reason for this is unclear.

Reasons for the inability of the affected lobe to deflate include:

- loss of elasticity
- structural airway defects
- partial obstruction of the airway by external compression.

Treatment of this condition involves respiratory support for the infant followed by surgery to remove the affected lobe.

REFERENCES

Abman S H, Griebel J L, Parker D K, Schmidt J M, Swanton D, Kinsella J P 1994 Acute effects of inhaled nitric oxide in children with severe hypoxaemic respiratory failure. Journal of Pediatrics 124(5):881–888

Altman D G 1991 Practical statistics for medical research. Chapman and Hall, London

Ashbaugh D G, Bigelow D B, Petty T L, Levine B E 1967 Acute respiratory distress in adults. Lancet 320:323

Beck Koff P, Eitzman D, Neu J 1993 Neonatal and pediatric respiratory care, 2nd edn. Mosby, St Louis

Davies H, Kitchman R, Gordon I, Helms P 1985 Regional ventilation in infancy: reversal of adult pattern. New England Journal of Medicine 313(26):1626–1628

Downham M A P S, Scott R, Sims D G, Webb J G K, Gardner P S 1976 Breast feeding protects against respiratory syncytial virus infections. British Journal of Medicine 2:274

Gozal D, Colin A A, Jaffe M, Hochberg Z 1990 Water, electrolyte and endocrine homeostasis in infants with bronchiolitis. Pediatric Research 27(2):204–209

Guy's, Lewisham and St Thomas' Hospital 1997 Paediatric formulary, 4th edn. Guy's & St Thomas' Hospital Trust, London

Heaf D P, Helms P, Gordon I, Turner H M 1983 Postural effects on gas exchange in infants. New England Journal of Medicine 308:1505

Martin J G, Shore S, Engel L A 1982 Effect of continuous positive airway pressure on respiratory mechanics and pattern of breathing in induced asthma. American Review of Respiratory Disease 126:812

Mulnier C, Evans T 1995 Acute respiratory distress in adults. Care of the Critically Ill 11(5):182–186

Prien T, Traber D L 1988 Smoke compounds and inhalation injury — a review. Burns 14(6):451–460

Qvist J, Anderson J B, Pemberton M, Bennike K A 1982 High levels of PEEP in severe acute asthma. New England Journal of Medicine 370:1347

Rogers M 1992 Textbook of pediatric intensive care, 2nd edn. Williams & Wilkins, Baltimore

Roitt I 1994 Essential immunology, 8th edn. Blackwell Scientific, Oxford

Singh N 1997 Manual of pediatric critical care. WB Saunders, Philadelphia

Swann H, Spafford N R 1951 Body salt and water changes during fresh and sea water drowning. Texas Reports on Biology and Medicine 9:356 (cited in Rogers 1992)

Thompson A H, Beardsmore C S, Firmin R, Leanage R, Simpson H 1990 Airway function in infants with vascular rings: pre-operative and post-operative assessment. Archives of Diseases of Childhood 65:1711

Thompson P B, Herndon D N, Traber D L, Abston S 1986 Effect of burn injury on mortality. Journal of Trauma 26(2):163–165

Tibbals J 1993 The role of nitric oxide (formerly endothelium derived relaxing factor — EDRF) in vasodilatation and vasodilator therapy. Anaesthetic Intensive Care 21:759–773

Tibbals J, Shann F A, Landan L I 1992 Placebo controlled trial of prednisolone in children intubated for croup. Lancet 340:745–748

van Steensel-Moll H A, Hazelet J A, van der Voort E, Neijens H J, Hackeng W H L 1990 Excessive secretions of antidiuretic hormone in infections with respiratory syncytial virus. Archives of Diseases of Childhood 65:1237–1239

Welliver R C, Wong D T, Sun M, Middleton E, Vaughan R, Ogra P 1981 The development of respiratory syncytial virus specific IgE and the release of histamine in nasopharyngeal secretions. New England Journal of Medicine 305:841

8

Cardiovascular anatomy and physiology in infants and children

Alan G. Magee

ANATOMY

An appreciation of normal cardiac anatomy is necessary to understand cardiac function, congenital cardiac abnormalities and the transitional circulation from fetus to neonate. Nowadays, the best approach to understanding cardiac anatomy is the segmental approach. This is based on the work of Anderson in the UK and Van Praagh in the USA (Freedom et al 1992). Using this method, the three cardiac segments are the atria, the ventricles and the great arteries, which are in turn connected at the atrioventricular and ventriculoarterial junctions. It is important to realise that the anatomy of the individual cardiac chambers is not defined by their position in the chest (e.g. right, left, superior or inferior) nor by their relationship one to another but by their intrinsic features.

The atria

Atria are defined as being anatomically 'right' or 'left' by the appearance of the atrial appendage. The right atrium has a broad triangular-shaped appendage and normally receives blood from the superior and inferior vena cavae and from the heart itself via the coronary sinus. The left atrium has a long narrow appendage and normally receives blood from the four pulmonary veins, two of which drain from each lung.

The usual arrangement (Fig. 8.1a), called *situs solitus*, consists of an anatomically 'right' atrium on the right hand side and anatomically 'left' atrium on the left hand side. Possible variations are inversion of the normal arrangement, which is

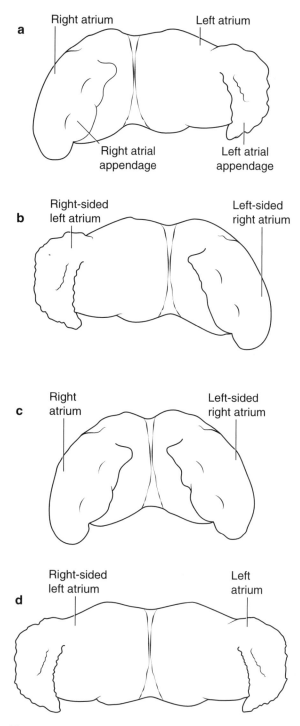

Figure 8.1 Varieties of atrial arrangement: (a) *situs solitus* (usual arrangement); (b) *situs inversus* (mirror image arrangement); (c) *situs ambiguus*, right atrial isomerism; (d) *situs ambiguus*, left atrial isomerism.

called *situs inversus* (Fig. 8.1b), or the presence of two 'right' atria or two 'left' atria which is called *situs ambiguus*. The presence of two 'right' atria is also termed right atrial isomerism (Fig. 8.1c), and two 'left' atria left atrial isomerism (Fig. 8.1d), and in each case there is usually symmetry of the lungs and abdominal organs. Therefore, right atrial isomerism is associated with absence of a spleen, which leaves the child prone to overwhelming pneumococcal infection and requiring lifelong antibiotic prophylaxis. In addition, pneumococcal vaccine should be administered after the age of 2 years. Conversely, left atrial isomerism is associated with multiple spleens and also with atresia of the intrahepatic bile ducts. In both types of isomerism there may also be malrotation of the bowel. However, isomerism of the atrial appendages is rare and accounts for only 4% of congenital heart malformations.

Between the atria is the atrial septum, which has a thin-walled central portion called the fossa ovalis; this is important when considering fetal circulation.

The ventricles

The ventricles constitute the bulk of the cardiac muscle, and each ventricle normally consists of three components:

- an inlet region beneath the atrioventricular valves
- a trabecular region extending towards the apex of the heart
- an outlet region extending towards the great arteries.

The trabecular region is so called because of the prominent muscle bars or trabeculations seen within this part of the ventricle. The definition of an anatomically 'left' or 'right' ventricle depends on the appearance of the trabeculations on the septal surface, with those of the left ventricle having a smoother appearance, and not on its position within the chest.

The great arteries

The normal aorta gives rise to the two coronary

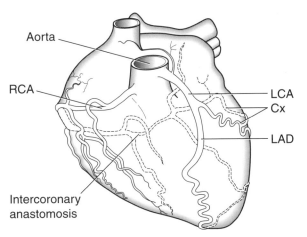

Figure 8.2 The arrangement of the proximal coronary arteries: RCA, right coronary artery; LCA, left coronary artery; LAD, left anterior descending; Cx, circumflex. Adapted from Andreoli et al (1986).

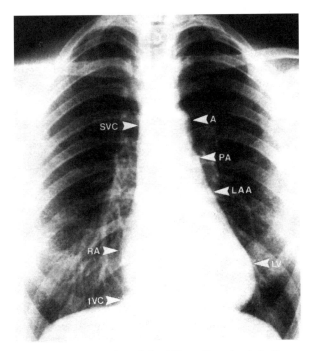

Figure 8.3 Normal frontal chest X-ray. From top to bottom, the left side of the cardiac silhouette is formed by the aorta, A; main pulmonary artery, PA; left atrial appendage, LAA; and left ventricle, LV. The right side comprises the superior vena cava, SVC; right atrium, RA; and inferior vena cava, IVC.

arteries supplying the heart (Fig. 8.2) and then ascends in the chest to become the aortic arch (Fig. 8.3). The first branch of the aortic arch is the

brachiocephalic (innominate) artery which in turn divides to form the right subclavian and right common carotid arteries. Beyond the brachiocephalic artery the arch turns posteriorly and to the left and gives rise to the left common carotid and left subclavian arteries. The arch terminates at the left side of the spine and then turns inferiorly to become the descending aorta which continues to the left of the spine and gives rise to the intercostal and bronchial arteries.

At the point where the aortic arch turns inferiorly it is connected to the bifurcation of the main pulmonary artery by the arterial ligament. This is the fibrous remnant of the arterial duct, which is discussed further under fetal circulation. The aortic arch may also be right sided and the aorta descend to the right of the spine. In this situation there is usually some form of congenital heart disease such as tetralogy of Fallot. The normal main pulmonary artery is a short vessel which crosses in front of the ascending aorta before dividing into the right and left pulmonary arteries. These branches extend into the hila of each lung before further subdividing.

Connections between segments

This refers to how the three segments described above are linked together. Normally, the right atrium connects through a tricuspid (three leaflet) valve to the right ventricle, which in turn connects through the pulmonary valve to the pulmonary artery. The left atrium connects through a mitral (two leaflet) valve to the left ventricle which in turn connects through the aortic valve to the aorta. The mitral valve is so named because of its likeness to a 'bishop's mitre'.

On the right side of the heart, the tricuspid and pulmonary valves are separated by a prominent muscle bar which mostly consists of the inner curvature of the heart produced by the folding of the primitive heart tube (see under Embryology). On the left side of the heart, the mitral and aortic valves are not separated, and indeed the anterior leaflet of the mitral valve is continuous with the aortic valve.

Both the arterial valves normally have three

leaflets or cusps and are termed semilunar. Above each leaflet is a slight outpouching, called the sinus of Valsalva, into which the leaflet is pushed during ventricular systole (when blood is ejected from the heart). Superiorly, the aortic sinuses merge with the ascending aorta at the sinotubular junction. The three leaflets of the aortic valve are the left, right and non-coronary leaflets depending on whether the left, right or neither coronary artery arises from the corresponding sinus.

The cardiac silhouette

Much information can be obtained from the cardiac silhouette as seen on a standard frontal chest X-ray (Fig. 8.3). Normally the diameter of the cardiac shadow makes up less than 50% of the diameter of the thoracic cage (60% in infants) and is therefore a useful indicator of cardiac enlargement. An outline of the various cardiac chambers is visible at the margins of this silhouette. At the top of the silhouette is the aortic arch which may be to the left or right of the spine. It is usually possible to tell which side the arch is on by its relationship to the air-filled midline trachea. On the left heart border an indentation is seen below the aorta, and below this is a bulge produced by the pulmonary artery. This bulge is enlarged with enlargement of the central pulmonary arteries, which occurs in pulmonary hypertension. However, it may disappear when the pulmonary artery is underdeveloped, which occurs in cyanotic congenital heart disease such as tetralogy of Fallot or pulmonary atresia.

Beneath the pulmonary artery a small bulge may be visible, produced by the left atrial appendage, and below this the silhouette extends outwards to the apex of the heart which is formed by the border of the left ventricle. The inferior border of the heart is formed by the right ventricle and atrium and extends along the diaphragm to the right side of the sternum. The right border of the heart is visible just to the right of the sternum and is formed by the right atrium together with the superior and inferior caval veins joining at its upper and lower edges.

Histology of the heart

The heart consists of three basic layers of tissue which are analogous to the three layers which line the major blood vessels. The innermost layer is the one-cell-thick endocardium, which presents a smooth non-adherent surface for the flow of blood. Next to this, the muscular myocardium comprises the bulk of cardiac tissue. Normally, left ventricular myocardium is thicker than right ventricular myocardium which in turn is thicker than atrial myocardium, reflecting the different pressure loads in the respective chambers. On the outside, the epicardium consists of a loose layer of connective tissue and fat cells and contains the major blood vessels and nerves which supply the heart. These blood vessels and nerves then give rise to perforating branches which supply the myocardium.

The pericardium is developmentally a separate structure and consists of a tough outer fibrous pericardium and a fine double membrane inner serous pericardium. The two layers of the serous pericardium are fused to the fibrous pericardium and the epicardial surface of the heart, respectively. Between the layers of serous pericardium is a thin film of fluid which acts as a lubricant and allows unimpeded movement of the heart during systole and diastole. The heart is fixed within the chest by the great vessels lying superiorly and posteriorly and by the fusion of the fibrous pericardium to the outer linings of these vessels. Fluid collecting in the pericardial space, for example blood following trauma or cardiac surgery or serous fluid due to pericardial inflammation, can eventually restrict filling of the heart and so reduce cardiac output. This process of pericardial tamponade requires urgent relief which may be performed by either opening the chest or by the insertion of a percutaneous drain.

Ultrastructure of cardiac muscle

The properties of cardiac muscle represent a cross between the smooth muscle found in the lining of the gut, airways and blood vessels and the striated muscle of the musculoskeletal sys-

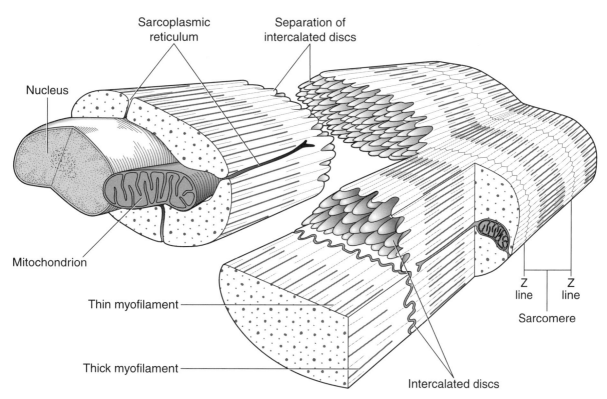

Figure 8.4 Diagram of a myocyte, based on electron microscopy. Adapted from Katz (1977).

tem. Smooth muscle contracts and relaxes slowly, can initiate contraction and does not tire. By contrast, skeletal muscle can contract and relax rapidly but is unable to initiate contraction and quickly tires.

The most common type of cell in the heart is the myocyte or myocardial cell which provides the force to eject blood from the cardiac chambers. The heart also contains fibrous tissue together with specialised conducting tissue which initiates and conducts the spread of electrical activity that causes contraction. Each myocyte is approximately 100 µm long and 15 µm wide (Fig. 8.4). The cells branch with adjacent cells and are joined at their ends by a specialised membrane called the intercalated disc which is able to transmit both the force of contraction and the electrical signals of conduction. In keeping with their high energy demand, myocytes contain large numbers of mitochondria and are surrounded by a rich network of capillaries.

The myocyte is made up of myofibrils which in turn consist of a series of sarcomeres which are the basic unit of contraction. Surrounding the myofibrils and spreading throughout the entire cell is the lace-like sarcoplasmic reticulum which acts as a reservoir for calcium. It is the coordinated shortening of the sarcomeres within each cell which produces contraction of the heart. Forming the ends of each sarcomere is the Z-line, and the alignment of sarcomeres and Z-lines in adjacent myofibrils produces the characteristic striated appearance of cardiac muscle under the microscope. The sarcomere is made up of interdigitating thick and thin filaments. The thick filament mainly consists of the protein myosin and the thin filament of the protein actin. The myosin molecule has a body consisting of two intertwining helical peptides called heavy chains and a head consisting of heavy chain material together with two further peptides called light chains. The myosin molecule heads extend

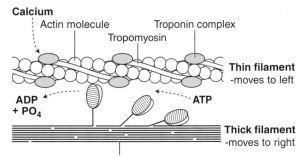

Figure 8.5 Diagram of thick and thin filaments. Contraction is produced by movement of the myosin heads on the thick filaments in relation to the thin filaments. This process requires the breakdown of ATP. Adapted from Julian et al (1996).

laterally and are staggered around the filament to interact with the actin molecules of the thin filaments (Fig. 8.5).

The thin filaments consist of two chains of small globular actin proteins forming a helix. Between the chains of the helix is a further molecule called tropomyosin which provides the skeleton of the thin filament. Attached to every seventh actin molecule is a complex molecule called troponin. This protein has three parts:

- troponin C, which binds calcium
- troponin I, which prevents the interaction between actin and myosin
- troponin T, which binds the protein complex to tropomyosin.

Contraction begins with the binding of calcium ions to troponin C, which then prevents troponin I from inhibiting the interaction between actin and myosin. The enzyme ATPase, which is situated on the myosin heads, causes the breakdown of ATP into ADP and phosphate which releases the energy required to change the angle at which the myosin head is attached to its body. This causes the two filaments to move relative to each other and shortens the myofibril. Contraction ceases when calcium is released from troponin C.

Blood supply to the heart

The precise definition of the proximal coronary artery anatomy in neonates has assumed greater importance in recent years with the development of the arterial switch operation for transposition of the great arteries (see next chapter). Considerable variations are possible which may cause technical difficulties during the crucial transfer of the coronary arteries. There are usually two coronary arteries arising from the mid point of two of the three aortic valve sinuses. The most common coronary arrangement is as shown in Fig. 8.2.

After leaving its sinus, the right coronary artery enters the atrioventricular groove and circles the tricuspid valve orifice giving branches to the right atrium superiorly and right ventricle inferiorly. The left coronary artery almost immediately divides to form the left anterior descending and circumflex branches. The left anterior descending runs in the anterior interventricular groove and supplies most of the anterior interventricular septum and adjacent left ventricle before turning past the apex to supply a small amount of the posterior interventricular septum. The circumflex runs in the left atrioventricular groove and supplies the leftwards margin and inferior surface of the heart. The posterior interventricular artery supplying the posterior interventricular septum arises as a branch of the right coronary artery in 90% of hearts and of the left coronary artery in 10%.

The majority of the venous drainage of the heart follows the course of the coronary arteries and terminates in the coronary sinus which lies in the posterior aspect of the left atrioventricular groove. This then empties into the inferior aspect of the right atrium. The remainder of the venous drainage of the heart is via the anterior cardiac veins which enter the right atrium and right ventricle and the Thebesian veins which enter both ventricles.

PHYSIOLOGY

The cardiac cycle

The two main phases of the cardiac cycle are:

- ventricular contraction or *systole*
- ventricular relaxation or *diastole*.

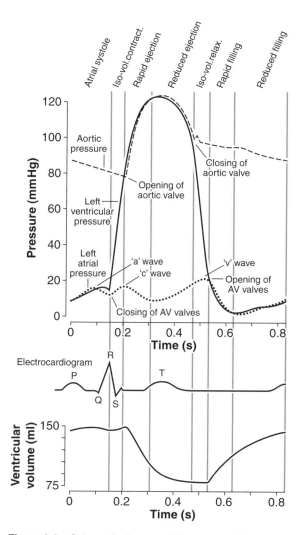

Figure 8.6 Schematic diagram of the events of the cardiac cycle. Ventricular systole is made up of 3 phases: isovolumetric contraction, rapid ejection and reduced ejection. Ventricular diastole is made up of 4 phases: isovolumetric relaxation, rapid filling, reduced filling and atrial systole. Adapted from Julian DG, Camm AJ, Fox KM, Hall RJC, Poole-Wilson PA Diseases of the heart. WB Saunders, London 1996.

These phases are controlled by the conducting system. A schematic diagram of the events of the cardiac cycle and the pressures in the various chambers is shown in Fig. 8.6.

The cardiac cycle begins with ventricular systole. Pressure in the ventricles rapidly rises above atrial pressure, which closes the atrioventricular valves producing the first heart sound. During the brief isovolumetric contraction period, both the atrioventricular and arterial valves remain shut, but once pressure in the great arteries is exceeded the arterial valves open and blood is rapidly ejected from the heart. As aortic and pulmonary pressure rises, ejection of blood slows and stops. At the end of systole, pressure in the ventricles falls to below great artery pressure, and the pulmonary and aortic valves close. This produces the second heart sound and marks the beginning of ventricular diastole. Ventricular pressure continues to fall rapidly and, once lower than atrial pressure, the atrioventricular valves re-open and the ventricles begin to fill. The brief period from closing of the arterial valves to opening of the atrioventricular valves is called the isovolumetric relaxation time. As blood has accumulated in the atria during ventricular systole, inflow from atria to ventricles is rapid at first but then slows for much of diastole until atrial systole. This event occurs during the last quarter of ventricular diastole and accounts for the last 25% of ventricular filling.

Cardiac output

The amount of blood ejected from the heart during each cardiac cycle is termed the stroke volume (SV). Cardiac output (CO) is the volume of blood ejected by the heart each minute and is the product of stroke volume and heart rate (HR):

$$CO = SV \times HR$$

where CO is in litres/min, SV is in litres and HR is in beats/min.

Cardiac output increases with age, as does stroke volume, while heart rate decreases (Fig. 8.7). In response to increased demand, infants have less scope to increase cardiac output by increasing stroke volume compared with older children and adults, and therefore must increase heart rate. Cardiac output may be corrected for patient size by dividing by the body surface area (BSA) to obtain the cardiac index (CI). The normal range for resting cardiac index is 3.5 ± 0.7 L/min/m^2 (Yang et al 1988).

$$CI = CO/BSA$$

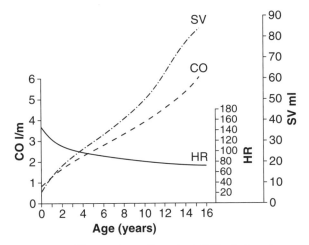

Figure 8.7 Changes in cardiac output (CO), stroke volume (SV) and heart rate (HR) with age. From Rudolph (1977), with permission.

where CI is in $L/min/m^2$ and BSA is in m^2.

The classical method for measuring cardiac output which is employed in most cardiac catheter laboratories is based on the Fick principle (Fick 1870). This states that flow through a vascular bed (e.g. the lungs) can be determined by the amount of oxygen entering the bloodstream during a given period of time divided by the difference in concentration of oxygen between the inflow and outflow of that vascular bed. Total body oxygen consumption must equal oxygen delivery during steady state conditions, giving the equation:

total body oxygen consumption = cardiac output × (arterial oxygen content – mixed venous oxygen content)

Rearrangement of this equation gives:

cardiac output = O_2 consumption/(arterial oxygen content – mixed venous oxygen content)

Oxygen consumption can be measured in spontaneously breathing children using a flow-through oxygen consumption computer connected to a clear plastic hood. Oxygen consumption can also be measured from analysis of oxygen and carbon dioxide in ventilator circuits or it can be estimated using tables of normal values. When indexed to body surface area, resting oxygen consumption varies from 160–180 $mL/min/m^2$ in infants

to 100–130 $mL/min/m^2$ for older children. The oxygen content of blood is the amount of oxygen carried by haemoglobin plus the amount of dissolved oxygen. The total binding capacity of haemoglobin is approximately 1.36 mL/g. Therefore the oxygen content of blood is given by the equation:

O_2 content = (1.36 × haemoglobin × O_2 saturation) + dissolved O_2

where the O_2 content is given in mL/L, haemoglogin is in mg/L and saturation as a fraction where 1 is fully saturated.

For children with a systemic arterial partial pressure of oxygen of less than 100 torr (mmHg), dissolved oxygen can safely be ignored, as the amount of dissolved oxygen is only 0.03 $mL/mmHg\ O_2/L$. However, if dissolved oxygen is not considered in the patient breathing 100% oxygen, the cardiac output will be greatly overestimated. The systemic arterial sample can be obtained from any peripheral arterial line. Mixed venous blood is best obtained from the pulmonary artery, at which point deoxygenated blood will be most thoroughly mixed, although a sample from a central venous line is usually adequate for clinical purposes.

Therefore, for a child breathing room air who has an oxygen consumption of 120 mL/min, a haemoglogin of 13.5 mg/dL (135 mg/L), a pulmonary artery saturation of 70% and an aortic saturation of 98%:

arterial oxygen content = 1.36 × 135 × 0.98 = 180 mL/L

mixed venous oxygen content = 1.36 × 135 × 0.7 = 129 mL/L

cardiac output = 120/(180 – 129) = 2.35 L/min.

Examination of the Fick equation enables practitioners to appreciate that a wide difference in arteriovenous oxygen saturations provides a quick bedside indication of a low cardiac output.

Other methods of estimating cardiac output use basically the same principle that flow through a vascular bed can be estimated by dividing a known amount of an indicator substance by the difference in concentrations upstream and downstream of that vascular bed. Instead of oxygen, the substance measured is a dye, in the indicator dilution method (indocyanin green), or cooled saline in the thermodilution technique.

This latter technique is the most commonly used method in the intensive care unit and is readily performed using a Swan–Ganz catheter (pulmonary artery thermodilution catheter). This catheter has multiple ports for injection and sampling as well as a balloon tip which facilitates positioning of the thermistor end of the catheter within the main pulmonary artery. A specific volume of saline at a specific temperature is quickly injected through the proximal port positioned in the right atrium, and the change in temperature of the blood passing the thermistor tip is used to calculate cardiac output.

Calculation of shunts

In most situations, the output from the right ventricle equals that from the left ventricle. However, in the presence of an intracardiac shunt this will not be the case. The output from the right side of the heart (pulmonary blood flow or Qp) and from the left side of the heart (systemic blood flow or Qs) can be calculated according to the Fick principle using the following equations:

$$\text{pulmonary blood flow (Qp)} = O_2 \text{ consumption}/(\text{pulmonary venous oxygen content} - \text{pulmonary arterial oxygen content})$$

$$\text{systemic blood flow (Qs)} = O_2 \text{ consumption}/(\text{aortic oxygen content} - \text{mixed venous oxygen content})$$

Systemic flow is the same as cardiac output. However, in the presence of a shunt, the mixed venous sample is usually taken from the superior vena cava or right atrium rather than from the pulmonary artery. One way of expressing the degree of intracardiac shunting is by the ratio of pulmonary to systemic flow, which is abbreviated to Qp/Qs. When no shunt is present the ratio is 1, but, in the presence of a left-to-right shunt the ratio is greater than 1, and in the presence of a right-to-left shunt the ratio is less than 1.

Pressures and resistances

The best-known indicator of overall circulatory function is the mean arterial pressure, which depends on cardiac output and systemic vascular resistance. Arterial blood pressure can be measured directly by using an invasive catheter attached to a fluid-filled manometer, or indirectly, using a non-invasive manual or electronic flow detection device (sphygmomanometer or DINAMAP™). For invasive pressure measurement, the transducer must be set at exactly the same level as the vessel or chamber being measured. In practice this means the midchest level for supine patients. Once in position, the transducer is zeroed using atmospheric pressure.

When a blood pressure cuff is inflated to greater than arterial pressure, the systolic pressure corresponds to the return of arterial pulsation in the artery, which can be detected by fingertip, by doppler probe or by listening for the appearance of the Korotkoff sounds. Auscultation can also detect the diastolic pressure which corresponds to the fourth Korotkoff phase when a distinct muffling of the sounds is heard. DINAMAP™ non-invasive blood pressure devices are based on the oscillotonometry principle, which means the detection of fluctuations in cuff pressure as the cuff is deflated. These devices display systolic, diastolic and mean arterial pressures. Mean arterial pressure (MAP) may also be calculated from systolic and diastolic pressure using the formula:

$$\text{MAP} = \text{diastolic pressure} + (\text{systolic pressure} - \text{diastolic pressure})/3$$

For any non-invasive method, correct cuff size is important. Too wide a cuff will produce falsely low readings and too narrow a cuff will produce falsely high readings. The correct size is around 20% wider than the diameter of the arm (Blumenthal 1977). Normal ranges for blood pressures in children are given in Fig. 8.8.

When mean pressures and flow rates are known, it is possible to calculate the resistance across a vascular bed. For the systemic vascular bed the systemic vascular resistance (SVR) is given by the equation:

$$\text{SVR} = \frac{\text{mean arterial pressure} - \text{mean right atrial pressure}}{\text{QS}}$$

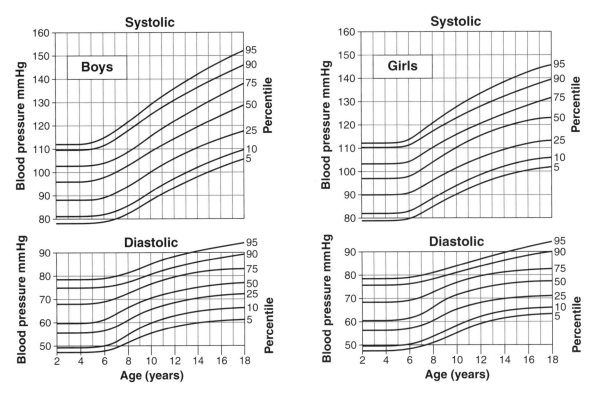

Figure 8.8 Blood pressure percentiles with age. Those for boys are on the left and for girls are on the right. From Blumenthal (1977). Reproduced with permission. From *Pediatrics*, Vol. 59, p 797, 1977.

and for the pulmonary vascular bed the pulmonary vascular resistance (PVR) is given by the equation:

$$PVR = \frac{\text{mean pulmonary artery pressure} - \text{mean left atrial pressure}}{Qp}$$

Both these values are usually indexed to body surface area. Normal indexed SVR is 15–20 mmHg/L/min/m^2 and normal indexed PVR is 1–2 mmHg/L/min/m^2. High pulmonary vascular resistance may indicate the presence of irreversible pulmonary vascular disease which will render congenital heart malformations inoperable. 100% oxygen and nitric oxide is often administered to such patients during preoperative cardiac catheterisation to assess reversibility of elevated pulmonary vascular resistance.

Typical haemodynamic pressures and oxygen saturations measured during cardiac catheterisation of a normal heart are shown in Fig. 8.9.

Normally the systolic pressure in the right ventricle is around one quarter of the systolic pressure in the left ventricle. The lower pressure value shown in the ventricles refers to the pressure at end diastole, which reflects preload.

Systolic function

The understanding of systolic cardiac function began with studies on isolated muscle preparations. The main concepts are preload, afterload and contractility. In the isolated preparation, preload refers to the resting length of the muscle prior to contraction. In the intact heart, the analogous measurement would be the end-diastolic volume. However, this is difficult and cumbersome to measure accurately (particularly for the right ventricle because of its shape), and for most practical purposes the end-diastolic pressure is used. In the intensive care situation, the end-diastolic pressure of the right ventricle can

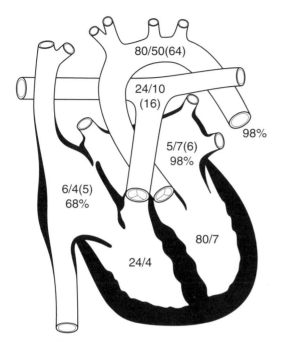

Figure 8.9 Typical haemodynamic pressures and percentage oxygen saturations measured during cardiac catheterisation of a normal infant. Mean pressures are in brackets.

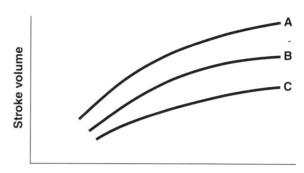

Figure 8.10 Relationship between stroke volume and end-diastolic volume or preload as first described by Starling: A, increased contractility; B, normal; C, reduced contractility. Adapted from Andreoli et al (1986).

usually be estimated from central venous pressure and of the left ventricule from left atrial or pulmonary capillary wedge pressure. One exception to these rules would be after a cavopulmonary shunt operation when the superor vena cava is no longer connected to the right atrium.

Afterload is defined as the force against which the isolated muscle or ventricle must contract. Clinically this can be estimated from the mean arterial pressure and the vascular resistance. Vascular resistance is better, as it is less affected by preload and contractility. Contractility refers to the intrinsic force-generating capacity of the myocardium and is independent of loading conditions but is affected by the action of inotropic drugs and autonomic activity.

The relationship between stroke volume and preload was first described by Starling using an isolated heart-lung preparation (Starling 1915). Stroke volume increases with end-diastolic volume until a plateau is reached beyond which further increases in filling volume result in a

decrease in stroke volume (Fig. 8.10). This is probably because of excessive stretching of the sarcomeres and is analogous to the situation in the failing heart with a high ventricular end-diastolic volume. Sympathetic activity shifts the stroke volume to ventricular end-diastolic volume to the left (positive inotropic effect), while parasympathetic activity shifts it to the right (negative inotropic effect).

Diastolic cardiac function

The importance of impaired diastolic function of the ventricle is being increasingly recognised. During ventricular filling, the change in ventricular volume for an increase in pressure is termed the compliance. This may be reduced by the stiffness of the ventricular wall or by forces exerted on the ventricle by the opposite ventricle or pericardium. Stiffness is increased by increases in wall thickness and by increased myocardial connective tissue content. In the postoperative cardiac patient, myocardial oedema reduces diastolic function, and this may be compounded by pre-existing myocardial hypertrophy and/or increased connective tissue. Reduced compliance means that the ventricle takes longer to fill and that filling is more dependent on atrial contraction. For these reasons avoidance of high heart rates (for example over 180/min) and maintenance of synchronous atrial and ventricular contraction is particularly important in the early post-bypass period. In addition a high filling pressure may be required.

Cardiopulmonary interactions

The heart and lungs display a complex interaction during both spontaneous and mechanical ventilation. To summarise events during spontaneous respiration, the negative intrathoracic pressure generated during inspiration causes increased systemic venous return and increased right heart filling. In addition, filling of the left heart is reduced during inspiration because of a tendency for blood to pool in the lungs. During expiration the opposite occurs: positive intrathoracic pressure reduces systemic venous return and increases pulmonary venous return, leading to increased left ventricular stroke volume and decreased right ventricular stroke volume.

The addition of positive end-expiratory pressure (PEEP) during mechanical ventilation, has the effect of reducing preload by reducing systemic venous return and of reducing effective afterload. A balance between these effects must be sought to optimise cardiac output.

THE CONDUCTING SYSTEM

Initiation and propagation of the cardiac impulse

In common with all nerve and muscle tissue, cardiac muscle cells have the ability to propagate an action potential (Fig. 8.11). This depends on the electrical properties of the cell membrane. In the resting state, the inside of the cell membrane is between 80 mV and 95 mV negative with respect to the outside. This resting membrane potential is produced by the concentration gradients for positively charged potassium and sodium ions. Within the cell, the concentrations for potassium and sodium are 140 and 10 mmol/L, respectively, and outside the cell concentrations for potassium and sodium are 5 and 140 mmol/L, respectively.

These concentrations are maintained by ion pumps in the cell membrane which force sodium ions out of the cell and allow potassium ions in. Potassium tends to move out of the cell along its

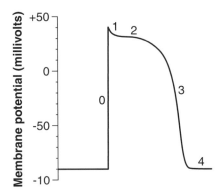

Figure 8.11   The myocyte action potential. Phase 0 (depolarisation) is due to the rapid influx of sodium ions, phase 1 to potassium ions moving out, phase 2 (plateau) to influx of calcium ions, phase 3 (repolarisation) to further outflow of potassium, and phase 4 is the resting membrane potential. RMP = resting membrane potential.

concentration gradient and, as the intracellular proteins which carry a negative charge are unable to cross the cell membrane, the inside of the cell becomes negative relative to the outside. An equilibrium is reached whereby the electrical forces trying to keep potassium within the cell are balanced by the tendency for it to diffuse out. This equilibrium potential occurs at −89 mV. The resting cell membrane is much more permeable to potassium than to any other ion, and therefore the equilibrium potential for potassium is mostly responsible for the membrane potential.

Electrical stimulation causes the inside of the membrane to become relatively more positive. Once a threshold of approximately −50 mV is reached, membrane channels open, allowing sodium ions to rush in and depolarise the cell, making the inside up to 30 mV positive with respect to the outside (phase 0). This is the beginning of the action potential which then causes depolarisation in the adjoining membrane and so spreads throughout the tissue.

Opening of the sodium channels is brief, and, almost immediately, potassium ions move out of the cell, making the inside more negative (phase 1). At this point, cardiac muscle cells differ from other types of excitable tissue in that their action potential has a plateau phase which keeps the membrane depolarised (phase 2). This is maintained by an influx of calcium ions, and during this period the membrane is refractory to further stimulation. At the end of the plateau phase, the calcium channels are inactivated and potassium conductance is increased, allowing a large outward flow of potassium ions (phase 3) which returns the membrane potential to the resting value (phase 4). This process is termed repolarisation.

The influx of calcium, during phase 2 of the action potential, triggers further release of calcium from the sarcoplasmic reticulum, and these changes in calcium concentration in the region of the myofibrils cause muscle contraction. Cells of the conducting system of the heart have the ability to depolarise spontaneously, producing action potentials. In other words they can act as pacemakers. The rate of depolarisation of the sinoatrial node normally exceeds that of other potential pacemakers and therefore initiates and maintains the cardiac rhythm. Damaged cells also have the ability to depolarise spontaneously and therefore may cause rhythm disturbances.

Anatomy of the conducting system

The sinoatrial node is located beneath the epicardium at the junction of the superior vena cava and right atrium (Fig. 8.12a). From there, electrical activity spreads over the atrial myocardium to reach the atrioventricular node. This structure is located just beneath the endocardium of the right atrium and directly above the insertion of the septal leaflet of the tricuspid valve. The atrioventricular node connects to the bundle of His which penetrates the central fibrous body of the heart. The central fibrous body is part of the fibrous skeleton of the heart and acts as an electrical insulator between atrial and ventricular muscle.

The bundle of His then divides into right and left bundle branches supplying each ventricle. The right bundle stays intact until it reaches the distal right surface of the ventricular septum, while the left fans into a series of fascicles across the left side of the ventricular septum. These conduction pathways are composed of specialized Purkinje cells which extend to form networks just beneath the endocardium of the left and

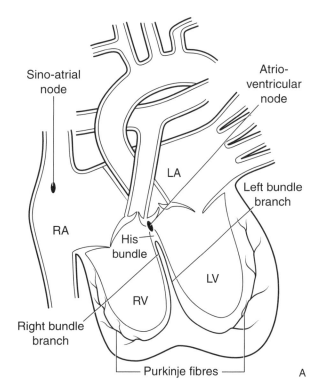

A

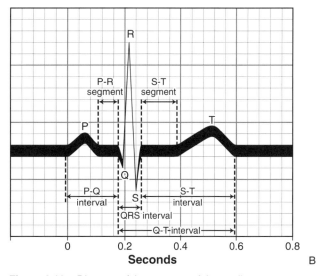

B

Figure 8.12   Diagram of the anatomy of the cardiac conducting system (a) and the corresponding surface ECG (b). Adapted from Larsen (1993), with permission.

right ventricle. From there, impulses pass more slowly from endocardium to epicardium and throughout the ventricular mass.

The electrocardium

This represents the sum of all the electrical activity of the heart as recorded on the body surface and is shown diagramatically in Fig. 8.12b. The P wave represents depolarisation across the atria, the first part being due to right atrial depolarisation and the second to left atrial depolarisation. Right atrial enlargement is reflected by a peaked P wave and left atrial enlargement by a broad or bifid (two peaked) P wave. The PR interval measures the time taken for the electrical impulse to travel from the region of the sinoatrial node to the ventricular mass. Most of the delay is caused by transit through the specialised cells of the atrioventricular node. This delay is necessary to allow the coordination of atrial and ventricular contraction, as described under 'The cardiac cycle'.

The QRS complex represents the spread of ventricular depolarisation. The contribution of each chamber changes with age, and this is reflected in the standard 12 lead ECG. Full-term neonates exhibit right ventricular dominance; this changes to left ventricular dominance by around 1 month of age and to an adult pattern by around 6 years. The T wave is produced by ventricular repolarisation, and there are marked changes in T wave orientation in the first week of life. For the first 3 to 4 days the T wave is positive or upright in lead V1. However, by 7 days of age most T waves in V1 are negative and remain so until adolescence, when they again become upright. Persistently upright T waves in an infant are a sign of right ventricular hypertrophy. The T wave is also a clinically useful indicator of the level of intracellular potassium. Hyperkalaemia causes a peaked T wave, while hypokalaemia causes a flattened T wave and possibly a U wave, which is a low-amplitude deflection seen just after the T.

The QT interval is measured from the beginning of the QRS complex to the end of the T wave and should measure less than 0.45 s when corrected for age. This is given by Bazett's formula:

$$\text{corrected QT interval (QT}_c) = \frac{\text{measured QT interval}}{\sqrt{\text{of the R to R interval of the previous 2 beats}}}$$

A prolonged QT interval may be caused by:

- hypocalcaemia
- hypokalaemia
- hypomagnesaemia
- antiarrhythmic drugs, e.g quinidine, amiodarone
- prolonged QT syndromes, e.g. Romano-Ward and Jervell Lange-Neilson.

In these dominantly inherited conditions, individuals are at risk of a specific form of ventricular tachycardia called 'torsades des pointes', which is life threatening if sustained. To prevent this arrhythmia, lifelong beta-blocker therapy is usually recommended. However, in situations when there has been a previous near-fatal collapse, insertion of an automatic implantable cardiodefibrillator (AICD) may be required. Unfortunately, asymptomatic affected family members may not always demonstrate clear ECG abnormalities, and, although genetic markers are being developed, it remains difficult to decide which relatives of a symptomatic patient also require treatment.

Neurological control of the heart

The heart is supplied by sympathetic nerve fibres from the sympathetic ganglia via the cardiac nerves and by parasympathetic fibres via the vagus nerve. These nerves also carry sensation from the heart. Parasympathetic fibres supply the atria, including the atrioventricular node, with a particularly rich supply to the sinoatrial node. Sympathetic fibres supply the atrioventricular node and to a lesser extent the sinoatrial node. Sympathetic fibres also form networks around the coronary arteries and spread into the ventricular myocardium. Sympathetic stimulation causes an increased rate of spontaneous discharge from the sinoatrial node and a reduction in the refractory period of the action potential, which speeds conduction particularly through the atrioventricular node. Parasympathetic stimulation has an opposite effect. As previously mentioned, sympathetic stimulation also enhances the strength of contraction by a direct effect on ventricular myocardium, while parasympathetic stimulation has a less profound effect to reduce the strength of contraction.

EMBRYOLOGY OF CARDIAC DEVELOPMENT

Embryology is a difficult topic to communicate and understand, but attempting to form some concept of cardiac development is extremely helpful in understanding the origins of congenital heart disease. In this discussion, the terms cephalic, caudal, dorsal and ventral will be used as orientation. Respectively these mean towards the head, towards the tail, towards the back and towards the front of the developing embryo.

Early development

The heart is one of the first organs to develop, and formation of the circulation itself is intimately associated with early fetal development. At around 16 days of gestation, cells leave the deep surface of the primitive embryonic streak and become the mesoderm or mesenchyme. The superior surface of the primitive streak becomes the ectoderm and the deep surface becomes the endoderm, thus forming the three primary germ cell layers. The heart develops from paired longitudinal endothelial channels from the cardiogenic region of the mesenchyme. These channels begin to fuse, and by the time that fusion is completed, blood is circulating and the heart is beating. This occurs around day 20 of gestation. From outside to inside, the cells of the heart then develop into epicardium, myocardium and endocardium.

Development of venous return

Venous return to the heart develops around the 4th week of gestation and includes the vitelline veins from the yolk sac, the umbilical veins from the chorion (which develops into the placenta) and the cardinal veins from the body of the fetus. These veins then drain into the sinus venosus, which is at the caudal end of the developing atrium. The cardinal venous system consists of two paired anterior (cephalic) veins and two paired posterior (caudal) veins which empty into a com-

mon cardinal vein before entering the sinus venosus. The paired anterior cardinal veins form the brachiocephalic vein and superior vena cava, while the posterior cardinal veins largely disappear, only contributing to the common iliac veins and part of the azygous vein. The vitelline veins will form parts of the hepatic and portal venous systems. The inferior vena cava has a complex origin, being formed from the hepatic veins and also from two further parallel venous systems, the subcardinal and supracardinal veins.

Development of the great arteries

At around the 4th week of gestation, paired ventral aortae arise from the truncus arteriosus at the cephalic end of the developing heart. These connect with paired dorsal aorta via the six pairs of aortic arches (Fig. 8.13). The ventral and dorsal aortae fuse caudally to form single vessels. Not all pairs of aortic arches are present at the same time: for example, by the time the third pair have formed, the first and second pairs have disappeared.

The segment of the ventral aortae between the 3rd and 4th arches becomes the common carotid artery on each side. The external carotid arteries develop from the cephalic ends of the ventral aortae beyond this, and the internal carotid arteries develop from the 3rd arch and the cephalic ends of the dorsal aortae. The right 4th arch gives rise to the origin of the right subclavian artery, while the ventral aorta proximal to the 4th arch on the right becomes the innominate artery. On the left side the 4th arch gives rise to the segment of the aortic arch between the left common carotid and left subclavian, and the ventral aorta proximal to the 4th arch becomes the area of the aortic arch between the innominate and left common carotid arteries. The 5th paired arches usually disappear. The proximal part of the 6th arch forms the origin of the pulmonary artery on each side, and the distal portion forms the arterial duct.

As the fetus grows, the heart migrates caudally and the brachiocephalic arteries elongate, the future subclavian arteries therefore travel in a cephalic direction. On the right side this vessel aligns with the origin of the right subclavian

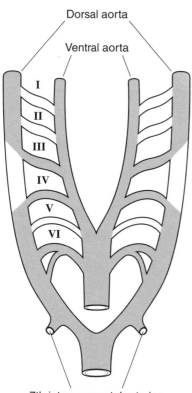

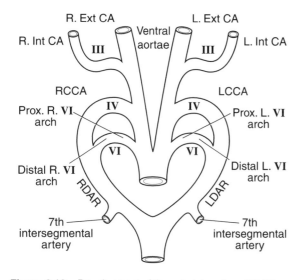

Figure 8.13 Development of the arterial system. RDAR, right dorsal aortic root; LDAR, left dorsal aortic root; Int CA, internal carotid artery; Ext CA, external carotid artery; RCCA, right common carotid artery; LCCA, left common carotid artery. From Moe in Freedom et al (1992).

artery, and on the left side it comes to lie between the ductus arteriosus and left common carotid artery. Malformations of the aortic arch arise when areas that would normally regress fail to do so or when areas regress that normally remain patent. This may result in interruption of the arch or in a vascular ring around the trachea and oesophagus, causing upper airway obstruction and/or difficulty swallowing solids.

Further development and septation

At this stage the heart consists of a tube which will become, from cranial to caudal ends:

1. the origin of the aortic arches
2. the truncus arteriosus
3. the bulbus cordis or outlet part of the ventricle
4. the inlet part of the ventricle
5. the atrium
6. the sinus venosus.

The regions between the atria and ventricles are known as endocardial cushions. Around day 23 the heart tube begins to bend. This is caused by differential rates of growth, with the cells of the bulbus cordis and ventricular areas growing faster than other regions, and eventually brings the atrium and sinus venosus to lie dorsal to the bulbus cordis and ventricle (Figure 8.14).

The next stage in development is septation of the heart into left and right sides, which is normally complete by the 6th week of gestation. The atria are separated by the downward growth of the septum primum until it fuses with the endocardial cushion tissue between atria and ventricles. As it grows, perforations develop within the septum primum which come together to form the foramen ovale. The septum secundum then develops from infolding of the posterosuperior wall of the atrium and overlaps the septum primum, forming the upper edge of the foramen ovale (Fig. 8.15). This upper edge or limbus helps to direct inferior vena caval blood across the foramen ovale in intrauterine life. Failure of the septum primum to join the endocardial cushion results in a partial atrioventricular septal defect, formerly known as an ostium primum atrial septal defect, while failure of the septum secundum to form

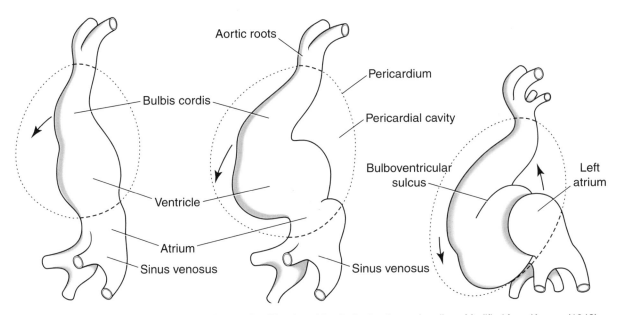

Figure 8.14   Folding of the primitive fetal heart tube. The dotted line indicates the pericardium. Modified from Kramer (1942).

results in an ostium secundum atrial septal defect. With separation of the atria, the left side of the sinus venosus becomes the coronary sinus, which drains blood from the heart, and the right side becomes incorporated into the right atrium.

The ventricular septum begins as a muscular ridge at the apex and fuses with a membraneous (fibrous) component and with the aorticopulmonary septum to completely separate the ventricles. The aorticopulmonary septum is a spiral structure that divides the bulbus cordis and the truncus arteriosus into the aorta and main pulmonary artery. Failure of fusion of the components of the ventricular septum results in ventricular septal defects, and failure of formation of the aorticopulmonary septum results in the defect known as truncus arteriosus.

FETAL AND TRANSITIONAL CIRCULATION

Fetal circulation

Well oxygenated blood (O_2 saturation 70%) returns to the fetus via the umbilical vein and passes either through the liver substance or through the ductus venosus, which bypasses the liver, to reach the inferior vena cava (Fig. 8.16). This blood then enters the right atrium where approximately one-third is directed across the foramen ovale to enter the left atrium and there mixes with the small amount of pulmonary venous return. This left atrial blood (O_2 saturation 65%) then enters the left ventricle and is pumped to the ascending aorta where it is distributed to the coronary, cerebral and upper limb circulations.

The remaining inferior vena cava blood mixes with blood from the superior vena cava (O_2 saturation 40%) and coronary sinus to enter the right ventricle and from there is pumped into the pulmonary artery (O_2 saturation 55%). As the deflated fetal lung has a high vascular resistance, only around 10% of blood in the pulmonary artery passes through the lung to return via the pulmonary veins, while the remainder passes through the patent arterial duct to enter the descending aorta. This blood supplies the remainder of the fetus and also returns to the placenta via the two umbilical arteries. Therefore the cerebral and coronary blood supply has a relatively high oxygen content compared with blood supplying the lower body.

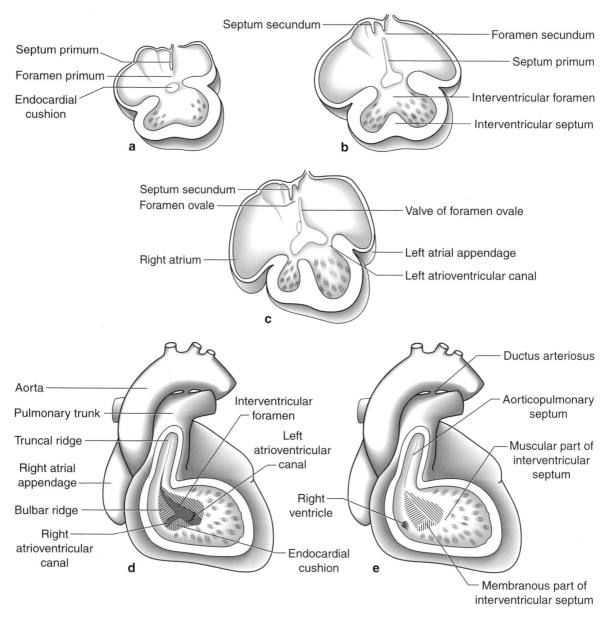

Figure 8.15 Drawings of the developing heart, illustrating partitioning of the primitive atrioventricular canal, atrium and ventricle. A, B and C are frontal sections of the embryonic heart during the fourth week; D and E are schematic drawings of the heart illustrating closure of the interventricular foramen and formation of the interventricular septum; D, five weeks: E, seven weeks. Note that the interventricular foramen is closed by tissues from three sources. (Modified from Moore KL. The developing human. Clinically oriented embryology. 4th ed. Philadelphia: WB Saunders 1988).

Transitional circulation

Understanding the transitional circulation is vital in the management of neonates presenting with congenital heart disease, severe asphyxia and/or with lung disease of prematurity. After delivery, the onset of respiration causes a rapid decrease in pulmonary vascular resistance. This is partly due to the process of ventilation but mostly to diffusion

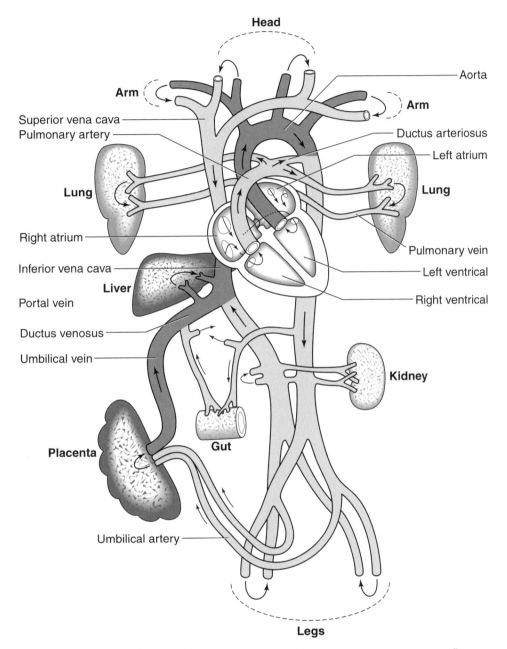

Figure 8.16   Fetal circulation. Relatively well-oxygenated blood from the inferior vena cava flows across the foramen ovale to left heart which preferentially perfuses the head and upper trunk. Superior vena caval blood together with some flow from the inferior vena cava enters the right ventricle and is ejected via the pulmonary artery and the arterial duct to the placenta and lower trunk.

of oxygen from the alveoli to the pulmonary capillaries. This fall in pulmonary vascular resistance leads to an increase in pulmonary blood flow.

The increasing oxygen concentration of the circulating blood also causes constriction and eventual closure of the arterial duct. This probably involves the decline in activity of the relaxant prostaglandin E2 which is necessary to maintain patency of the arterial duct throughout gestation. Prostaglandins are derived from a polyunsaturated fatty acid called arachidonic acid. The first step in their production involves the enzyme cyclo-oxygenase whose action is inhibited by non-steroidal antiinflammatory drugs such as indomethacin. In babies born with congenital heart disease and duct-dependent lesions, exogenous prostaglandin E2 is often administered to keep the duct open (Olley & Coceani 1981). Conversely, in premature babies with acute or chronic lung disease and persistent patency of the arterial duct, indomethacin is used to close the duct and therefore reduce harmful left-to-right shunting of blood to the lungs. Normally the duct is completely functionally closed by the end of the first day of life.

Increasing pulmonary venous return raises pressure in the left atrium and closes the flap valve of the foramen ovale. Decreased flow in the inferior vena cava after separation of the placenta probably contributes to this process. Finally, the ductus venosus gradually closes by a passive process due to the cessation of umbilical venous return.

AETIOLOGY OF CONGENITAL HEART DISEASE

Introduction

In order to understand how often congenital heart disease appears in the population, it is useful to re-examine some commonly used terms in epidemiology. Incidence refers to the number of new cases of a disease in a specified time period and prevalence to the frequency of that disease in a defined population. These terms were originally applied to infectious diseases, and it is difficult to apply them to birth defects. This is because birth defects do not suddenly occur at the time of birth but at some time during embryonic and fetal development, and their incidence at each stage of development is not fully known. Some birth defects are determined at the time of conception, some in early embryonic life and so on,

and some may lead to fetal loss. Therefore a better way to describe birth defects, such as congenital heart disease, is the prevalence of a defect at the time of livebirth.

For congenital heart disease, the first major study into prevalence was the New England Regional Infant Care Program (Fyler et al 1980). This established a prevalence of cardiovascular malformations of 8/1000 live births. More recently, the Baltimore–Washington Infant Study (Ferencz et al 1985) established a prevalence of 4.34/1000 live births. These studies were only possible with the improved accuracy of diagnosis and by the development of regional transport to large tertiary referral centres. The most common lesions in decreasing order of frequency are:

1. ventricular septal defect
2. pulmonary valve stenosis
3. atrioventricular septal defect
4. atrial septal defect
5. tetralogy of Fallot
6. transposition of the great arteries
7. coarctation of the aorta
8. hypoplastic lcft heart syndrome
9. patent arterial duct
10. complex cardiac defects.

Management of these lesions is discussed in the next chapter. Overall the number of cases that require some form of intervention during infancy is 3.5/1000 live births (Benson 1989).

Aetiology

As can be seen from the discussion of cardiac development, the heart has completely formed by around the 7th week of gestation. Therefore factors which cause structural heart disease must act within the first 2 months of pregnancy. Chromosomal and single-gene defects are thought to account for around 13% and 5%, respectively, with environmental and maternal factors accounting for 9%. For the remainder the cause is unknown and these are termed multifactorial in origin. As defects tend to cluster in families, these multifactorial cases probably represent an interaction between genetic and environmental factors.

Table 8.1   Major chromosomal defects associated with congenital heart disease

Syndrome	Cardiac defect
Trisomy 21 (Down's)	Atrioventricular septal defect
Trisomy 18	VSD, ASD, PDA
Trisomy 13	VSD, ASD, PDA
Turner syndrome (XO)	Coarctation of the aorta, aortic stenosis

ASD, atrial septal defect; PDA, patent ductus arteriosus; VSD, ventricular septal defect.

Table 8.2   Gene defects associated with cardiac lesions.

Lesion	Sites of genetic defect
Hypertrophic cardiomyopathy	14q1, 1q3, 15q2, 11q11
Prolonged QT syndrome	11p15.5
Mitochondrial muscle disorders	Mitochondrial DNA
Marfans syndrome	15q21.1 (gene for fibrillin)
Williams syndrome	7q11- (gene for elastin)
Noonans and Holt–Oram syndromes	12q
Total anomalous pulmonary venous return	4p13-q12
'Catch 22' syndrome	22q1.2-

Key: the first number is the chromosome, p is the short arm, q is the long arm and the second number indicates the site on the chromosome where either a mutation or a deletion (indicated by the symbol –) has occurred.

Chromosome abnormalities associated with congenital heart defects are shown in Table 8.1. The most important is Trisomy 21 (Down's syndrome) which affects 1 in 700 children and is associated with heart disease in 40% to 50% of cases. The most frequently associated lesion is atrioventricular septal defect. However, ventricular septal defect, atrial septal defect, tetralogy of Fallot and patent ductus arteriosus are also found in decreasing order of frequency. The incidence of Down's syndrome and other additional chromosome conditions increases with increasing maternal age, being 1:2000 at 20 years and 20–50:1000 above 40 years. It is important to remember that most children with Down's are born to younger mothers, as the birth rate falls with increasing maternal age. Other trisomies have a higher rate of spontaneous abortion and few survive beyond 1 year of age.

Associations between single- or multiple-gene defects and cardiac diseases are now being recognised (Table 8.2). For example, a number of cardiac conditions have been linked to a partial deletion at position 11 of the long arm of chromosome 22; these include truncus arteriosus, tetralogy of Fallot and interrupted aortic arch. This syndrome may also include characteristic facial features (the velocardiofacial syndrome), partial or complete absence of the thymus gland and parathyroid glands. Complete absence of the thymus is called diGeorge syndrome, and affected individuals have no T cell immunity. Partial absence is also thought to impair immune function, and absence of the parathyroid glands causes neonatal hypocalcaemia. This defect is detected by in-situ hybridisation of chromosome material from the patient's white cells. Some other recently discovered associations between gene defects and cardiac disease are listed.

REFERENCES

Andreoli T E, Carpenter C C J, Plum F, Smith L H Jr 1986 Cecil essentials of medicine. Saunders, Philadelphia

Benson Jr D W 1989 Changing profile of congenital heart disease. Pediatrics 83(5):790–791

Blumenthal S 1977 Report of the task force on blood pressure control in children. Pediatrics 59 (Suppl.):797–820

Ferencz C, Dubin J D, McCarter R J et al 1985 Congenital heart disease: prevalence at livebirth: The Baltimore–Washington infant study. American Journal of Epidemiology 121:31–36

Fick A 1870 Uber die Messung Des Blutquantums in den Herzventrikeln. Sitz der Physik-Med Ges Wurtzberg

Freedom R M, Benson L N, Smallhorn J F (eds) 1992 Neonatal heart disease. Springer-Verlag, London

Fyler et al 1980 Report of the New England Regional Infant Care Program. Pediatrics 65:375–461

Hazinski M F 1992 Nursing care of the critically ill child, 2nd edn. Mosby, St Louis

Julian D G, Camm A J, Fox K M, Hall R J C, Poole-Wilson P A 1996 Diseases of the heart. Saunders, London

Katz A M 1977 Physiology of the heart. Raven Press, New York

Kramer T C 1942 The partitioning of the truncus and conus and the formation of the membraneous portion of the interventricular septum of the human heart. American Journal of Anatomy 71:343

Larsen W J 1993 Human embryology. Churchill Livingstone, Edinburgh

Marian A J, Roberts R 1995 Recent advances in the molecular genetics of hypertrophic cardiomyopathy. Circulation 92:1336–1347

Moore K L 1988 The developing human. Clinically-oriented embryology. WB Saunders, Philadelphia

Olley P M, Coceani F 1981 Prostaglandins and the ductus arteriosus. Annual Review of Medicine 32:375–385

Rudolph A M 1977 Congenital diseases of the heart. Year Book Medical Publishers

Starling E H 1915 The Linacre lecture on the law of the heart (Cambridge University). Longmans, Green, London, 1918

Tortora G J, Anagnostakos N P 1990 Principles of anatomy and physiology, 6th edn. HarperCollins, New York

Yang S S, Bentivoglio L G, Maranhão V, Goldberg H (eds) 1988 From cardiac catheterization data to haemodynamic parameters, 3rd edn. Davis, Philadelphia

9

Care and management of infants and children requiring cardiac surgery

Eiri Jones   Bernie Steer

INTRODUCTION

To manage the care of infants and children requiring cardiac surgery, it is important to have an understanding of normal anatomy and physiology and how this is altered with congenital cardiac defects. Over the past fifty years, since the development of cardiopulmonary bypass (CPB) techniques, cardiac surgery has evolved rapidly. Intricate and complex cardiac surgery has become the norm in the neonatal and paediatric age groups as CPB, cardiology and cardiac surgical techniques have improved. Development of paediatric intensive care services has resulted in early detection, prompt management of pre- and postoperative complications, improved survival and better quality of life.

This chapter discusses the principles of managing care for infants and children with congenital heart disease (CHD), CPB, the most commonly presenting defects, their altered physiology and the acute aspects of their pre- and postoperative management.

When planning the care and management of children with CHD, it is useful to categorise defects according to results of sequential analysis (normally used to provide an understanding of cardiac anatomy) interpreted in terms of alterations to blood flow. Most defects fall into one of four categories:

- increased pulmonary blood flow
- decreased pulmonary blood flow
- decreased systemic blood flow
- altered circulation.

Surgical management of infants and children presenting with cardiac defects may be either palliative or corrective. Whilst the surgical procedure performed depends on the type and severity of the defect, early correction should be the treatment of choice where possible (Norwood 1989). If this is not possible, treatment options include:

- early palliation with later correction
- palliation only
- transplantation
- no treatment.

Corrective surgery aims to restore the anatomy to produce normal blood flow. This is possible when the structure of the heart and vessels is either fundamentally normal or potentially easily correctable. Palliative surgery, which is usually staged, aims to relieve symptoms caused by the defect, whilst allowing for growth and development.

PREOPERATIVE MANAGEMENT

Infants and children requiring cardiac surgery often present in one of two ways. Children who present with non-life-threatening defects will be referred to a paediatric cardiologist and will be reviewed regularly and managed medically until surgery is required. The second group present as emergencies either in the newborn period, infancy or childhood. The symptoms most commonly seen during emergency presentations are severe heart failure or cardiogenic shock. Both heart failure and cardiogenic shock can be defined as the inability to deliver adequate oxygen supply to the peripheral vascular bed and eliminate the waste products of cellular metabolism. This can be with or without pulmonary oedema.

Oxygen in the lungs diffuses into the bloodstream via the alveolar/capillary membrane. Oxygenated blood enters the heart prior to being pumped around the body to the vital organs and the peripheries. The volume of blood circulating around the body is termed cardiac output (CO) which can be affected by changes in the following:

- preload
- afterload
- heart rate
- stroke volume
- contractility.

Clinical presentation of heart failure usually occurs when the pulmonary vascular resistance (PVR) has started to fall after the newborn period. In this instance, there is often a left-to-right shunt making ventricular function hyperdynamic. Symptoms commonly seen include:

- failure to thrive and poor weight gain
- sweating around head during feeding
- tachycardia at rest
- tachypnoea, especially with subcostal and/or intercostal recession
- hypotension
- cool peripheries/mottling
- poor urine output
- central and/or peripheral oedema
- palpable liver (hepatomegaly).

If heart failure does present in the neonatal period, this is classified as a medical emergency and the baby should be admitted to an intensive care area. If untreated it can rapidly progress to cardiogenic shock requiring resuscitation and cardiovascular support. Maximising myocardial function becomes the priority prior to diagnosis and treatment of the cause of the collapse. Cardiovascular collapse in the neonatal period may be caused by:

- congenital heart disease
- primary respiratory disease
- metabolic disorder
- sepsis.

To establish the presence of CHD, oxygen and a pulse oximeter are required. If PaO_2 remains < 20 kPa during administration of 100% oxygen, the most likely cause of cardiovascular collapse is CHD. With defects such as truncus arteriosus and hypoplastic left heart syndrome, the infant will deteriorate whilst receiving oxygen, as pulmonary and systemic blood flow are dependent on vessel diameter. Administration of oxygen may increase flow to the lungs whilst compromising systemic circulation, leading to collapse. Therefore, with this group of infants, air should be used instead of oxygen for resuscitation. Once stabilised further investigations will include:

- cardiac ECHO
- chest X-ray
- blood gas analysis and electrolyte and full blood count (FBC) assessment.

The chest X-ray can indicate the types of cardiac defect by the size and shape of the heart. Assessment of the lung fields can confirm the presence of high or low blood flow and pulmonary oedema.

POSTOPERATIVE MANAGEMENT

Postoperative management of an infant or child following cardiac surgery, irrespective of the defect involved, has common principles. Initial management takes place in the PICU and can be explored using a systematic approach:

- safety
- airway and breathing
- cardiovascular
- fluid balance (input and output)
- temperature control
- neurological
- pain management
- nursing care
- family care
- dying.

Only the aspects specific to management of CHD will be discussed here.

Airway and ventilation

Following cardiac surgery, most children are ventilated artificially using positive pressure ventilation. Frequent assessment of ventilation is important to evaluate changes and use appropriate interventions. Observations recorded on return from theatres are:

- ventilation rate
- peak, end expiratory and mean airway pressures

- tidal and minute volume (in volume control mode)
- inspired oxygen concentration (FiO$_2$)
- Oxygen saturations.

Once these observations are charted and a baseline obtained, they should be recorded at regular intervals, e.g. hourly, and when significant changes occur. The child should also be observed for colour, chest movement and breath sounds.

Investigations performed include:

- chest X-ray
- blood gas analysis.

Potential therapeutic interventions include:

- endotracheal (ET) suction
- chest physiotherapy

Possible complications include:

- ET tube blockage or displacement
- lung collapse or consolidation
- infection
- pulmonary oedema
- pleural or pericardial effusions
- pnemo or haemothorax
- pulmonary hypertension
- pulmonary haemorrhage.

Management of pulmonary hypertension

Where high pulmonary blood flow was present preoperatively, postoperative management is likely to include control of the resulting pulmonary hypertension. Arterial blood sampling enables symptoms such as acidosis, hypoxia or hypercapnia to be detected and treated. Any of these factors may precipitate constriction of the pulmonary vasculature, causing pulmonary hypertension (Fig. 9.1). Clinical signs exhibited are systemic hypotension and decreasing oxygen saturation. If manual hyperventilation is performed, the practitioner may have difficulty acquiring good chest movement, indicating non-compliant lungs in the presence of a clear ET tube. Recovery from an episode of pulmonary hypertension requires a reduction in pulmonary vascular pressure.

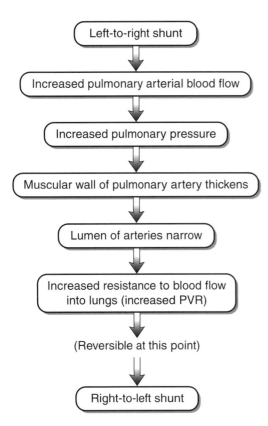

Figure 9.1 Development of pulmonary vascular disease.

vasodilators such as epoprostenol and glycerine trinitrate (GTN) have failed. The significant effect of inhaled NO is that it acts locally by relaxing smooth muscle, reducing pulmonary pressure and increasing pulmonary blood flow, without any effect on the systemic circulation. As intravenous vasodilators reduce both systemic and pulmonary pressure, the selective action of inhaled NO makes it a suitable treatment option for cardiovascularly unstable infants and children. Care should be taken in the initial 30 min following commencement, as the general consensus is that the effect should be apparent by this time. Arterial blood gases should be taken to determine changes. As NO binds with haemoglobin to form methaemoglobin, regular monitoring of metHb is required; a level of > 10 can significantly reduce the child's oxygen-carrying capacity.

The weaning process may begin when all expected parameters are stable and the child is showing signs of waking and making respiratory effort. Gradual reduction of rate, pressure or volume, with reassessment of arterial blood gases, chest movement, oxygen saturation and skin colour, enables early extubation.

Hyperventilation with 100% oxygen will reduce $PaCO_2$ and dilate the pulmonary vascular bed. The infant may require sedation with or without a paralysing agent such as vecuronium at a therapeutic range of 50–200 µg/kg/h (Guy's and St. Thomas' and Lewisham 1997). A vital element of nursing care is to avoid hypoxia, so procedures such as suctioning should only be performed after pre-oxygenating the infant prior to rapid, effective suction technique. Agitation may cause changes in pulmonary pressure, so minimal handling with appropriate sedation and pain control are essential.

Over the last decade, inhaled nitric oxide (NO) has been used successfully in treating pulmonary hypertension. As a relatively new treatment for pulmonary hypertension, little research is available relating to its use in the postoperative cardiac child. However, many believe it should be considered as a treatment when intravenous

Cardiovascular

There are many potential cardiovascular problems following cardiac surgery. An understanding of expected physiological parameters is required, to interpret changes and implement appropriate management. As soon as the child is admitted to the ICU he is connected to a monitor. The most essential parameters to record are heart rate, oxygen saturation and arterial blood pressure, but others may be available. Parameters recorded following more complex surgery include:

- heart rate (HR)
- arterial blood pressure (ABP)
- right atrial pressure/central venous pressure (RAP/CVP)
- left atrial pressure (LAP)
- pulmonary artery pressure (PAP)
- oxygen saturation content (SaO_2).

Table 9.1 Most common arrhythmias exhibited postoperatively in neonates and children

Arrhythmia	Cause	Treatment
Supraventricular tachycardia (HR: babies > 240 bpm; older children > 200 bpm)	• AV node not functioning • Reduced diastolic filling time • Reduced cardiac output • Reduced coronary artery filling time • Increased myocardial oxygen demands	• Synchronised cardioversion • Drug therapy: adenosine then digoxin • Vagal stimulation • Override pacing • Cooling to 35°C centrally
Nodal rhythm	• Sinoatrial node not participating • Reduced cardiac output (15–20%)	Atrial pacing (to replace atrial firing)
Heart block	• Usually transient as a result of conductive tissue damage • Reduced cardiac output	• Ventricular or AV sequential pacing • Isoprenaline
Sinus tachycardia	• Hypovolaemia • Pain • Pyrexia	• Fluid administration • Analgesia • Antipyretics/cooling
Bradycardia (<100 bpm neonate; < 80 bpm infant)	Reduced cardiac output	• Isoprenaline • Atrial pacing

Essential investigations performed are:

• chest X-ray
• arterial blood gas
• full blood count and clotting screen
• renal, bone and liver profile
• 12-lead ECG
• echocardiography.

Several factors contribute to a reduction in cardiac output in the postoperative period. These are:

• long bypass time
• complex surgery
• arrhythmias as a result of conduction tissue oedema or damage.

Potential complications following surgery include:

• arrhythmias
• poor ventricular function
• bleeding and hypovolaemia.

Arrhythmias

Deviation from the normal heart rate and rhythm is fairly common in the postoperative period. In infancy and childhood this is often insignificant and is usually a temporary disturbance that does not cause long-term problems. In the postoperative phase, identifying the site of surgical repair can help in detecting the potential risk of arrhythmias. Despite care, arrhythmias are not uncommon (Table 9.1). For example, many infants/children following repair of ventricular septal defects exhibit bundle branch block, tachycardias or ectopic beats due to localised oedema. However, most resolve in the postoperative period.

Arrhythmias can be induced by factors other than surgical damage. These include:

• electrolyte imbalance which can be detected early by regular measurement and correction of potassium, calcium and magnesium
• vagal stimulation during endotracheal suctioning, inducing hypoxia — a major cause of sinus-bradycardia in the neonate and infant
• decreased stroke volume which occurs following cardiac surgery. It is important to remember that neonates have a restricted ability to increase stroke volume; as the neonatal heart possesses more non-contractile than contractile tissue, ventricular diastolic compliance is reduced. Therefore, although small amounts of volume may enhance preload, cardiac output is rate dependent, and sinus tachycardia of 180–200 bpm is consequently often well tolerated in the immediate postoperative period.

Ventricular function

When surgical repair causes interruption of myocardial tissue, the efficiency of ventricular function may be compromised (e.g. Fallot's repair or ventricular septal defects). Small amounts of volume may be given cautiously to increase preload. If CVP is >8 mmHg then inotropic support may be needed (Tritschler 1993). Inotropic and vasoactive drugs that may be considered include:

- dopamine 5–10 µg/kg/min
- dobutamine 5–20 µg/kg/min
- adrenaline
- noradrenaline
- enoximone
- milrinone
- glycerine trinitrate
- sodium nitroprusside.

Dopamine is a naturally occurring catecholomine. In small doses (<5 µg/kg/min) it stimulates dopamine receptors, which increases renal and splanchnic blood flow and urinary output and allows coronary and cerebral artery dilatation. In higher doses, because it stimulates beta receptors, it can increase HR and contractility. Dobutamine infused at 5–20 µg/kg/min affects B_1 and B_2 receptors, resulting in improved myocardial perfusion allowing more efficient contractility, with some peripheral vasodilation. If cardiac output is poor, some vasodilator agents may be introduced to aid peripheral dilation. Glycerine trinitrate or sodium nitroprusside at 0.1–5 µg/kg/min may be used. Vasodilators reduce afterload by dilating arteries and veins in both systemic and pulmonary vascular systems. This therapy may in addition require colloid administration to maintain CVP at 5–8 mmHg. Glycerine trinitrate (GTN) dilates both arteries and veins but primarily affects peripheral vessels. Sodium nitroprusside (SNP) relaxes smooth muscle and therefore acts similarly to GTN. However, there is a risk of toxicity if prolonged usage occurs. SNP is broken down to cyanide; therefore it should be protected from light and used for limited periods only. When administering vasodilator agents and inotropes, these should be infused in separate lines to avoid purges of any one of these agents.

Extracorporeal membrane oxygenation

Extracorporeal membrane oxygenation (ECMO) or extracorporeal life support (ECLS) is used as a method of cardiac and/or pulmonary support. Whilst initially used when maximal conventional therapy had failed, established centres now use it when conventional therapy is not improving the haemodynamic status of a critically ill child. Based on the principles of cardiopulmonary bypass, ECMO can be used in a variety of conditions. Two types of pumps are available: the centrifugal (vortex) pump and the roller (occlusive) pump. The multicentre research trial of ECMO used in neonates has shown that it is a valuable therapy, but also that there are some conditions where it should not be used, e.g. diaphragmatic hernia. Some early success was shown when ECMO was used for cardiovascular support for children with meningococcal septicaemia.

When used in the presence of congenital heart disease the important principle to remember is that ventricular or respiratory dysfunction should be reversible. Occasionally it has been used as a bridge to transplant, but limited availability of donor organs can influence its use in this group of children. It is also essential to assess the possibility of irreversible brain damage prior to commencing ECMO, particularly if there has been a history of cardiac arrest or instability. Established centres providing ECMO as a regular treatment either provide or have access to an established training programme. Without adequately trained and experienced personnel the use of ECMO can be unsafe. Even in very experienced centres, ECMO remains a high-risk intervention.

There are three obvious phases to the therapy:

- setting up
- running the circuit
- weaning or discontinuation.

In each stage there are important principles to follow.

Setting up

This should be done either in the operating theatre or preferably in the intensive care unit as moving the child from theatres to the PICU on ECMO is a high-risk situation. Essential personnel include surgeon, perfusionist or ECMO specialist, intensivist and PICU nurse. Appropriate equipment is important. Most centres have an ECMO trolley readily available on the PICU to facilitate cannulation and priming of the circuit as quickly as possible. The circuit itself consists of:

- circuit tubing (sized according to the child's weight)
- venous reservoir (only with a roller pump)
- pump (roller or centrifugal)
- oxygenator
- heater
- control console.

It is also necessary to inform other departments including blood transfusion, the haematology and chemistry laboratories and the portering service that this treatment is to be commenced. This ensures that essential supplies of blood products and results are available promptly. Cannulation is achieved using a cut-down method to isolate the major neck vessels, the internal jugular vein and the common carotid artery. These are the vessels of choice for all ages. Occasionally, following cardiac surgery, the child may be cannulated through the sternotomy incision, with the drainage cannulae inserted in both the right and left atria to empty and rest the heart completely. Arterial blood is then returned into the descending aorta. This type of ECMO is known as veno-arterial support. Where ECMO is used to support the respiratory system, it is possible to use veno-venous ECMO where one double-lumen catheter is used. Both types have advantages and disadvantages (Table 9.2).

As with cardiopulmonary bypass, it is neccessary to heparinise the child before cannulation, with a loading dose of 100 units/kg.

Running the circuit

The principles of running the circuit are the same as those of cardiopulmonary bypass. Each child on ECMO is usually allocated two nurses: one to care for the child and family, the other to manage the circuit. Large ECMO centres have a specialist team of trained nurses who can run the circuit and troubleshoot any problems. An understanding of the principles of gas exchange and blood flow on ECMO is essential. Routine observations of the circuit are done to check the blood flow, gas flow and pressures and to observe potential sites where clots or leaks may occur (full flow is usually between 80 and 150 mL/kg depending on weight). A heparin infusion is used to prevent the circuit and cannulation sites from clotting. The amount of heparin required varies from child to child but is usually in the range of 20–60 units/kg/h. The heparin rate is recorded and blood samples taken to measure the activated clotting time (ACT). This is usually maintained at 180–200 s, with the heparin infusion titrated according to ACT value.

Regular blood samples are taken to assess gas exchange whilst on ECMO. Gas exchange takes

Table 9.2 Comparative advantages and disadvantages of veno-arterial and veno-venous ECMO

	Advantages	Disadvantages
Veno-arterial	• Supports heart and lungs • One surgical site • Excellent oxygenation • Not dependent on cardiac function	• Particles, bubbles, emboli within arterial circuit go directly to brain • Carotid ligation required • Hyperoxia to brain
Veno-venous	• No haemodynamic instability • No carotid ligation required • Particles, bubbles, emboli go to the lungs first • Hyperoxygenated blood goes to lungs — decreases pulmonary arterial pressure	• High flows required for adequate oxygenation • Dependent on cardiac output • Requires IJV cannulation • Need to wean conventional ventilation slowly

place in the oxygenator by a counter-current mechanism. Blood flows in one direction, with gas (a potential mixture of air, oxygen and carbon dioxide) flowing in the opposite direction. Between them lies a silicone layer through which the gases diffuse from high to low concentration. Thus oxygen enters the blood and carbon dioxide is extracted. Pre-oxygenator gases give the mixed venous saturation level, which provides an indication of oxygen delivery (DO_2) to the tissues. Post-oxygenator gases are checked less frequently and give an indication of oxygenator function.

Whilst on ECMO, conventional ventilation is reduced to a resting rate and pressure setting. Maintaining the airway with the ventilator in place allows for quick re-introduction of conventional ventilation in the presence of pump failure or circuit disruption. Full blood count, clotting screen and electrolyte values also need to be checked regularly and treated according to any deleterious change. The use of blood products during ECMO is an essential part of circuit care. Haemoglobin and platelet levels are maintained by transfusing in alloquots of 10 mL/kg. In addition, if there is any indication of bleeding, fresh frozen plasma can be given and cryoprecipitate may also be needed if fibrinogen levels fall. Due to the administration of heparin, bleeding is a major potential complication; however, the heparin should never be stopped, because of the risk of clot formation; the coagulopathy should be treated with the appropriate agent.

There are many potential complications whilst on ECMO. The circuit complications are:

- oxygenator failure
- raceway or tubing rupture
- pump failure
- clots.

The patient complications are:

- cannula site haemorrhage
- gastrointestinal bleed
- surgical site bleed
- cerebral haemorrhage or infarct and fitting
- pneumothorax
- sepsis
- death.

Whilst on ECMO, it is important to ensure that the child is adequately sedated and if necessary paralysed.

Weaning or discontinuation

Throughout each 24 h period the child will be assessed to evaluate whether there has been any improvement in cardiac or respiratory function. Transoesophageal echo can be performed with the ECMO flow reduced to assess ventricular function. Patient arterial blood gas analysis with reduced ECMO flow and increased conventional ventilation will also indicate whether respiratory function has improved. If improvement is evident then the circuit flow is weaned slowly. For cardiac ECMO, inotropic support may be required as part of the weaning process, and for respiratory ECMO a return to back-up ventilator rates will be needed. At times it becomes apparent that the child's cardiac or respiratory function is not going to recover or that the child has suffered a major cerebral insult. At this point, discussion with the parents recommending the withdrawal of treatment should be considered.

Bleeding and hypovolaemia

The child may be hypovolaemic following by-pass and will need fluid replacement with colloid or crystalloid to maintain an adequate circulating volume as evidenced by acid–base balance and circulatory pressures. An estimated volume can be calculated according to weight, as infants have 80 mL/kg circulating volume.

A potential postoperative complication is bleeding. If a 3 kg infant is bleeding 5 mL/kg/h, a large proportion of circulatory volume is lost and therefore CO will fall. Assessment in the immediate postoperative period includes measurement of chest drainage at 15–30 min intervals, with the frequency reducing as drainage lessens. Losses may be replaced with blood products, the choice of which will depend on haemoglobin and clotting results. Products commonly used are:

- packed red cells

- fresh frozen plasma
- platelets
- cryoprecipitate.

Protamine sulphate is prescribed if the bleeding is caused by bypass heparin. If large volumes continue to be lost, the surgeon will need to re-explore the chest to rule out a specific bleeding point.

Following the initial blood loss, a drainage of 5–10 mL/h can be expected from chest drains. Occasionally, cardiac tamponade occurs whereby drainage has been impaired, causing blood to collect inside the chest cavity and form a clot which compresses the heart, resulting in reduced cardiac output. This is a surgical emergency, which should be treated by reopening the chest and removing the clot. It may be necessary to ligate bleeding points and reposition the chest drain. The child may exhibit the following signs:

- increasing CVP and decreasing BP with reduction in pulse pressure difference, due to compression of the ventricle leading to reduced cardiac output
- a compensatory increase in heart rate, to improve cardiac output
- low saturations (SaO_2) due to the reduced cardiac output and poor oxygenation. This causes poor peripheral and eventually central perfusion.

Fluid balance

On return from theatres, fluid balance is calculated by recording hourly input and output including:

1 Input
   - crystalloid
   - colloid
   - drugs
   - enteral feeds

2 Output
   - urine
   - nasogastric
   - drain losses.

Crystalloid fluid is restricted until the heart and kidneys have recovered, to prevent pulmonary oedema and overstressing the myocardium. If the chest is clear, urinary output >1 mL/kg/h and fluid balance negative or equal for the 24–48 h following surgery, the infant is allowed fluids at normal requirements. Feeding should be re-introduced once bowel sounds are audible and bowel function evident. Care should be taken prior to starting feeds in neonates and infants, as necrotising entercolitis (NEC) can occur in this age group. In particular, neonates with previously obstructed systemic flow, where there has been reduced blood flow to the gastrointestinal tract, have a higher risk of developing NEC.

Temperature control

Rewarming commences with weaning of CPB. A rebound hyperpyrexia can occur due to hypothalamic insult or as a result of immaturity in the neonate. Cool peripheries may result from a cold environment and exposure but can also indicate hypovolaemia or poor cardiac output

Neurological

Early assessment of the postoperative neurological response is essential. CPB carries a significant risk of neurological damage due to anticoagulation, temperature changes and risk of air emboli. Sedation should be initiated only after a response is observed unless the child is haemodynamically unstable.

SURGICAL OPTIONS
Non-bypass surgery

Some surgical options do not require the use of cardiopulmonary bypass. These are normally palliative procedures (e.g. shunts) or extracardiac repairs (e.g. PDA ligation). If the site of operation is outside the heart, the heart may then continue to beat efficiently whilst the surgery is performed. This type of surgery is known as closed heart surgery.

Cardiopulmonary bypass

The main principle of CPB is to circulate and oxygenate the blood for the patient, redirecting it away from the heart and lungs to facilitate surgery within the heart. Many developments in CPB techniques since its inception in the 1960s have allowed more complex surgery to be performed on a non-beating heart while maintaining tissue viability and perfusion of the major organs. CPB is now routine, and many recent manipulations of the circuit and its components allow it to be a relatively safe and simple procedure when used by experienced technicians. The individual components of CPB are discussed below.

The circuit

The circuit comprises an oxygenator, heat exchanger and pump. This allows blood to be drained from the patient via a venous cannula into a circuit which pumps blood through an oxygenator and heater and back to the patient via the arterial cannula. The basic principle of the circuit is to carry out the normal work of the heart and lungs. However, the circuit is non-pulsatile, and, as blood circulates, cells are broken down, increasing the risk of embolism. Initially, adult CPB circuits were used and adapted for paediatric surgery. More recently, paediatric circuits have improved volume and flow control and decreased the risk of cell breakdown and embolism.

Haemodilution

The circuit is primed with isotonic Ringer lactate (Hartmann's solution) and one unit of blood, maintaining the haematocrit at 25–30% (normal = 40%) during CPB. Previously, circuits were primed with blood only but infants and children were found to exhibit capillary leak syndrome postoperatively. CPB is a non-physiological procedure, which triggers a severe inflammatory response in the infant/child. This response results in production of powerful vasoactive chemicals including bradykinin and histamine, which increase cellular permeability. The use of isotonic haemodilution reduces the degree of inflammatory response, reducing the extent of capillary leak. Additionally, the inflammatory response produces vasoconstriction and shock. By minimising this process, peripheral vascular resistance is not increased, enhancing end organ perfusion.

Anticoagulation

Anticoagulation is used during CPB to inhibit the normal clotting cascade mechanism and reduce the risk of clotting. Heparin is normally used at 300 u/kg, to maintain ACTs at greater than 200 s (normal 80 s). The anticoagulation effect is reversed as the child comes off CPB with protamine sulphate 1 mg/100 units heparin (Guy's and St Thomas' and Lewisham Hospitals 1997).

Hypothermia

This mechanism is used to preserve and maintain tissue viability while using CPB. Normally, both superior and inferior vena cava (SVC and IVC) are cannulated to divert venous return from the body into the circuit. The ascending aorta is cannulated to return the circulating volume to the body. The ascending aorta is used to maintain cerebral perfusion and allow efficient cross-clamping of the aorta.

Cooling is used to reduce oxygen requirements to 50% of normal and reduce haemolysis by allowing CPB flow rates to be decreased, therefore reducing the risk of neurological damage. Two methods of cooling are used:

- surface cooling, where the head and heart are packed with ice
- core cooling is achieved via the heat exchanger in the circuit.

Body temperature is measured at four sites, including nasopharynx, oesophagus, skin and rectum. Measuring temperature at these sites gives an indication of perfusion to these areas. Asystole occurs at 22–24°C, allowing complex surgery to be performed on a non-beating heart.

Table 9.3 Periods of ischaemia allowable for heart surgery at varying degrees of hypothermia

Temperature	Ischaemic time
Mild hypothermia 37–32°C	10 min
Moderate hypothermia 32–28°C	20 min
Deep hypothermia 23–18°C	40 min
Profound hypothermia < 18°C[a]	Variable

[a]Rarely used, as more harmful than preserving.
For each 7°C drop in temperature below 37°C, oxygen requirements are reduced by 50%.

The degrees of cooling increases the time available for actual repair while maintaining appropriate perfusion to major organs and tissues using CPB, reducing the risks of damage to the body (Table 9.3).

Neonates requiring complex heart surgery will be cooled to 20°C and below to minimise damage to the rest of the body, as cross-clamp time is often around 60 min. As a safety precaution and to ensure the heart is completely still, a cardioplegic solution is infused into the heart, via the coronary arteries. This procedure ensures the heart arrests quickly and remains still. Crystalloid cardioplegia using St Thomas' solution and normal saline is used in most cases, although blood cardioplegia is occasionally used with the additional bonus of oxygenation. The solution may be administered at frequent intervals if the repair is complex.

Rewarming

The final stage of CPB is to rewarm the patient. This is done using the heat exchanger on the circuit (it is important for professionals to remember that, whilst the child is rewarming, he/she is still being supported by CPB). The process requires the heart to be refilled with blood to ensure all air is vented. As this is taking place, the myocardial incision is closed, and if there is no bleeding from this site the aortic cross-clamps are removed. CPB flow is increased to allow an increase in the blood flow into the heart, and as core temperature begins to rise to normothermia the heart should begin to eject. This is the time when poor ventricular function or high ventricular or pulmonary pressures may become evident. If a problem arises, the child may be cooled again and supported by CPB to allow for further investigation. If there are no problems, the surgeon and perfusionist prepare to take the child/infant off CPB. The venous drainage is gradually decreased, allowing more blood flow into the heart. As ejection occurs the venous cannula is clamped and inotropic drugs may be introduced to support the ventricle.

Potential complications of CPB (Weiland & Walker 1996) which may be exhibited in the immediate postoperative period are:

- altered blood profile (volume and flow)
- altered clotting
- altered cardiac output
- altered thermoregulation.

CONGENITAL CARDIAC DEFECTS

Cardiac defects are catergorised according to the alterations in blood flow and circulation.

Increased pulmonary blood flow

Defects in this category include:

- persistent arterial duct (PDA)
- atrial septal defect (ASD)
- ventricular septal defect (VSD)
- atrioventricular septal defect (AVSD).

These defects cause a high pulmonary blood flow. Infants present with congestive heart failure usually after the first few weeks of life when the pulmonary vascular resistance (PVR) has fallen. If unresponsive to conventional medical management, using diuretics and an angiotensin-converting enzyme inhibitor (ACE inhibitor) such as captopril, early surgery or interventional cardiac catheterisation is indicated. Infants and children with high flow defects who are undiagnosed or poorly managed risk developing irreversible pulmonary hypertension and lung disease.

Persistent arterial duct

This defect is a communication between the pul-

Persistent
arterial
duct

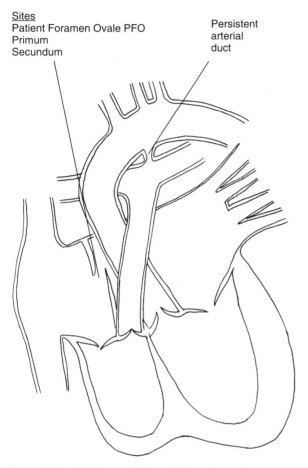

Figure 9.2a Atrial septal defect (ASD) with persistent arterial duct (PDA). Sites: patent foramen ovale (PFO); primum; secundum.

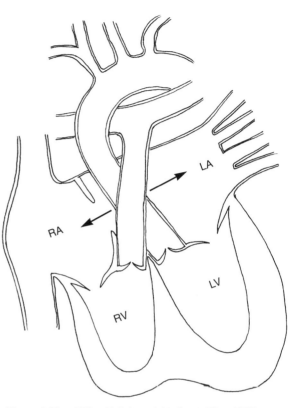

Figure 9.2b ASD with left-to-right shunt. Sites: PFO; ostium primum; ostium secundum.

monary artery and the aorta (Fig. 9.2a). In utero, the duct diverts blood from the lungs into the descending aorta causing a right-to-left shunt. Shortly after birth, the ductal tissue constricts (Tynan 1993) due to the combined effect of the tissue structure itself, respiration, increased oxygenation and reduction in levels of prostaglandin E_2 in the mature, well neonate. This contractile duct or tissue is only present in intrauterine life from 25 weeks; therefore premature infants have a high incidence of PDA, as failure of this tissue to develop or the presence of hypoxia can inhibit the duct from closing.

The severity of presentation depends on the size of the ductus. Small ducts cause no symp-

toms, whilst a large duct can cause all the symptoms of heart failure. There are two treatment options: either surgical repair or transcatheter occlusion. Surgery is performed normally via a thoracotomy, and the duct is ligated using two ligatures or clipped. This operation normally carries a 1% mortality risk. The child requires a short stay in hospital and is discharged home within 3–7 days. For premature neonates who are ventilator dependent because of a persistent duct, this procedure can be undertaken at a specialist centre as a day case with return to their Special Care Baby Unit (SCBU) for postoperative recovery.

Transcatheter occlusion is a less invasive choice of treatment than surgery. This is achieved by passing the duct occluder via a venous catheter to either end of the duct, where umbrella-like devices are released to occlude blood flow. This method is commonly used, as it presents fewer risks than surgical repair.

Sites
Subpulmonary infundibulum
Infundibular muscular
Perimembranous
Perimembranous inlet
Anterior Trabecular
Mid Trabecular
Inlet Trabecular (posterior)

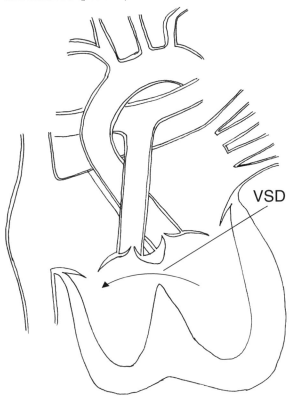

VSD

Figure 9.2c   Ventricular septal defect (VSD) with left-to-right shunt. Sites: subpulmonary infundibulum; infundibular muscular; perimembranous; perimembranous inlet; anterior trabecular; mid trabecular; inlet trabecular (posterior).

Atrial septal defect

An ASD (Fig. 9.2b) is a communication between the right and left atrium which persists after birth. There are two types: primum and secundum. The primum defect is at the lower end of the atrial septum near the atrioventricular (AV) valves, whilst the secundum defect is in the upper part of the atrial septum near the SVC.

Treatment is dependent on the type of defect. At birth, the right and left ventricular pressures are equal, and the ventricles have walls of similar thickness. As pulmonary vascular resistance (PVR) falls, the right ventricular pressure is reduced, allowing blood to shunt from left to right through the ASD. Children with this defect may not be symptomatic unless the defect is large, causing a significant shunt. If undiagnosed, pulmonary hypertension and congestive heart failure may develop later in life.

Secundum ASD is the most common type of ASD. Frequently the child may be asymptomatic and closure is indicated to reduce the risk of pulmonary hypertension. As with duct occlusion, the non-surgical method involves occluding the defect with an umbrella-like device during a cardiac catheter procedure (Magee & Qureshi 1997). Surgery requires a short period of CPB to repair the defect either with a direct suture or a patch (Kirklin & Barratt-Boyes 1993)

Primum ASDs can be more complicated because of the defect's close proximity to the AV valves. If AV valve function is affected by the defect the condition then becomes a partial atrioventricular septal defect, which is discussed later in this chapter.

Ventricular septal defect

The effect of this defect (Fig. 9.2c) is dependent on the size and site. It is the commonest congenital heart defect in childhood, accounting for approximately 30% of all cardiac defects (Ferencz et al 1985). VSDs can occur at any site along the ventricular septal wall and vary in size, which is reflected in the clinical presentation. Larger defects result in increased pulmonary blood flow and signs of congestive heart failure (CHF). VSDs are classified as:

- subpulmonary infundibulum
- infundibular muscular
- perimembranous
- perimembranous inlet (near the AV valves)
- anterior trabecular
- mid trabecular
- inlet trabecular (posterior).

Large VSDs allow significant volumes of blood to shunt from the left to the right ventricle and result in higher than normal right ventricular pressure. This results in an increased pulmonary artery blood flow and pressure, which will cause irreversible pulmonary hypertension if left untreated. Small defects may close spontaneously as the child grows.

Pulmonary artery banding has commonly been used to reduce increased pulmonary blood flow, although current practice includes early closure if medical management fails to control symptoms. Banding is currently recommended only in the presence of multiple VSDs (Stark & de Leval 1994). Closure of the VSD may be performed transatrially via the tricuspid valve using a suture or patch technique, or via a ventriculotomy. Potential complications following this surgery include pulmonary hypertension, arrhythmias due to conductive tissue oedema or damage, and decreased cardiac output due to the temporary myocardial insult following ventriculotomy.

Atrioventricular septal defects

This is a communication at the lower end of the atrial septum and the upper end of the ventricular septum, which accounts for 5% of all congenital heart defects. The atrioventricular valves are no longer separate (Fig. 9.3), producing clinical symptoms similar to those of children presenting with ventricular septal defects. Often the mitral valve is regurgitant or incompetent, producing signs of heart failure and failure to thrive at an early age. The defect may be partial or complete, partial being a primum ASD with mitral valve involvement and complete being primum ASD with VSD and both left and right AV valve involvement.

Complete AVSD usually presents with severe congestive heart failure early in life and needs medical management as previously described. Both partial and complete defects are commonly associated with Down's syndrome. A complete defect carries a much higher risk of pulmonary vascular disease. Surgery is performed once congestive heart failure has been controlled, although intervention may be necessary for infants in severe heart failure despite maximum medical management. Studies reviewed for elec-

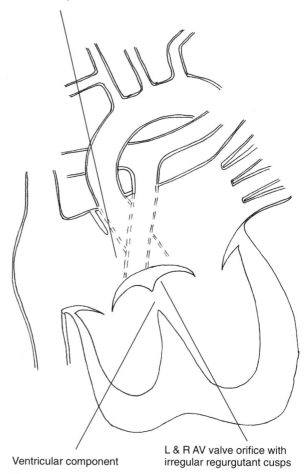

Atrial component

Ventricular component

L & R AV valve orifice with irregular regurgutant cusps

Figure 9.3 Atrioventricular septal defect (AVSD) with parachute-type valve showing right and left AV valve incompetence.

tive operation concluded that mortality rates were below 6%, with poor cardiac function being the main causative factor (Stark & de Leval 1994). Outcome is dependent on AV valve incompetence, with a percentage of children requiring reoperation for valve repair or replacement.

Infants with complete AVSD may require surgical repair in the first year of life, as pulmonary vascular disease remains a high risk in this group. If the defect is not repaired early, PVR continues to rise, making the child's condition inoperable.

Surgery consists of patch repair of the interventricular and interatrial communications, with attachment of the crest of the AV valve to the patch. The surgeon may also directly suture the commissure to decrease the possibility of valvular incompetence. Postoperative problems include pulmonary hypertension, ventricular dysfunction, AV valve incompetence and arrhythmias due to damage to the conductive tissue.

Reduced pulmonary blood flow

These defects include:

- pulmonary stenosis
- pulmonary atresia
- Fallot's tetralogy·
- tricuspid atresia.

Infants and children with these defects mainly present with cyanosis.

Pulmonary stenosis

This defect may be:

- valvular stenosis
- infundibular stenosis
- absent pulmonary valve.

Pulmonary stenosis accounts for approximately 8% of all CHD. The right ventricular outflow tract is narrowed, causing an increased pressure gradient from the right ventricle to the pulmonary artery, with decreased blood flow. In the case of absent pulmonary valve, mixing occurs, giving cyanosis with a high pulmonary blood flow. The stenosis may be

- valvular — the valve cusps are malformed, restricting normal valve function
- infundibular or absence of the pulmonary valve — the severity of the stenosis varies and consequently determines the increase in muscular mass of the right ventricle.

Initially, valvular stenosis can be treated with a balloon dilatation via cardiac catheter which allows the valve to be widened without surgery. In some cases the valvular ring is hypoplastic, a defect often seen in Noonan's syndrome.

Infundibular stenosis, often associated with Fallot's tetralogy, requires surgical intervention.

As with many of the other cardiac defects, principles of management depend on the symptoms. A small number of children with pulmonary stenosis are asymptomatic and may not require treatment for a few years. Neonates who present with cyanosis will need some palliative treatment as the patent ductus closes and cyanosis worsens. Initially blood flow can be maintained or increased using an infusion of prostaglandin E_2, maintaining patency of the duct until a systemic–pulmonary shunt can be performed. This is usually a right modified Blalock Taussig shunt, which is performed by dissecting the right subclavian artery and anastomosing this to the right pulmonary artery with a Gortex conduit. This palliative procedure increases pulmonary blood flow and enables growth prior to further surgery being performed.

Infundibular stenosis with valvular obstruction is normally repaired with a transannular patch, using CPB. The patch may be made from pericardium, dacron or Gortex. Normally the incision is performed across the pulmonary valvular ring, the pulmonary valve being partially excised; the patch is then inserted and sutured into place along the right ventricular outflow tract and into the main pulmonary artery. If replacement of the valve is required, then an aortic or pulmonary homograft is used.

Pulmonary atresia

This defect (Fig. 9.4) is characterised by the absence of blood flow from the right ventricle to the pulmonary artery and can be associated with both VSD or intact ventricular septum. Where there is a VSD the structure of the pulmonary arteries varies from having good sized main and branch pulmonary arteries to no central pulmonary trunk and small distal pulmonary arteries. In pulmonary atresia with intact ventricular septum there is a main pulmonary artery with flow through the duct. Occasionally, multiple aortopulmonary collateral vessels (MAPCAS) are present which can cause episodes of high pulmonary flow. The right ventricle is usually small

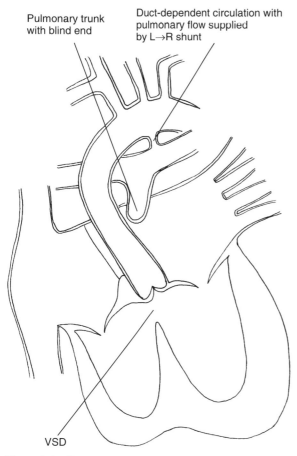

Figure 9.4 Pulmonary atresia with VSD.

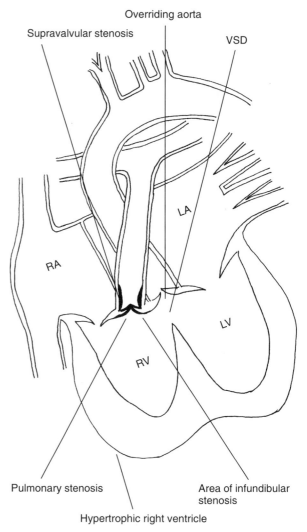

Figure 9.5 Tetralogy of Fallot.

and often hypoplastic with a hypoplastic, dysplastic or regurgitant tricuspid valve, as seen in Ebstein's Anomaly (Stark & de Leval 1994). Surgical management is similar to that of pulmonary stenosis, with early palliation and later reconstructive surgery. In some instances interventional cardiology has a role to play, with insertion of stents in small PAs or occlusion of collaterals.

Tetralogy of Fallot

This defect consists of four potential anomalies (Fig. 9.5):

- pulmonary stenosis
- ventricular septal defect
- overriding aorta
- right ventricular hypertrophy.

The complete defect accounts for 5% of all children with CHD. Clinical presentation depends on the severity of the pulmonary stenosis and the size of the VSD. The infant is usually pink at birth, but becomes more cyanosed as the outflow tract stenosis becomes more significant (Anderson et al 1988).

Prior to the 1980s, palliative shunts were performed to increase pulmonary blood flow. Current practice in many centres consists of complete repair at an early age and usually before 2 years. Infants who present with severe pulmonary stenosis may exhibit 'spelling'. These are hypercyanotic episodes that prevent blood flow from the right ventricle to the pulmonary artery. These appear to occur when the infant is irritable and crying. Because of greater energy and oxygen requirements, the infant becomes increasingly cyanosed and breathless, eventually losing consciousness. This enables the blood flow from the right ventricle to resume, and the child regains consciousness. If the spell is prolonged, intervention is needed to prevent death. First line treatment includes positioning the child with knees flexed towards the chest, oxygen and morphine administration. The use of a beta-blocker such as propranolol can prevent spells occurring but early surgery may be indicated if severe or frequent.

Postoperative care of a child following a Fallot's repair. Complete repair of this defect consists of closure of the VSD and resection of infundibular stenosis with or without a transannular patch to the right ventricular outflow tract.

Specific problems observed postoperatively may include low cardiac output and arrhythmias. Cardiac output reduction may be a particular problem if closure of the VSD is performed via a ventriculotomy or if the right ventricle is non-compliant. Total recovery with this operation is good, with a less than 5% mortality rate.

Tricuspid atresia

In this defect, there is no blood flow from the right atrium to the right ventricle, resulting in a small hypoplastic chamber. Venous return via the IVC and SVC flows into the right atrium and through the foramen ovale into the left atrium. At ventricular level, blood may flow left to right through a VSD to supply the lungs. If no VSD is present, duct patency must be maintained until palliative surgery can be performed.

Infants with this defect usually present early in life because of the presence of cyanosis. Some infants have tricuspid atresia as well as other defects, e.g. VSD, TGA, pulmonary valve stenosis.

Primary palliative surgery may be a modified Blalock–Taussig shunt. Definitive surgery consists of redirecting the systemic venous return to the pulmonary artery either through a bidirectional Glenn procedure, or a total cavopulmonary connection (TCPC).

Reduced systemic blood flow

Infants and children with poor systemic blood flow have poorly oxygenated tissues and normally present as emergencies early in life, usually when the persistent arterial duct closes. Examples of these defects include:

- coarctation of aorta (COA)/interrupted aortic arch
- aortic stenosis
- hypoplastic left heart syndrome (HLHS).

Coarctation of aorta

This defect (Fig. 9.6a) is a narrowing of the aorta occurring at the junction of the duct and accounts for approximately 8% of congenital heart defects (Anderson et al 1988). The typical clinical presentation is 3–10 days after birth. The initially well baby suddenly becomes breathless, grey and cool to touch. As the PDA closes, systemic circulation is reduced because of the narrowed aorta, causing poor systemic perfusion with associated reduced renal, liver and GI function. Femoral pulses may be weak or absent. As the systemic blood flow is obstructed, the left heart fails with a clinical presentation of cardiogenic shock.

Older children presenting with coarctation of aorta are normally asymptomatic and sometimes present because of reduced physical fitness, diagnosed during routine school examination. They exhibit weak or absent femoral pulses, with upper extremity hypertension. Balloon dilatation is presently used for many older children and performed via cardiac catheterisation. Using this technique a balloon catheter is passed into the femoral artery after an arterial catheter has measured the gradient across the narrowing. The balloon catheter (the size used is dependent on the severity of the narrowing)

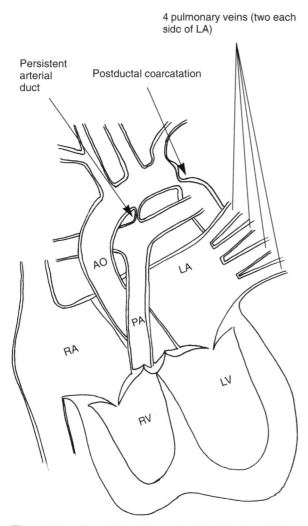

Figure 9.6a Coarctation of the aorta with PDA. Coarctation sites: preductal; postductal; ductal.

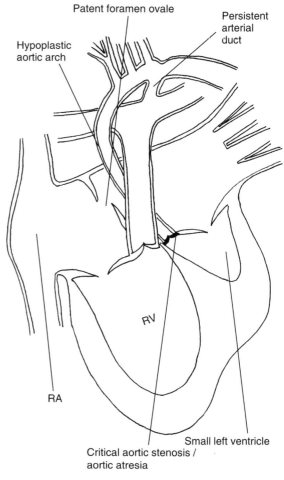

Figure 9.6b Hypoplastic left heart syndrome (HLHS) demonstrated here with critical aortic stenosis.

is passed into the aorta, across the narrowed segment. The balloon is inflated at this segment until the waist is abolished.

The operation of choice is usually resection of the narrowed segment and end-to-end anastomosis of the remaining aorta via a thoracotomy incision.

Older children may have developed a collateral circulation, and, if these vessels are considered large, some may be ligated during surgery. Postoperative care should include assessment of femoral pulses and upper and lower extremities

blood pressure to assess perfusion. Recoarctation is the main postoperative risk.

Specific postoperative management includes reduction of hypertension whilst ensuring adequate filling.

Aortic stenosis

This defect accounts for approximately 5–10% of the total number of congenital heart defects, but isolated aortic stenosis is about four times as common in boys than in girls (Jordan & Scott 1989). The stenosis may occur at three sites:

- *Valvular* — This is the commonest type (Fig. 9.6b). The valve leaflets are thickened, and sometimes a fibrous ridge is present on one or both cusps. In the majority of cases the valve is bicuspid, but some may be tricuspid. In the case of tricuspid aortic valves, the valve produces a closure with a central orifice, which may be stenotic. This type is quite favourable to valvotomy (Stark & de Leval 1994). This defect is associated with Turner's syndrome.

• *Supravalvular* — An area above the valve is narrowed. The narrowing may extend into the ascending aorta and arch. Mostly associated with Williams' syndrome.

• *Subvalvular* — A crescent or fibrous ring beneath the valve.

Neonates presenting with aortic valve stenosis are usually in congestive heart failure (CHF). Echocardiography should be performed to rule out coarctation.

The narrowing (regardless of which site) obstructs blood flow from the left ventricle. As with coarctation, the symptoms are dependent on the severity of obstruction. This defect may be isolated or associated with others such as septal defects or coarctation.

Neonates and infants presenting with symptoms should be promptly treated. Often, as in coarctation of the aorta, these infants require mechanical ventilation, with fluid and electrolyte management in addition to prostaglandin therapy to maintain duct patency. Surgical repair is normally via a valvotomy, the valve orifice may be enlarged, or the commissures (bundles of nerve fibres) present at the valve site are incised.

In infants valvotomy for aortic stenosis is a palliative procedure, as a degree of stenosis normally remains and the child may require further valve surgery in later years. In older children, many centres adopt the Ross procedure as the repair of choice. This technique involves the transfer of the child's own pulmonary valve to the aortic position (pulmonary homograft), with reconstruction of the right ventricular outflow tract using a homograft (Stark & de Leval 1994).

Hypoplastic left heart syndrome

This defect (Fig. 9.6b) accounts for 2% of all cardiac defects. The main feature is a small left ventricle with aortic stenosis or atresia and/or mitral stenosis or atresia. The aorta may also be hypoplastic. The ascending aorta and arch are normally a branch of the ductus arteriosus. If the defect is not diagnosed antenatally and provision made for treatment (if that is the parents' wish following counselling), these babies usually present with poor systemic perfusion and are critically ill. Many die in the first few days of life.

If the decision to treat is made, clinical stabilisation is required. This means re-establishing the fetal circulation with prostaglandin E_2 and in some instances mechanical ventilation. It is important to remember that the parents also have the choice to take their baby home without treatment. If this is the decision, support for the family in the community should be organised. However, if surgery is the choice, two options are available: a staged reconstruction (palliative) known as Norwood's repair, or a heart transplant (Norwood 1989). Due to limited availability of donor organs, particularly in this age group, the latter is not always a realistic option. The staged reconstruction consists of separating the pulmonary and systemic circulations so that the right ventricle becomes the systemic ventricle. Stage I involves the anastomosis of the main pulmonary artery to the ascending aorta, the Damus–Kaye–Stansel operation with the creation of a systemic-to-pulmonary shunt and atrial septectomy. After this, systemic venous return will flow into the RA, pulmonary venous return into the LA and shunt into the RA, via the ASD. Mixed blood will then flow into the RV via the tricuspid valve and into the neo-aorta. Blood flow will shunt from the ascending aorta via the Blalock–Taussig shunt into the main pulmonary artery (Mosca et al 1995). Stage II, a bidirectional Glenn or hemi-Fontan procedure, consists of creating a cavopulmonary connection, thus increasing pulmonary flow. At this stage the B–T shunt is taken down. The Fontan procedure constitutes Stage III of the palliation. Systemic venous return flows into the RA and into the pulmonary circuit via the right pulmonary artery. Pulmonary venous return will flow into

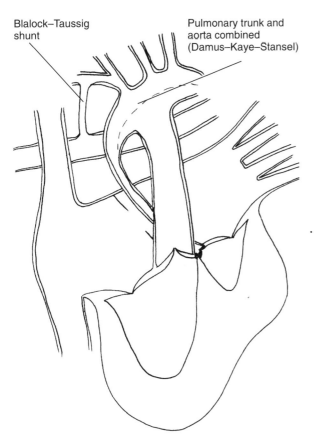

Figure 9.6c HLHS Norwood, Stage I.

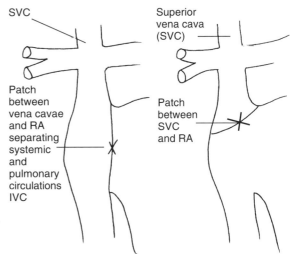

Figure 9.6d Norwood Stages II and III (hemi-Fontan and Fontan).

the LA, shunt into the RA via the ASD, and into the right ventricle and aorta.

Modifications of surgery for this condition will vary, but the main principle of a single ventricle and separate systemic and pulmonary blood flow will be the end result. Due to the critical condition of these neonates, the initial stage has a high mortality risk. Most centres demonstrate increasing survival with increased experience. Major postoperative problems occur with the regulation of pulmonary and systemic blood flow patterns (Figs 9.6c and 9.6d).

Postoperative care following Nørwood's Procedure for HLHS. Assessing and controlling pulmonary blood flow is a vital element of postoperative care, to maintain balance between systemic and pulmonary blood flows. The clinical practical indicators are as follows:

- if acidosis is persistent
- saturation > 85%
- PaO$_2$ is 6 kPa or above (i.e. 40–50 mmHg)
- systemic hypotension exists.

In order to control pulmonary blood flow and consequently balance both systemic and pulmonary flows, low oxygen concentrations should be administered.

Care following cavopulmonary connection. Care following a Glenn procedure or Fontan requires maintaining appropriate preload to enhance pulmonary blood flow. The maintenance of adequate filling is essential, as it should be high enough to ensure blood flow to the lungs without precipitating the complications of pleural effusions and ascites. The CVP is maintained at a higher than normal pressure (> 10 mmHg). Early extubation is indicated to reduce the effect of positive pressure ventilation on the venous return.

Altered circulation

These defects include:

- transposition of the great arteries (TGA)
- total anomalous pulmonary venous connection (TAPVC)
- truncus arteriosus.

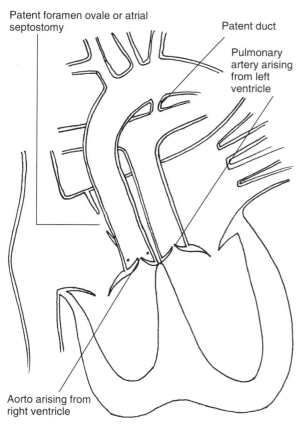

Patent foramen ovale or atrial septostomy

Patent duct

Pulmonary artery arising from left ventricle

Aorto arising from right ventricle

Figure 9.7   Transposition of the great arteries (TGA) with PFO.

Transposition of the great arteries

This defect (Fig. 9.7) presents as the second most common cyanotic lesion (Jordan & Scott 1989). The aorta arises from the right ventricle and the pulmonary artery from the left ventricle. If no other defect is present, including PDA, ASD, VSD, this is incompatible with normal life, as two circulatory systems are operating independently of each other, inhibiting any mixing of oxygenated and deoxygenated blood flow. At birth the ductus arteriosus allows some mixing; however, as it closes, the infant will deteriorate. If this defect is suspected, an infusion of prostaglandin E_2 at 5–20 nanogram/kg/min should be commenced until a definite diagnosis is reached. Palliative measures can be used such as balloon atrial septostomy (balloon dilatation of foramen ovale), which allows mixing of blood at atrial level. Previously two palliative procedures were used for this defect, namely the Senning and Mustard operations. Neither of these is corrective, and they produce long-term sequelae of their own. Over the last decade the corrective operation of choice for TGA is the arterial switch. Early results for this repair are promising. Recent data for this group show a mortality of less than 5%. The technique consists of dissecting the main pulmonary artery and aorta and switching both to the anatomically correct positions. As the coronary arteries arise from the aorta close to the aortic valve, they are re-implanted separately. It is important to know the coronary anatomy before surgery is performed, as some TGAs may not be suitable for the switch repair in the neonatal period. Another problem is subvalvular stenosis. This small percentage may therefore be banded palliatively and switched at a later date. If the arterial switch is possible, this is normally performed in the first few days or weeks of life.

Postoperative care and management following a switch repair of TGA.   Infants born with TGA have been used to the left ventricle pumping blood into the pulmonary circuit, and postoperative recovery is dependent on the ability of the ventricle to maintain adequate systemic circulation and function. Specific postoperative management therefore consists of maintaining and supporting adequate cardiac output and left ventricular function.

Total anomalous pulmonary venous connection

This anomaly is a rare defect, occurring in approximately 1–2% of infants. As the name suggests, there is an abnormality with the drainage of the pulmonary veins, and this may be partial or total. The anomalous drainage can occur in several sites:

- supracardiac — at site of SVC innominate vein
- cardiac — drainage into right atrium/ coronary sinus
- infracardiac — portal vein or IVC
- partial — combination of one or more types
- total.

The neonate normally presents in the first few

days of life with heart failure. Half of all oxygenated blood from the lungs flows into the right side of the heart, at some site, allowing oxygenated blood from lungs to go to the right atrium then right ventricle, then main pulmonary artery and back to the lungs. Sometimes the venous drainage is obstructed at the site of the venous connection. Neonates with TAPVC are critically ill. The right heart and pulmonary artery are working at systemic pressures, and gas exchange is often affected. These neonates need medical management in ITU with fluid balance and electrolyte monitoring and artificial ventilation. If the TAPVC is obstructed, corrective surgery is undertaken; if non-obstructed, many centres will maintain medical management with balloon atrial septostomy until corrective surgery is performed. The presence of an ASD or PDA allows shunting from right to left atrium, which is vital. A vital element of nursing management with these infants is observation of pulmonary hypertension in the postoperative period. Pulmonary vascular obstructive disease is an important entity in the pathophysiology of this lesion. Even in infants without pulmonary venous obstruction, advanced fibrotic changes in the pulmonary vasculature can occur early. Therefore, surgical correction is recommended at the time of diagnosis regardless of the presence or absence of pulmonary venous obstruction (Callow 1991). Surgical repair of TAPVC obviously depends upon the type of pulmonary venous drainage present. In the partial variety, a combination of techniques may be used. All are performed using CPB and deep hypothermia to 20°C.

Postoperative care of total anomalous pulmonary venous connection. Problems experienced following TAPVC repair relate to pulmonary and systemic pressures. The preoperative circulation was one of high pulmonary flow and consequently raised pulmonary pressures. Specific postoperative management consists therefore of preventing and/or treating pulmonary hypertensive episodes. Whilst surgery has corrected the altered blood flow it can take time for the vasculatures to adapt to this change. Whilst adaptation takes place, these infants may require ECMO support.

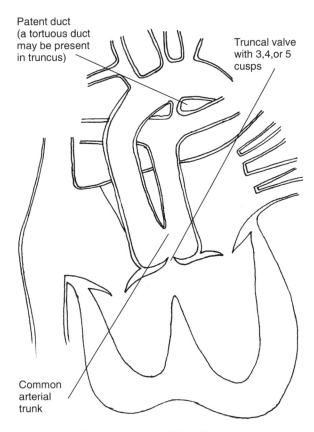

Patent duct (a tortuous duct may be present in truncus)

Truncal valve with 3,4,or 5 cusps

Common arterial trunk

Figure 9.8 Truncus arteriosus (Type 1).

Truncus arteriosus

This defect is rare, accounting for approximately 3% of all CHD. A single arterial vessel arises from the ventricles and comprises pulmonary, systemic and coronary circulations. The defect occurs as the trunk in fetal life fails to divide into main pulmonary artery and aorta. Three types of the defect are described:

- Type 1 — right and left pulmonary arteries arise from truncus and have a common stem (Fig. 9.8)
- Type 2 — right and left pulmonary arteries separate, but behind truncus
- Type 3 — right and left pulmonary arteries separate, arising from side of trunk.

In approximately 50% of cases, the truncal valve is tricuspid; bicuspid accounting for about 30% and the remainder being quadricuspid. Most have two coronary arteries, but some infants may present with only one (Stark & de Leval 1994). A significant proportion of infants with truncus arteriosus have DiGeorge syndrome, which consists of aplasia (complete) or hypoplasia (partial) of the thymus and parathyroid glands. This can cause postoperative complications with calcuim imbalance and an increased risk of infection.

Infants present with a variety of features. Clinical symptoms usually occur around 14–21 days following birth as pulmonary vascular resistance falls, increasing pulmonary blood flow. The infant may be breathless and in congestive heart failure.

Treatment.   Control of heart failure is attempted but, if this is unsuccessful, early surgery is performed. If possible, many surgeons will want at least 2–3 weeks to allow pulmonary vascular resistance to fall before operating. The repair consists of three steps (Stark & de Leval 1994):

1. detachment of the pulmonary artery or arteries from the truncus and repair of the aorta
2. closure of the VSD
3. establishment of continuity between the right ventricle and pulmonary artery or arteries.

The pulmonary artery or arteries are separated from the trunk and the defect in the aorta patched. If pulmonary arteries are separated then they are joined together and the confluence may be enlarged, using a patch. The VSD is closed via a right ventriculotomy. The patch is used to isolate the right ventricle, and a conduit is usually inserted between right ventricle and pulmonary artery. Valve replacement is avoided in infancy. Mortality risk associated with this repair is high at approximately 10–20%. Where there is preoperative pulmonary hypertension, this risk is even greater.

Transplantation.   Where no other surgery is feasible or the child had irreversible cardiac or respiratory failure, heart or heart-lung transplantation is a treatment option (Van Trigt et al 1996). Acceptance onto a transplant programme entails assessment of clinical status, psychosocial evaluation and an educational programme. The waiting time for transplant is dependent on the

child's condition and donor availability. Demand for organs continues to outweigh supply even though compatibility is only neccessary in terms of ABO grouping and heart size. A child with cardiomyopathy may be given a heart up to three times his own size.

The immediate post-transplant management is similar to that for CPB. Specific issues are:

- immunosuppression
- prevention of infection
- management of cardiac denervation using isoprenaline or pacing
- disease-specific management, e.g. for cystic fibrosis.

The commonest post-transplant problems are rejection, which is treated with high-dose steroids, and infection. Little advance has been made in recent years in controlling rejection episodes (Addonizio 1996). Death is usually from rejection or infection.

Complex lesions

As already discussed, the majority of defects fall into the above categories. Occasionally, however, a baby is born with a more complex alteration in flow. Examples of these include:

- right atrial isomerism
- left atrial isomerism
- double inlet left ventricle
- anomolous connections and drainage vessels whose origins or end points are difficult to isolate.

Very rarely is the management of these defects straightforward. The principle used is therefore to palliate in order to minimise the symptoms and altered flow caused by the defect.

In right atrial isomerism, for example, there may be any of the following components: AVSD, TGA, PAPVD or TAPVD, pulmonary stenosis, tricuspid atresia with either asplenia or polysplenia. This example typifies the problems faced in the clinical management. Initial surgery may be needed to repair the total or partial anomalous drainage, and if the PS is not significant a PA band may also be needed to restrict pulmonary flow. At a later stage the pulmonary blood supply will need to be augmented, usually using a Glenn or TCPC. Throughout this group's care, sepsis remains a major problem due to the absence or poor functioning of the spleen.

In left atrial isomerism, the added complication of potential heart block or bradyarrhythmia is present as there is no normal sinus node. In addition to the presence of an AVSD and pulmonary stenosis there is likely to be a coarctation of the aorta which has to be repaired at an early stage. The pulmonary artery may also be banded at this operation if there is concern about high pulmonary flow.

Other diseases of the cardiovascular system that may need a period of intensive care include Kawasaki syndrome, cardiomyopathies which may require transplant, and viral myocarditis. Whilst these children do not have altered flow they can present with severely reduced myocardial function requiring ventilation and pharmacological support.

REFERENCES

Addonizio L J 1996 Current status of cardiac transplantation in children [review]. Current Opinion in Pediatrics 8(5):520–526

Anderson R H, McCartney F J, Shinebourne E A, Tynan M 1988 Paediatric cardiology. Churchill Livingstone, London

Callow L B 1991 Post-operative nursing management of the infant with total anomalous pulmonary venous connection. Dimensions of Critical Care Nursing 10(3):140–149

Ferencz C, Rubin J D, McCarter R J, Brenner J L, Neill C A, Perry L N, Hepner S I, Downing J W 1985 Congenital heart disease: prevalence at live birth: the Baltimore–Washington Infant Study. American Journal of Epidemiology 1(121): 31–36

Guy's and St Thomas' and Lewisham Hospitals 1997 Paediatric formulary, 4th edn. London

Jordan S C, Scott O 1989 Heart disease in paediatrics, 3rd edn. Butterworth, London

Kirklin J W, Barratt-Boyes B G B 1993 Cardiac surgery, 2nd edn. Churchill Livingstone, New York

Magee A G, Qureshi S A 1997 Closure of atrial septal defects by transcatheter devices. Paediatric Cardiology 18: 326–327

Mosca R S, Bove E L, Crowley D C, Sandhu S K, Shork M A, Kulik T J 1995 Hemodynamic characteristics of neonates following first stage palliation for hypoplastic left heart syndrome. Circulation 92(Suppl. II):267–271

Norwood W I 1989 Hypoplastic left heart syndrome [review]. Cardiology Clinics 7(2):377–385

Norwood W I, Piggott J D 1988 Recent advances in congenital cardiac surgery [review]. Clinics in Perinatology 15(3):713–719

Stark J, de Leval M 1994 Surgery for congenital heart defects, 2nd edn. Saunders, Philadelphia

Tritschler I 1993 Cardiology update: drug therapy. Nursing Standard 8(8):52

Tynan M 1993 The ductus arteriosus and its closure. New England Journal of Medicine 329(21):1570–1572

Van Trigt P, Davis R D, Shaeffer G S, Gaynor J W, Landolfo K P 1996 Survival benefits of heart and lung transplantation. Annals of Surgery 223(5):576–584

Weiland A P, Walker W E 1996 Physiologic principles and clinical sequelae of cardio-pulmonary bypass. Heart and Lung 15(1):34–39

FURTHER READING

Bailey L, Gundry S 1990 Hypoplastic left heart syndrome. Pediatric Clinics of North America 37(1)

Nisco S J, Reitz B A 1994 Developments in cardiac transplantation [review]. Current Opinion in Cardiology 9(2):237–246

Qureshi S A 1997 Practical interventional paediatric cardiology. In: Grech D E, Ramsdale D R (eds) Practical interventional cardiology. Martin Dunitz, London

Stark J, Pacifico A D (eds) 1989 Reoperations in cardiac surgery. London

10

Care and management of infants and children with neurological dysfunction

Yvette Arendse   Alison Green
Carol Williams   Yvonne Hill
Petra Shroff

INTRODUCTION

The neurological system is closely integrated with the endocrine and musculoskeletal systems. Therefore, it influences both voluntary and involuntary functions of the body and is seen as the system responsible for coordination and control. At birth, this system is immature, but rapid maturation takes place during the first 2 years of life, with further development throughout childhood. Disorders affecting the neurological system are not uncommon during infancy and childhood. These are commonly associated with trauma and infection, but could occur as a result of metabolic and electrical dysfunction, congenital anomalies, space-occupying lesions and hypoxic-ischaemic damage. Therefore, this chapter will address the development of the neurological system, disorders commonly seen in paediatric intensive care, and management issues.

EMBRYOLOGICAL DEVELOPMENT

The nervous system originates from the neural plate, which is a thickened area of ectoderm that develops early within the third week of life. A groove develops within the centre of this structure (the neural groove) with neural folds on each side. These folds begin to fuse by the end of the third week to form the neural tube (Fig. 10.1).

The neural tube develops into the brain and spinal cord. Around the third week, the neural tube is open at the rostral and caudal ends, which close on or before day 26 and at the end of the

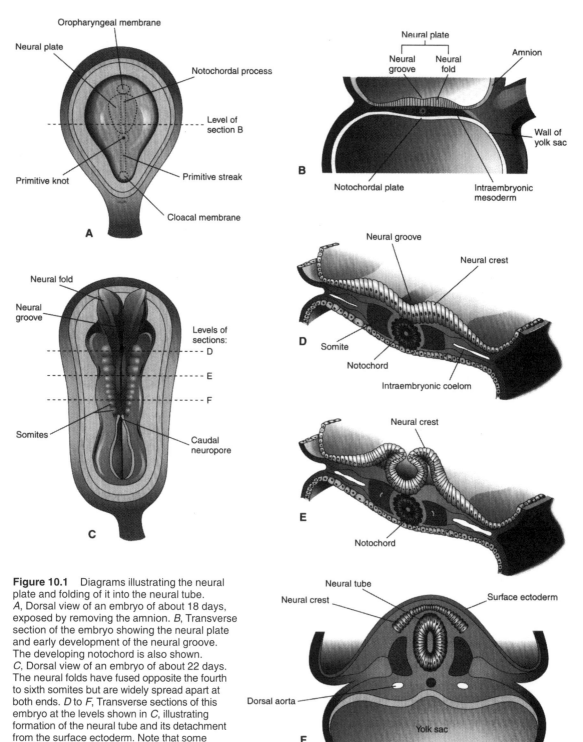

Figure 10.1 Diagrams illustrating the neural plate and folding of it into the neural tube. *A*, Dorsal view of an embryo of about 18 days, exposed by removing the amnion. *B*, Transverse section of the embryo showing the neural plate and early development of the neural groove. The developing notochord is also shown. *C*, Dorsal view of an embryo of about 22 days. The neural folds have fused opposite the fourth to sixth somites but are widely spread apart at both ends. *D* to *F*, Transverse sections of this embryo at the levels shown in *C*, illustrating formation of the neural tube and its detachment from the surface ectoderm. Note that some neuroectodermal cells are not included in the neural tube but remain between it and the surface ectoderm as the neural crest. Moore (1998).

fourth week, respectively. It is the neural folds at the rostral end which eventually thicken to form the brain. Cells from the neural folds combine to form a neural crest, and from this the spinal ganglia, cranial ganglia and autonomic ganglia develop.

The spinal cord develops from three layers of cells forming the neural tube:

- ventricular zone (inner layer)
- intermediate zone (middle layer)
- marginal zone (outer layer).

Neuroblasts, which form future nerve cells, and glioblasts, which form future glial cells, develop from the ventricular zone. These cells complete their differentiation in the intermediate zone.

On each side of the neural tube, ventral and dorsal to the sulcus limitans there is a group of cells. Those placed dorsally are called the alar plate, which predominantly develops into afferent or sensory neurons. Those placed ventrally are called the basal plate and develop into efferent or motor neurons. Cells in the alar plate give rise to the dorsal horn of grey matter, and cells in the basal plate develop into the ventral horn of grey matter.

During the first 12 weeks of development the spinal cord and vertebral column grow at the same rate, to allow the nerve roots to pass directly into the intervertebral foramina. This changes during postnatal development, when the growth of the vertebral column is greater than that of the spinal cord. Whilst the cranial end of the spinal cord is attached to the brain, the tail end of the spinal cord ascends in the vertebral canal. This is why the spinal cord ends at the third lumbar vertebra in the newborn infant. The brain develops from three primary brain vesicles — hindbrain, midbrain and forebrain — which form from the thickened neural folds of the rostral neuropore. Table 10.1 outlines the mature brain structures into which each vesicle develops.

During the fifth week the forebrain area develops outgrowths called optic vesicles, which develop into the eyes, and cerebral vesicles which develop into the cerebral hemispheres. Thickening of nerve cells in the floor of the lateral wall develops into the corpus striatum. The thal-

Table 10.1 Development of the brain from the embryonic brain vesicles

Primary brain vesicles	Secondary brain vesicles	Region of mature brain
Hindbrain vesicle	Myelencephalon	Medulla
	Metencephalon	Pons and cerebellum
Midbrain vesicle	Mesencephalon	Midbrain
Forebrain vesicle	Diencephalon	Thalamus, hypothalamus
	Telencephalon	Cerebral hemispheres

From Moore (1988), p. 162.

amus originates from thickening of the lateral walls of the diencephalon. There is little change in the midbrain vesicle except increased thickening of its walls due to the growth of large nerve fibre tracts, which become the cerebral aqueduct. Neuroblasts in the basal plates of the midbrain form the nuclei of two motor cranial nerves: the oculomotor and trochlear nerves.

The hindbrain divides into the myelencephalon and metencephalon, forming the medulla and cerebellum, respectively. From cells in the basal plates in the myelencephalon the motor nuclei of cranial nerves IX, X, XI and XII are formed. The sensory nuclei of cranial nerves V, VIII, IX and X develop from the alar plates. Lastly the dorsal parts of the walls of the metencephalon develop into the grey matter of the brain known as the cerebellum.

DEVELOPMENTAL ANATOMY AND PHYSIOLOGY

The bones of the skull and spinal column protect the central nervous system (CNS). During infancy the cranial bones are incompletely fused and are connected at their margins by membranous tissues. These allow the skull to reduce in size during passage through the birth canal. Membranes between adjacent bones can be extensive and are called fontanelles.

- The anterior fontanelle is present in the skull's midline, where the frontal and parietal bones are separated. Extension of ossification into the membrane results in the closure of the fontanelle at approximately 18 months of age.
- The posterior fontanelle lies between the

occipital and parietal bones and is closed by 3 months of age.

Palpation of the anterior fontanelle in a resting infant can provide useful information about fluid status and can provide an indicator of CNS infection or coarctation of the aorta.

If the brain does not grow, the bones may fuse early, resulting in microcephaly. Likewise, craniosynostosis or premature fusion of the cranial bones can result in microcephaly as brain growth is inhibited. At birth, the normal brain is 25% of the eventual adult size. Rapid growth during the first 2 years of life increases this size to 75% by the end of the second year. Head circumference is used as one of the parameters to assess growth from birth through early childhood. The cranium continues to grow until approximately 7 years of age, when cerebral development is near completion. Ossification is complete by 8 years of age, although sutures are not completely fused until approximately 12 years, when the cranium becomes a fixed structure, which does not expand with increases in intracranial pressure.

The brain comprises three key areas:

- cerebrum
- cerebellum
- brainstem.

The cerebrum

The cerebrum is the largest subdivision of the brain, containing two hemispheres, the basal ganglia, hypothalamus, thalamus, olfactory and optic nerves. Each hemisphere is divided into lobes by deep grooves or fissures. The lobes are named according to the overlying bones:

- frontal lobe
- parietal lobe
- temporal lobe
- occipital lobe.

Each hemisphere's surface consists of numerous convolutions or 'gyri' folding on one another, increasing the surface area. The cerebral cortex comprises relatively thin (2–5 mm) grey matter, composed of six layers of cell bodies and fibres

Table 10.2 Infant reflexes

Reflex	Age at which this is normal
Stepping	Birth to 6 weeks
Moro	Birth to 3 months
Sucking	Birth to 4 months awake (7 months asleep)
Rooting	Birth to 4 months awake (7 months asleep)
Palmar grasp	Birth to 6 months
Plantar grasp	Birth to 10 months
Tonic neck reflex	2 to 5 months
Landau reflex	3 to 24 months
Neck righting	4 to 24 months
Parachute	9 months onwards

Adapted from McCance & Heuther (1994).

containing billions of neurons. The cerebral cortex is involved in the higher sensory and motor functions and continues to develop beyond childhood. Infant neurological function is primarily subcortical, with infant reflexes originating from the brainstem and spinal cord. As motor function progresses and movement becomes voluntary, early reflexes disappear. Persistence of these reflexes beyond specific points in development suggests neurological damage (Table 10.2). Damage to the cortex in older children can be predicted by neurological deficits. The dominant hemisphere normally becomes apparent by 3 years of age. If this hemisphere is damaged in children, the other hemisphere can be taught to control dominant functions.

The corpus callosum joins the two hemispheres at their base. This complex area of nerve fibres connects every part of one hemisphere with the corresponding part of the other hemisphere.

- Commissural (transverse) fibres connect one area of a hemisphere with its counterpart in the other, thereby forming pathways that are essential for maintaining the unity of the higher sensory and major functions of the cerebral cortex (Hickey 1992).
- Projection fibres connect the cerebral cortex with the lower portion of the brain and spinal cord.
- Association fibres connect various areas within the same hemisphere.

The basal ganglia consist of grey matter deep within each cerebral hemisphere, partially surrounding the thalamus. These structures, collectively known as the corpus striatum, include:

- the caudate nucleus
- the putamen
- the globus pallidus.

and may also include the subthalamic nucleus and substantia nigra.

The basal ganglia control transmission of impulses between the motor cortex and the thalamus, inhibiting unintentional motor movement. Regulation of the extrapyramidal system allows messages from lower motor pathways to be selected and projected upwards towards the cerebral cortex. Disorders of the basal ganglia are usually bilateral and give rise to motor disorders or dyskinesias. High bilirubin levels during infancy stain this area, leading to kernicterus resulting in cerebral palsy.

The remaining structures within the cerebrum include the thalamus and hypothalamus and are collectively called the diencephalon. The thalamus consists of groups of grey matter located on either side of the third ventricle. Large numbers of axons conduct impulses into the thalamus from the spinal cord, brainstem, cerebellum, basal ganglia and parts of the cerebrum. These axons synapse in the thalamic nuclei, from where impulses are conducted to virtually all areas of the cerebral cortex. Basic roles of the thalamus include:

- relay of sensory impulses to the cerebral cortex, with the exception of olfactory information
- recognition of sensations of pain, temperature and touch
- responsibility for emotions by associating sensory impulses with feelings of pleasantness and unpleasantness
- alteration of arousal mechanism
- contribution to the production of complex reflex movements.

The hypothalamus is a complex structure located in the basal region of the diencephalon, forming part of the third ventricle. It includes several other structures:

- the optic chiasma, where the optic tracts cross
- the stalk of the pituitary, which connects the pituitary gland with the hypothalamus
- the mamillary bodies, which relay cortically originating limbic data to the thalamus.

The hypothalamus is involved in the subcortical integration of sympathetic and parasympathetic activity. It is the source of two hormones:

- vasopressin (ADH)
- oxytocin.

These hormones are synthesized by the hypothalamus, transmitted in the nerve tract to the posterior pituitary gland and released as required.

Functions of the hypothalamus include:

- regulation of body temperature
- regulation of water metabolism
- regulation of appetite
- regulation of visceral and somatic activities through the autonomic nervous system
- regulation of sleep–wake cycle
- regulation of thirst
- mediation of visible physical expressions in response to emotions, e.g. blushing, clammy hands
- control of hormones released by the anterior pituitary gland.

There are few activities in the body that are not influenced by the hypothalamus. Damage to the hypothalamus causes a wide variety of endocrine disorders and fluid and electrolyte imbalances.

The brainstem

The brainstem reaches from the base of the diencephalon to the base of the skull, where it extends into the spinal vertebrae to become the spinal cord. The brainstem comprises the midbrain, the pons and the medulla.

The midbrain is located between the diencephalon and the pons, consisting mainly of white matter with some internal grey matter around a cerebral aqueduct. It is responsible for assimilating sensory information relating to consciousness, arousal and sleep and visual and auditory reflexes. It also provides the origin of cranial nerves III and IV.

The pons connects the medulla and cerebellum with higher centres and consists mainly of fibres of white matter. The reticular formation from the medulla extends into the pons to form the pneumotaxic centre responsible for controlling respiratory rate. Cranial nerves V to VIII also originate from the pons.

The medulla lies between the spinal cord and pons, at the level of the foramen magnum. Nerve fibres from the spinal cord cross in the medulla before impulses are transmitted to the cortex. It is composed of white matter, the reticular formation (interlaced white and grey matter) and grey matter or nuclei forming vital centres:

- respiratory centre
- vasomotor centre
- cardiac centre.

Cranial nerves IX to XII originate here. Damage to the medulla can result in loss of swallow and gag reflexes and causes decorticate and decerebrate posturing.

The cerebellum

The cerebellum is situated beneath the occipital lobe of the cerebrum. It is attached to the medulla, pons and midbrain by cerebellar peduncles. It has a similar structure to the cerebrum, with outer grey matter overlying white matter. It also has two hemispheres divided by a longitudinal fissure. The cerebellum is responsible for spatial awareness, balance, fine movements and dexterity.

The meninges

Although protected by the skull and spinal vertebrae, the central nervous system gains additional protection from the meninges. These are:

- the dura mater
- the arachnoid
- the pia mater.

The dura mater is a tough, inelastic membrane

lining the interior of the skull. Folds in the dura mater provide additional support and stabilisation of the major structures and their hemispheres.

- The falx cerebri lies between the cerebral hemispheres.
- The tentorium cerebelli covers the upper surface of the cerebellum, supporting the occipital and temporal lobes and preventing pressure on the cerebellum. It also acts as an important anatomic landmark, as lesions are often described as supra- or infratentorial.
- The falx cerebelli separates the cerebellar hemispheres.

The dura comprises two fused layers, which separate at the bases of the three dural folds to form venous sinuses, draining blood and CSF from the brain into veins exiting the skull. The inner layer of the dura continues with the spinal cord lining to the level of the second or third sacral vertebrae, protecting spinal nerves and blood vessels.

The arachnoid is a thin membrane loosely following the surface of the brain and spinal cord to the end of the spinal cord. The arachnoid is separated from the dura by the subdural space, which is crossed by blood vessels. These can rupture easily during serious head injury, resulting in subdural haemorrhage and potential compression of vital centres. The subarachnoid space contains cerebral spinal fluid (CSF), a clear fluid containing water, oxygen, carbon dioxide, sodium, potassium, chloride, glucose and a few lymphocytes. It performs several functions:

- acts as a shock absorber for the brain and spinal cord
- provides nutrients
- drains unwanted substances away from the brain cells.

CSF is primarily formed from collections of capillaries called the choroid plexus. This is found mainly on the floors of the lateral ventricles, but also in the third and fourth ventricles. In addition, CSF is produced by ependymal cells lining the ventricles and meninges and by blood vessels throughout the CNS. CNS infection and trauma during infancy and early childhood can obstruct the flow of CSF, resulting in hydrocephalus.

The pia mater is a fine, mesh-like membrane, rich in minute blood vessels, which closely follows the surface of the brain. The pia mater of the spinal cord is thicker, firmer and less vascular than that covering the brain.

The blood–brain barrier is highly impermeable, comprising capillaries enclosed by glial cells. During infancy the glial cells are immature, making the barrier incomplete and thus permeable to toxic substances such as bilirubin. Once mature, the brain is protected from changes in pH and toxic substances. However, many drugs, including antibiotics, do not cross this barrier, making CNS infection difficult to treat.

NEUROLOGICAL ASSESSMENT

Serial assessment of conscious level acts as an indicator of changes in the child's condition. This is commonly undertaken using a coma scale. In the UK, the most commonly used tool for assessing level of consciousness is the Glasgow Coma Scale (GCS). While this scale is useful in older children, its interpretation is difficult in infants and young children, as it makes no allowance for a child's motor or verbal immaturity. Modifications of the GCS used in Britain include:

- the Adelaide Scale (Simpson & Reilly 1982) (Tables 10.3 and 10.4)
- the Modified Glasgow Coma Scale (Table 10.3)
- the James Adaptation of the Glasgow Coma Scale (Tatman et al 1997) (Table 10.5).

This last tool is considered appropriate for use with intubated children, as a grimace score rather than verbal response is used to complete the assesment (Tatman et al 1997).

Interpretation of a coma scale score

The coma score reflects central nervous system function, with low scores indicating diffuse dysfunction rather than damage to a specific area. It will indicate decreased activity of the cerebral cortex, or decreased communication between the cortex, brainstem, thalamus and reticular activat-

Table 10.3   Coma scales commonly used with children

Modified Glasgow Coma Scale		Adelaide Coma Scale	
Eyes open		**Eyes open**	
spontaneously	4	spontaneously	4
to speech	3	to speech	3
to pain	2	to pain	2
none	1	none	1
Best verbal response		**Best verbal response**	
orientated	5	orientated	5
confused	4	words	4
inappropriate words	3	vocal sounds	3
incomprehensible sounds	2	cries	2
none	1	none	1
Best motor responses		**Best motor responses**	
obeys commands	5	obeys commands	5
localise pain	4	localise pain	4
flexion	3	flexion	3
extension	2	extension	2
none	1	none	1

Adapted from Allan (1994).

Table 10.4   Adelaide Scale: normal score for age

Birth to 6 months	9
6 months to 1 year	11
1–2 years	12
2–5 years	13
>5 years	14

Adapted from Williams (1992).

ing system (Teasdale 1975). Neurological assessment of the non-paralysed child can elicit valuable information. However, accurate assessment is difficult in the child who is sedated with or without paralysing agents, making it necessary to consider additional forms of assessment such as continuous EEG.

When undertaking neurological assessment, it is important to increase the level of stimulus in an incremental manner to determine level of consciousness and provide an accurate assessment of response. Therefore, before approaching a child, it is important to observe his/her wakefulness and posture and to determine whether he/she is responding in any way to his/her family. Once this observation is made, the child's response to movement, speech, touch, gentle pressure and painful stimulus should be assessed to determine the least stimulus to produce a response. The assessment should be based

Table 10.5 James' adaptation of the Glasgow Coma Scale

	Adult or child > 5 years	Child < 5 years
	Eye opening response	
E4	Spontaneous	Spontaneous
E3	To verbal stimulus	To verbal stimulus
E2	To pain	To pain
E1	No response to pain	No response to pain
	Verbal response	
V5	Orientated	Alert, babbles, coos, words or sentences to usual ability
V4	Confused	Less than usual ability or spontaneous irritable cry
V3	Inappropriate words	Cries to pain
V2	Incomprehensible sounds	Moans to pain
V1	No response to pain	No response to pain
VT	Intubated	Intubated
	Grimace	
G5	Spontaneous normal facial/oromotor activity, e.g. suck, cough	
G4	Less than usual spontaneous ability or only responds to touch	
G3	Vigorous grimace to pain	
G2	Mild grimace or some change in facial expression to pain	
G1	No response to pain	
	Motor response	
M6	Obeys commands	Normal spontaneous movements or withdraws to touch
M5	Localises to pain stimulus	
M4	Withdraws from pain	
M3	Abnormal flexion to pain	
M2	Abnormal extension to pain	
M1	No response to pain	

on the child's level of development prior to the illness.

Eye opening

Spontaneous opening of the child's eyes when approached (if not deeply asleep), implies an intact reticular activating system. In cases of flaccid ocular muscles, where the eyes remain open or where the child is blind, the arousal system should still be intact. When assessing eye opening, ocular movements should also be assessed, as abnormal movements can provide indication of underlying pathology (Downey & Leigh 1998). Failure to open the eyes when stimulated implies marked depression of the arousal system.

Verbal response

Verbal response is difficult to assess in the child requiring assisted ventilation. However, facial expression or grimace may assist practitioners to obtain accurate assessments of neurological status (Tatman et al 1997).

Best motor response

Motor responses should be tested on both arms and the best response documented. With spinal injury, motor responses should not be confused with a spinal reflex. In the child with reduced level of consciousness, pressure on the nail bed may produce a spinal response. In order to provide an accurate assessment of motor response, a central stimulus should be used (Teasdale 1975, Lower 1992). Teasdale (1975) recommends that the child is not asked to squeeze the examiner's hand, as touching the child's hand may induce a grasp reflex. If used, the test must be repeated several times.

The child subjected to painful stimuli should try to purposefully remove it. The most frequently used stimuli are application of pressure to the supra orbital notch or pinching the trapezius muscle. The application of pressure to the sternum should be used with caution in children, as it can cause intrathoracic damage (Teasdale 1975, Stewart 1996). Care should be taken if the child has coagulopathy or is thrombocytopenic.

Normal flexion involves brisk removal of the limb from the painful stimulus. This is a natural protective reflex. Abnormal flexion occurs when the response is sluggish or hyper-reflexive. Extension of the limb involves straightening towards the noxious stimulus. This may be accompanied by inward rotation of the limb to the midline with fingers straightened. This abnormal movement indicates loss of protective motor responses. If limbs adopt this posture without stimulation, it is grossly abnormal.

Complete flaccidity is an extremely abnormal sign.

Babinski's reflex indicates grossly abnormal motor function in children who have learnt to walk. When the sole of the foot is stroked with an upward movement the toes fan out. The normal response in an adult or walking child is for the foot to flex at the ankle, moving away from the stimulus and for the toes to curl.

Vital signs

It is important to record vital signs when assessing neurological function, as these may indicate abnormal pathology or assist identification of the cause of coma, such as hypothermia or infection. In addition, it is important to monitor blood glucose and arterial O_2 and CO_2 as abnormalities could independently cause coma.

When intracranial pressure (ICP) is monitored, measurement of mean arterial pressure (MAP) is required for calculation of the cerebral perfusion pressure (CPP). If the CPP is not maintained, blood flow to the cerebral tissue is compromised, resulting in ischaemia. A rising systolic arterial pressure, widening pulse pressure and bradycardia occur as an attempt to increase CPP. This is known as Cushing's reflex and is a late sign of cerebral ischaemia when brain herniation is imminent (Hickey 1986). Warning signs such as tachycardia and erratic arterial pressure should be detected and treatment instituted to prevent brainstem herniation. Hypotension occurs after the Cushing reflex is exhausted.

Pupil responses

Pupils are normally equal in size and constrict briskly in response to a bright light. This demonstrates a functioning ocular motor nerve. If both pupils are dilated and fail to react to light this is a late sign of raised intracranial pressure, with some degree of irreversible brain damage. If just one pupil fails to respond to light there is likely to be an enlarging mass such as an haematoma (Teasdale 1975). The size of the pupils should be recorded in millimetres along with a note of a positive or negative reaction.

Certain pharmaceutical agents affect pupil size: for example, opiates reduce pupil size and catecholamines and sympathetic agonists dilate pupils.

Limb movement

The best motor responses are sufficient for assessing motor function if the child has proven diffuse brain dysfunction. If localised injury is suspected, the function of only one limb or one side of the body may be affected, so it may be necessary to document individual limb function.

COMA

Coma is characterised by reduction in the level of consciousness to a level where the child becomes unresponsive to vocal and painful stimuli. Causes of coma can be largely divided into two groups: acute and diffuse injury. Specific causes include:

- trauma
- space-occupying lesions
- arteriovenous malformation
- toxins (alcohol)
- hypernatraemic dehydration
- fulminant liver failure
- CNS infection
- respiratory obstruction with hypercarbia
- hypoglycaemia
- obstructive hydrocephalus
- status epilepticus
- hypoxic-ischaemic injury
- uraemia
- diabetic ketoacidosis
- hypothermia.

All of these disorders cause coma, as they cause changes in the volume of the intracranial contents. Normal intracranial contents comprise:

- brain tissue   80%
- CSF   7–10%
- blood   7–10%.

Change in volume of any of these compartments will cause raised intracranial pressure, cerebral oedema, reduced cerebral blood flow and a reduction in the level of consciousness. Cerebral requirements for oxygen and glucose are high, therefore the brain requires a constant oxygenated blood supply to meet its needs. For this reason, the brain receives approximately 15% of the cardiac output when at rest and uses the Circle of Willis to ensure that the blood supply is continuous.

RAISED INTRACRANIAL PRESSURE

Raised intracranial pressure in children results from any of the disorders listed above. Intracranial pressure is generated from the pressure of the intracranial contents on the skull (Stewart-Amidei 1998). This is a normal phenomenon where transient rises occur as a response to a variety of everyday activities such as sneezing and coughing. These transient rises are not dangerous in themselves, as the body is designed to accommodate them, with pressures returning to normal following the activity. However, uncompensated rises are dangerous and potentially life threatening.

The intracranial volume must remain relatively constant, as the skull provides a solid barrier to expansion. Intracranial pressure can be defined in terms of the Monro–Kellie hypothesis (Robinson 1997), which states that ICP is proportional to the sum of the volumes of the cerebral contents. Therefore, cerebral compliance is determined by the relationship between ICP and intracranial volume. Compensation occurs through autoregulatory mechanisms, whereby an increase in one of the components causes a reduction in another, e.g. redirection of CSF into the spinal space or a fall in cerebral blood volume. Autoregulatory mechanisms are effective at maintaining ICP within normal limits (0–15 mmHg). However, loss of autoregulation will result in fluctuations in both ICP and cerebral blood flow (CBF), causing cerebral ischaemia and cell death. The ability of the body to compensate will depend on pathology, as a slow-growing tumour may not present signs of raised ICP until it has reached a significant size. However, a rapid intracranial bleed would cause an acute rise in ICP, as compensatory mechanisms are unable to

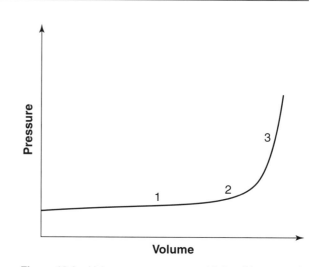

Figure 10.2 Volume–pressure curve. (1) Small increases in volume produce small rises in pressure. (2) Autoregulation begins to fail as small increases in volume cause significant rises in ICP. (3) Small volume increases result in uncompensated rises in ICP and loss of autoregulation. Adapted from Germon (1994).

respond quickly. This is better understood by referring to the volume–pressure curve (Fig. 10.2). This demonstrates how changes in intracranial volume will influence intracranial pressure, with poor compliance leading to decompensation.

In infants and children with neurological problems, the primary aims are to determine and treat the cause of the problem whilst preventing secondary neurological damage associated with raised ICP. Therefore, when considering ICP, assessment should also be made of mean systemic arterial pressure (MAP), cerebral perfusion pressure (CPP) and cerebral blood flow (CBF). CBF is influenced by MAP and ICP, but is best assessed by calculation of CPP:

$$CPP = MAP - mean\ ICP$$

There is considerable debate in the literature regarding the optimal values for both ICP and CPP. CPPs of between 40 and 80 mmHg have been recommended (Prendergast 1994), whilst 60 to 100 mmHg is considered a normal range (Germon 1994). It has been suggested that the actual value of the ICP is not important, but its contribution to CPP is the important consideration. However, an ICP greater than 40 mmHg has been responsible for severe damage even when CCP has been maintained (Robinson 1997). Therefore, maintenance of ICP within a normal range is important. It is suggested that the ICP in children should be stabilised below 25 mmHg, with CPP at least 50 mmHg; in neonates, ICP should be 10 mmHg or less, with a CPP greater than 30 mmHg.

Measurement of intracranial pressure

ICP measurement has been described since the 1960s (Germon 1994). Current methods of monitoring involve placing a monitor under the skull in one of five sites (Germon 1994):

- epidural — between the skull and dura
- subdural — between the dura and the arachnoid
- subarachnoid — in the subarachnoid space
- intraparenchymal — into brain tissue
- intraventricular — into a lateral ventricle.

The accuracy of the readings obtained from the different type of monitors will vary, as those lying nearer the skull provide less direct measurements of ICP. Therefore, epidural and subdural monitors may be most useful for observation of trends in readings and responses to interventions. The intraventricular catheter is considered the most accurate method of monitoring, as readings are taken from deep within the brain, whilst the other methods reflect pressures at the top of the brain. In the child who is in the process of coning, pressures from the top of the brain may be misleadingly low (Germon 1994). Whichever method of monitoring is used, there is an associated risk of infection and haemorrhage. Therefore, the use of invasive ICP monitors should be carefully considered in relation to individual children. Non-invasive monitors are not currently available, but research is being carried out into their use.

Examination of the waveform produced by invasive ICP monitors has shown that each pulse waveform comprises three distinct peaks, which become progressively lower in amplitude during each pulsation, when ICP is normal (Germon

1994). However, it has been suggested that elevation of the middle peak is an early indication that autoregulation is failing and decompensation will occur, producing neurological deterioration (Stewart-Amidei 1998). The clinical relevance of this is not currently apparent, and further research is required.

Management of raised intracranial pressure

The aims of management are to:

- maintain optimum cerebral perfusion
- maintain ICP below 25 mmHg
- provide oxygen and glucose
- maintain cardiorespiratory stability

(Prasad & Tasker 1990).

Airway management and ventilation

Intubation and mechanical ventilation are essential for the child who is neurologically compromised and unable to maintain his or her own airway. Oxygen and carbon dioxide levels influence cerebral blood flow and should be controlled to contribute to management of ICP. When severe hypoxia occurs, cerebral vessels dilate in an attempt to increase oxygen delivery, which in turn raises intracranial pressure (ICP) by increasing cerebral blood flow (CBF). Therefore, it is important to maintain PaO_2 within the normal range. Maintenance of $PaCO_2$ within the normal range (4.0–6.0 kPa) ensures adequate blood flow to the brain when autoregulation is intact. Reduction in $PaCO_2$ below normal has been shown to reduce blood flow to the brain and has previously been used as a treatment to reduce CBF and thus ICP. Hyperventilation to a $PaCO_2$ of 3.5 to 4.0 kPa has been routinely used to reduce ICP. However, concerns that continuous hyperventilation causes cerebral ischaemia have led to current recommendations for management being maintenance of $PaCO_2$ between 4.0 and 4.5 kPa (Prendergast 1994, Fisher 1997), with further reduction used for controlling sudden increases in ICP.

The use of positive end expiratory pressure

(PEEP) is controversial. The associated increase in intrathoracic pressure and reduction in cardiac output can impede venous return, increasing ICP (Robinson 1997). However, when oxygenation is difficult, PEEP may be required. In this case, it is important to support the arterial blood pressure by maximising circulating volume and administering inotropes as required.

Physiotherapy and suctioning will be required to maintain a patent airway. The increased stimulation associated with these procedures may cause rises in ICP. This can be minimised by additional boluses of sedation prior to treatment (Prasad & Tasker 1990), by limiting the number of suction catheters passed each time suction is required and by allowing the ICP to return to baseline prior to further intervention. Preoxygenation, prior to suction, can reduce the incidence of ICP spikes (Prendergast 1994) and reduce the risk of hypoxia with rises in ICP. There is some evidence that intravenous or endotracheal lignocaine can reduce sudden increases in ICP associated with endotracheal suction (Prendergast 1994).

Sedation and paralysis

The agitated child will require sedation and muscle relaxants to reduce cerebral oxygen requirements and consumption. The use of these drugs will interfere with the ability to assess the child neurologically. However, they will reduce the child's responses to stimulation and suction, contributing to the control of ICP. Reflexes such as coughing and gagging will increase intrathoracic pressure and stress, which both elevate ICP.

The use of sedatives may contribute to a fall in systemic pressure. Therefore, it is important to observe and monitor blood pressure, and it may be necessary to administer inotropes and additional fluid to maintain cardiac output (Fisher 1997).

Diuretics

Diuretics can be used to reduce ICP by reducing the fluid volume within the brain. Mannitol, an osmotic diuretic, reduces free brain water, which

is thought also to reduce blood viscosity and potentially improve blood flow to the cerebral tissue (Robinson 1997). Monitoring of serum osmolality is essential, as large doses of mannitol or repeated doses over a long period of time can lead to rebound rises in ICP. Loop diuretics such as frusemide may also be used, as they reduce or inhibit CSF production from the choroid plexus.

Pharmacological coma

Induction of coma may be necessary when other therapies have been unsuccessful at reducing ICP. The barbiturate thiopentone will lower ICP, reduce metabolic rate and oxygen consumption by inducing 'brain silence', in turn improving cerebral perfusion (Prasad & Tasker 1990). Although this is invaluable, there are a number of undesirable side effects such as respiratory infections, hypokalaemia, and renal and hepatic dysfunction. Therefore its use should be carefully considered. Storage and excretion of the drug makes it difficult to assess the child once treatment has ceased. Serum thiopentone levels should be assessed prior to neurological assessment.

Fluid and electrolyte management

Electrolyte imbalances are common with brain injury, with hyponatraemia causing most problems. Three main causes are:

- syndrome of inappropriate antidiuretic hormone secretion (SIADHS)
- cerebral salt wasting syndrome
- overhydration.

Therefore, fluid restriction with cautious replacement of both sodium and volume is necessary. Other common electrolyte disturbances include:

- hypo/hyperglycaemia
- diabetes insipidus
- hypokalaemia.

Therefore, electrolytes should be assessed twice daily and when changes are made to fluid therapy or if the child's condition deteriorates. Fluid restriction to two thirds normal requirements is often advocated to control intracranial pressure. However, this may contribute to electrolyte and hormonal disturbances, and fluid balance should therefore be monitored closely.

Temperature control

Temperature control is known to influence cerebral metabolism: for every 1°C rise in body temperature, cerebral metabolism may rise as much as 19% (Fisher 1997). Therefore, it is necessary to maintain normothermia by actively treating pyrexia with antipyretics, ice packs, or a cooling mattress. If there is a known cause of raised temperature, such as infection, appropriate treatment should be given. However, if the pyrexia originates from hypothalamic dysfunction, all treatments may be ineffective. The use of artificially induced hypothermia remains debatable. It is thought to reduce cerebral oxygen demand and provide protection to cerebral cells (Robinson 1997). Induction of systemic hypothermia to 32°C within the first 6 h of head injury is thought to protect the brain from ischaemia and the release of glutamate (see Head Injury, below). Cooling is undertaken using paralysing agents and cooling blankets with or without cold gastric lavage and is limited to a period of 48 h (Prendergast 1994). It is important that the temperature is not allowed to fall below 30°C, as clotting disorders and ventricular dysrhythmias may occur. More research is required into the use of hypothermia, as it also affects white cell function, causing the child's neurological condition to be complicated by pneumonia and other infections. Its use has not been shown to improve neurological outcome in children.

Patient position

Children should be nursed supine with the head in the midline position, to prevent jugular venous obstruction and maximise venous return. Venous return can be improved further by nursing the child on a head-up tilt of up to 30°. However, research into this practice has produced conflicting results (Prendergast 1994). Head elevation can result in a fall in mean arterial pressure, reducing CPP, but in some patients the ICP is lower when the head is elevated. Therefore, the use of head elevation should be assessed for individual children at regular intervals throughout their treatment.

A policy of minimal handling can prevent overstimulation and harmful rises in ICP. Clustering care at regular intervals can also overstimulate individual children. Extra sedation may be given prior to nursing intervention, or care can be staggered to prevent excessive stimulation. The response to stimulation should be assessed for individual children.

Stimulation can be positive, reducing stress, which may otherwise contribute to raised ICP. The effect on ICP of intervention from members of the child's family and use of familiar music should be assessed.

HEAD INJURY

Young children are at greater risk of sustaining head and neck injuries than adults, because of the higher ratio of head size to that of the rest of the body. An infant's brain constitutes 15% of total body weight, whilst an adult's brain in only 3% (Fisher 1997). The progressive fusion of the skull suture lines and thinner, pliable bones in infants often lead to local rather than global brain injuries.

Brain injury varies with age: in school aged children, road traffic accidents are often the primary cause for severe head injury, whereas infants and preschool age children commonly sustain injury from falls and non-accidental trauma. Males have a higher incidence of head injury irrespective of age.

Children often recover with only minor neurological deficits when compared with adults with similar severity of injury. This is largely because the brain continues to develop until approximately 7 years of age; therefore, more aggressive intensive care management can produce a good outcome.

Pathophysiology

The pathophysiological changes associated with

head injury can be divided into primary and secondary injuries. Primary injuries result from the biochemical effects of trauma to the brain. These injuries can be diffuse or focal, but the immediate effects occur as a direct result of the initial injury. Secondary injury occurs due to complications of the primary insult. Non-accidental injury should always be considered, especially if there is no satisfactory explanation of the injury.

Types of injury

Head injuries are classified according to the location, extent and severity of the injury as follows.

Scalp injury. This may be subdivided into:

- abrasion — break in the top layer of the skin, which may cause bleeding
- laceration — tear in scalp tissue, with a tendency to bleed profusely. Blood loss from these wounds should not be underestimated.

Skull injury. The type of skull fracture is dependent on the velocity, direction and momentum of impact. Fractures are classified as follows.

- Linear fracture is the most common type seen in children. The fracture is not displaced, and the dura mater remains intact
- Comminuted fracture results from fragmentation of bone or multiple fracture lines.
- Depressed fracture features inward depression of bone fragments below the normal contour of the cranium, without a tear to the dura.
- Basal skull fractures often involve dural tears with associated leakage of CSF, and the risk of meningitis. Haemorrhage or the development of an aneurysm/fistula may also occur if there is a fracture around the foramen magnum, where the internal carotid arteries enter the skull.

Brain injury. This is categorised as diffuse or focal.

Diffuse injuries. These include the following.

- *Contusion* is localised bruising of the brain resulting from a blow to the head or a shearing rotational injury of the brain. A coup injury occurs from damage to the cortex beneath the site of impact. A contre coup injury results from dam-

age due to the brain rebounding on the opposite side of the skull to the initial injury.

- *Hypoxic-ischaemic injury* is caused by impaired cerebral perfusion following a head injury. Autoregulation may be impaired during episodes of hypotension, causing reduced cerebral perfusion pressure.
- *Diffuse axonal injury* occurs as a result of mechanical shearing following acceleration/deceleration at the time of impact between the skull and hard object. The solid skull and semi-solid intracranial contents move at different speeds, causing tearing and disruption of axons.

Focal injuries. These include the following.

- *Cortical contusions and lacerations* may occur at the site of impact or immediately opposite. Contusions do not directly contribute to a decrease in conscious level, except in the presence of a haematoma. A cerebral laceration on the cortical surface may cause similar effects to cortical contusions.

Haemorrhage

Intracranial haemorrhage can be classified as:

- *extradural* — normally associated with a fracture of the temporal bone. There is often a rapidly expanding haematoma due to damage to the middle meningeal artery, requiring surgical intervention
- *intradural* — these are often a combination of subdural and intracerebral haematomas. These are often slow to develop and can be managed medically. If associated with retinal haemorrhages, non-accidental injury should be suspected.

Subarachnoid haemorrhages are not commonly seen in children; they may occur following severe head injury but can also occur spontaneously.

Intraventricular haemorrhages can occur as a result of rapid acceleration/deceleration injury, often associated with violent shaking or impact of a child's head against a solid object. This is also often seen in newborn infants with unstable blood pressure or following hypoxic episodes.

Secondary brain damage

Secondary brain damage may occur at any time following the initial injury. Causes include:

- hypercapnia
- hypoxia
- infection
- ischaemia
- brain swelling
- raised intracranial pressure
- reperfusion injury
- systemic hypotension
- electrolyte imbalance.

Although the initial impact is unavoidable, secondary brain damage is often preventable with the correct intervention and management.

Assessment and nursing management

Initial assessment and management concentrates on airway, breathing, circulation and disability.

Airway and breathing. In children with a severe head injury, with a GCS score of < 8, intubation is required to maintain an adequate airway. Care must be taken not to hyperextend the neck, causing cervical damage. Artificial ventilation to establish adequate respiration and optimisation of cerebral perfusion is of paramount importance. Oral intubation is often undertaken, as a head injury may have produced a cranial vault opening via a basilar skull fracture. Until basal skull fracture is excluded, an orogastric tube is also advocated to prevent further damage or infection.

Circulation. Circulatory assessment is specifically aimed at controlling bleeding and maintaining an adequate circulating volume to produce a mean arterial pressure at the upper end of the normal limits for age.

Disability. All children who have sustained a head injury should be suspected of having a spinal cord injury until excluded. A hard collar is used to immobilise the cervical spine to maintain neutral alignment. Log rolling or straight lifting is used to move the child. Close monitoring of neurological status and vital signs is important to detect or reduce the risk of secondary injury. Ongoing management is based on the care of a child with raised ICP (see above), with nursing priorities relating to the assessment and monitoring of neurological status. Prediction of long-term neurological outcome is extremely difficult, but the consequences of a head injury can be devastating. Therefore, families should be prepared for all potential outcomes.

SPINAL CORD INJURY

Spinal injuries occur as a result of excessive force from acceleration/deceleration events, resulting in:

- hyperextension
- deformation
- hyperflexion
- axial loading
- excessive rotation.

It is often the mechanism of injury that assists in determining the degree of stability.

Pathophysiology

Relative to the child's body, the head is large and heavy. Therefore, if a child sustains a head injury, it is more likely that hyperextension or flexion of the neck will result in a cervical spinal injury. The ligaments along the cervical vertebrae are relatively loose, with incompletely formed paraspinous muscles. The facet joints of the cervical vertebrae are relatively flat, enabling movement during the application of force. Therefore, during injury the vertebrae may shift.

Spinal cord injuries occur when vertebral bodies are fractured or when subluxation (partial dislocation) of the vertebrae occurs. The degree of neurological deficit is dependent on the severity of the subluxation. The spinal cord can be injured by:

- contusion
- concussion
- laceration
- transection

- haemorrhage
- damage to the vessels that supply the cord.

In most cases, the spinal cord is not severed at the time of injury but bruised or compressed. However, chemical and vascular changes occur relatively soon after the initial injury, causing the spinal cord to initiate an intrinsic process of self destruction. Children, however, often develop a delayed onset of symptoms, so repeated clinical evaluation of their movement and sensation should occur. The most consistent sign of spinal cord injury is loss of movement and sensation below the level of the injury. When all sensation and movement is lost, complete injury results, with partial injury causing parasthesis or transient weakness.

Investigation

Diagnosis can be made from lateral, cervical, thoracic and anteroposterior X-rays. Oblique views may also be taken to demonstrate the intervertebral foramina. CT and MRI scans can aid further with diagnosis, but the stability of the child will dictate the investigations carried out.

Assessment and management

Spinal injury must always be considered at the scene of any accident. The cervical spine should be immobilised, with log rolling or straight lifting used when assessment or transportation is required. On examination, the development of respiratory depression or neurogenic paradoxical breathing (indrawing of chest on inspiration due to absent intercostal activity) are indications of cervical spinal cord injury. Additional clinical signs are the absence of limb reflexes in flaccid limbs and unresponsiveness to painful stimuli.

Management depends on the stability and site of the lesion. However, the basic rules are:

- decompression
- stabilisation
- realignment.

An unstable injury risks further spinal cord damage, so stabilisation through operative fixation (spinal fusion) or immobilisation (plaster jacket, halo traction) is indicated. Decompression is mainly carried out when a patient with normal cord function, or with incomplete cord lesion, progressively deteriorates. Realignment of the vertebral column is often associated with decompression. Traction or surgical intervention may be required depending on the type of problem. Steroid therapy within 8 h of injury has been shown to be of benefit in reducing oedema and inflammation. However, it is not known whether this significantly improves functional outcome (Lyndsay et al 1997).

Long-term respiratory support may be required if respiratory muscles are involved. Therefore, aims of management include prevention of secondary problems such as infection and loss of skin integrity. In addition, it is important to maximise the child's quality of life, involving the family in decision-making and management and returning the child home, if this is possible.

CENTRAL NERVOUS SYSTEM INFECTION

Infection of the central nervous system is a common cause of neurological deterioration and deficit in infancy and childhood. Early diagnosis and treatment can reduce the risk of permanent neurological disability. The increase in foreign travel makes isolation of specific organisms difficult. Therefore, when assessing a child with possible central nervous system infection, it is important to determine whether he or she has travelled abroad. Common infections include encephalitis and meningitis, but focal neurological signs can result from cerebral abscess.

Encephalitis

Encephalitis is caused by inflammation of the brain associated with invasion of either toxic or infectious agents, including:

- viruses
- bacteria
- fungi

- parasites
- chemicals.

Neurological deterioration results from cerebral oedema and tissue damage. Encephalitis may occur during an acute viral illness or following vaccination (such as measles). Toxic encephalopathy (neurological disorder of unknown or noninfectious cause) may develop during a viral illness, in which inflammation is not a pathological feature, as seen in Reye's syndrome (Lyndsay et al 1997). It is more common in school age children than the younger age group.

Signs and symptoms

The signs and symptoms of viral encephalitis vary depending on the invading organism and the area of the brain involved. However, common signs include:

- headache
- fever
- neck stiffness
- nausea and vomiting
- seizures
- changes in level of consciousness
- visual, auditory and speech disorders.

On examination, CSF may be almost normal with slightly elevated protein and white cell count. CSF culture will be negative, but viruses may be detected.

Aims of management

Management is primarily supportive and symptomatic, as the underlying cause is often not detected. Neurological assessment is maintained in order to detect any signs of neurological deterioration, which could indicate further inflammation or an increase in intracranial pressure. Depending on local guidelines, prophylactic antibiotics and antiviral agents may be prescribed until bacterial, viral and mycoplasma infections are ruled out. Common drugs used include cefotaxime, acyclovir and erythromycin to cover all types of infection.

The herpes simplex virus is a rare but serious cause of encephalitis in infants and children. When untreated, it can cause devastating neurological damage with a high mortality rate. When treated early, outcome is improved. Therefore, there may be some benefit to administering acyclovir prior to confirmation of diagnosis in children with encephalitis (Cameron et al 1992).

Bacterial meningitis

Meningitis is much more commonly seen in infants and children than encephalitis. The highest incidence is seen in the first year of life, with increasing numbers of infections between 1 and 5 years and relatively few in school age children and adolescents (Fortnum & Davis 1993). Mortality is highest in the first year of life and in those infants and children affected by *Neisseria meningitidis* and *Haemophilus influenzae* (Fortnum & Davis 1993). A significant number of children have neurological sequelae ranging from hearing deficits to both mental and physical disability. In the UK, meningitis is a notifiable disease, to enable monitoring of incidence. However, the incidence is likely to be higher than recorded, as a significant number of cases are not notified to Public Health Authorities (Fortnum & Davis 1993).

Bacterial meningitis is an acute infection involving the meninges, particularly the pia and arachnoid space. Bacteria from the upper respiratory tract reach the subarachnoid space and meninges indirectly via the nasal mucosa, from where they enter the bloodstream. Alternatively, organisms can enter directly from connecting structures such as sinuses, skull fractures, or head wounds. In children, the most common causative organisms of bacterial meningitis change with age:

- neonates: — *E. coli*
        — Group B haemolytic *Streptococcus*
        — *Listeria*
        — others

- 1–11 months: — *Neisseria meningitidis*

— *Haemophilus influenzae*
— *Streptococcus pneumoniae*

- 1–5 years:
  — *Neisseria meningitidis*
  — *Haemophilus influenzae*
  — *Streptococcus pneumoniae*

- 5–16 years:
  — *Neisseria meningitidis*
  — *Streptococcus pneumoniae*
  — others.

Pathophysiology

The presence of bacteria within the subarachnoid and pia-arachnoid space triggers an inflammatory response. The underlying brain, although not invaded by bacteria, becomes congested, oedematous and ischaemic. The inflammation may cause cerebral vascular endothelial damage producing arteritis, venous thrombophlebitis or infarction of cerebral tissue. Oedema or scarring of the third ventricle can result, with stenosis of the Sylvian aqueduct leading to obstructive hydrocephalus.

Signs and symptoms

Clinical signs of meningitis will vary with age. In infants and young children the signs and symptoms are often non-specific and difficult to differentiate from other childhood illnesses affecting the upper respiratory tract and ears. Early signs include:

- fever
- headache
- irritability
- lethargy
- vomiting.

Later signs facilitate diagnosis, but indicate more critical illness. These include:

- neck stiffness and photophobia from meningeal irritation
- purpuric or petechial skin rash indicates meningococcal disease
- Kernig's sign — pain associated with the flexion of the upper leg and then extension of the knee, caused by the inflammation of the meninges and the spinal root

- Brudzinski's sign — a positive Brudzinski's sign is flexion of the knees and hips in response to flexion of the neck and head
- convulsions
- raised intracranial pressure
- reduction in conscious level and coma.

Other symptoms include:

- coagulopathies, especially associated with septicaemia
- endocrine disorders such as SIADH and diabetes insipidus.

Diagnosis

Diagnosis is made from examination of the CSF following lumbar puncture. This procedure should not be undertaken in the child with raised intracranial pressure, because of the risk of coning and brainstem death. In addition, children requiring assisted ventilation and those with loss of skin integrity in the lumbar region would be put at risk from lumbar puncture. These children should be treated for the most likely causative organisms.

CSF is examined for:

- bacterial culture
- microscopy
- rapid antigen detection
- protein and sugar
- staining for acid-fast bacilli.

In addition, viral and fungal cultures, serology and cytology should be undertaken to differentiate from other causes of meningitis. Blood cultures may also indicate the causative organism and should be taken, as CSF cultures are often negative. If bacterial meningitis is present, the following will be seen:

- high white cell count ($> 100 \times 10^6$/L)
- increased protein levels (> 0.6 g/L)
- reduced glucose (< 2.2 mmol/L).

Aims of management

Management includes treatment of the cause and prevention of secondary complications.

Therefore, it is important to administer antibiotics relevant to the most likely causative organism for the age of the individual child. Neurological assessment is essential to detect signs of deterioration of conscious level and rising ICP. In addition, cardiovascular and respiratory monitoring is essential, as severe shock is often associated with meningococcal meningitis, and respiratory depression is associated with reducing levels of consciousness.

Reye's syndrome

Reye's syndrome is a rare form of encephalopathy mainly confined to children. It is associated with fatty changes in the liver and other viscera. Although the cause is unknown, American studies in the 1970s and 1980s suggested that there was a higher incidence of Reye's syndrome amongst children who had been given salicylates (aspirin) during the course of an acute viral infection. Since the recommendation that salycilates should no longer be given to children under the age of 12 years, this syndrome is rarely seen in the 1990s.

Pathology

Liver cellular mitochondrial damage interrupts the normal pathways for detoxification of waste products. Thus, hyperammonaemia occurs along with fatty infiltration of the liver, kidneys and myocardium and cerebral oedema.

Signs and symptoms

Acute deterioration occurs in the days following the viral infection. The initial symptoms are recurrent vomiting and developing encephalitis.

The liver becomes infiltrated with small lipid drops, whilst the mitochondria of both the liver and the brain become enlarged. A decreasing level of consciousness ensues as a result of the developing encephalopathy, cerebral oedema and raised ICP.

Hepatic enzymatic activity is decreased, resulting in reduced conversion of toxic ammonia to urea. The high levels of ammonia exacerbate the developing encephalopathy.

Aims of management

Management aims primarily to maintain and support vital functions and treat underlying infection:

- correct coagulapathies
- reduce ammonia levels
- monitor ICP and CBF.

STATUS EPILEPTICUS

Status epilepticus is a medical emergency which, if untreated, can lead to irreversible brain damage and death. Seizures occur at such a rate that the body does not have time to recover between episodes, preventing a return to consciousness. Status epilepticus is defined as a period of 30 min or more of continuous seizure activity or repeated seizures with reduced level of consciousness between seizures. Tonic-clonic status epilepticus is the most common and life-threatening form. It may be caused by:

- head trauma
- metabolic abnormalities
- rapid growth spurts in children with epilepsy, or withdrawal from anti-epileptic medication
- alcohol
- central nervous system infection
- fever.

Pathophysiology

The exact trigger is unknown. Electrical disturbance caused by repeated firing of neurons in the brain increases the metabolic demands of cerebral cells, with a resulting reduction in essential nutrients and potential cell death. This activity may be confined to a small area of neurons and remain localised, resulting in focal seizures. However, involvement of a larger area of neurons leads to generalised tonic-clonic seizures.

Cerebral blood flow is increased to maximise oxygen and glucose for increased cellular activity. In addition, the constant rapid contraction and relaxation of muscles increases tissue oxygen requirements. Therefore, oxygen requirements can be significantly increased.

Signs and symptoms

When seizure activity is sustained during status epilepticus, rapid depletion in glucose and ATP levels occurs. Hypoxia and hypercapnea are common due to laryngospasm and the chest wall being maintained in tonic inspiration. An increase in sympathetic activity results in systemic hypertension and the potential for cardiac arrhythmias. If the body is unable to sustain an adequate CBF to maintain oxygenation, then cellular exhaustion, cerebral ischaemia and cell destruction occur with the potential for brain death if seizure activity continues.

It is important to recognise that myoclonic or tonic-clonic seizure activity will be suppressed in the child receiving paralysing agents. Therefore, observation of vital signs for tachycardia, pupil dilatation, fluctuations in blood pressure and poor systemic perfusion is required. Cerebral function analysing monitors (CFAM) can be used to provide a constant recording of the EEG, enabling detection of prolonged seizures.

Aims of management

The management of status epilepticus requires maintenance of vital functions, cessation of seizure activity, monitoring of neurological status, prevention of complications and treatment of the underlying cause of the seizure activity.

- Maintenance of airway involves positioning to avoid aspiration, and adequate oxygenation. Although facial oxygen may be sufficient, airway intubation is often necessary in severe status.
- Observation and monitoring of cardiorespiratory signs. Hypotension and bradycardia can result in inadequate systemic and cerebral perfusion and should, therefore, be treated by maximising circulating volume and providing inotropic support when hypotension is severe.
- Signs of increased ICP should be treated as described above. However, reduction in seizure

activity often reduces ICP and should therefore be the treatment priority.
- Core temperature should be monitored to eliminate febrile convulsions as the cause of seizures. Tepid sponging and antipyretic therapy should be administered if pyrexia is apparent.
- Metabolic screening should occur to correct any derangement, which could be the focus for seizure activity.
- Once seizure activity has been controlled, then all efforts should be taken to determine the underlying diagnosis.

Anticonvulsant therapy

Anticonvulsant agents are essential to stop seizure activity, but many can have significant side effects. First line drugs include:

- intravenous or rectal diazepam — can cause respiratory depression and hypotension
- rectal paraldehyde.

These may stop or reduce seizure activity in the short term, but alternative drugs may be required to halt seizure activity in the long term.

- Phenytoin — serum levels should be monitored, as side effects include hypotension and cardiac dysrhythmias. Enteral feeds should be stopped 30 min before administering phenytoin into the stomach, as these reduce absorption. In status, doses are most effectively delivered intravenously, with ECG monitoring.
- Phenobarbitone — may be required in doses which cause respiratory depression and reduced level of consciousness. Serum levels should be monitored, particularly when used in conjunction with other anticonvulsants such as phenytoin, carbamazepine and sodium valproate.
- Heminevrin — cardiovascular and respiratory depression are common with high doses and prolonged infusion. Once seizures are controlled, the dosage should be reduced. Assisted ventilation may be required with high doses.
- Clonazepam — can cause increased salivary and respiratory secretions. Serum levels should be monitored, and respiratory depression is associated with intravenous infusion.
- Midazolam — has been shown to rapidly

control seizure activity when given by continuous infusion, with little respiratory depression (Koul et al 1997).

- Lorazepam — given intravenously or rectally as a single dose, has been suggested as a good alternative to diazepam due to a reduced incidence of respiratory depression (Appleton et al 1995).
- Propofol — used to produce coma in refractory status epilepticus. Requires continuous EEG monitoring, but the short half life of propofol facilitates the process of waking the patient (Borgeat et al 1994).
- Thiopentone — used to produce coma in refractory status epilepticus. Requires continuous EEG and cardiovascular monitoring, as hypotension is common, often requiring inotropic support to maintain systemic blood pressure. In addition, the drug is excreted slowly, with recovery of conscious level taking several days in many patients.

BRAIN TUMOURS

These are abnormal masses arising from any tissue in the body that has undergone uncontrolled cell division. Two-thirds of all childhood brain tumours are located in the posterior fossa region, with medullablastomas and cerebellar astrocytomas being the most common.

Classification of brain tumours as benign or malignant can be misleading. A tumour that is histologically benign and well differentiated may be surgically inaccessible, and therefore continued growth of the tumour will cause a rise in ICP, herniation and death.

Classification of intracranial tumours can be made according to location, histologic features and degree of malignancy. In 1979, the World Health Organization (WHO) agreed an international classification of intracranial tumours based on the tissue of origin (Lyndsay et al 1997).

Types of brain tumour

Supratentorial tumours involve the cerebral hemispheres and structures above the tentorium cerebelli:

- *Astrocytomas* arise from abnormal proliferation of the cerebral astrocytes and often contain a cyst filled with fluid rather than solid tissue. They are the most common supratentorial brain tumours in children. Their growth may be slow or rapid, spreading into the surrounding tissues. They can be found in all areas of the brain; therefore symptoms are related to the specific region involved.
- *Craniopharyngioma* arises from the growth of displaced neuroepithelial cells and lies close to the pituitary stalk. It is a nodular tumour with cystic areas containing cellular and calcified material. Obstruction of the pituitary gland, optic pathways and hypothalamus will occur as the tumour increases in size. Therefore, symptoms depend on the degree of obstruction. It is predominantly present in children and young adults.

Infratentorial tumours involve the brainstem and cerebral structures below the tentorium cerebelli:

- *Medulloblastomas* arise from the cerebellar vermis extending into the fourth ventricle. They occur predominantly in children, with a peak age of 5 years old (Lyndsay et al 1997). They are highly malignant, with rapid growth leading to spread throughout the CSF pathways.
- *Brainstem tumours* are cysts that compress the vital centres of the brain. They develop mainly in children and young adults (Lyndsay et al 1997). The prognosis is very poor, as surgical removal is not often possible. Chemotherapy is often of no value, thus radiotherapy is the treatment of choice.

Treatment

Chemotherapy aims to destroy the cancer cells, but may affect normal tissue. Therefore each child's treatment is specific to the type of tumour, age of the child, amount of surgical removal and the child's general health. The main side effects are:

- hair loss
- marrow suppression
- nausea and vomiting.

Radiotherapy is a painless form of treatment that is used to destroy tumour cells. Irradiation is often the treatment of choice for tumours that are surgically inaccessible or the remains of a tumour that cannot be totally excised. As with chemotherapy, the dosage of radiation is calculated for each individual child's needs and is given in divided doses, which can often mean weeks of treatment. The main side effects are:

- hair loss
- sore/dry skin
- bone marrow suppression.

Aims of management

- Maintain the airway, with ventilatory support when required. Ensure adequate physiotherapy and suction are given. Neurological assessment is important to observe for signs of increased intracranial pressure. Treatment of raised intracranial pressure is described above.
- Following surgical intervention to remove the tumour, it is important to observe for signs of haemorrhage and excessive fluid loss if a wound drain is in situ. In addition, observation for orbital oedema is important, particularly if tarsorrhaphy has been used. The suture between the eyelids may need cutting if orbital oedema becomes excessive.
- Intravenous fluids will be prescribed until the patient is extubated and has adequate cough and gag reflexes. Once enteral feeds are commenced, vomiting may be a sign of or lead to increased ICP.
- Urine output and specific gravity are monitored for signs of diabetes insipidus and SIADH. Diabetes insipidus is most common following removal of a craniopharyngioma, due to its close location to the pituitary gland.
- Hypo/hyperthermia may occur postoperatively. Persistent pyrexia may indicate infection.
- Adequate analgesia is essential, and codeine may be the drug of choice to facilitate accurate neurological assessment.

DIABETES INSIPIDUS

Diabetes insipidus (DI) is characterised by a fluid imbalance occurring as a result of:

- decreased production of antidiuretic hormone (ADH) (vasopressin) — central or neurogenic DI
- reduced responsiveness of the kidneys to ADH — nephrogenic DI.

The following section will focus on central DI, as two-thirds of patients developing this have sustained a head injury, a CNS infection, intraventricular haemorrhage or have undergone neurosurgery. This can develop quickly or appear up to 14 days after surgery/insult. Central DI can be divided into four subcategories (Parobek & Alaimo 1996):

- Type 1 — resulting from failure of the pituitary to produce/release ADH — the classic DI seen in head injuries
- Type 2 — high plasma osmolarity fails to stimulate ADH release, due to defective osmoreceptors
- Type 3 — ADH release is only stimulated when plasma osmolarity is abnormally high due to alteration of the pituitary gland's sensitivity following cerebral insult
- Type 4 — ADH secretion is inadequate in relation to serum osmolarity.

Pathophysiology

ADH is normally released in response to:

- increased extracellular osmolality
- decreased circulating volume.

Large volumes of dilute urine are produced in DI, because of the lack of ADH acting on the renal collecting tubules, thus resulting in insufficient reabsorption of water. The child's circulating volume becomes depleted, causing hypernatraemia as a result of haemoconcentration. The osmotic gradient causes fluid to move from the intracellular to the intravascular space, which is quickly lost from the circulation. Intravascular hypovolaemia stimulates aldosterone secretion from the adrenal cortex, leading to reabsorption of water and sodium from the proximal renal tubule. This increases serum sodium, but the water reabsorbed has little effect on serum osmolality or on intravascular volume.

An alert child may compensate by drinking large volumes of fluid. However, the child only receiving intravenous fluids may become hypovolaemic and hypernatraemic with serum hyperosmolality.

Signs and symptoms

These include:

- normal to impaired level of consciousness
- increased serum sodium level (> 145 mEq/L)
- low urine sodium
- serum hyperosmolality (> 295 mOsm/kg)
- urine specific gravity < 1.005
- polyuria — up to 200–300 mL/h
- high blood urea nitrogen (BUN)
- decreased extracellular fluid
- reduced body weight.

If untreated, signs of hypovolaemic shock may develop. Diagnosis can be made on these clinical symptoms and by eliminating other possible underlying pathology.

Management

Management aims to:

- replace lost intravascular volume
- correct electrolyte imbalances
- administer vasopressin.

Intravenous access is essential to administer fluids and to measure central venous pressure (CVP). Hourly urine volumes are replaced with crystalloid over the following hour. Replacement fluid depends on assessment of serum and urine electrolytes and osmolality, monitoring of sodium levels is essential. Hypovolaemic shock is treated with 10–20 mL/kg boluses of 5% dextrose or dextrose saline administered over 15–20 min.

In acute situations, vasopressin may be given by intravenous infusion, with dosage dependent on urine output. In less extreme cases, adminis-

tration is by subcutaneous or intramuscular injection, although absorption may be slow and irregular. A positive response is indicated by a decrease in urine volume (1 mL/kg/h) and a rise in specific gravity (> 1.010) and osmolality. During the vasopressin infusion, the child should be closely monitored for side effects, including:

- ↑↓ heart rate
- ↑↓ blood pressure
- signs of hypersensitivity
- abdominal cramps.

If the child responds to vasopressin, replacement intravenous fluids must be tapered off as urine output reduces, to prevent water intoxication. DI is usually transient following cranial insult, resolving within days or weeks. Permanent DI only develops if over 80% of ADH-producing nuclei of the hypothalamus or proximal end of the pituitary are destroyed (Parobek & Alaimo 1996).

SYNDROME OF INAPPROPRIATE ANTIDIURETIC HORMONE SECRETION

SIADH is characterised by an abnormally high or continuous secretion of antidiuretic hormone (ADH). In children this usually occurs as an acute event, but can be a chronic problem. Injury to the hypothalamus or pituitary gland significantly increases the risk of the child developing SIADH. It is most commonly seen in children following:

- head injuries
- intracranial haemorrhage
- encephalitis
- meningitis
- Guillain Barré syndrome
- neurosurgery
- hydrocephalus
- increased intracranial pressure
- ADH-secreting tumours.

Pathophysiology

The hypothalamus produces the hormone

arginine vasopressin, or ADH. This is transported to the posterior pituitary gland, from where it is released in response to differences between extracellular and intracellular osmolality.

ADH acts directly on the distal renal tubules and collecting ducts to increase permeability, allowing water to be reabsorbed into the intravascular space. Less water is lost in the urine, reducing urine volume and increasing concentration. Increased absorption of water decreases the serum osmolality and increases the blood volume, which decreases secretion of ADH. However, in SIADH, the hormone continues to be secreted and the ADH levels remain elevated. Thus, water continues to be reabsorbed, resulting in hyponatraemia and serum hypo-osmolality. Urine output remains reduced but with elevated osmolality and sodium concentration.

Signs and symptoms

The first sign is usually low urine output, less than 1 mL/kg/h, associated with weight gain. Urine sodium concentration and osmolality remain high, while serum sodium and osmolality are low. Additional fluid intake fails to increase urine output, and water continues to be absorbed. If the situation continues, water intoxication may occur, with water passing from the intravascular space into the cerebral tissue, producing lethargy and stupor progressing to seizures and coma.

Management

Renal and adrenal disease need to be excluded prior to confirming SIADH when the child responds to fluid restriction and correction of hyponatraemia. Fluid intake is restricted to 30–75% of maintenance. Fluid input and output are assessed hourly. The aim is to increase fluid output and decrease urinary sodium and osmolality. Twice daily weights also assist in assessment of fluid loss. Monitoring of serum and urine electrolytes is required, including:

- sodium
- potassium

- chloride
- osmolality.

Close monitoring of the child's neurological state enables detection of water intoxification. Treatment may include administration of intravenous hypertonic saline and a loop diuretic such as frusemide. This increases serum sodium concentration and eliminates excess intravascular water.

Occasionally the child may develop chronic ADH secretion requiring permanent therapy, usually lithium carbonate or demeclocydine to inhibit the effect of ADH on the renal collecting tubules. The underlying cause of SIADH must be treated.

MYASTHENIA GRAVIS

Definition

Myasthenia gravis is thought to be an autoimmune disorder affecting transmission at the neuromuscular junction. Unless occurring during the neonatal period, it is a chronic disorder causing weakness of skeletal and facial muscles, which in extreme cases can lead to respiratory failure.

Pathophysiology

There is neuromuscular dysfunction caused by:

- a decreased number of acetylcholine receptor sites at the myoneural junction
- blockage of the remaining receptor sites by acetylcholine antibodies which are present in the synaptic cleft. Thus, acetychloline is inactivated before it has an opportunity to reach the limited number of receptor sites. Diagnosis is made by titres for acetylcholine receptor antibodies, electromyogram (EMG) and a tensilon test.

Tensilon test. Tensilon (edrophonium) is a short-acting anticholinesterase drug given intravenously. The child will almost immediately show a dramatic, temporary increase in muscle strength.

Classification

There are three types of myasthenia gravis seen in children.

- Neonatal — occurs in infants born to myasthenic mothers. It involves muscles associated with the distal cranial nerves, causing dysphonia and dysphagia. It resolves spontaneously within the first 5 days of life.
- Congenital — onset occurs within the first few days of life. Mothers of these infants rarely have myasthenia gravis, but it may be present in siblings. Respiratory failure is very unusual, but the infants will be poor feeders, and extraocular muscles will be affected.
- Juvenile — may be present after the age of 2 years, but is most commonly present during adolescence. It first presents in muscles supplied by the lower cranial nerves. This is the form of myasthenia gravis seen in adults.

Signs and symptoms

The muscles controlling ocular movement are most often affected first. The eyelids droop, with ptosis and double vision. The muscles of the face and neck become affected, causing bulbar palsy with difficulty eating, chewing and speaking. As the disease progresses there may be sudden paralysis of the respiratory muscles, causing a *myasthenic crisis*. Severe respiratory failure is often diagnosed before this stage, requiring intubation and artificial ventilation. The most common cause of myasthenia crisis is insufficient medication.

Management

Management of acute myasthenia gravis includes assessment and treatment of immediate problems – specifically, respiratory failure and assessment of effectiveness of medication. Treatments include the following:

- Anticholinesterase drugs inhibit acetylcholinesterase in the synaptic cleft. The availability of acetylcholine for binding with receptor sites consequently increases, reversing the muscle weakness or paralysis. Medications most commonly used are neostigmine and pyridostigmine. This medication must be taken according to a strict regime and must not be stopped abruptly.
- Immunosuppression is thought to complement anticholinesterase therapy by reducing the production of acetylcholine receptor antibodies. Prednisolone is most commonly used but, in severe cases, azothioprine and cyclophosphamide can also be administered.
- Plasmapheresis can give temporary remission in a myasthenic crisis, as acetylcholine receptor antibodies are protein bound.
- Thymectomy may improve muscle strength either immediately or months following surgery for some children, as the thymus gland may increase the development of acetylcholine receptor antibodies. Thymectomy may have long-term implications for the development of the immune system in children.

Cholingeric crisis is caused by overmedication producing the opposite of myasthenic crisis. Signs of excessive parasympathetic activity include:

- tear production
- salivation
- diarrhoea
- abdominal cramps
- nausea and vomiting
- bradycardia.

There will also be a negative tensilon test. Symptoms will respond to the withdrawal of anticholinesterase therapy. Severe symptoms require intravenous atropine or glycopyralate. Both cholinergic and myasthenic crises are life threatening and require intensive care.

Drugs for intubation

Suxemethonium should not be used for children with myasthenia gravis as prolonged scoline apnoea can occur. Non-depolarising muscle relaxants such as atracurium, should be used in low doses with extreme caution.

Other less common neurological problems

encountered within the PICU include cerebral abscess and Guillain–Barré syndrome. Children following near drowning episodes can also require management of raised intracranial pressure. The principles of management of children with these problems are the same as outlined above and will not be addressed individually in this text.

COMMON DIAGNOSTIC TESTS

The developments in X-ray techniques, computerised tomography and magnetic resonance imaging allow detailed and non-invasive investigations to aid diagnosis in children with neurological dysfunction. Common investigations include the following.

Skull and spinal X-rays. These provide specific information regarding:

- size and shape of skull
- bone abnormalities
- abnormal calcification or erosion
- fractures.

This investigation is often used in conjunction with other diagnostic tests.

Lumbar puncture. This aids diagnosis of:

- intracranial and intraventricular haemorrhage
- infection.

If increased intracranial pressure is suspected then this procedure should not be undertaken, as transtentorial herniation can occur, causing irreversible damage to vital centres in the brainstem.

Computerised axial tomography (CAT) scan. This allows non-invasive visualisation of the cross sections of the brain at regular intervals between the cervical spine and the crown of the head. This can be enhanced using intravenous radioisotope contrast. This is useful for diagnosing:

- cerebral oedema
- haemorrhage
- space-occupying lesions
- cerebral atrophy
- hypoxic-ischaemic damage
- alterations in CSF circulation.

Magnetic resonance imaging (MRI) scan. This enables non-invasive visualisation of soft tissue and can also be enhanced using intravenous contrast. A magnetic field is applied around the child, therefore metallic objects should be placed outside the scan to prevent injury. MRI gives more detailed pictures of the brain that clearly outline the anatomy.

Cerebral angiography. This provides visualisation of intracranial and extracranial blood vessels by injection of radioisotope contrast into the cerebral arterial system or through catheterisation of the carotid or vertebral arteries. This assists diagnosis of:

- aneurysms
- arterial venous malformations.

Electroencephalography (EEG). This provides intermittent or continuous recording of cerebral electrical activity, and can detect abnormal function not visualised by scanning. Deviation from normal electrical activity is recognised by means of:

- frequency
- location
- form
- amplitude
- functional properties.

An EEG specifically aids the diagnosis of epilepsy. It also assists in the diagnosis of brain death, usually demonstrating the absence of brain waves. Brainstem evoked potentials can also be measured by applying specific sensory stimuli and recording the electrical activity created. The three brainstem sensory pathways tested are:

- auditory
- visual
- somatosensory.

BRAINSTEM DEATH AND ORGAN DONATION

Definition of brainstem death

Pallis defines brainstem death as 'the irreversible loss of capacity for consciousness, combined with the irreversible loss of capacity to breathe' (British Paediatric Association 1991, p. 2).

Diagnosing brainstem death

In 1968, the Harvard Medical School produced a set of criteria to confirm the definition of irreversible coma to guide medical practitioners. More recently the conference of the Royal Medical Colleges produced further guidelines, since revised in 1991. These guidelines identify three essential preconditions for brainstem testing), as follows.

1. The patient's condition is due to irreversible structural brain damage. If the primary diagnosis is unclear then the patient does not fulfil these criteria.
2. The patient requires ventilatory support as a result of inadequate spontaneous respiration. The use of muscle relaxants must be eliminated as a cause of respiratory failure. As muscle relaxants block nerve impulses at the neuromuscular junction, the reversal of neuromuscular blockades must be demonstrated by the presence of peripheral reflexes or by response to a nerve stimulator (BPA 1991). Narcotic drugs induce respiratory and central nerve depression; therefore, serum barbiturate levels should be measured prior to brainstem testing (Stephenson 1987).
3. The patient is deeply comatose. Factors shown to affect neurological function are hypothermia, drug interaction, metabolic and endocrine abnormalities.

As core temperature falls below 33–35°C, the thermoregulatory system becomes ineffective, with loss of consciousness occurring at 30°C. Hypothermia in critically ill children commonly occurs, slowing responses and metabolism, thus mimicking brain death (Stephenson 1987). Therefore it is essential to ensure the child is normothermic prior to brainstem testing.

Metabolic and endocrine disorders can also alter level of consciousness. It is essential that serum glucose, electrolytes and acid–base balance are within normal parameters prior to testing. Severe acidosis and abnormal electrolytes, such as severe hyponatraemia, are specific causes

of metabolic coma. Blood glucose level below 2.2 mmol/L can induce hypoglycaemic coma.

With the dramatic improvements in technology in the care of infants, including the very premature, the issue of discontinuing ventilation in the presence of irretrievable brain damage generates much debate. In 1988, the Council of the British Paediatric Association formed a working party to review the diagnosis of brainstem death in infants and children. It recommended that children over the age of 2 months fulfilled the same criteria identified by the Conference of Royal Medical Colleges in 1976. The exception is that one of the assessors carrying out the brainstem tests should be a paediatrician.

In the case of infants between 37 weeks gestation and 2 months of age, the working party concluded 'that given the current state of knowledge it is rarely possible confidently to diagnose brainstem death at this age' (BPA 1991, p. 1). In infants below 37 weeks gestation, the working party acknowledged that the concept of brain death was inappropriate. Therefore, decisions regarding continuation of treatment are based on discussion with the family and medical assessment of the child's likely outcome.

Confirmatory investigations

Additional tests to assess brainstem function include:

- electroencephalogram (EEG)
- cerebral angiography
- cerebral blood flow measurements.

The BPA (1991) reviewed the use of these investigations and concluded that these additional investigations were useful in diagnosing brainstem death.

Brainstem death tests

Brainstem tests must be carried out by two senior clinicians, one of whom should be involved primarily with the child's care. The BPA recommends that one of these clinicians should be a paediatrician and the other a consultant.

The tests are divided into two catergories:

- brainstem and cranial nerve function — to fulfil the criteria of brainstem death, all brain reflexes should be absent (Box 10.1).
- assessment of apnoea.

Box 10.1 Signs of brainstem death

1. pupils fixed with no response to light
2. absent corneal reflex
3. no vestibulo-ocular reflex
4. no motor response to painful stimuli within the cranial nerve distribution
5. no gag or cough reflex to tracheal stimulation
6. no respiratory movement when respiratory centre is stimulated by $PaCO_2$ > 6.6 kPa

Adapted from Tatman et al (1997).

Pupillary response to light. If the brainstem is intact, the pupils react to light by constricting briskly and consensually. If the child is brainstem dead, the pupils will be fixed, unresponsive and often fully dilated.

Corneal reflex. An intact brainstem elicits an automatic blink reflex when an object approaches the eye. If brainstem function is absent, this reflex will be apparent when a piece of cotton wool is stroked across the cornea.

Vestibulo-ocular reflex (cold water calorics). The child's head is tilted to a 30° angle and approximately 10 mL of iced water is injected into the ear canal. When the vestibulo-ocular reflexes are intact, a slow horizontal nystagmus towards the stimulus, followed by a rapid nystagmus away from the stimulus is apparent. Absent reflexes are indicated by no eye movement in response to this test. The tympanic membrane must be intact and clearly accessible.

Motor response to pain. If brainstem death is indicated, there will be no motor response from cranial nerves when a central painful stimulus is applied. Peripheral stimuli may produce limb reflexes.

Cough or gag response. This reflex is tested by inserting a catheter into the endotracheal tube, or the back of the throat, to stimulate the mucosa. Brainstem death is indicated when no cough or gag reflex is elicited.

Apnoea. This is demonstrated when no respiratory effort is made, despite a rise in $PaCO_2$ to greater than 6.6 kPa in the presence of a normal PO_2 (BPA 1991). However, the Taskforce for the Determination of Brain Death in Children (1987) recommended that a rise in $PaCO_2$ to greater than 7.92 kPa is required to establish a respiratory drive.

The criteria required for apnoea testing are constantly debated. Outwater & Rockoff (1984) established that the $PaCO_2$ in children rises by approximately 0.54 kPa/min during apnoea. They therefore suggest that 5 minutes of apnoea is sufficient time to allow stimulation of the respiratory effort.

Apnoea testing requires preoxygenation with 100% oxygen prior to ventilator withdrawal and oxygenation for the duration of the testing with a continuous flow of 100% oxygen. Arterial blood testing is required to establish that a rise in $PaCO_2$ is sufficient to establish an adequate respiratory stimulus.

An observational period then follows prior to repetition of the test. No specific observation time is recommended, but the procedure needs to be approached in an unhurried manner, ensuring that all the stated preconditions are satisfied. However, a prolonged period of time may cause emotional hardship for the family and possible detrimental effects on organs for possible donation.

If there is no response to the second set of tests and organ donation is inappropriate, reconnection to the ventilator is inappropriate. However, this may be necessary to allow the child's family time to prepare for discontinuation of therapy.

Organ donation

Early explanation of organ donation is essential if a child is considered as a possible donor. This is a stressful and a difficult decision for families, but media coverage has increased awareness and many families will raise the issue themselves.

Following parental consent and completion of the first set of brainstem tests, the transplant coordinator will be contacted, who will be able to answer questions from the family. The child will be electively ventilated until organ donation occurs. Ethically this is difficult for both staff and the child's family, especially if PIC bed usage is under pressure.

Nursing implications

It is essential that the nurse caring for the child has significant knowledge of brainstem testing and organ donation, in order to support the family. If the tests are negative, then the aim of care

may change to facilitating a dignified death and possibly organ donation.

Families have often had little time to adjust to the child's illness and require significant support, particularly if organ donation is being considered. The family should be given an opportunity to say goodbye to their child before and after surgery to remove the organs. Acceptance of death is often only achieved when the family is able to see and hold the child without ventilatory and technical support.

REFERENCES

Allan D 1994 Paediatric coma scale. Surgical Nurse 7(3):14–16

Appleton R, Sweeney A, Choonara I, Robson J, Molyneux E 1995 Lorazepam versus Diazepam in the acute treatment of epileptic seizures and status epilepticus. Developmental Medicine and Child Neurology 37:682–688

Borgeat A, Wilder-Smith O H G, Jallon P, Suter P M 1994 Propofol in the management of refractory status epilepticus: a case report. Intensive Care Medicine 20:148–149

British Paediatric Association 1991 Diagnosis of brain stem death in infants and children. Working Party Report. BPA, London

Cameron P D, Wallace S J, Munro J 1992 Herpes simplex virus encephalitis: problems in diagnosis. Developmental Medicine and Child Neurology 34:134–140

Conference of Medical Royal Colleges and Faculties in the UK 1976 Diagnosis of brain death. British Medical Journal 2 (Nov):1187–1188

Downey D L, Leigh R J 1998 Eye movements: pathophysiology, examination and clinical importance. Journal of Neuroscience Nursing 30(1):15–23

Fisher M D 1997 Pediatric traumatic brain injury. Critical Care Nursing Quarterly 20(1):36–51

Fortnum H M, Davis A C 1993 Epidemiology of bacterial meningitis. Archives of Disease in Childhood 68:763–767

Germon K 1994 Intracranial pressure monitoring in the 1990s. Critical Care Nursing Quarterly 17(1):21–32

Hickey J V 1996 The clinical practice of neurological and neurosurgical nursing. Philadelphia, JP Lippincott

Hickey J 1992 The Clinical Practice of Neurological and Neurosurgical Nursing, 3rd edn. Philadelphia, JB Lippincott

Koul R L, Aithala G R, Chacko A, Joshi R, Elbualy M S 1997 Continuous midazolam infusion as treatment of status epilepticus. Archives of Disease in Childhood 76:445–448

Lindsay K, Bone I, Callander R 1997 Neurology and neurosurgery illustrated, 3rd edn. Churchill Livingstone, New York

Lower J S 1992 Rapid neuro assessment. American Journal of Nursing (June):38–45

Moore K L 1998 Essentials of human embryology. Blackwell Scientific, Oxford

McCance K L, Heuther S E 1994 Pathophysiology. St Louis, Moshy

Outwater K M, Rockoff M A 1984 Apnea testing to confirm brain death in children. Critical Care Medicine 12(4):357–358

Parobek V, Alaimo I 1996 Fluid and electrolyte management in the neurologically impaired patient. Journal of Neuroscience Nursing 28(5):322–328

Prasad A, Tasker R 1990 Guidelines for the physiotherapy management of critically ill children with acutely raised intracranial pressure. Physiotherapy 76(4):248–250

Prendergast V 1994 Current trends in research and treatment of intracranial hypertension. Critical Care Nursing Quarterly 17(1):1–8

Robinson A L 1997 Focus on paediatric intensive care—The management of raised intracranial pressure in children. Current Anaesthesia and Critical Care 8:8–13

Simpson D, Reilly P 1982 Pediatric coma scale. Lancet ii (8295):450

Stewart N 1996 Neurological observations. Professional Nurse 11(6):377–378

Stewart-Amidei C 1998 Neurological monitoring in the ICU. Critical Care Nursing Quarterly 21(3):47–60

Stephenson C 1987 Brain death in children. Focus on Critical Care 14(1):49–56

Taskforce for the determination of brain death in children 1987 Guidelines for the determination of brain death in children. Pediatric Neurology 3(4):242–243

Tatman A, Warren A, Williams A, Powell J E, Whitehouse W 1997 Development of a modified paediatric coma scale in intensive care clinical practice. Archives of Disease in Childhood 77(6):519–521

Teasdale G 1975 Acute impairment of brain function — 1: Assessing conscious level. Nursing Times 71(24):914–917

Williams J 1992 Assessment of head injured children. British Journal of Nursing 1(2):82–84

FURTHER READING

Buzea C 1995 Understanding computerised EEG monitoring in the intensive care unit. Journal of Neuroscience Nursing 27(5):292

Conference of Medical Royal Colleges and Faculties in the UK 1995 Criteria for the diagnosis of brain stem death: a working party report. Journal of the Royal College of Physicians of London 29 (Sept/Oct):381–382

Price T E 1996 An evaluation of neurological assessment tools in the intensive care unit. Nursing in Critical Care 1(7):72–77

Rodrigo E, Murray M, Mejia P et al 1995 Variability in brain stem death determination practices in children. JAMA 274(17):550–553

Staworn D et al 1994 Brain death in pediatric intensive care unit patients: incidence, primary diagnosis and the clinical occurrence of Turner's triad. Critical Care Medicine 27(8):1301–1305

Teasdale G, Galbraith S, Clarke K 1975 Acute impairment of brain function — 2: Observation record chart. Nursing Times 71(25):972–973

11

Care and management of infants and children with renal dysfunction

*Karen Lockhart   Rachelle Lowe
Judith Harris*

Renal failure is seen in paediatric intensive care in association with a variety of problems, including sepsis, trauma and following cardiopulmonary bypass. When detected early and managed effectively, the majority of cases of acute renal failure (ARF) in children are reversible (Maxwell et al 1992). This chapter will address normal renal physiology and provide an overview of the diagnosis and management of ARF.

The developing renal system

Embryological development of the kidneys begins during the first week of gestation (Bissinger 1995). The mesonephric duct produces urine between 6 and 10 weeks gestation, but ceases this function at around 10 weeks to become part of the developing sex organs in boys (Larsen 1993). The metanephros develops from the mesonephric duct during week 5 (Fig. 11.1) as the ureteric bed and produces urine which contributes to the amniotic fluid at 9 weeks. This structure will eventually develop into the definitive kidney at around the 32nd to 36th week of gestation (Fig. 11.2).

Nephron formation commences at 8 weeks and is complete between 32 and 36 weeks, after which further development involves only growth and maturation. Cortical nephrons develop later than the juxtamedullary nephrons as development of the kidneys occurs outwardly from the centre.

The developing kidneys ascend from the pelvis to the lumbar region by the 9th week of

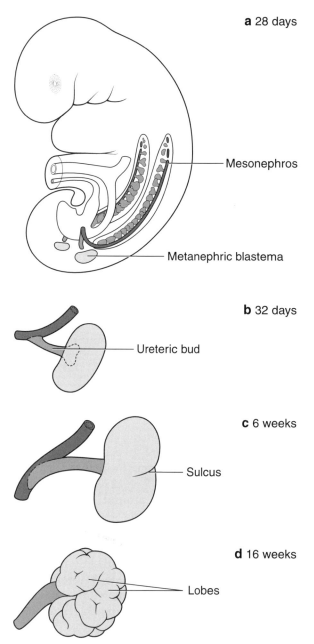

a 28 days

Mesonephros

Metanephric blastema

b 32 days

Ureteric bud

c 6 weeks

Sulcus

d 16 weeks

Lobes

Figure 11.1 Origin of the metanephric kidneys.
(A) A metanephric blastema develops from intermediate
mesoderm on each side of the body axis early in the 5th
week. (B) Simultaneously, the metanephric ducts sprout
ureteric buds that grow into each metanephric blastema.
(C) By the 6th week, the ureteric bud bifurcates, and the two
growing tips (ampullae) induce superior and inferior lobes in
the metanephros. (D) Additional lobules form during the next
10 weeks in response to further bifurcation of the ureteric
buds. From Larsen (1993), with permission.

gestation. At this time they are separate and in
the adult position, above the waist, against the
posterior abdominal wall, outside the peritoneum and partially protected by the ribs.

Renal blood supply

Blood supply is from the renal arteries, which
contribute to both glomerular and peritubular
capillary networks. Blood leaves the glomerulus
via the efferent arteriole, which in turn supplies
the peritubular capillary network. From this network, blood drains into the venous system to be
removed via the renal vein.

Pressure within the glomerular capillaries is
high, facilitating constant filtration through the
glomerular capsular membrane. In contrast, peritubular capillaries form a low-pressure system
around the renal tubules, which contain approximately 2% of the cardiac output (Bissinger 1995).
This arrangement facilitates reabsorption of water
and solutes and, thus, concentration of urine.

Mature kidneys receive 20–25% of the cardiac
output. At birth, this may be as low as 5%, due to
high renal vascular resistance (Bissinger 1995).
This increases to 15% in the neonatal period and
continues to rise during the first year of life.
Renal vascular resistance is high in infancy
because of the high levels of circulating renin and
immaturity of the sympathetic nervous system
which adjusts the diameter of renal vessels
(Gluckman & Heymann 1993, McCance &
Heuther 1994).

Functions of the kidney

The kidney is primarily involved in the homeo-
static control of the volume and content of the
blood, fulfilling the following functions:

- excretion of waste products of metabolism,
  including urea, creatinine and ammonia
- regulation of solutes, including sodium,
  potassium, chloride, calcium, phosphate and
  magnesium
- regulation of plasma pH through hydrogen
  ion secretion and bicarbonate reabsorption
  and generation

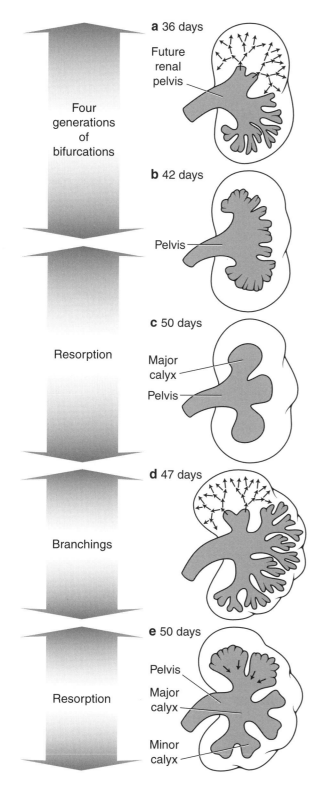

a 36 days

Future renal pelvis

b 42 days

Pelvis

c 50 days

Major calyx

Pelvis

d 47 days

e 50 days

Pelvis

Major calyx

Minor calyx

Four generations of bifurcations

Resorption

Branchings

Resorption

Figure 11.2 Development of the renal pelvis and calyces. (A–C) The first bifurcation of the ureteric bud forms the renal pelvis, and the collapse of the next four generations of bifurcations produces the major calyces. (D,E) The next four generations of bifurcation collapse to form the minor calyces of the renal collecting system. From Larsen (1993), with permission.

- regulation of blood pressure by secreting renin from the juxtaglomerular apparatus (JGA)
- activation of Vitamin D to 1,25 dihydroxycholecalciferol, which influences calcium and phosphate balance
- production of erythropoietin which stimulates red blood cell production from the bone marrow.

RENAL PHYSIOLOGY

The functional unit of the kidney is the nephron, of which there is a full complement of 1 to 1.5 million at birth. Each nephron is made up of a Bowman's capsule and glomerulus and renal tubules (Fig. 11.3). Large volumes of glomerular filtrate are filtered at the Bowman's capsule, but only small volumes of urine are produced through reabsorption and secretion.

Two types of nephron have been identified:

- cortical nephrons
- juxtamedullary nephrons.

Cortical nephrons make up approximately seven-eighths of the total number and are found in the outer and midcortical regions. These nephrons have short loops of which only a small segment lies within the medulla. Perfusion is poor at birth, but increases rapidly as renal vascular resistance falls. Adult values for assessing renal function are seen when the cortex is mature. Cortical nephrons are thought to be salt losing, as blood flow to this area is increased when serum sodium is high.

In contrast, juxtamedullary nephrons are thought to be associated with sodium balance and concentration of urine. The glomeruli of these nephrons lie deep in the cortex, with long loops extending deep into the medulla. These nephrons are more mature at birth, with greater blood flow than cortical nephrons (Bissinger

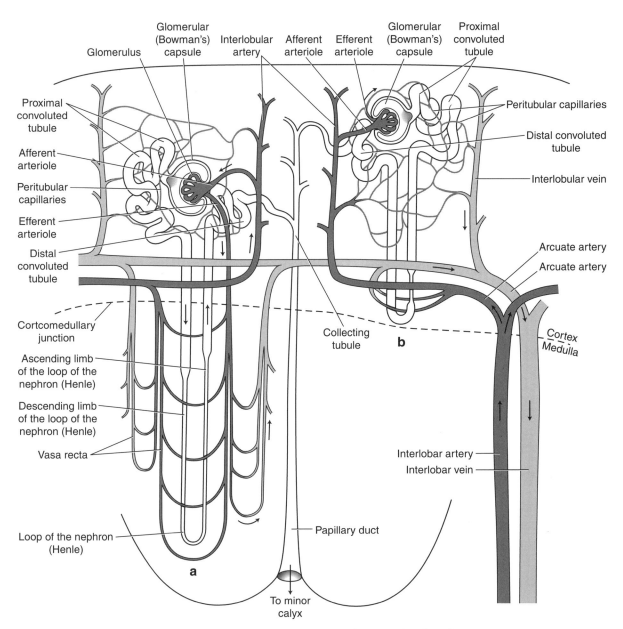

Figure 11.3 Nephrons: (a) juxtamedullary; (b) cortical. From Tortora & Anagnostakos (1990).

1995). However, the loops are short during infancy, resulting in production of dilute urine with low urea content as this is conserved to produce a concentration gradient within the renal medulla.

Urine production involves three processes:

- glomerular filtration
- tubular reabsorption
- tubular secretion.

Glomerular filtration

Filtration occurs across the glomerular–capillary membrane as a result of the interplay between

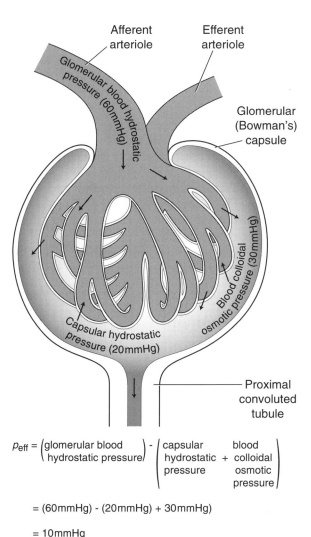

$$p_{eff} = \begin{pmatrix} \text{glomerular blood} \\ \text{hydrostatic pressure} \end{pmatrix} - \begin{pmatrix} \text{capsular} & & \text{blood} \\ \text{hydrostatic} & + & \text{colloidal} \\ \text{pressure} & & \text{osmotic} \\ & & \text{pressure} \end{pmatrix}$$

$$= (60 \text{mmHg}) - (20 \text{mmHg}) + 30 \text{mmHg}$$

$$= 10 \text{mmHg}$$

Figure 11.4 Forces involved in effective filtration pressure (P_{eff}). From Tortora & Anagnostakos (1990).

the pressures within the capillaries and the Bowman's capsule (Fig. 11.4). Glomerular capillary hydrostatic pressure (GCHP) approximately equals systemic arterial pressure and contributes to movement of fluid out of the capillaries into the capsule. This is opposed by blood colloidal oncotic pressure (BCOP), which is generated by proteins and other large molecules in the blood, and tubular hydrostatic pressure (THP) or the pressure of filtrate in the capsule. The resultant net filtration pressure (NFP) forces water and solutes across the membrane:

$$NFP = GCHP - (BCOP + THP)$$

Net filtration pressure, and thus GFR, can be altered by changes in cardiac function, circulating volume and passage of urine along the tubules. However, autoregulatory mechanisms controlling the diameter of the afferent and efferent arterioles ensure that GFR is maintained across a wide range of systemic blood pressures. The 10th to 12th thoracic nerves and the vagus nerve provide sympathetic and parasympathetic innervation of the vessels respectively. These ensure that blood flow is increased during periods of mild hypotension and restricted during hypertension to maintain effective excretion of fluid and solutes.

The glomerular–capillary membrane acts as a sieve, preventing large molecules and formed elements of the blood passing into the renal tubules. The glomerular basement membrane is negatively charged, repelling the plasma proteins which may be small enough to pass through the sieve. The ultrafiltrate has an ionic content similar to plasma, containing water, glucose, vitamins, amino acids, electrolytes and nitrogenous waste.

Tubular reabsorption

Tubular reabsorption involves movement of water and solutes from the renal tubules to the peritubular capillaries, using both active and passive processes. Passive processes require no energy, as movement of water and solutes occurs along electrical and concentration gradients. For example, water moves by osmosis from an area of low solute concentration to an area of high concentration. Active processes require energy, as movement occurs against an electrical or concentration gradient. Substances reabsorbed actively include sodium (Na^+), chloride (Cl^-), glucose and bicarbonate (HCO_3^-).

As much as 99% of the filtrate can be reabsorbed into the blood, with as little as 1% excreted as urine. Water and solutes are removed at different points along the tubules, with fine balance of water and sodium controlled by antidiuretic hormone (ADH) and aldosterone, respectively.

The proximal convoluted tubule is the primary site for reabsorption of water and many filtered solutes. 100% filtered glucose and amino acids are reabsorbed here, with between 80% and 90% of the sodium and potassium. Active transport of substances such as glucose and phosphate requires a carrier molecule. These molecules are often involved in the transport of more than one substance, but are available in large enough amounts that this does not prevent effective reabsorption during normal conditions. When glucose appears in large quantities in the blood, as in diabetes or during extreme stress, it may also be found in small amounts in the urine. This occurs because each substance has a renal threshold above which some of the substance will remain in the urine. However, reabsorption will continue until all carriers are saturated and the transport maximum has been reached. At this point the carrier molecules are unable to transport any more of the substance and large quantities will be found in the urine. For those substances, like phosphate, which are regulated by the kidney, the renal threshold and transport maximum will be similar to the quantity of filtered substance. Other substances requiring a carrier molecule include sulphates and nitrates. These substances are also found in the urine when large quantities occur in the blood.

The Loop of Henle provides a countercurrent mechanism for concentration of urine. It has a thin-walled descending limb, which is highly permeable to water but relatively impermeable to solutes such as urea and sodium. Therefore, the filtrate becomes more concentrated as it passes down the Loop. The ascending limb is impermeable to water but chloride is actively reabsorbed, facilitating the passive movement of sodium. The vasa recta provides a countercurrent exchange mechanism to maintain a concentration gradient between the filtrate, interstitium and blood. This is achieved by the movement of water from the vessels to the interstitium in exchange for Na^+ and Cl^-. Together with reabsorption of urea, this contributes to the countercurrent mechanism, which concentrates the filtrate to make it hypertonic in the thick-walled ascending limb of the Loop (Fig. 11.5).

Within the distal convoluted tubule, the filtrate becomes hypotonic, as the wall of the tubule is relatively impermeable to water but permeable to solutes, including sodium, chloride, potassium, bicarbonate, calcium and magnesium. The proximal portion of the distal tubule contacts with the afferent arteriole of the glomerulus at an area within the juxtaglomerular apparatus called the macula densa. Together with the juxtaglomerular cells, this is responsible for regulating renal blood flow, glomerular filtration and renin secretion. The permeability of the wall of the latter portion of the tubule is controlled by ADH, which regulates water loss.

The collecting ducts are involved in the acidification of urine by reabsorbing sodium, potassium, hydrogen and bicarbonate.

Tubular secretion

Secretion involves active or passive movement of substances from the blood into the tubules to be excreted in the urine. Secreted substances include ammonia, creatinine, potassium, urea, hydrogen and drugs. This process plays an essential part in the control of blood pH. Neonates have restricted ability to excrete acids in the urine. This is not generally a problem unless the infant becomes unwell, as infants are anabolic, using protein for growth. As the protein content of the diet is increased during infancy, renal acid excretion is increased.

Immature renal transport mechanisms and poor response to ADH make fluid and electrolyte balance easily compromised during illnesses such as gastroenteritis and infection during the first 2 years of life. In the neonatal period, approximately 9% of energy expenditure relates to reabsorption of sodium and water (Seaman 1995). The control of sodium reabsorption in response to rapid changes in serum sodium is poorly developed, which may be due to lack of aldosterone receptors in the distal convoluted tubules or lower transportation thresholds. In addition, neonates have lower serum bicarbonate levels, as they are unable to reabsorb large quantities of bicarbonate, because of immaturity of proximal tubular transport mechanisms (Gluckman & Heymann 1993).

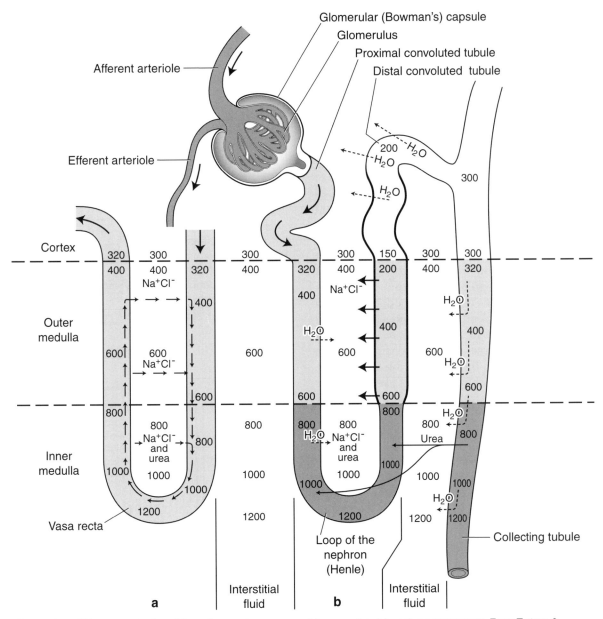

Figure 11.5 Urine concentration: (a) cardiovascular component (vasa recta); (b) nephron component. From Tortora & Anagnostakos (1990).

Mechanisms controlling renal blood flow and glomerular filtration

Glomerular filtration rate (GFR) is maintained at a normal level by autoregulatory mechanisms controlling renal blood flow within a wide range of systemic arterial pressures. The mechanisms involved are controlled by the juxtaglomerular apparatus, an area of specialised cells between the distal convoluted tubule and the afferent arteriole of the glomerulus. The area of tubular cells in contact with the arteriolar wall is called the macula densa. This is responsible for monitoring the sodium and chloride content within the tubule and adjusting the diameter of the afferent arteriole to regulate blood flow. For example, when circulating blood volume is increased, blood pressure is raised, which in turn increases afferent arteriolar pressure. This will increase the NFP, raising the volume of fluid filtered at the glomerulus, leading to ineffective tubular function. This is detected by the macula densa, which causes the afferent vessel to constrict, reducing blood flow and the rate of filtration.

A reduction in blood flow or volume through the afferent vessels stimulates the release of renin from the juxtaglomerular cells within the apparatus. Renin is present from 13 weeks gestation (Seaman 1995) and is responsible for arterial blood pressure regulation, sodium and potassium balance and regional blood flow. Once released into the blood, it stimulates angiotensin from the liver and kidneys to form angiotensin I. This is converted to angiotensin II in the lungs. Angiotensin II stimulates the adrenal cortex to release aldosterone and causes the efferent vessels to constrict, thus maintaining GFR (Fig. 11.6).

Renin, aldosterone and ADH release are all suppressed by the hormone atrial natriuretic factor (ANF), released from the atria in response to stretch of the atrial walls. Therefore, when there is a high circulating volume, ANF acts on the tubules as a potent diuretic to promote sodium and water loss.

Glomerular filtration rate

GFR has traditionally been measured using calculation of creatinine clearance:

$$GFR = \frac{\text{urine creatinine} \times \text{volume urine/minute}}{\text{plasma creatinine}}$$

However, in infants and young children, this can be an inaccurate method of measuring GFR, because of the difficulties associated with collecting total urine volume in this age group. Therefore, a more accurate method involves the administration of intravenous inulin, which is a substance neither metabolised nor absorbed by

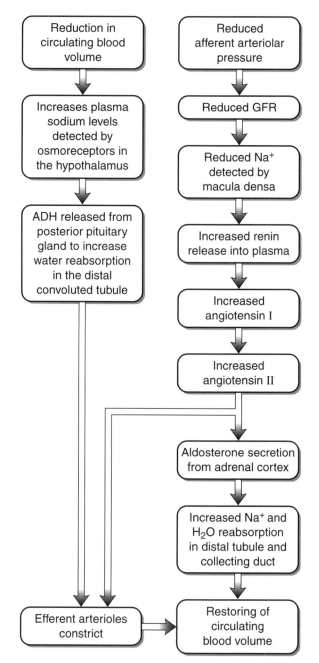

Figure 11.6 Mechanisms controlling arterial blood pressure and renal blood flow. Adapted from Seaman (1995).

the body, but is totally excreted by the kidneys. Three to five blood samples are taken over a 4 h period following the administration of inulin. GFR is calculated using a single-injection plasma

Table 11.1 Glomerular filtration rates in infancy

Age	GFR
Premature infant	12 mL/min/1.73 m^2
Term infant	20 mL/min/1.73 m^2
2 weeks	40 mL/min/1.73 m^2
2 years	125 mL/min/1.73 m^2
Adult	125 mL/min/1.73 m^2

Source: Bissinger (1995).

disappearance curve. The faster the rate of disappearance, the higher the GFR in mL/min.

Normal GFR in older children and adults is 125 mL/min/1.73 m^2. This is much lower in the neonatal period and increases to adult values by the age of 2, when renal vascular resistance will be normal (Table 11.1).

Acid–base balance

Acid–base balance refers to regulation of H$^+$ ions. Maintaining pH within normal limits (7.35 to 7.45) is a complex process which involves chemical buffers, the lungs and kidneys. Hydrogen is produced from the metabolism of proteins, fats and carbohydrates required by the body. Maintenance of H$^+$ levels within normal limits is essential for the function of proteins such as enzymes. To achieve this, the body uses three systems:

- buffer system — effective immediately
- respiratory system — effective in minutes
- renal system — effective in hours to days.

The focus here will be on the role of buffers and the renal system in this process, which involves reclaiming HCO$_3^-$ and excreting H$^+$ and fixed acids.

The buffer system

Buffers are pairs of chemicals which respond to changes in hydrogen ion concentration, preventing significant changes in pH. Within each chemical pair, an acid is responsible for releasing H$^+$ when levels fall, and the base combines with it when levels rise. The most commonly assessed buffer pair is the bicarbonate:carbonic-acid system important in intra- and extracellular fluid. This system uses the enzyme carbonic anhydrase to produce rapid H$^+$ ion exchange prior to excretion either through the lungs or renal system:

$$H_2O + CO_2 \rightleftharpoons H_2CO_3 \rightleftharpoons H + HCO_3$$

The renal system

The kidneys play an important role in acid–base balance by buffering and eliminating fixed acids, regulating H$^+$ secretion and reabsorbing HCO$_3^-$ to maintain the HCO$_3^-$:H$_2$CO$_3$ buffer system. The lungs are only able to excrete hydrogen ions if the kidneys regenerate HCO$_3^-$ for use within the buffer system.

80–90% of HCO$_3^-$ is passively reabsorbed in the proximal convoluted tubule, along a concentration gradient. Within the tubule cell, carbonic acid is broken down into H$^+$, which is excreted into the filtrate in exchange for Na$^+$ and HCO$_3^-$ which is reabsorbed. In the filtrate, H$^+$ combines with HCO$_3^-$ prior to conversion to CO$_2$ and H$_2$O. The CO$_2$ diffuses into the cell to contribute to the cycle of reclamation of HCO$_3^-$. This process is dependent on the continuous exchange of H$^+$ for Na$^+$ (Fig. 11.7).

In the distal convoluted tubule, H$^+$ excretion is achieved through the phosphate buffer system, due to the limited amount of HCO$_3^-$ available:

$$H^+ + HPO_4^- \rightarrow H_2PO_4$$

This process promotes H$^+$ excretion, preventing filtrate pH rising above 4.5 (Fig. 11.8).

Hydrogen ions are also excreted in combination with ammonia. Ammonia combines with H$^+$ in the tubule to form ammonium, which is positively charged and thus unable to diffuse back into the cell (Fig. 11.9):

$$H^+ + NH_3 \rightarrow NH_4^+$$

This mechanism is important in conditions where chronic acidosis is a problem.

Assessment of acid–base balance involves analysis of pH, CO$_2$, base deficit or excess and HCO$_3^-$ levels in the blood. After the neonatal period, normal values equate to those seen in adults.

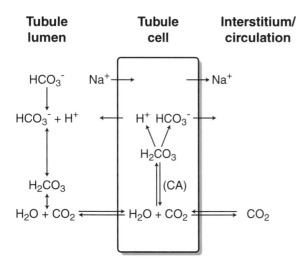

CA = carbonic anhydrase

Figure 11.7 Reabsorption of bicarbonate in the renal tubules. Adapted from Seaman (1995).

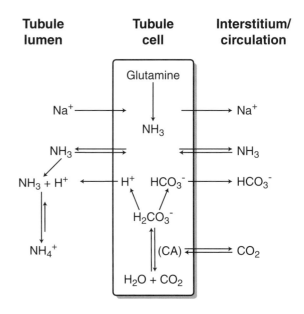

CA = carbonic anhydrase

Figure 11.9 Hydrogen excretion with ammonia. Adapted from Seaman (1995).

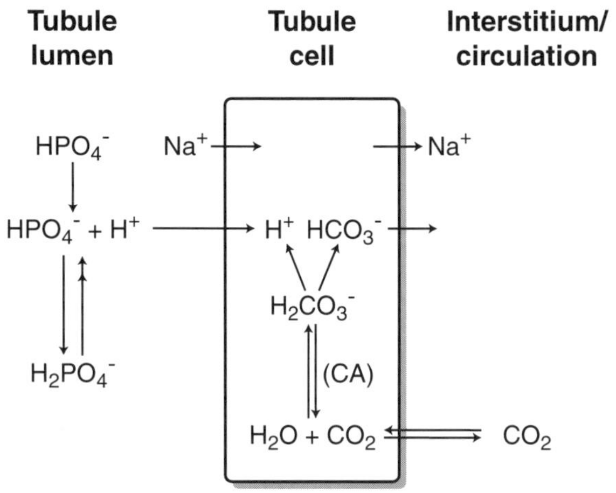

Tubule lumen | **Tubule cell** | **Interstitium/ circulation**

HPO_4^- $Na^+ \longrightarrow$ $\longrightarrow Na^+$

$HPO_4^- + H^+ \longrightarrow$ H^+ $HCO_3^- \longrightarrow$

$H_2CO_3^-$

(CA)

$H_2PO_4^-$ $H_2O + CO_2 \longrightarrow CO_2$

CA = carbonic anhydrase

Figure 11.8 Hydrogen excretion with phosphate buffer. Adapted from Seaman (1995).

ACUTE RENAL FAILURE

Acute renal failure (ARF) results from a sudden decrease in renal function accompanied by retention of nitrogenous wastes and disturbance of water, electrolyte and acid–base balance. A sudden decrease in GFR or increase in serum creatinine is often sufficient to cause symptoms, which are frequently reversible. Onset is rapid and often secondary to an identifiable cause. Complete recovery often occurs when ARF is detected and treated early.

ARF should be anticipated following:

- cardiac or other major surgery
- episodes of shock
- multiple trauma
- thermal injury
- birth asphyxia, hypotension or RDS in neonates
- episodes of hypoxia
- multiple organ system failure
- chemotherapy
- administration of nephrotoxic agents, e.g. aminoglycosides
- transfusion reactions
- episodes of illness in children with chronic renal failure or renal transplant
- investigations requiring IV contrast

(Toro-Figueroa et al 1992).

Classification of ARF

ARF can be classified into three groups by cause:

- pre-renal
- intrinsic
- post-renal.

Pre-renal causes

This is the commonest and least severe form of ARF, caused by reduced perfusion of the kidneys:

- a reduction in circulating volume due to either loss or redistribution of volume, e.g. haemorrhage, septic shock or anaphylaxis
- a reduction in cardiac output, e.g. congestive cardiac failure
- renal artery obstruction
- asphyxia.

Reduced circulating volume results in poor renal blood flow causing a reduction in filtered sodium and water and stimulation of angiotensin release. Unless reduced perfusion is prolonged, renal function returns with correction of the problem.

Intrinsic causes

Intrinsic renal failure results from damage to parts of the nephron (glomeruli, tubules or vessels). This can be secondary to chronic pre-renal or post-renal causes, toxins or infections. In addition, acute tubular necrosis (ATN) can develop following:

- severe cardiovascular instability
- hypoxia
- sepsis
- ingestion of drugs or toxins.

Specific causes include:

- nephrotoxins (aminoglycosides, NSAIDs, ACE inhibitors, myoglobin, IV contrast)
- coagulation disorders (DIC, haemolytic uraemic syndrome)
- diseases of the kidney and vessels (glomerulonephritis)
- ATN

- congenital disorders (polycystic disease, renal hypoplasia)
- infections
- tumours
- prolonged electrolyte disorders
- systemic illness (systemic lupus)
- renal transplantation.

Acute tubular necrosis is the commonest cause of ARF in critically ill children. Toxins and reduced renal blood flow cause necrotic damage to the tubule epithelium. This damage is reversible, as these cells are able to regenerate. Damage to the glomerular basement membrane produces areas of fibrosis, as epithelial cells are unable to regenerate in this area. Recovery time can be prolonged, making it difficult to assess the degree of permanent damage.

Post-renal causes

Obstruction to urine flow can be caused by a variety of problems:

- extrarenal mass (Wilm's tumour, neuroblastoma)
- blood clots
- calculi
- inflammation/oedema
- posterior urethral valves
- posterior insertion of ureters.

Relief of the obstruction usually involves surgery, which often results in return to normal renal function. An initial increase in urine output called post obstructive diuresis may occur before homeostasis is achieved with intravascular volume and electrolyte imbalance corrected.

Diagnosis

Anticipation and early detection of failing renal function may enable clinicians to prevent ARF, by treating underlying causes. Close monitoring of serum electrolytes in children at risk of developing ARF will enable clinicians to observe trends in creatinine and urea levels. Creatinine may be the best indicator of failing kidneys, with rising levels reaching above 132 µmol/L. High urea levels may not be an indicator of ARF, as this is linked to factors such as diet. However, high urea may be an indication for dialysis, as untreated uraemia will lead to severe neurological problems and death.

Clinical signs that also contribute to the diagnosis include:

- rising serum potassium and phosphates
- falling serum sodium, bicarbonate, calcium and pH
- oliguria (< 1 mL/kg/h), although polyuria and normal urine output do occur
- pulmonary oedema
- peripheral oedema
- high CVP
- changes in urine osmolarity and sodium.

A fluid challenge with 10 mL/kg of normal saline may increase the CVP in a child with ARF. The additional administration of up to 5 mg/kg of frusemide may produce a diuretic response. However, if urine output remains minimal, fluid intake should be restricted to 35 mL/kg/24 h in infants, 15–20 mL/kg/24 h or 300 mL/m^2/day in children. Additional fluids may be given to replace urinary losses.

Aims of management

- Maintain fluid balance.
- Maintain urea and electrolytes within the normal range.
- Provide adequate nutrition in order to prevent catabolism.

This usually involves dialysis as a replacement for renal function until the child's kidneys recover.

RENAL REPLACEMENT THERAPIES

Chemical indications for acute dialysis are:

- hyperkalaemia (greater than 6 mmol/L)
- uraemia (greater than 40 mmol/L)
- hypervolaemia
- acid–base imbalance.

Children may require renal replacement therapy for one or a combination of the above factors. However, renal replacement therapies may be indicated in other situations:

- children following prolonged bypass time during surgery for correction of congenital heart defects, who are at great risk of developing acute renal failure due to acute tubular necrosis; those with poor cardiac output may be dialysed early to facilitate improved fluid management before acute renal failure is well established
- children with chronic renal failure
- children with inborn errors of metabolism who have lost the ability to compensate for their defect through viral illness or dehydration.

Clinical indications for renal replacement therapies are:

- acute renal failure not responding to conservative management
- chronic renal failure
- drug poisoning
- fluid overload with multisystem failure
- metabolic disorders: hyperammonaemia, pyruvate dehydrogenase deficiency
- need for high calorie intake with major fluid restriction.

Principles of dialysis

Dialysis involves the transportation of solutes and water molecules across a semipermeable membrane. In peritoneal dialysis the peritoneum acts as the semipermeable membrane, whereas in haemofiltration or haemodialysis a synthetic membrane is used. Diffusion and ultrafiltration are the main principles involved in movement of solutes and water across these membranes. Convection plays an important part in haemofiltration.

Diffusion. Diffusion is the movement of solutes along a concentration gradient from an area of high concentration to an area of low concentration. Diffusion of solutes will continue until equilibrium is reached. In dialysis, waste products and electrolytes diffuse from the blood into the dialysate, and solutes such as calcium, magnesium and potassium diffuse from the dialysate into the blood.

Ultrafiltration. Ultrafiltration is the movement of fluid through a membrane, caused by a pressure gradient. This can result from hydrostatic or osmotic pressure.

Convection. Convection is the movement of solutes with water, which has been referred to as 'solvent drag'. The greater the movement of water the larger the volume of solute transported.

A range of therapies is available for the child in PICU requiring renal replacement therapy:

- peritoneal dialysis
- haemofiltration
- haemodialysis.

Peritoneal dialysis

Peritoneal dialysis (PD) is used as a treatment for acute or chronic renal failure, and is particularly useful for small children and infants, who have a relatively large peritoneal surface compared with adults. This allows more rapid diffusion of solutes than would be achievable with adults; therefore, it is frequently considered as the treatment of choice in infants and young children.

Ultrafiltration caused by osmosis is the main principle involved in movement of solutes in peritoneal dialysis. The glucose used in dialysis fluid generates a high osmotic pressure which induces ultrafiltration from the blood and prevents absorption of the dialysate (Levine 1991). Osmotic pressure combined with the permeability of the peritoneum affects ultrafiltration rates.

Contraindications to peritoneal dialysis are:

- diaphragmatic hernia, gastroschisis and necrotising enterocolitis
- damage to the peritoneal membrane from trauma, surgery or peritonitis (abdominal surgery in itself is not a contraindication if the peritoneum remains intact)
- inborn errors of metabolism — slow removal of solutes and toxic metabolites render it unsuitable for these children.

The peritoneum is the largest serous membrane of the body and consists of a layer of simple squamous epithelium with an underlying supporting layer of connective tissue. The two layers of the peritoneum line the inside wall of the abdominal cavity and cover the abdominal organs. Potential space between the layers is referred to as the peritoneal cavity, and it contains serous fluid and surfactant. The rich blood supply of the peritoneum facilitates effective dialysis.

In peritoneal dialysis, warmed fluid is instilled into the peritoneum via a soft or rigid peritoneal catheter, allowed to dwell and then drained out. The dialysate fluid used consists of glucose with calcium, sodium, magnesium chloride and lactate. Potassium is not included by the manufacturers but can be added on the basis of the child's serum potassium level (Box 11.1).

Box 11.1 Composition of peritoneal dialysis fluid (mmol/L)	
Glucose	1.36%, 2.27%, 3.86%
Na^+	132
K^+	0
Ca^+	1.75
Mg^+	0.75
Cl^-	102.0
Lactate	35

Cooled dialysis fluid has been used with success in the hyperpyrexial child to reduce body temperature.

Lactate is the buffer of choice for most manufacturers. This is metabolised by the body to generate bicarbonate. Children unable to tolerate lactate because of hepatic failure or severe lactic acidosis may require a solution containing bicarbonate (Box 11.2). This fluid will not include calcium or magnesium, because of the resultant precipitation of salts. These electrolytes may need to be administered concurrently according to the needs of the child.

Diffusion and ultrafiltration take place within the peritoneal cavity, removing excess electrolytes, fluid, waste products and correcting acid–base imbalance. The time allowed for dwelling of dialysate fluid and the concentration and quantity of fluid affects the degree of fluid and solute removal. For example, a long dwell time allows equilibration to take place, whereas a shorter dwell period enhances fluid and solute removal.

Box 11.2 Composition of bicarbonate dialysis fluid

NaCl 0.9%,	650 ml
Dextrose 5%,	300 ml
Dextrose 50%,	10 ml
NaHCO$_3$ 8.4%,	40 ml

Gives

Na$^+$	140 mmol/L
Dextrose	2%
Bicarbonate	40 mmol/L

This solution has been used in the PICU at Guy's Hospital, London, produced by pharmacy in 3 litre bags.

Peritoneal dialysis can be achieved by manual or automated methods. Some machines can perform fluid exchanges as small as 50 mL, and with the use of special neonatal administration sets the priming volume can be just 5 mL in the patient line.

Usually 30 mL/kg of dialysis fluid is used for each cycle, but 20–50 mL/kg can be effective. Larger volumes may cause a degree of respiratory compromise due to diaphragmatic splinting during the dwell phase. In some instances cardiovascular instability can occur with changes in blood pressure during the dwell and the drain periods.

A typical peritoneal dialysis cycle would be:

- fill — 5 min
- dwell — 15 min
- drain — 10 min.

Dwell times of 10–15 min enhance the efficiency of solute clearance and ultrafiltration. Extended dwell times reduce the rate of solute and fluid loss, which may be desirable when the child is more stable. Dwell times in excess of 10 min are advocated to allow diffusion to take place (Lowrie & Stark 1990). Drain times should be long enough to allow for complete emptying after each cycle.

However, in some institutions, two dialysis catheters are inserted in the peritoneal cavity and fluid is constantly administered through one catheter and constantly drained through the other. Anecdotal evidence suggests that, although this method does not appear to utilise a dwell time, the efficacy of the treatment is unaffected. This might be explained by the fact that filling of the peritoneum would inevitably have to take place before the process of filling and concurrently draining could take place. The chosen fill volume would then be topped up and drained constantly, thus allowing fresh dialysis fluid to enter the peritoneum and dialysate to be drained.

Heparin (500 iu/L dialysate) is frequently added to dialysate to prevent clotting and fibrin formation in the catheter. There is no systemic anticoagulation from a dose of this size (Lowrie & Stark 1990). Potassium is added to dialysate as required, but it is important to remember that, because solutes diffuse along the concentration gradient, solutes can be lost from the child into the dialysate or absorbed from the dialysate into the child. If the child has a normal serum potassium, then the addition of up to 4 mmol/L potassium chloride should allow the child to maintain a normal serum potassium. When calculating the required additives, it is advis-able to identify the amount of potassium supplement present in any enteral or parenteral fluids.

Complications of peritoneal dialysis

Splinting of the diaphragm and respiratory compromise may necessitate a reduction in cycle volume. Elevating the child's head can help to reduce the intra-abdominal pressure compromising the diaphragm. The application of PEEP (positive end expiratory pressure) has been advocated as a method of reducing respiratory compromise (Huchison & Gokal 1995).

Pleural effusion may be caused by leakage of fluid through a structural deformity of the diaphragm or following thoracic surgery. Severe acute respiratory compromise may occur, requiring the cessation of dialysis, support of respiratory function and drainage of the pleural cavity.

Peritonitis can occur as a result of the introduction of microorganisms into the peritoneal cavity, through contaminated fluid, contaminated site or circuit break. Signs and symptoms include:

- cloudy dialysate
- pyrexia
- abdominal pain and tenderness
- vomiting
- paralytic ileus
- septicaemia.

Prevention of peritonitis involves adherence to aseptic principles when inserting the catheter and breaking the circuit. Keeping the drainage bag below the level of the abdomen prevents backflow into the peritoneum. Antibiotics can be added to the dialysate if > 50 white cells per litre or organisms are seen. Fungal peritonitis usually warrants removal of the catheter and treatment with systemic antifungal agents. Alternative renal replacement therapy must be initiated. Gentamicin is the drug of choice for *Staphylococcus aureus* peritonitis. 5 mg gentamicin/L dialysis fluid for 5 days is recommended (Guy's and St Thomas' and Lewisham Hospitals 1997).

Catheter obstruction may result from:

- mechanical obstruction in the circuit or catheter
- improper placement of the catheter
- constipation
- dehydration
- blockage of the catheter by omentum or fibrin and debris.

Repositioning of the child and or catheter may relieve the obstruction. Prevention of dehydration and constipation is important. The catheter may be flushed aseptically and forcefully with 5–10 mL NaCl 0.9% to remove debris. Fibrin blockage may be removed by flushing the catheter with urokinase 5000 iu with NaCl 0.9% to the priming volume of the catheter (Guy's and St Thomas' and Lewisham Hospitals 1997). This should be left in situ for 4 h and then aspirated to remove the urokinase solution.

Haemofiltration/haemodiafiltration

When peritoneal dialysis is contraindicated or insufficient to produce the results required, intermittent dialysis or continuous haemodialysis or haemofiltration must be considered. Intermittent dialysis may be considered for those children in chronic renal failure who are unable to tolerate peritoneal dialysis, or for those with acute renal failure who can tolerate the rapid solute shifts that occur during the dialysis process.

For those children who are unable to tolerate this process, or for those who do not require dialysis but require removal of fluid alone, continuous treatments are more appropriate. Continuous treatments are particularly useful for children who are cardiovascularly unstable or have severe electrolyte derangement or metabolic acidosis and hence may not tolerate intermittent dialysis. Children with pulmonary oedema or multisystem failure who are not yet in established renal failure may also benefit from continuous haemofiltration to facilitate desired fluid management.

It has been suggested by some that there is a role for haemofiltration in removing the mediators of inflammatory response particularly in meningococcal disease and acute respiratory distress syndrome. There is, however, no consensus as to the exact role of haemofiltration in the removal of inflammatory mediators. Continuous treatment provides a more gentle method of removing waste products than intermittent treatments and therefore is tolerated better.

Continuous treatments

Continuous treatments are:

- slow continuous ultrafiltration (SCUF)
- continuous arteriovenous haemofiltration (CAVH)
- continuous arteriovenous haemofiltration with dialysis (haemodiafiltration) (CAVHD)
- continuous venovenous haemofiltration (CVVH)
- continuous venovenous haemofiltration with dialysis (haemodiafiltration) (CVVHD).

For both continuous and intermittent treatments, access to the circulation is required. Continuous haemofiltration removes fluid and solutes from the child by processes of ultrafiltration and convection. Blood flows along one side of a highly permeable membrane allowing water and solutes of molecular weight up to 20 000 to pass across it (Forni & Hilton 1997). Urea, creatinine and phosphates are cleared at similar rates. Heparin, insulin, myoglobin and vancomycin are cleared efficiently by haemofiltration but not haemodialysis.

Arteriovenous systems (including SCUF) require both arterial and venous access, and the system is driven by the patient's own blood pressure and blood flow from the arterial catheter. Limitations of this system include:

- difficulty in obtaining adequate arterial access for optimal flow rates
- poor blood pressure will reduce the efficiency of the filter
- disconnection may lead to rapid exsanguination
- low blood flows increase the likelihood of clot formation in the filter.

Despite these difficulties, arteriovenous treatments are successfully used for adults and children.

SCUF is the simplest form of arteriovenous continuous treatment. Using the same circuit as for CAVH, small amounts of fluid are constantly removed from the patient. No replacement fluid is given. This simple system can create enough space to allow increased calorific intake. Like CAVH, it is dependent upon good arterial access, good flow and good pressures. The risks are the same as for CAVH.

In contrast, venovenous systems rely upon a pump to remove venous blood and pump it through a filter before returning it to the patient. Air and pressure detectors are an integral part of the equipment (Fig. 11.10). Provided that the venous access is not restrictive, high flows can be used to facilitate excellent solute and water removal.

Inherent risks associated with intravenous catheter insertion include haemorrhage, pneu-

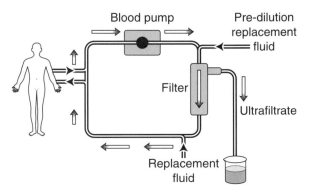

Figure 11.10 CVVH circuit principles.

Table 11.2 Circuit volumes available

Filter type/SA[a]	FH22 (0.16 m^2)	FH22 (0.16 m^2)	FH66 (0.6 m^2)
Filter volume	11 mL	11 mL	43 mL
Blood lines	14 mL neonatal	25 mL large neonatal	56 mL paediatric
Total circuit volume	25 mL	36 mL	99 mL

[a]Surface area
The maximum dialysate flow rate achievable through the FH22 filter is 1000 mL/h, and through the FH66 is 2000 mL/h.

mothorax, cardiac arrhythmias from vagal stimulation and infection.

Selecting circuits and flow rates. Prior to commencing treatment the most appropriate size of circuit and filter must be chosen so that the total volume of blood filling the extracorporeal circuit does not exceed 8% total circulating volume:

$$\text{maximum extracorporeal volume} = (\text{weight in kg} \times 80 \text{ mL}) \times 8\%$$

Larger children will tolerate this well and might tolerate up to 10% as an extracorporeal volume. However, small children and infants may have difficulty tolerating the volume of the smallest available circuit. The surface area of the filter should not exceed that of the child (Table 11.2 and Box 11.3). The surface area of the child can be calculated by plotting the height (cm) and weight (kg) on a nomogram.

Blood flow rates should not exceed 8% circulating volume/min or 6.4 mL/kg/min.

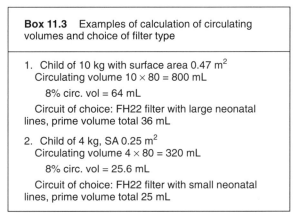

Box 11.3 Examples of calculation of circulating volumes and choice of filter type

1. Child of 10 kg with surface area 0.47 m^2
   Circulating volume 10 × 80 = 800 mL

   8% circ. vol = 64 mL

   Circuit of choice: FH22 filter with large neonatal lines, prime volume total 36 mL

2. Child of 4 kg, SA 0.25 m^2
   Circulating volume 4 × 80 = 320 mL

   8% circ. vol = 25.6 mL

   Circuit of choice: FH22 filter with small neonatal lines, prime volume total 25 mL

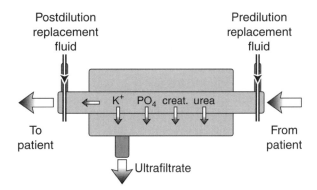

Figure 11.11 Positions where replacement fluid might be added to the haemofiltration circuit.

Factors affecting filtration efficiency are:

- adequate blood flow
- size of extracorporeal circuit
- fluid state of the patient
- cardiovascular stability of the patient
- size of the haemofilter
- blood viscosity
- transmembrane pressure.

$$\text{Transmembrane pressure TMP} = \frac{PA + PV}{2} - PN$$

where PA = arterial (prefilter) pressure in mmHg; PV = venous (postfilter) pressure in mmHg; PN = absolute value of any applied vacuum on the ultrafiltrate outlet, in mmHg.

Increases in transmembrane pressure will increase the efficiency of filtration up to a point. The maximum transmembrane pressure that can be borne by the filter is 600 mmHg (Gambro GmbH).

Haemofiltration treatment. Cannulation of internal jugular, subclavian or femoral vessels can provide adequate flows for filtration systems. Blood flows from one of the two venous lumen via the extracorporeal circuit to the pump which then pumps the blood through the haemofilter and then returns blood to the patient via the second lumen of the catheter. Large volumes of fluid may be removed to facilitate solute removal (Fig. 11.11). Some or all of the fluid removed may be replaced by a physiological solution after the filter and before the return to

the patient. Heat loss may become a significant problem because of the large surface area of the filter, requiring replacement fluid to be warmed prior to addition to the circuit.

Commencing and maintaining treatments. The circuit should be primed and filled according to the manufacturer's instructions, using heparinised priming solution throughout the entire circuit and filter to remove all the ethylene oxide from the filter, to remove air and to coat the filter membrane and tubing with heparinised fluid to minimise platelet adhesion when the treatment commences. Infants and small children who have proportionally larger extracorporeal volumes than older children may benefit from the circuit's being primed with albumin or blood immediately prior to connection to the patient to ensure that the risk of developing clots in the circuit is minimised. Usually an anticoagulant is used to minimise the risks of clotting within the circuit. Heparin and epoprostenol have both been used to good effect in the following doses:

- heparin 10–30 iu/kg/h
- epoprostenol 1–2 nanogram/kg/min (5 ng/kg/min recommended by the manufacturers for circuits on adults).

Anecdotal evidence suggests that heparin doses can be adjusted to achieve an activated clotting time (ACT) of 120–150 s to ensure circuit patency. The administration of blood products will inevitably require an adjustment of the heparin dose, as will dehydration or an increased haematocrit.

When the patient is sufficiently stable to connect to the extracorporeal circuit, flow rates should be built up slowly as tolerated. Although 8% circulating volume per minute is the desired flow rate, it may be advisable to commence treatment at one quarter to one third of this until the patient is stable on the pump. Once the patient is stable with the desired flow rate, fluid removal can commence. Volumetric pumps can be used to regulate the volume of fluid removed from the patient. All or some of this volume can then be replaced using a haemofiltration fluid which has similar composition to the crystalloid component of plasma.

Removal of fluid and salts results in an increase in the viscosity of blood and a high colloid osmotic pressure at the distal end of the filter. Instilling the replacement fluid distally to the filter helps to redress the balance before the blood is returned to the patient. Because of this it is important to keep the filtration rate at less than 30% of the blood flow rate: e.g. if the blood flow rate is 100 mL/min, maximum ultrafiltrate rate is 33 mL/min or 1980 mL/h.

It is possible, however, to use a predilution technique such that the replacement fluid is added to the circuit before the pump and the filter. This reduces the risk of the increased viscosity in the filter causing clot formation within the filter and the venous line, but it does reduce slightly the efficiency of the filter and does lead to an increase in cost through increased usage of dialysis fluid. Despite this the advantages of the predilution technique in terms of prolonged filter life and better clearance of urea are felt to outweigh the disadvantage of slightly increased cost. Optimal predilution fluid infusion rates are 0.5 mL/kg/min.

By manipulating the amount of dialysate removed from the child and the amount of replacement fluid administered, it is possible to provide for increased calorific or drug requirements. A child with multisystem failure in a severely catabolic state can receive good nutritional support if undergoing effective continuous haemofiltration to achieve the desired fluid balance.

Standard haemofiltration fluid contains sodi-

Table 11.3 Fluids used for CAVH(D)/CVVH(D)

	Haemofitrasol 21	Haemofitrasol 22	Lactate-free solution
Na^+	140	140	110
Ca^+	1.6	1.6	1.75
Mg^+	0.75	0.75	0.75
K^+	1.0	0	0
Cl^-	100	100	100
Lactate	45	45	0

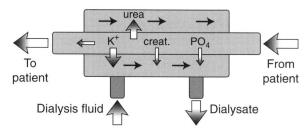

Figure 11.12 CVVHD solute movement.

um, calcium, magnesium and chloride in predominantly physiological proportions. Solutions are available with added potassium if required. Lactate is the buffer in standard fluid preparations (Table 11.3). It is possible to use fluid with lactate removed for those children with severe lactic acidosis or lactate intolerance. Bicarbonate-based solutions can be prepared by pharmacy departments with appropriate manufacturing facilities, but these solutions will not contain calcium or magnesium. These electrolytes must then be given enterally or parenterally as required.

Continuous venovenous haemodiafiltration. This is a continuous treatment in which blood flows along one side of a semipermeable membrane, with dialysis fluid flowing countercurrent on the other side of the membrane, allowing water and solutes of molecular weight up to 20 000 to pass across the membrane by diffusion and ultrafiltration (Fig. 11.12). Higher clearance rates of small solutes can be achieved with this treatment than with continuous haemofiltration, but the removal of larger molecules by convection is reduced.

Continuous diafiltration may be the treatment

of choice for the child with hyperammonaemia or other severe metabolic derangement who is unable to tolerate intermittent haemodialysis.

Intermittent haemodialysis

Unstable patients with multisystem failure do not tolerate intermittent dialysis well, because of the rapidity with which the treatment removes solutes and water. Using an extracorporeal circuit, blood is removed from the child, pumped through the dialyser/artificial kidney and returned to the child. Treatment frequency may vary from child to child.

Haemodialysis removes fluid and solutes from the patient by processes of diffusion and ultrafiltration. Blood flows along one side of a highly permeable membrane, dialysis fluid flows in a countercurrent on the other side of the membrane, allowing water and solutes of molecular weight up to 20 000 to pass across the membrane by diffusion and ultrafiltration. Urea,

creatinine and phosphates are not present in the dialysis fluid and therefore are removed by diffusion at varying rates. Small molecular weight molecules such as urea (60 daltons) are cleared well, but larger molecules such as creatinine (113 daltons) are cleared less well. Heparin, insulin, myoglobin and vancomycin are cleared efficiently by haemofiltration but not by haemodialysis.

Initially it is advisable that the filter used has a surface area which is no greater than two-thirds the surface area of the child. If a dialyser with a high clearance is used it can lead to a rapid deterioration of the child's condition by causing hypotension and disequilibrium. Disequilibrium syndrome is caused by the rapid removal of solutes, particularly urea. This condition can occur during or immediately following a dialysis treatment and it has been suggested by Bloe (1990) that this results from the slow removal of urea from the brain relative to the rest of the body, causing cerebral oedema.

REFERENCES

Bissinger R L 1995 Renal physiology, part I: structure and function. Neonatal Network 14(4):9–19

Bloe C G 1990 Peritoneal dialysis. Professional Nurse, April:345–349

Carter B 1993 Manual of Paediatric Intensive Care Nursing. Chapman and Hall, London

Forni L G, Hilton P J 1997 Continuous hemofiltration in the treatment of acute renal failure. New England Journal of Medicine 336:1303–1309

Gluckman P D, Heymann M A 1993 Perinatal and pediatric pathophysiology. Edward Arnold, Boston

Guy's and St Thomas' and Lewisham Hospitals 1997 Paediatric formulary, 4th edn. Whitstable Litho Printers, Kent

Huchison A J, Gokal R 1995 Peritoneal dialysis in the ICU: what is its role? Care of the Critically Ill 11(3):111–113

Levine D Z 1991 Care of the renal patient, 2nd edn. Saunders, Philadelphia

Larsen W J 1993 Human embryology. Churchill Livingstone, New York

Lowrie L, Stark J E 1990 A practical guide to paediatric intensive care, 3rd edn. Mosby Yearbook, St Louis

McCance K L, Heuther S E 1994 Pathophysiology: the biologic basis for disease in adults and children. Mosby, St Louis

Maxwell L G, Colombani P M, Fivush B A 1992 Renal, endocrine and metabolic failure. In: Rogers M C (ed) Textbook of paediatric intensive care, 2nd edn. Williams & Wilkins, Baltimore

Seaman S L 1995 Renal physiology, part II: fluid and electrolyte regulation. Neonatal Network 14(5):5–11

Toro-Figueroa L O, Levin D L, Morris F C (eds), 1992 Essentials of pediatric intensive care manual. Quality Medical Publications, St Louis

Tortora G J, Anagnostakos 1990 Principles of anatomy and physiology, 6th edn. HarperCollins, New York

12

Care of the critically ill child with infectious disease

Simon Nadel   Rebecca Brownlie

Infections constitute a significant threat at all ages, but particularly at the extremes of life, such as infancy and childhood. Severity of infection and immunological status of the child contribute to the downhill spiral leading to critical illness. This chapter will address the important common infectious diseases which may present in paediatric intensive care.

Humans are protected against infection by complex defence mechanisms (Table 12.1), resulting from the numerous biochemical and molecular pathways of the immune response. These lead to alterations in physiological processes which produce pathological changes. Anticipation of these changes is essential to recognise and treat the disordered physiology.

Host responses similar to those of acute infection are also seen following other acute insults, including trauma, surgery and metabolic derangements (Box 12.1). Generalised responses are determined by several factors which significantly influence outcome (Miller & Ackerman 1996):

Table 12.1   Non-specific immune-response to infection

Protective factor	Where found
Lysozyme	Mucosal surfaces
Complement	Plasma
Mannose binding protein	Plasma
Neurophil-derived proteins	Neutrophil
Reactive oxygen and nitrogen species	Neutrophil, macrophage endothelium
Histamine	Eosinophil and mast cells
Kinins	Inflammatory cells, plasma
Interferons	Lymphocytes, other cells
Prostaglandins	Many cells

Box 12.1 Non-specific clinical features seen following infection, surgery, trauma and miscellaneous other conditions (e.g. acute pancreatitis, acute metabolic derangement, acute autoimmune phenomena and acute drug toxicity)

- fever
- tachycardia
- tachypnoea
- leucocytosis
- cytokine release: e.g. tumour necrosis factor-alpha (TNF-α), interleukin1-beta (IL1β) and interleukin 6 (IL6)
- increased immunoglobulins

- age and sex of the child
- presence of genetic resistance or susceptibility traits
- nutritional status
- presence of significant underlying disease
- severity and duration of the infectious process.

Additionally, systemic responses may result from localised infection in certain anatomic sites or organs. For example, central nervous system (CNS) infection may affect airway control and respiratory function, leading to respiratory failure; bloodstream infection may cause septic shock and multisystem failure due to inadequate supply of oxygen and nutrients to the tissues.

This chain of events is caused by the host response to invading microorganisms. The control of these defence mechanisms influences the magnitude of the inflammatory response. If it is too aggressive it will be harmful to the host, but an inadequate host response may lead to increased susceptibility to severe infection.

IMMUNE SYSTEM RESPONSE TO INFECTION

From birth we are exposed to many invading organisms, which become part of our normal flora, or cause mild infection to severe infection. The type of response an infecting organism elicits once it has colonised the host depends on:

- characteristics of the infecting organism
- host's ability to respond to the invading organism
- control of the host's response.

Table 12.2 Protective effects of various components of the immune system

Agent	Mechanism
Skin and mucous membranes	Barrier function
Complement	Opsonisation and lysis of bacteria
Mannose binding protein	Opsonisation of bacteria and fungi
Immunoglobulin	Opsonisation and neutralisation of viruses (e.g. Enterovirus), bacteria and parasitic organisms
Neutrophils	Phagocytosis
Eosinophils	Protection against parasites
Monocytes/Macrophages	Phagocytosis
B-lymphocytes	Secrete immunoglobulin
T-lymphocytes	Protection against viruses, fungi and protozoa

N.B. All of these elements have extremely important interactions. Therefore, dysfunction of one of them may cause dysfunction of other elements.

Development and control of the human immune system is genetically determined. We possess many genes governing the pattern of responses following microbial invasion. Understanding the control of these genes and their protein products has been the subject of much research into the pathophysiology of infectious disease. The mechanisms which determine immune-responsiveness to invading organisms are also responsible for the immunological identity of the 'self' (Table 12.2).

Human Chromosome 6 contains a set of genes that code for cell surface proteins determining a 'cellular fingerprint'. These genes, called the major histocompatibility complex (MHC) are important in determining the recognition and response of the host to foreign antigens and define the extent of antibody or cell-mediated immune responses (Krensky & Clayberger 1994). At least two products of MHC genes have been identified: Class I and Class II proteins.

Class I proteins are primarily involved in self-recognition and are therefore important in transplant rejection and cytotoxic T-cell activity. This latter function is antibody-independent, resulting in attacks on infected cells, which is critical for limiting the spread of viruses by destroying cells producing new viral particles.

Class II proteins are found mainly on macrophages and B cells and aid interaction with the helper/suppressor T-cell system, controlling T-cell-dependent antibody production. Macrophages ingest invading foreign antigens and present specific antigen-derived peptides on their surface to activate specific T-cells. These T-cells then interact with specific B cells to 'turn on' antibody production, initiating and amplifying the immune response.

Proliferation of stimulated cells induces long-term memory for the antigen, producing rapid and intense immune responses on subsequent encounters with the same or similar antigens. Suppressor T-cells modulate and help to control this response to achieve an immunological balance (Bellanti et al 1994).

Invading organisms have evolved mechanisms to overcome the host's hostile response. Many bacteria secrete proteases to inactivate host-protective antibodies; specifically, staphylococci produce enzymes which cause plasma to clot, thus isolating the organism from the usual bloodborne host inflammatory response. These organisms are efficient producers of localised infections such as abscesses. Streptococci produce enzymes which break down host tissue barriers and protective inflammatory barriers allowing dissemination of infection along tissue planes and into the bloodstream (Gaur et al 1994).

FACTORS AFFECTING IMMUNE FUNCTION

Age

Extremes of age are associated with poor outcome from critical illness. Specific immune responses involve both antibody production (B-cell mediated) and cellular immune responses (T-cell mediated). These are antigen-specific and require previous immunological experience of that particular antigen and the presence of immunological memory for a complete response. The relative lack of exposure to foreign antigens

in neonates causes susceptibility to a number of microorganisms, as specific immune responses are impaired. Non-specific mechanisms of host defence include the complement system, opsonic and chemotactic chemicals and phagocytic cells. Newborns are deficient in all measurable products of complement activation (Drew & Arroyave 1980). They have deficient opsonisation, in particular for Gram-negative organisms and the group B streptococci. Phagocytic cells of the newborn have decreased motility, adherence and chemotaxis with normal bactericidal activity except when the neonate is stressed (Anderson et al 1974). This explains why newborn and premature infants are more susceptible to infections by Gram-negative coliforms (such as *Escherichia coli*) and group B streptococci. Organisms that require production of specific antibodies to induce protection, particularly the encapsulated organisms such as *Haemophilus influenzae* type b (Hib), pneumococcus and meningococcus are the most frequent causes of serious bacterial infection in young children. Immunisation using purified capsular polysaccharide vaccine has proved that immune responses to these antigens are poorly developed in children under 2 years. Therefore, a new class of vaccine has been developed whereby the capsular polysaccharide is conjugated with a protein antigen, dramatically enhancing the immune response to polysaccharide. An example is the significant decline in the incidence of Hib infection following production of a conjugate vaccine. Similar vaccines are under evaluation for pneumococcal and meningococcal infection (Kroll & Booy 1996).

Many viral infections produce less serious illness in infants and young children because cell-mediated immune responses are well developed by the time of birth. However, infections such as Herpes simplex virus (HSV) types 1 and 2, Varicella zoster virus (VZV) and Cytomegalovirus (CMV), are particularly serious in the neonate, probably because of the relative imbalance in T-cell helper and suppressor functions (Durandy et al 1979).

Mucosal immunity, which requires presence of secretory immunoglobulin A (sIgA), is also deficient in the neonate and infant. Secretory IgA

Table 12.3 Effect of major anaesthetic agents on immune function

Agent	Effect
Halothane	Reduced phagocytosis, chemotaxis and antibody synthesis
Nitrous oxide	Bone-marrow depression, reduced phagocytosis and lymphocyte function
Barbiturates	Neutropenia, reduced phagocytosis and lymphocyte function
Opiates	Reduced phagocytosis and lymphocyte function

is not detected in significant quantities until 1–2 years. Diseases requiring this antibody for protection, such as viral respiratory infections and infectious diarrhoea, are therefore prevalent throughout infancy.

Trauma, surgery and anaesthesia

Many children are admitted to PIC following surgery or trauma, which are major physiological stresses affecting immune function, the nature of which varies with age, type of injury and presence of underlying illness. The associated anaesthesia (Table 12.3) and breach of host defence barriers caused by endotracheal intubation, mechanical ventilation and insertion of intravenous and urinary catheters are major contributors to the development of infection.

A non-specific stress response with an acute increase in the circulating neutrophil count occurs in response to a surgical wound and trauma (Lennard & Browell 1993). Other effects include alteration in B- and T-cell function and activation of the complement pathway.

The second commonest cause of death in the child surviving acute trauma is nosocomial infection (Allgower et al 1980), the risk of which increases with severity of injury. This is greatest following blunt or penetrating abdominal trauma with associated bowel perforation.

Head trauma and basal skull fracture may cause disruption of the dura and communication between the subarachnoid space and the external or middle ear, nasal cavity or sinuses, creating a risk of subsequent intracranial infection. Such injuries are rare in children; however, in adults, post-traumatic meningitis is seen in up to 25% of cases following such injuries (Helling et al 1988).

Thermal injury

Thermal injury has well-described effects on host defence (Alexander 1990):

- suppressed phagocytosis, chemotaxis, opsonisation and bactericidal activity
- activation of complement and suppression of immunoglobulin (Ig) level
- reduction of T-helper cells and increased T-suppressor cell numbers
- increased levels of prostaglandins, which inhibit lymphocyte proliferation.

Apart from immunosuppressive effects of the injury itself, the wound provides an excellent culture medium for colonising organisms. Nosocomial infection is a major cause of death in survivors of the initial insult.

Debridement of devitalised tissue and administration of topical disinfectants or organism-specific antimicrobials, are vital in prevention of sepsis. Infecting organisms include:

- Pseudomonas
- Enterococcus
- fungi, e.g. *Candida albicans*
- toxin-producing staphylococci.

Malnutrition

Malnutrition has significant effects on immune status. The extreme protein-calorie malnutrition seen in the developing world causes increased susceptibility to infection, particularly with viruses, mycobacteria and fungi (Chandra & Kumari 1994). Such children were uncommon in the developed world, but improved survival of children with severe underlying illness such as malignancy and acquired immunodeficiency syndrome (AIDS) has made malnourished children more prevalent in PICUs. This is often due to critical illness, when inadequate protein-calorie intake occurs, however, greater emphasis is being placed on ensuring adequate dietary intake for these children.

Immunosuppressive therapy

Numerous medical conditions are treated with agents that suppress immune function, including:

- organ transplantation
- malignant disease
- nephrotic syndrome
- connective tissue disease
- asthma.

Suppression of immunity is essential when managing these conditions, but this significantly increases the risk of overwhelming infection. In addition, management of chronic disease often necessitates long periods in hospital using devices such as central venous catheters for parenteral nutrition or intravenous drugs, increasing the risk of nosocomial infection.

Steroids and other immunosuppressive agents

Immunity is impaired by steroid usage. Their antiinflammatory action may mask manifestations of infection, delaying diagnosis. Other commonly used immunosuppressants include cyclophosphamide, azathioprine and cyclosporin A. These drugs increase the risk from viral infections such as CMV and Epstein Barr virus (EBV). Known risk factors should be reduced: for example, blood products should be screened for pathogens, and isolation may be required according to local policy.

UNDERLYING IMMUNODEFICIENCY

Severe infection in PIC is both a primary and secondary problem, but not all children with severe infection will have any underlying immunodeficiency. However, if immunodeficiency is apparent, a comprehensive search for both common and unusual infections is required. Possible underlying immunodeficiency may be indicated by:

- recurrent serious bacterial infection
- systemic fungal infection
- serious infection with a relatively benign organism
- unusual presentation of infection with a common organism
- neutropenia
- recurrent skin infection or mouth ulceration
- recurrent fever without any obvious source
- chronic diarrhoea
- failure to thrive
- recurrent or persistent meningoencephalitis
- congenital heart disease with hypocalcaemia (DiGeorge syndrome)
- family history of immune or autoimmune disease
- asplenia.

Primary immunodeficiency

Primary immunodeficiency most commonly presents in infants or young children and involves any component of the immune system. Severe Combined Immunodeficiency (SCID) presents the most serious disturbance of immune function. This group of genetically determined disorders, with X-linked or, more rarely, autosomal recessive inheritance, are characterised by a severe defect of cellular immunity, together with abnormal level of immunoglobulin. Children with SCID may present with overwhelming infection in the first few months of life, typically associated with declining level of maternally derived antibody. The classical course is failure to thrive, chronic diarrhoea, oral candidiasis and chronic respiratory disease (Hague et al 1994).

These children may present acutely with respiratory failure due to infection with organisms of low virulence in the normal host, such as *Pneumocystis carinii* or CMV, which are highly pathogenic in the presence of impaired immunity. However there are many potential pathogens that must be excluded. Therapy for these children is symptomatic and directed at identified organism(s), with prophylactic cotrimoxazole or pentamidine to prevent *Pneumocystis carinii*. Without effective bone marrow transplantation, these children often die by 2 years of age.

Prevention of nosocomial infection is essential, including the use of CMV-negative blood-products when required. In addition, these children often lack the ability to destroy foreign blood cells; therefore, all blood products must be irradiated to prevent development of transfusion-associated graft-versus-host disease (GVHD).

Acquired immunodeficiency, in particular HIV infection

Children with human immunodeficiency virus (HIV) face similar problems to those with other causes of acquired immunodeficiency, but there are certain clinical characteristics unique to HIV infection.

In the USA it is estimated that 2% of all HIV infection occurs in children, with AIDS being the 9th commonest cause of death in children aged 1–4 years (Centers for Disease Control 1994).

In the absence of universal prenatal HIV screening, most children with HIV infection will not be identified until they present with features of AIDS, or an AIDS-defining illness (Gibb & Newell 1992):

- *Pneumocystis carinii* pneumonia (PCP)
- unusual or recurrent infection
- neurological disorder/developmental delay
- wasting syndrome
- failure to thrive
- haematological disorders
- generalised lymphadenopathy
- hepatosplenomegaly
- oral and perineal candidiasis poorly responsive to commonly used topical antifungal agents.

A significant proportion of children with HIV infection will be diagnosed within PICU. In the developed world, nearly all children with HIV are infected vertically from their mother during pregnancy, delivery or in the postpartum period. The transmission rate from HIV-infected mothers to their offspring is 13–40%. Risk of transmission is dependent on:

- the population studied
- maternal immune-status

- mode of delivery
- whether the child was breast fed
- if the mother received antiretroviral therapy during the latter part of pregnancy

(Farley et al 1996). HIV infection may be acquired from transfusion of infected blood products; however, this is now rare following the introduction of universal screening of blood products in the mid 1980s.

Pulmonary disease

Pulmonary disease occurs in the majority of children with HIV infection. It may be acute or chronic, infectious or non-infectious and is the most common cause of death (Hauger 1991) (Box 12.2).

Box 12.2 Lung disease in children with HIV infection

Infectious	• viral: respiratory syncytial virus, influenza, parainfluenza, adenovirus, measles, cytomegalovirus, varicella zoster virus • bacterial: *Streptococcus pneumoniae, Haemophilus influenzae, Staphylococcus aureus, Pseudomonas aeruginosa* • mycobacteria: *Mycobacterium tuberculosis, Mycobacterium avium* • fungal: *Cryptococcus neoformans, Candida* spp., *Aspergillus* spp. • parasitic: *Pneumocystis carinii, Toxoplasma gondii.*
Non-infectious	• lymphocytic interstitial pneumonitis • bronchiectasis • Kaposi's sarcoma • lymphoma.
N.B. Several of these conditions may coexist.	

Pneumocystis carinii causes disease in the immunocompromised host with T-cell immunodeficiency. It is the most common reason for admission of an HIV-infected child to PIC, occurring in infants less than 3 months of age.

Pneumocystis carinii pneumonia (PCP) is the initial HIV-related illness in over 50% of children progressing to AIDS in the first year of life. Associated mortality during infancy is 40–60% (Hughes 1994). Common presentation of PCP includes:

- dyspnoea
- tachypnoea
- cough
- fever.

These symptoms may progress over several days, or present acutely. Chest X-ray may show hyperinflation, diffuse infiltrates or reticulonodular shadowing. The cardinal clinical finding in PCP is hypoxic, normocarbic respiratory failure. Definitive diagnosis is by isolation of organisms in lower respiratory tract secretions. Specimens are usually obtained by non-bronchoscopic bronchoalveolar lavage (BAL). Pneumocysts are demonstrated in BAL fluid by special stains such as Grocott or Gomorri stain. This method is less invasive than open-lung biopsy. Children with HIV infection may have infection with several pathogens; therefore specimens should be sent for full virological, bacteriological, mycobacteriological, fungal and histological examination. Specific antimicrobial therapy of intravenous high-dose cotrimoxazole or pentamidine is commenced as soon as the diagnosis is suspected. There is now evidence for the use of adjunctive corticosteroid therapy once the diagnosis of PCP is confirmed. However, children with PCP may be co-infected with other pathogens, which may be exacerbated by steroid therapy.

PCP may take several days to respond to treatment. During this period, children may require aggressive ventilatory support to maintain normal blood gases, including therapy for acute respiratory distress syndrome (ARDS). Treatment with artificial surfactant, inhaled nitric oxide (NO) and high-frequency oscillating ventilation (HFOV) may significantly reduce volutrauma and barotrauma and enable more rapid weaning from the ventilator.

PCP may be prevented by the administration of prophylactic cotrimoxazole or pentamidine. The usual criteria for administration of prophylactic therapy in HIV-infected adults is: CD4 count $< 200/mm^3$. However in children and infants with HIV infection, PCP has occurred with CD4 cell count $> 1000/mm^3$. Therefore, PCP prophylaxis should be given to all infants < 1 year of age if HIV status is indeterminate or positive and all patients who conform to the recommendations of the Centers for Disease Control (1995).

Lymphocytic interstitial pneumonitis (LIP) affects approximately 50% of children with HIV infection (Connor & Andiman 1994). It is characterised by diffuse lymphocytic infiltration of alveolar septae. Children with LIP usually have evidence of generalised lymphoid proliferation with widespread lymphadenopathy, parotitis and hepatosplenomegaly. LIP is often associated with peribronchial lymphoid infiltration together with hilar lymphadenopathy. This results in restrictive and obstructive lung disease, eventually causing hypoxaemia.

The aetiology of LIP is unclear but there may be an association with EBV infection. LIP may progress to hypoxic respiratory failure with secondary corpulmonale. Symptoms include:

- tachypnoea
- wheezing
- cough
- exercise intolerance.

The diagnosis is suggested by its chronic nature and lack of acute symptoms. Chest radiography reveals widespread reticulonodular shadowing.

Deterioration in lung function may occur acutely due to superimposed bacterial infection with consequent bronchiectasis. Lung biopsy is required if the diagnosis is in doubt, or if progression to lymphoid malignancy is suspected. Treatment is supportive with supplemental oxygen therapy, bronchodilators and inhaled steroids. Systemic steroid therapy is beneficial in advanced cases, when opportunistic infections have been excluded.

Cardiac disease

Cardiac dysfunction is common in HIV infection (Lipshultz 1994). Dilated cardiomyopathy is the most common manifestation and may progress to congestive cardiac failure. Intercurrent infection or anaemia may precipitate acute decompensation. Symptoms of cardiac failure may be mistaken for acute pulmonary or liver disease, or systemic sepsis. Children may develop dysrrhythmias or suddenly die. The aetiology of cardiac involvement is unclear, but may be associated with:

- direct HIV infection of cardiac muscle
- chronic viral myocarditis
- nutritional deficiency, particularly of selenium or zinc
- antiretroviral therapy.

Treatment is with diuretics and inotropes, replacement of trace elements and antiarrhythmic agents.

Renal disease

HIV-nephropathy presents with proteinuria, electrolyte anomalies, uraemia, haematuria and hypertension (Wigfall 1994). Renal replacement therapy may be indicated if an acute precipitant, such as drug-toxicity, is identified as a cause of decompensation. The prognosis of the underlying disease is a major determinant of the suitability for dialysis. Renal dysfunction may be exacerbated by recurrent infection, immune-complex nephropathy and drug-induced renal damage.

Haematological disturbance

Haematological abnormalities are common in children with HIV infection, as a consequence of the disease itself, the complications and treatment (Mueller 1994). HIV infection suppresses the bone marrow, causing:

- anaemia
- leucopenia
- thrombocytopenia
- immune-mediated destruction of blood cells
- neutropenia due to treatment with antiretroviral agents, ganciclovir and septrin
- coagulation factor abnormalities causing thrombosis or bleeding.

Therapy is supportive, although some of the abnormalities may be corrected by antiretroviral therapy.

Neurological disease

HIV encephalopathy occurs in > 50% of infected children. It may present in the first year of life, with developmental delay, neurological regression and spasticity. Other neurological complications may be superimposed on this background, producing acute deterioration including:

- CNS lymphoma
- bacterial, viral or cryptococcal meningitis
- encephalitis
- acute haemorrhagic or thrombotic strokes.

Intensive care may be required for coma, status epilepticus or raised intracranial pressure (Brouwers et al 1994).

Other infections

Although the main target of HIV infection is the T-cell, all aspects of immune function are affected, including production of functional antibody and neutrophil function. In addition, immunity is affected by antiretroviral, antiviral and antibiotic therapy. Bacteraemia occurs in up to 50% of HIV-infected children, most commonly with:

- *Streptococcus pneumoniae*
- *Staphylococcus aureus*
- enterococcus
- salmonellae.

Bacteraemia should be considered a likely possibility in all HIV-infected children with fever. Antimicrobial treatment should be broad-spectrum to ensure that all likely organisms are covered (Krasinski 1994).

Prophylactic use of intravenous immunoglobulin (IVIG) for prevention of invasive bacterial infection has been shown to be of benefit in certain groups of patients with HIV disease (NICH-HDIISG 1991).

Special precautions for the child with HIV infection in the PICU

Children with HIV infection are often undiagnosed prior to admission to PIC; therefore, universal precautions are essential when caring for all children. Potential sources of infection to health care workers are by direct inoculation with blood by accidental needle puncture, or by contact of mucous membranes with blood or secretions. Approximately 80% of accidental occupational acquisition of HIV infection in health care workers is by needle-stick injury, rather than by exposure to infected secretions. The risk of acquiring HIV infection following needle-stick injury from an infected individual is approximately 1%. In the event of a needle-stick injury or significant exposure, it is recommended that zidovudine (AZT) or a combination of anti-retroviral drugs is administered as soon as possible, in line with local policy. This has been shown to reduce the risk of seroconversion.

Other infections occurring in immunocompromised children

Viral infections are common in patients with T-cell immunodeficiency and HIV infection, usually by those associated with upper respiratory infections:

- respiratory syncytial virus (RSV)
- parainfluenza viruses
- adenovirus
- influenza viruses.

These infections may be more severe and protracted in the immunocompromised child. Infections with CMV, measles or Varicella zoster virus (VZV) may produce pneumonitis and systemic infection which are extremely difficult to treat and commonly fatal. CMV infection is common in immunodeficient children, but, as degree of immunosuppression progresses, latent CMV may reactivate to cause symptoms. Most commonly it causes retinitis, which may lead to blindness, or infection of the gastrointestinal tract. Treatment for viral infections should be organism-directed. For example, if RSV is demonstrated, inhaled ribavirin may be indicated. Pneumonitis due to other respiratory viruses has no specific therapy, but anecdotal use of ribavirin, amantidine and IVIG has been reported.

Bacterial pneumonia occurs frequently in children with immunodeficiency, particularly those with immunoglobulin deficiency or with abnormal leucocyte function or number, and may progress to respiratory failure. Therefore, antimicrobial therapy should be broad spectrum to cover common organisms, including:

- *Streptococcus pneumoniae*
- Hib
- *Pseudomonas aeruginosa*
- tuberculosis (TB).

Atypical mycobacteria such as the Mycobacterium avium complex (MAC) or BCG are important pathogens to be considered in severely immunocompromised children. These organisms often cause systemic infection rather than isolated pneumonia. If suspected, treatment with antimycobacterial therapy should be initiated whilst awaiting results of microbiological investigation (Farley et al 1996).

HOSPITAL-ACQUIRED INFECTION

Any infection acquired in the community can be transmitted to other children in PICU, but nosocomial or hospital-acquired infection is a significant problem. Nosocomial infections occur during hospitalisation and are not present or incubating at the time of admission; they include infections acquired in hospital but not apparent until after discharge. Nosocomial infection may be caused by organisms originating from the patient's own flora or from the hospital environment. As patients acquire commensal organisms from their environment, the two routes of infection may overlap. Surgically related infections are those involving a surgical wound, where deep tissues or organs have been exposed or manipulated during surgery. Infections occurring in the postoperative period, distant from the site of surgery — for example, postoperative pneumonia or urinary tract infection — are nosocomial.

Colonisation implies presence of an organism on a mucosal or skin surface, or in tissue or body fluid, without evidence of adverse effects. Infection implies presence of an organism at these sites, together with local or systemic evidence of inflammation. Unless there is reason to suspect specimen contamination, any organism isolated from a normally sterile site should be considered pathogenic. For organisms cultured from sites which contain 'normal flora', pathogenicity is suspected only if evidence of infection exists.

Children in PIC are at risk of nosocomial infection, which increases with length of stay due to the number of invasive procedures. Up to 1.2% of nosocomial infections lead directly to death, and 3.5% contribute to death. Nosocomial bacteraemia occurs in 33% of admissions to adult ICU, probably because of the severity of the patient's underlying condition and the high number of invasive procedures (Merritt & Green 1996).

Illness, hospitalisation and antibiotic therapy alter normal oral and upper respiratory tract flora. Broad-spectrum antibiotics also disturb the balance of normal flora, increasing the likelihood of colonisation with pathogenic and antibiotic-resistant organisms. Hospitals are colonised by antibiotic-resistant bacteria because of the frequent use of these drugs. Therefore, strict hand washing between patients and sterilisation of equipment is essential.

Children admitted with community-acquired respiratory infection are well-recognised sources of hospital-acquired respiratory disease. In particular the transmission of RSV bronchiolitis, where up to 40% of infants visiting hospital may contract the disease (Filippell & Rearick 1993). Transmission by droplets, or on the hands of staff, is a major factor in outbreaks of RSV infection in hospital. Infants with congenital cardiac disease, chronic lung disease and immunodeficiency are at risk of developing serious RSV infection. Reduction of cross infection from RSV is best achieved by isolating infants in separate areas away from children with these chronic conditions.

Pneumonia

Approximately 15% of all nosocomial infection

occurs in the lung. Tracheal intubation increases the likelihood of pneumonia by the following mechanisms.

- Passing endotracheal (ET) tubes through the upper airway carries non-sterile material into the trachea and lower airway.
- The ET tube obliterates glottic protective mechanisms and allows seepage of oral secretions into the trachea, even with a cuffed tube. The incidence of aspiration is 7 times higher with a non-cuffed tube.
- The tube or cuff may damage the tracheal mucosa, increasing likelihood of local infection.
- Presence of the ET tube impairs mucociliary function and cough reflex, inhibiting clearance of bronchial secretions and making the child dependent on relatively inefficient tracheal suction for removal of secretions.

Treatment with antacids or H_2 antagonists causes an increased risk of colonisation of gastric contents with Gram-negative bowel flora and subsequent colonisation of the oropharynx and trachea (duMoulin et al 1982).

Additional factors associated with increased risk of respiratory infection include the following.

- Contaminated respiratory equipment generates bacterial aerosols directly into the patient's lungs.
- Passage of the tracheostomy tube through the skin breaches normal protective function.
- Normal warming and filtration of inspired gas by the upper airway is absent.
- Effective coughing is impaired.
- Prolonged periods of mechanical ventilation associated with tracheostomy are likely to lead to colonisation with hospital-acquired organisms. Therefore there is a higher incidence of respiratory infections, caused by enteric Gram-negative organisms, Pseudomonas species and anaerobes (Brook 1979).

Infections from intravascular catheters and other percutaneous devices

Invasive monitoring necessarily involves passage

of a device through the skin. Skin flora consist of a range of Gram-positive and Gram-negative aerobes, anaerobes and fungi, with more pathogenic organisms found in hospitalised patients. The most densely populated areas are the groin, thighs, axillae, umbilicus, head and scalp. Any device breaching the skin becomes colonised with these organisms. A fibrin sheath forms around all transcutaneous materials, promoting growth and migration of bacteria along the device and beneath the skin. Intravascular devices may also become infected from contamination of the materials being infused, or from bacteria derived from other infected sites within the body.

Peripheral venous catheters

The duration of catheter placement and colonisation with pathogenic bacteria are directly linked. Organisms present in inflamed skin are often found in the intravascular segment of the catheter. In neonates, peripheral venous catheters are three times more likely to be colonised if in place for > 3 days than those present for < 3 days, or if sited in leg veins rather than arm or scalp veins (Cronin et al 1990). Splints and bandages used to secure peripheral catheters have also been implicated in catheter-associated sepsis, particularly aspergillus infection (McCarty et al 1986).

Arterial catheters

Intra-arterial pressure monitoring has associated complications of thrombosis, embolism and infection. There is a similar association between local inflammation and infection as with peripheral venous catheters, with a significant incidence of bacteraemia. Infection risk of arterial catheters is not site-related and incidence overall is approximately 5% (Ducharme et al 1990). Another cause of bacteraemia associated with arterial catheters is colonisation of transducers or blood gas syringes. Both Serratia and Flavobacterium have been associated with colonisation of transducer chamber-dome fluid. Use of disposable systems have shown a reduction in colonisation if used for < 4 days (Luskin 1986).

Central venous catheters

Central venous catheters (CVCs) may be placed surgically or percutaneously. There is a strong association between organisms colonising the insertion site and those contaminating the catheter (Guidet et al 1994). If a CVC is inserted during a period of sepsis, it often becomes colonised with the causative organism and may become a focus for continued bacteraemia. Duration of insertion is correlated with likelihood of colonisation. Risk of colonisation is significantly increased in the presence of bacteraemia, tracheostomy and thermal injuries, with up to 80% of CVCs in such patients causing bacteraemia (Pruitt et al 1980). However, it is estimated that < 5% of CVCs become infected if present for < 3 days, with no site-related differences. There is no difference in infection rates between single- and multilumen catheters, but any device that traverses cardiac valves may damage the endocardium. Autopsies from patients with PA catheters have shown a high incidence (> 50%) of both infected and non-infected endocardial vegetations (Rowley et al 1984). These are also noted in neonates with umbilical catheters extending into the right atrium (Noel et al 1988).

Prolonged central venous access

Prolonged CV access is required for parenteral nutrition or extended antimicrobial therapy. Since the introduction of total parenteral nutrition (TPN) in the 1960s it has become evident that infection rates can only be minimised by:

- antiseptic catheter insertion
- inhibiting use of additional infusions
- avoidance of line breakages
- avoidance of blood-sampling
- use of sterile dressings
- use of dedicated catheter care teams

(Merritt & Green 1996). Over 50% of TPN-related infections are due to Gram-positive organisms, mainly coagulase-negative Staphylococci, *Staphylococcus aureus* and Enterococci. However, fungal infection is also significant (30%), with

Candida and Torulopsis species. *Malessezia furfur* is particularly associated with use of lipid solutions (Powell et al 1984). Gram-negative organisms and, rarely, mycobacteria cause the remainder of TPN-associated infection.

The decision to remove or replace a catheter may be extremely difficult, as it is often desirable to leave the catheter in place to ease management. Quantitative bacterial culture taken through the catheter, with simultaneous peripheral blood culture, can determine whether the CVC is infected. Other indications of infection include erythema or pus at the catheter site.

If a CVC is infected there is a 50–80% chance of clearing the infection with appropriate antimicrobial therapy, particularly in Gram-positive infections (Johnson et al 1986). However, if there is ongoing sepsis, shock, line-associated suppurative thrombophlebitis or fungal infection the line requires urgent removal.

Broviac and Hickman catheters are made of silicone rubber and designed to be tunnelled subcutaneously. The use of tunnelling procedures and Dacron cuffs for tethering the catheter reduce catheter infection. Implantable devices, such as Portacaths have similar rates of colonisation to non-implantable devices (Morris et al 1990).

Extracorporeal circuits

Devices used for haemofiltration, haemodialysis and extracorporeal membrane oxygenation (ECMO) may lead to infection from colonisation of the dialysis membrane or fluid in addition to the mechanisms previously described. Pseudomonas infection is particularly common in patients on dialysis (Cheesbrough et al 1986). Children on ECMO have a similar incidence of infection as those with CV and arterial catheters in situ (Merritt & Green 1996).

Urinary tract infections

The cumulative risk of urinary tract infection (UTI) of catheterised patients in PIC is approximately 30% (Kasian et al 1988). The presence of a urinary catheter may obscure symptoms of dysuria or frequency and may cause pyuria from mechanical irritation. The colony count of organisms in the urine is a sign of UTI, with $> 10^5$ organisms/mL indicating UTI in a clean-catch specimen. However, in the presence of a urinary catheter, counts as low as 10^2/mL may indicate infection (Stark & Maki 1984). Despite closed urinary drainage systems, bacteruria occurs in most patients catheterised for > 30 days. Females are four times more likely to develop bacteruria than males, because of the shorter urethra. In short-term catheterisation (< 3.5 days) Gram-positive organisms (coagulase-negative Staphylococci and Enterococci) are more commonly found, with Gram-negative enteric organisms becoming more prevalent over time (Kunin & Steele 1985). Fever is the most common symptom, but approximately 30% of patients will be asymptomatic.

Intracranial devices

Intracranial pressure monitoring or drainage devices pierce the skin, scalp, skull, meninges and brain. Frequent interruptions in the system and prolonged placement significantly increase the risk of infection. Whilst many organisms are implicated, Staphylococcus is most commonly isolated. Non-specific symptoms such as fever and peripheral blood leucocytosis make definitive diagnosis difficult. This is further complicated as specific CSF leucocytosis is not seen in up to 25% of device-associated CNS infections where cultures are negative. Suspected CSF infection should be treated by removing the device and adminstering broad-spectrum antibiotics known to penetrate the blood–brain barrier. Nosocomial CNS infection has a poor prognosis. Often empyema, abscess or ventriculitis will develop with associated neurological sequelae.

TREATMENT OF LIFE-THREATENING INFECTION

Prior to establishing a definitive diagnosis, the basic principles of resuscitation and stabilisation apply whether the child has an overwhelming infection, cardiogenic shock or multiple trauma. A history including the following signs and symptoms would suggest an infectious aetiology:

- prodromal illness
- fever
- rash
- haemodynamic collapse
- meningeal irritation
- respiratory impairment
- altered mental status and focal neurological signs.

Further information which may assist differential diagnosis includes:

- history of recent foreign travel
- contact with individuals with infectious disease
- contact with potentially infectious animals
- ingestion or contact with possibly infected water sources or foodstuffs
- recent insect bites
- immunisation status.

Initial investigations include:

- full blood count
- clotting studies
- erythrocyte sedimentation rate (ESR)
- electrolytes
- renal function
- hepatic function
- urinalysis
- analysis of CSF
- rapid antigen tests for bacteria in blood or CSF
- initial radiology.

Many signs and symptoms of sepsis may be imitated by diseases such as acute cardiac failure, cerebrovascular accident, metabolic abnormalities, drug or toxin ingestion.

The initial antibiotic regimen is determined by knowledge of the most likely offending organism. This is determined by:

- age of the child
- presence of serious underlying condition
- presence of invasive devices
- presenting signs and symptoms of the current illness.

The aim of the antibiotic regimen is to eradicate the offending organism, with minimal risk of toxicity.

Bacteraemia may be caused by a variety of Gram-negative and Gram-positive organisms, but a similar clinical picture is seen with viraemia or fungaemia. Bacteraemia may lead to focal infections such as meningitis, pneumonia, endocarditis or osteomyelitis which are often a consequence rather than the cause. Occasionally, bacteraemia is transient and self-limiting, only detected following investigation for fever. In this case, positive blood culture is reported even though the child may have made a complete recovery on follow-up assessment. This may be followed by significant focal infection if not appropriately treated (McGowan et al 1973).

The most common causes of bacteraemia in normal children outside the neonatal age group are:

- *Neisseria meningitidis*
- *Streptococcus pneumoniae*
- Salmonella species
- *Staphylococcus aureus*
- *Haemophilus influenzae* type b (prior to the introduction of Hib vaccine).

Immunosuppressed children or those with invasive devices are particularly vulnerable to infections with:

- coagulase-negative Staphylococci
- Enterococci
- Pseudomonas
- coliforms
- Candida
- Aspergillus.

The major clinical consequence of bacteraemia is septic shock, characterised by inadequate end-organ perfusion and multisystem failure. The incidence of septic shock in children is unclear, but occurs in approximately 20–50% of children with bacteraemia, with 10–98% mortality dependent on cause of bacteraemia and presence of underlying disease (Kaplan 1987).

In Gram-negative infection, clinical presentation is related to the level of endotoxin (lipopolysaccharide, LPS) in the circulation. Endotoxin is derived from the cell wall of Gram-negative bacteria. Isolated LPS when injected into experimental models reproduces all the systemic complications of Gram-negative bacteraemia.

The presence of LPS in the bloodstream causes activation of many humoral and cellular factors, including activation of the complement and coagulation pathways, neutrophils, monocytes, platelets and endothelial cells, with the end result of widespread endothelial cell dysfunction and damage, leading to multisystem organ failure and death (Nadel et al 1995).

A similar clinical picture is also seen in Gram-positive infections such as Streptococcal and Staphylococcal bacteraemia and toxic-shock syndrome (TSS), which is characterised by:

- high fever
- erythroderma
- encephalopathy
- diarrhoea
- shock
- evidence of colonisation or infection with toxin-producing Staphylococci or Streptococci.

Importantly, Staphylococcal TSS is not associated with Staphylococcal bacteraemia, but is usually associated with minor focal infection such as occurs in a thermal or surgical wound. Therefore the features of septic shock may be present without bacteraemia, but may be due to toxins released into the bloodstream (Kaplan 1987).

Other non-infectious conditions such as multiple trauma and acute pancreatitis may produce a similar clinical picture, termed 'systemic inflammatory response syndrome' (SIRS), regardless of the underlying pathology (Vincent 1994).

SEPTIC SHOCK
Pathophysiology

Entrance of an organism into the bloodstream remains poorly understood, but once there, bacterial and host factors may be important in allowing bacterial survival and proliferation, including:

- absence of specific antibody
- deficiency in complement components
- immunosuppression due to severe illness or therapy
- presence of invasive devices.

Products released by bacteria, including endotoxin and peptidoglycan from the bacterial cell wall and exotoxins, trigger a host inflammatory response. Endotoxin is one of the most important bacterial components contributing to the inflammatory process. Endotoxin plasma levels correlate with severity of meningococcal disease and with the development and release of several inflammatory mediators. These include the cytokines tumour necrosis factor (TNF) and interleukin 1 (IL 1) and complement components, which trigger activation of macrophages, neutrophils and platelets. Activation of the coagulation system occurs with:

- increased tissue factor expression on monocytes and endothelium
- platelet activation
- depression of the anticoagulant proteins: antithrombin III, proteins C and S
- elevation of plasminogen activator inhibitor.

The degree of inflammatory cell activation and level of these mediators correlates with clinical severity.

While the link between endotoxin and inflammation is well established, the mechanisms by which bacteria and the inflammatory process induce clinical manifestations of disease are less well understood.

Clinical pathophysiology

Few medical conditions present with such complex clinical problems as those found in children with septic shock. Although cardiorespiratory failure is the dominant clinical problem, this coexists with:

- multiple organ failure
- coagulopathy
- complex metabolic derangement, with acidosis, electrolyte disturbance and abnormalities in intermediary metabolism.

Although the precise sequence of events is not well understood, most of the abnormalities are explained by four processes:

1. severe capillary leak causing loss of circulating volume
2. dysregulation in vascular tone
3. intravascular thrombosis
4. myocardial dysfunction.

Capillary leak

Early septic shock is characterised by increased vascular permeability. Leakage of albumin and other plasma proteins into the extravascular space causes hypovolaemia, diminished venous return and reduced cardiac filling, causing diminished cardiac output. Compensatory sympathetic responses to hypovolaemia initially maintain cardiac output by increasing heart rate and contractility, maintaining blood pressure and vital organ perfusion by intense vasoconstriction in the skin, splanchnic and renal vessels. Therefore children in the early stages of septic shock may have well-maintained blood pressure, the only signs being tachycardia and diminished skin perfusion. As shock progresses and severe hypovolaemia develops, compensatory mechanisms fail, cardiac output falls and hypotension ensues. If the vasoconstriction is sustained, hypoxia occurs in underperfused tissues and organs. Anaerobic metabolism in hypoxic tissues causes increasing acidosis. Myocardial function is further depressed by hypoxia, acidosis and reduced coronary perfusion due to hypotension. Once profound acidosis, hypoxia and hypotension are present, reversal of shock becomes increasingly difficult.

Disordered vascular tone

Vasoconstriction occurs early in children with septic shock; vasodilated or 'warm shock' commonly seen in adults is uncommon in children. Children have cold peripheries, stagnant capillary refill and diminished peripheral pulses. However, once circulatory volume is restored and myocardial function improved by correction of metabolic abnormalities and acidosis, and addition of inotropes, a different picture may emerge which more closely resembles 'warm shock'. Peripheral vasodilation, wide pulse pressure, hypotension and progressive acidosis develop despite an elevated cardiac output.

Mechanisms responsible for disordered vascular tone are poorly understood. Vasoconstrictor substances, including catecholamines, renin, aldosterone, thromboxane A2 and endothelin, are increased and, together with reduced cardiac output, this may explain the intense vasoconstriction. Reduction of the endothelially derived vasodilator prostacyclin may contribute to platelet activation and consumption, together with vasoconstriction and small-vessel thrombosis. Mediators of vasodilation seen later in the illness, or occasionally from the onset of the disease, are less well defined. Excess production of nitric oxide by endothelial cells and macrophages may have a role, but this requires further evaluation in children with septic shock.

Coagulopathy and intravascular thrombosis

Coagulopathy occurs early in septic shock, including:

- thrombocytopenia
- prolonged clotting time
- reduced plasma fibrinogen
- elevation of fibrin degradation products

This indicates the presence of disseminated intravascular coagulation (DIC). This is supported by elevated fibrinopeptide A and depletion of coagulation pathway factors. Reduction in the coagulation inhibitors antithrombin III, proteins C and S and extrinsic pathway inhibitor are commonly seen on admission in meningococcal disease. Extreme depletion of these factors is associated with severe disease. Defective fibrinolysis with reduced plasminogen and alpha 2 antiplasmin and increased plasminogen activator inhibitor is also seen.

Mechanisms responsible for the coagulopathy of sepsis are incompletely understood. Endotoxin induces tissue factor expression on endothelial cells and circulating monocytes, congenital deficiency of proteins C or S causes purpuric lesions similar to those in meningococcal disease, suggesting that depletion of these proteins is involved in the pathogenesis of purpura in septic shock. Endothelial prostacyclin production is also diminished. Defective endothelial thromboresistance may therefore coexist with upregulation of endothelial procoagulant activity.

The coagulopathy of septic shock may progress to purpura fulminans. Children may develop extensive confluent areas of skin necrosis. Lesions are sharply demarcated and mainly affect the peripheries. Although usually purpura is confined to the skin, sometimes major vessel thrombosis occurs, causing gangrene. This is often seen in children with profound shock and intense vasoconstriction. The limbs are initially cold, white and bloodless. This may be followed by venous and arterial occlusion with progressive gangrene. Infarction of other organs is rare, but occasionally thrombosis is seen at postmortem in the lungs and kidneys. Areas of thrombosis may coexist with haemorrhage, which for unknown reasons is most common in the adrenals: Waterhouse-Friedrickson syndrome.

Myocardial failure

Myocardial depression is an early finding in septic shock. End-diastolic and end-systolic volumes are elevated and ejection fraction reduced. A gallop rhythm is often audible with elevated CVP and PA pressures and liver engorgement.

Myocardial depression is multifactorial: coronary artery perfusion may be impaired due to hypotension, and myocardial contractility may be depressed by hypoxia, acidosis and metabolic abnormalities. Deranged glucose and fatty acid metabolism is recognised in sepsis and may adversely affect myocardial function, possibly because of inadequate energy provision for cardiac myocytes. Endotoxin, TNF and NO directly depress myocardial function. Also, poorly characterised myocardial depressant factors are detected in septic shock. These mediators and metabolic abnormalities alone or together cause myocardial dysfunction and failure.

Other organ dysfunction

Children with septic shock develop multiorgan dysfunction. Respiratory failure is common with pulmonary oedema resulting from the capillary leak syndrome and myocardial depression. Pulmonary microvascular thrombi containing platelets, thrombin and neutrophils contribute to the picture of ARDS. Early findings are tachypnoea, chest wall retraction and hypoxaemia. Initially, increased respiratory effort maintains oxygen saturation with low/normal arterial concentration of carbon dioxide ($PaCO_2$). Pulmonary oedema may supervene suddenly with acute respiratory failure.

Oliguria occurs early in septic shock. Initially this is prerenal in origin with concentrated urine, low urine sodium concentration and elevated urine/plasma-urea ratio. If shock persists, renal vasoconstriction causes vasomotor nephropathy. Renal dysfunction may be reversible if cardiac output and renal perfusion are restored, but acute tubular or cortical necrosis is seen with prolonged shock.

In the absence of meningitis, neurological dysfunction is usually due to impaired cerebral perfusion and metabolism secondary to hypotension, hypoxia and acidosis. Prolonged hypotension and hypoxia may precipitate coma and hypoxic/ischaemic encephalopathy. The presence of meningitis may compound the neurological deficit induced by hypoperfusion.

Management of septic shock

Recognition and initial therapy

To improve prognosis, infection must be quickly recognised and treated. Any febrile child, particularly with a petechial rash or clinical features suggestive of sepsis, should be considered to have impending septic shock, and presumptive treatment should be commenced. When the child presents to hospital, blood cultures should be obtained, intravenous access established and broad-spectrum antibiotics administered promptly.

Initial assessment, observation and detection of complications

Children with bacteraemia may not initially

appear severely ill but may rapidly deteriorate. In meningococcal disease, 20% of cases are associated with shock. Several clinical scoring systems have been developed to identify those at greatest risk of a poor prognosis. Any shocked child, especially without meningitis, with low peripheral WBC and a rapidly progressive purpuric rash, is likely to become critically ill. Admission to a PICU should be arranged and appropriate management commenced prior to transfer of the child. The presence of hypotension is a pre-terminal sign and therefore is not necessary to diagnose shock in children; diagnosis is based on evidence of impaired end-organ perfusion, including:

- cold peripheries
- delayed capillary refill
- tachycardia
- tachypnoea
- oliguria
- metabolic acidosis
- restlessness indicating poor cerebral perfusion or hypoxaemia.

Monitoring of the following is essential:

- blood pressure
- pulse
- skin perfusion
- urine output
- measurement of core/peripheral temperature gradient
- oxygen saturation.

A temperature gradient above 4°C indicates underperfusion, if the ambient temperature is normal.

Resuscitation

Children with septic shock require immediate resuscitation to restore circulating volume. Supplemental oxygen by face mask or endotracheal tube should be administered, even if the transcutaneous oxygen saturation is normal. Vascular access must be obtained; the intraosseous route should be used if this is difficult. The degree of hypovolaemia is often underestimated; therefore boluses of colloid should be given over 10–30 min. If perfusion improves, a further bolus can be given over the next hour. If the child fails to respond to 40 mL/kg of colloid, or if continued deterioration occurs, transfer to PICU is indicated. Commonly, children with septic shock require large volumes of colloid: up to 200 mL/kg in the first 24 h of illness. Such volumes should only be given with monitoring of CVP or pulmonary wedge pressure, along with continuous clinical assessment. Children receiving large volumes of fluid are at risk of developing pulmonary oedema. Therefore, they should be electively intubated and ventilated even if they appear alert and are ventilating adequately, as sudden deterioration may occur. Elective ventilation allows the child to be appropriately sedated and, where necessary, paralysed to reduce the effort of breathing and myocardial workload. In children who are intravascularly depleted, certain anaesthetics may exacerbate hypotension: for example, thiopentone is a vasodilator and myocardial depressant. Prior volume loading and early commencement of an inotrope is recommended.

Strategies to improve tissue perfusion in septic shock include:

- optimising preload
- decreasing afterload
- improving myocardial contractility.

In hypotensive children or those who remain underperfused despite aggressive volume replacement, inotropes should be started early, together with continued volume expansion. Low-dose dopamine (5–10 μg/kg/min) or dobutamine (5–10 μg/kg/min) can be administered peripherally with caution prior to gaining CV access. When CVP or PA pressure monitoring is established, further volume expansion can be undertaken to optimise intravascular volume. If shock persists, additional inotropic support with higher doses of dobutamine, adrenaline or noradrenaline may be required.

In children with peripheral vasoconstriction despite adequate CVP and blood pressure, vasodilation is effective in improving perfusion and reducing afterload. Prostacyclin and nitroprusside are commonly used and are particularly indicated in children with severe vasoconstriction and impending peripheral gangrene. Vasodilators should be administered cautiously to children in shock, as severe hypotension may result if cardiac filling is inadequate. Prostacyclin also inhibits platelet aggregation and TNF release; however, there have been no controlled trials in children with septic shock.

Respiratory failure

There are two main causes of respiratory failure in septic shock. Children may develop pulmonary oedema in the initial 24–48 h. Management priorities include positive pressure ventilation, with high positive end expiratory pressure (PEEP), correction of coagulopathy and improvement of left ventricular function.

ARDS may occur later, indicated by increased oxygen requirement and reduced pulmonary compliance. In non-ventilated children, there is progressive tachypnoea with increased work of breathing. In ventilated children, increased oxygen requirement and increased ventilation pressure are noted. Improved management of circulatory failure has led to more children surviving the acute phase of septic shock and developing ARDS which may cause delayed mortality.

Management of ARDS includes improvement of myocardial function, removal of extravascular fluid accumulation using dialysis or haemofiltration, and ventilatory strategies such as:

- permissive hypercapnoea (tolerance of higher than normal $PaCO_2$)
- pressure-limited ventilation
- reversed inspiratory to expiratory time ratios
- increased PEEP.

Recent therapies used in the treatment of ARDS include:

- high-frequency oscillation ventilation (HFOV)
- inhaled NO therapy
- extracorporeal membrane oxygenation (ECMO).

However, the effectiveness of these requires further evaluation.

Renal function and fluid management

Optimal intravascular volume is difficult to maintain with continual capillary leakage. Colloid or crystalloid is administered according to CVP, peripheral and end-organ perfusion. Extravascular fluid accumulation may be reduced by restriction of crystalloid to 50–75% of maintenance requirements. Shocked children often develop renal dysfunction, and replacement therapy should be instituted early to effectively reduce extravascular fluid accumulation and normalise electrolyte and acid–base balance.

Metabolic abnormalities

Children with septic shock may have complex derangements of electrolytes, acid–base balance and metabolism, including:

- metabolic acidosis due to tissue underperfusion
- hyponatraemia, which may be present if severe vomiting occurs early in the illness
- hypokalaemia, despite metabolic acidosis which would be expected to cause movement of potassium from the intracellular compartment into the plasma
- hypocalcaemia
- hypophosphataemia
- hypomagnesaemia
- hypoglycaemia early in the illness
- hyperglycaemia and glucose intolerance, which may occur following initial resuscitation, particularly with high-dose inotropes.

Electrolyte and acid–base balance should be monitored and imbalances corrected. Correction of the metabolic derangement may be hampered by oliguria or anuria, requiring renal replacement therapy.

Central nervous system involvement

Cerebral oedema and raised intracranial pressure (ICP) may occur in septic shock, particularly with associated meningitis. Elective ventilation, control of $PaCO_2$, optimising cardiac output and therefore cerebral perfusion pressure, are important aspects of treatment. If raised ICP is suspected, a loop diuretic such as frusemide should be used initially to establish diuresis and reduce intracranial water content. Mannitol (0.25–0.5 g/kg) may be considered if the child is not anuric.

Management of disseminated intravascular coagulation

Many children with septic shock have evidence of disseminated intravascular coagulation (DIC). While there is insufficient evidence to recommend heparinisation for all children with septic shock, individual children, particularly those with impending peripheral gangrene, may benefit from low-dose heparin (10 units/kg/h) together with fresh-frozen plasma (FFP). This is unlikely to exacerbate bleeding problems, since it has been demonstrated that low-dose heparin has little, if any, effect on measurable coagulation indices but may tip the clinical balance towards anticoagulation. FFP may also restore depleted levels of antithrombin III and proteins C and S.

Tissue plasminogen activator (tPA), protein C and antithrombin III concentrates have theoretical advantages for reversal of DIC. There is anecdotal evidence to suggest benefit in children with purpura fulminans. However, there may be associated haemorrhagic complications, and they should be used cautiously. None of these treatments has been subjected to controlled clinical trials in children with sepsis.

MENINGITIS

Meningitis is the most common form of intracranial infection. Acute bacterial meningitis remains a significant cause of morbidity and mortality throughout the world. The current morbidity and mortality is dependent on the causative organism and the duration of symptoms prior to therapy. Children with this disease will be more likely to require intensive care management.

The incidence of bacterial meningitis in the developed world is 3–5/100 000 per year, with a higher rate in infants. Approximately 75% of all cases occur in children under 15 years of age, and it is one of the most common life-threatening infections. Neonatal meningitis is usually caused by organisms acquired from the female genital tract during labour — for example, group B Streptococci and *Escherichia coli* — or acquired by the fetus transplacentally: *Listeria monocytogenes*. Most children with bacterial meningitis acquire the infection following bacteraemia.

Until the introduction of Hib vaccine, this organism was the commonest cause in children under 5 years. Currently, *Neisseria meningitidis* and *Streptococcus pneumoniae* are the commonest causes in children following the neonatal period (Table 12.4).

In older children and adults, nosocomial meningitis accounts for an increasing proportion of infections, often associated with recent neurosurgery or trauma. *Pseudomonas aeruginosa*, Enterococci, *Staphylococcus aureus* and coagulase-negative Staphylococci are the most common causative organisms (Table 12.5).

Pathophysiology

To cause meningitis, bacteria must colonise and penetrate the nasopharyngeal or oropharyngeal mucosa, cause bacteraemia and penetrate the blood–brain barrier.

Table 12.4 The most likely causes of acute bacterial meningitis according to age

Age	Organism
0–2 months (neonate)	Group B β haemolytic streptococcus, enteric bacilli (e.g. *Escherichia coli, Klebsiella pneumoniae, Proteus,* spp.), *Listeria monocytogenes*
2–4 months	Group B β haemolytic streptococcus, *Streptococcus pneumoniae, Neisseria meningitidis, Haemophilus influenzae* type b[a]
4 months–5 years	*Streptococcus pneumoniae, Neisseria meningitidis, Haemophilus influenzae* type b[a]
5–50 years	*Streptococcus pneumoniae, Neisseria meningitidis*

[a]In countries which have adopted the Hib vaccine, infections in infants and young children from *Haemophilus influenzae* type b have been virtually eradicated.

Table 12.5 Organisms associated with development of meningitis according to different underlying conditions

Underlying condition	Organism
Basilar skull fracture	*Streptococcus pneumoniae* *Neisseria meningitidis* *Haemophilus influenzae* type b *Staphylococcus aureus* *Streptococcus pyogenes* Gram-negative bacilli
Postneurosurgical procedure	Coagulase-negative staphylococci *Staphylococcus aureus* Gram-negative bacilli
With cerebrospinal fluid shunt	Coagulase-negative staphylococci *Staphylococcus aureus* Gram-negative bacilli Corynebacteria (Diphtheroids) *Propionibacteria acnes* Bacillus species
Nosocomial (without neurosurgery)	*Staphylococcus aureus* Gram-negative bacilli Enterococci Candida species
Immune deficiencies[a] (including hyposplenism)	*Streptococcus pneumoniae* *Neisseria meningitidis* *Haemophilus influenzae* type b *Listeria monocytogenes* Salmonella species *Cryptococcus neoformans* Nocardia species Gram-negative bacilli Enteric bacilli *Pseudomonas aeruginosa*

[a]These organisms also cause other infections in immunocompromised children.

Colonisation and penetration of the nasopharyngeal mucosa

Infection occurs following colonisation, usually in the upper respiratory tract. Pathogenic bacteria are transferred between individuals by droplet spread. Most individuals are asymptomatic following colonisation. It appears that invasion is more common following viral upper respiratory infections.

Secretory IgA on the respiratory mucosa is superior to other immunoglobulin isotypes in protection from viral and bacterial mucosal pathogens. However, pathogenic bacteria colonising the nasopharynx produce enzymes which inactivate secretory IgA. Attachment of bacteria to nasopharyngeal epithelial cells is determined by the presence of bacterial virulence factors such as fimbriae and pili.

The organisms commonly causing meningitis possess a polysaccharide capsule which is a potent virulence factor. The capsule inhibits complement-mediated phagocytosis and inhibits lysis of the organism. Non-encapsulated strains are less virulent and rarely cause invasive disease in the immunocompetent host. The alternative complement pathway plays an important role in prevention of infection by encapsulated organisms, particularly *S. pneumoniae*.

The spleen is vital for removal of non-opsonised material from the circulation, particularly in non-immune individuals without specific antibodies. Therefore, individuals without a functional spleen, for example in sickle-cell disease and congenital asplenia, are at high risk of invasion by encapsulated organisms.

Penetration of the blood–brain barrier

Once in the bloodstream, the organism may be neutralised by circulating antibodies, complement and phagocytic cells, or may survive and proliferate. Meningitis usually follows primary bacteraemia and secondary infection of the meninges. The mechanisms of penetration of the blood–brain barrier and seeding the CSF remain unclear. High-grade bacteraemia (> 10^2 organisms/mm^3 of blood) appears to be necessary.

Organisms causing meningitis exhibit tropism for the meninges. This may be due to bacterial adhesive structures which bind them to receptors on the choroid plexus and cerebral capillary endothelial cells facilitating bacterial translocation into the CSF. After penetrating the blood–brain barrier, bacteria may multiply rapidly, as the CSF is a poor immune environment. The CSF contains low concentrations of specific antibody and complement and thus has poor bactericidal activity.

The CSF inflammatory response

Once the organism has invaded the CSF, a number of bacterial components, particularly endotoxin and peptidoglycan, cause meningeal inflammation. Direct inoculation of endotoxin into the CSF of experimental animals causes an inflammatory reaction, with influx of leucocytes, increase in protein and lactate and reduction of CSF glucose concentration. These changes occur several hours after inoculation of bacteria or cell wall constituents into the CSF of experimental animals. Therefore it appears that elaboration and release of mediators such as TNF-α and IL1β are the cause of CSF inflammatory changes. This precedes cellular influx and protein exudation. These cytokines stimulate the inflammatory cascade, including platelet activating factor (PAF), interleukin 8 (IL8) and interferon-gamma (IFNγ), causing upregulation of adhesion molecules. This causes attraction, attachment and migration of leucocytes into the CSF where they degranulate, releasing proteolytic enzymes, cationic proteins and reactive oxygen species. These further alter the integrity of the blood–brain barrier.

Increased blood–brain barrier permeability results in leakage of albumin and other proteins into the CSF, causing vasogenic oedema. The presence of anaphylotoxins (C3a, C5a) in the CSF due to the leak, further encourages passage of leucocytes into the CSF, thus accentuating the inflammatory process. Toxic products of activated neutrophils and other inflammatory cells cause cytotoxic oedema and damage to surrounding cells.

Direct inoculation of TNF-α, IL1β and IFNγ into CSF induces inflammatory changes similar to those seen following endotoxin inoculation. In addition, the inflammatory response to endotoxin can be reduced by simultaneous inoculation of antibodies to TNF-α and IL1β. However, use of these antibodies does not completely stop the inflammatory response, suggesting that other mediators also play an important role.

In addition to proinflammatory cytokines, antiinflammatory cytokines, (e.g. IL10) are also present in the CSF of children with bacterial meningitis. The significance of IL10 and other host-produced antiinflammatory agents is not yet clear.

Cerebral oedema and thrombosis

Apart from vasogenic and cytotoxic oedema, interstitial oedema is caused by impaired reabsorption of CSF by arachnoid villi. The consequence of increased CSF secretion, diminished CSF reabsorption and breakdown of the blood–brain barrier, is an increase in brain water content and CSF volume, causing cerebral oedema, hydrocephalus and increased ICP. If the increased ICP is severe, cerebral blood flow (CBF) is reduced. In experimental meningitis, CBF at first increases due to local vasodilatation induced by oxygen-free radicals and local NO production from leucocytes, vascular smooth muscle, vascular endothelium and glial cells. Cerebral blood volume therefore increases and causes raised ICP. This is paralleled by increased CSF lactate level, indicating tissue hypoxia. Increased lactate contributes to increased CBF as acidosis causes vasodilation.

Following this initial stage, CBF then decreases, presumably due to raised ICP. Changes in CBF may also be due to loss of cerebrovascular autoregulation, which has been demonstrated in bacterial meningitis. CBF is normally maintained at constant levels irrespective of systemic arterial pressure. Once autoregulation is lost, CBF is dependent on systemic pressure. Inadequate CBF may occur if hypotension occurs. Increased ICP and hypotension, which is common in bacterial sepsis, may cause cerebral hypoperfusion.

All patients with bacterial meningitis have raised ICP. In one study the mean opening pressure at lumbar puncture was $18 \pm 7 \, \text{cmH}_2\text{O}$, more than twice the upper limit of normal. ICP is an important determinant of cerebral perfusion pressure (CPP). Morbidity and mortality is highest in those with CPP of < 30 mmHg. Reduction of CPP is more a consequence of increased ICP than of systemic hypotension. Vasculitis, vascular spasm and thrombosis occur in intracerebral arteries and veins in bacterial meningitis. As these blood vessels lie over the surface of the brain and are bathed in CSF containing cytokines, other mediators, bacterial products and leucocytes, they are particularly susceptible to damage. Another aspect of CNS disturbance is alteration in cerebral metabolism, with increased CSF lactate and reduced CSF glucose concentration.

This is probably due to increased metabolism of glucose by leucocytes and bacteria, and disturbance of glucose transport into CSF.

Clinical features

Children with bacterial meningitis present with:

- headache
- fever
- photophobia
- vomiting
- neck stiffness
- altered mental status.

Cranial nerve palsy, focal neurological signs and seizures occur in up to 30% of cases. With disease progression, signs of raised ICP such as coma, hypertension, bradycardia and altered respiratory status with focal brain involvement become more likely.

Clinical features of meningitis may be non-specific, especially in infants and young children. Neonates and infants may present with poor feeding, lethargy, listlessness, diarrhoea and vomiting. Fever may not be present.

Approximately 50% of patients with meningococcal meningitis, and most patients with meningococcal septicaemia, with or without meningitis have a petechial or purpuric rash which may initially be maculopapular and progress to haemorrhagic.

Seizures occur in 20–30% of patients with bacterial meningitis. Generalised seizures are not associated with severe outcome, but focal seizures are more likely to be associated with persistent neurologic sequelae, as are focal neurological signs and cranial nerve palsies.

Postneurosurgical meningitis may present with subtle alterations in mental status without any other signs.

Diagnosis

The diagnosis of bacterial meningitis is made by obtaining CSF, either by lumbar puncture, subarachnoid or ventricular drainage.

Lumbar puncture is usually safe but there are several recognised contraindications:

- signs of raised ICP
- infection of skin at the lumbar puncture site
- coagulopathy
- cardiovascular compromise.

In considering risk of lumbar puncture, particularly in those with presumed meningococcal disease, additional factors should be considered, including the presence of septic shock. Performing a lumbar puncture causes increased respiratory and cardiovascular workload due to stress and positioning of the child and may result in acute deterioration. The airway may become obstructed and respiratory function compromised by limiting chest expansion. Position of the child may interfere with venous return and cardiac output. These children are likely to have DIC with raised ICP and reduced CPP due to hypotension. In children with septic shock, lumbar puncture is contraindicated until cardiovascular compromise is adequately treated.

Elevated ICP occurs in virtually all patients with bacterial meningitis. Signs of raised ICP include:

- altered level of consciousness
- altered pupillary responses
- hyper- or hypotension
- bradycardia
- altered respiratory pattern
- papilloedema — a late sign.

If any of these features are present the risk of cerebral herniation following lumbar puncture is considerable and the procedure should be deferred. Diagnosis of raised ICP is based on clinical assessment rather than cranial imaging, as this is an insensitive method of predicting raised ICP. CNS imaging is not routinely required in the management of patients with meningitis.

In bacterial meningitis the CSF WBC count is usually > 1000/μL, with a neutrophil predominance. About 10% of patients have a lymphocytic CSF, especially in neonatal Gram-negative meningitis and in *L. monocytogenes* meningitis. Patients with low CSF WBC have a worse prognosis. Reduction of CSF glucose concentration to < 30% of simultaneously measured serum glucose is found in 70% of cases. CSF protein concentration is often elevated. CSF Gram stain is positive for organisms in 60–90% and is very specific. However, the sensitivity is only 40–60% and is dependent on the observer and whether the patient has received prior antibiotic treatment. CSF culture is positive in up to 85% of patients, but this falls to < 50% if patients have received prior antibiotic therapy. In children with bacterial meningitis, CSF is sterilised within 24–36 h of commencing appropriate antibiotic therapy, without significant change in other CSF indices.

In patients with typical CSF findings, but with a negative Gram stain, latex agglutination testing of CSF for bacterial antigen improves identification rate of the causative organism. Tests are available to detect Hib, *S. pneumoniae*, N. *meningitidis*, *E. coli* K1 and group B Streptococci. The sensitivity of the test is 50–100% dependent on the organism, but the specificity is high.

Polymerase chain reaction (PCR), for detection of bacterial DNA, has recently proved useful for identification of meningococcal meningitis.

Differential diagnosis

The main differential diagnosis from bacterial menigitis is acute viral meningitis or encephalitis. Although in its early stages viral meningitis may be associated with a neutrophil-predominant CSF, the CSF becomes lymphocyte-predominant in 12–24 h. Other causes of CSF pleocytosis include:

- chemical meningitis from intrathecal administration of chemotherapeutic agents
- carcinomatous meningitis
- parameningeal foci of infection.

In these, the CSF WBC is usually lower than in bacterial meningitis. However, patients should be assumed to have bacterial meningitis and treated until it is excluded. If the diagnosis is unclear, lumbar puncture should be repeated 12–24 h later to assess whether the CSF findings have changed. In bacterial meningitis, CSF findings are similar despite initiation of appropriate therapy, whereas in viral meningitis the CSF becomes lymphocyte predominant.

Alternative diagnoses in children presenting with focal neurological signs or papilloedema include:

- brain abscess
- intracranial haemorrhage
- cerebral tumour
- chronic meningitis such as tuberculosis or cryptococcal meningitis.

Lumbar puncture should not be performed in these patients until a space-occupying lesion has been excluded by CT or MRI scan. If there is suspicion of bacterial meningitis, presumptive antibiotic therapy should be started following blood culture and the patient should be reviewed by a neurosurgeon to decide on appropriate management, including obtaining CSF by ventricular drainage.

Antimicrobial therapy

Appropriate antimicrobial therapy for bacterial meningitis should be commenced within 30 min of presentation even if delay in obtaining CSF is unavoidable. In this situation, choice of antimicrobial therapy is empiric and based on the most likely causative organism for the patient's age. Antimicrobial therapy should not be delayed whilst awaiting imaging studies in the case of patients with focal neurological signs or papilloedema. Even if lumbar puncture is delayed after the start of antimicrobial therapy, CSF findings may still be diagnostic, and a microbiologic diagnosis may be obtained by latex agglutination or PCR.

In patients who are immunosuppressed, postsurgical or with a CSF leak, broad-spectrum antimicrobial therapy should be administered.

Recommendations on empiric antimicrobials in bacterial meningitis have recently been adapted to account for changing antimicrobial susceptibility patterns of commonly isolated organisms. Despite reports of penicillin-resistant meningococci in certain countries, these have not proven to be a serious clinical problem in the UK or USA. Other organisms have recently developed much more serious antimicrobial resistance patterns. β-lactamase-producing Hib account for 30% of all

Hib isolates, and chloramphenicol-resistant Hib account for > 50% of isolates in some parts of the world. Fortunately, the incidence of Hib meningitis has dramatically decreased since the widespread introduction of Hib vaccine.

A serious recent development has been the growing incidence of high-level penicillin resistance of *S. pneumoniae*, with up to 60% incidence in eastern Europe. In the UK in 1992, this figure was approximately 2%, but current estimates would be higher. There are also recent reports of high-level cephalosporin resistance, conferring resistance of *S. pneumoniae* to third-generation cephalosporins. Most authorities in Europe and North America now recommend third-generation cephalosporins (cefotaxime or ceftriaxone) as first-line treatment for bacterial meningitis. These have the advantage of activity against all common meningeal pathogens (except *Listeria monocytogenes*), lack of resistance in common organisms (apart from rarely *S. pneumoniae*), excellent penetration into CSF and ease of administration. If *S. pneumoniae* meningitis is suspected, there is a case for inclusion of vancomycin until antimicrobial susceptibility patterns are known. Vancomycin penetrates CSF adequately in the presence of meningeal inflammation, and combination of vancomycin with a third-generation cephalosporin may be synergistic for meningitis caused by high-level penicillin-resistant *S. pneumoniae*.

If *L. monocytogenes* is suspected, addition of penicillin or ampicillin is indicated. The cephalosporins have limited activity against this organism, but vancomycin is active and is adequate initial therapy while culture results are pending.

In the postneurosurgical patient, initial therapy must cover Gram-negative organisms (including coliforms and *P. aeruginosa*), skin flora and community-acquired organisms.

Duration of antimicrobial therapy is dependent on age and immune-status of the patient, organism and clinical course or development of complications. There is no universally accepted standard (Table 12.6). Duration of therapy may need to be extended due to complications such as brain abscess or subdural empyaema,

Table 12.6 Suggested treatment duration for acute bacterial meningitis

Causative organism	Duration of therapy
Meningococcus	7 days of antibiotics or less
Hib	10 days
Pneumococcus	14 days
L. monocytogenes	14 days (21 days in the immunocompromised child)
Neonatal Gram-negative	At least 21 days following CSF sterilisation

prolonged fever, or development of nosocomial superinfection.

Antiinflammatory treatment

The risk of morbidity and mortality remains high despite appropriate antimicrobial therapy. Powerful bactericidal antibiotics trigger the release of bacterial constituents which damage the brain because of the host inflammatory response. Therefore, injury may be reduced by antiinflammatory treatment. In experimental animals, the inflammatory process is reduced by agents which:

- neutralise endotoxin
- block binding of endotoxin to macrophages: for example, bactericidal permeability-increasing factor (BPI) and anti-CD14 antibodies
- block cytokine mediators
- stop neutrophil adhesion
- inhibit neutrophil and macrophage activation: for example, steroids, pentoxiphylline, or non-steroidal antiinflammatory agents.

Convincing evidence of the beneficial effect of steroids in humans has now emerged. There is reduction in severity of neurological sequelae, particularly deafness, in studies of children who had Hib or *S. pneumoniae* meningitis (Tunkel & Scheld 1995). Firm conclusions about efficacy of steroids in reducing neurological damage following meningococcal meningitis is lacking. However, the pathophysiology of meningococcal meningitis is unlikely to differ significantly from other forms of bacterial meningitis. There is no good data on the use of adjunctive steroid therapy in neonatal meningitis or in postneurosurgical meningitis.

The benefit of steroids is greatest if administered early, preferably prior to antibiotic administration. Current recommendation is: dexamethasone 0.15 mg/kg, 6 hourly for 4 days, starting prior to, simultaneously or shortly after the first dose of antibiotics.

On the basis of animal studies, a variety of other antiinflammatory agents may be beneficial in reducing brain injury, but there have been no clinical studies on which to base recommendations for routine use.

Management of raised intracranial pressure

The primary therapeutic objective in raised ICP is to preserve oxygen and nutrient delivery to the brain. Simple interventions to optimise respiration and cardiac output, and to prevent metabolic abnormalities, may be as important as direct reduction of ICP.

In patients who are comatose, obstruction of the airway, cessation of respiration or convulsions may result in hypoxia and hypercapnia, which alter cerebral perfusion and exacerbate cerebral oedema. Therefore, maintenance of the airway, elective ventilation and control of convulsions are important interventions.

Direct measurement of ICP is often advocated and may help to define required therapeutic interventions. However, no studies indicate that ICP monitoring reduces mortality from meningitis.

Simple measures to reduce ICP include nursing the child in a quiet environment, with head midline and elevated to 20–30°. Other interventions include use of osmotic agents, fluid restriction and control of cerebro-vascular tone by manipulation of $PaCO_2$.

Extravascular fluid accumulation and ICP is reduced by osmotic agents such as mannitol. Mannitol (0.25–1 g/kg) causes rapid movement of fluid from the extravascular to the intravascular space and may be associated with a prompt reduction of ICP. Because of its rapid action, mannitol may be life-saving in patients with impending cerebral herniation and is often valuable while other measures (e.g. airway control, artificial ventilation and fluid restriction) are being initiated.

In areas of brain with extensive vascular injury, mannitol may accumulate extravascularly, worsening brain oedema. Repeated doses may cause a hyperosmolar state, which may impair cardiac output in the child who is fluid restricted. Mannitol should therefore be used cautiously.

In patients with pupillary changes, hypertension/bradycardia, signs of respiratory insufficiency or Glasgow Coma Score (GCS) < 8, urgent tracheal intubation and artificial ventilation should be instituted, both for airway protection and to prevent an acute rise in ICP resulting from increasing $PaCO_2$.

Hyperventilation as treatment for raised ICP is controversial. Based on the linear correlation between $PaCO_2$ and CBF, hyperventilation to reduce $PaCO_2$ may decrease intracranial blood volume, therefore reducing ICP. It is not clear, however, whether reduction in CBF is beneficial, as blood supply to critically dependent areas may be reduced. In addition, cerebral autoregulation and CO_2 reactivity are impaired or absent in injured brain. Hyperventilation to reduce raised ICP should be used cautiously and with careful monitoring. Modest reduction in $PaCO_2$ to 3.5–4.5 kPa is advocated and should be monitored by repeated blood gases or by end-tidal CO_2. More extreme hyperventilation should only be undertaken in impending brainstem herniation.

Children with meningitis are often fluid restricted. However, they may have been vomiting and febrile, or had reduced fluid intake in the days preceding admission. Further restriction of fluid intake may reduce circulating volume and cardiac output, which could lead to renal failure.

Inappropriate secretion of antidiuretic hormone (SIADH) has lead to fluid restriction in patients with meningitis, even in the face of hypovolaemia. Recent studies indicate, however, that the increased level of antidiuretic hormone seen in patients with meningitis is an appropriate response to dehydration. With rehydration, this level returns to normal. Correction of hypovolaemia improves cardiac output and possibly CBF. In patients with shock the use of inotropes, together with fluid resuscitation, is important to optimise cerebral perfusion.

Sedation and control of convulsions

Children with reduced level of consciousness due to bacterial meningitis should not be sedated, even if irritable or combative. They may have cerebral hypoxia resulting from reduced respiratory drive. Use of hypnotic or transquillising agents may precipitate acute respiratory failure or respiratory arrest and cause a further rise in ICP. Simple analgesics or antipyretic agents should be used. Children who require endotracheal intubation and artificial ventilation should receive infusions of analgesics, hypnotics and sedatives, occasionally with muscle relaxants. Barbiturates are used to treat raised ICP that is refractory to other forms of therapy. However, high doses of agents such as thiopentone are cardiodepressant and should only be used in stable patients with careful monitoring. Thiopentone is particularly useful for induction of anaesthesia prior to endotracheal intubation in patients with raised ICP.

In children with raised ICP, seizures cause increased metabolic demands and CBF which can precipitate further rises in ICP. The use of anticonvulsants in self-ventilating children may precipitate respiratory arrest. Careful observation of respiration should be undertaken during the treatment of seizures. Short-acting agents such as diazepam or paraldehyde are used for acute seizure control, with barbiturates or phenytoin for longer-term control. Convulsions are difficult to detect in children who are pharmacologically paralysed for artificial ventilation. In such children cerebral function monitoring should be used to detect seizure activity.

Complications

Complications of bacterial meningitis vary according to causative organism, duration of symptoms prior to initiation of therapy and age and immune status of the child.

Some children suffer severe and permanent neurological sequelae. Although focal neurological signs such as hemiplegia and quadriplegia can develop early in meningitis, they are more common later. Vasculitis and thrombosis may explain these clinical findings; therefore, awareness of conditions that require acute neurosurgical intervention is necessary. These include subdural empyaema, brain abscess and acute hydrocephalus. Subdural effusions are more common after Hib meningitis, but can occur with any organism. They usually resolve spontaneously, but persistent neurological symptoms, including seizures, paresis, raised ICP and development of empyaema, are indications for drainage. Other causes of focal neurology include development of ischaemic areas or infarction. Cerebral abscess must be considered in any child with persistent fever who deteriorates following the acute phase of bacterial meningitis.

Fever persisting beyond the 10th day is considered prolonged, whereas new fever following defervescence for 24 h is considered to be secondary or recurrent. Most commonly, recurrent fever is due to nosocomial infection such as thrombophlebitis, but subdural empyaema or disseminated sepsis (e.g. osteomyelitis, peri- and endocarditis) must also be considered. It is unusual for fever to be caused by persistence of the organism in the meninges. However, with emergence of drug-resistant organisms, it cannot be assumed that persistent or recurrent fever is not due to continued presence of live bacteria within the CSF.

Prevention

Morbidity and mortality are reduced when prevention of infection is addressed by using immunisation or chemoprophylaxis. This has been accomplished in the case of Hib in children as young as 2 months by introduction of Hib-conjugate vaccine. This has virtually eliminated Hib as a cause of bacterial meningitis in areas with high vaccine uptake.

Although Meningococcus is now the most

common cause of bacterial meningitis, routine use of meningococcal vaccine is not widespread. Reliable vaccines are available against serogroups A, C, Y and W135. However, these are polysaccharide vaccines which are ineffective in young children, the group most at risk. A conjugate vaccine against these serogroups is currently being evaluated, with promising results.

There is no reliable vaccine against *N. meningitidis* group B. However, several experimental meningococcal group B vaccines are currently being evaluated. Of increasing importance is prevention of pneumococcal meningitis because of increasing prevalence of resistant *S. pneumoniae*. A polysaccharide vaccine is currently available for individuals at risk of invasive pneumococcal disease, such as individuals with:

- cardiac, respiratory, hepatic or renal disease
- diabetes
- sickle cell disease
- certain immunodeficiencies
- certain malignancies
- lymphoma
- functional or anatomic asplenia.

It is not useful in children < 2 years of age, who are at most risk. Several conjugate pneumococcal vaccines are currently being evaluated.

It is recommended that patients with a CSF leak should receive vaccination with all these available vaccines.

Chemoprophylaxis may prevent transmission and development of invasive meningococcal and Hib infection in susceptible individuals who are close contacts of an index case. 50% of the increased risk of meningococcal infection in household contacts occurs within 7 days of presentation of the index case, and half of this occurs within 48 h. Therefore decisions regarding administration of chemoprophylaxis should not be delayed by waiting for microbiological confirmation.

Fear and anxiety within the family, school or community frequently follows a case of meningitis. Careful handling of the family and the contacts is required, with close collaboration between primary physicians and those responsible for community and public health.

CONCLUSION

Recent years have seen enormous advances in our understanding of the pathophysiology of infectious disease. This has lead to important improvements in therapy, both antimicrobial and supportive. However, new challenges, such as the emergence of multidrug-resistant bacteria, will inevitably mean that medical and nursing staff working in intensive care will continue to be faced with the management of potentially life-threatening infections.

REFERENCES

Alexander J W 1990 Mechanism of immunologic suppression in burn injury. Journal of Trauma 30:S70–S75

Allgower M, Durig M, Wolff G 1980 Infection and trauma. Surgical Clinics of North America 60:133–144

Anderson D C, Pickering L K, Feigin R D 1974 Leukocyte function in normal and infected neonates. Journal of Pediatrics 85:420–425

Bellanti J A, Kadlec J V, Escobar-Gutierrez A 1994 Cytokines and the immune response. Pediatric Clinics of North America 41:597–621

Brook I 1979 Bacterial colonization, tracheobronchitis and pneumonia following tracheostomy and long-term ventilation in pediatric patients. Chest 76:420–424

Brouwers P, Belman A L, Epstein L G 1994 Central nervous system involvement: manifestations and evaluation. In: Pizzo P A, Wilfert C M (eds) Pediatric AIDS: the challenge

of HIV infection in infants, children and adolescents, 2nd edn. Williams and Wilkins, Baltimore, pp 318–335

Centers for Disease Control 1994 HIV/AIDS Surveillance Report 6:2

Centers for Disease Control 1995 revised guidelines for prophylaxis against Pneumocystis carinii pneumonia for children infected with or perinatally exposed to human immunodeficiency virus. MMWR 44:RR-4

Chandra R K, Kumari S 1994 Nutrition and immunity: an overview. Journal of Nutrition 124:S1433–S1435

Cheesbrough J S, Finch R G, Burden R P 1986 A prospective study of the mechanisms of infection associated with hemodialysis catheters. Journal of Infections Diseases 154:579–589

Connor E M, Andiman W A 1994 Lymphoid interstitial pneumonitis. In: Pizzo PA, Wilfert CM (eds) Pediatric

AIDS: the challenge of HIV infection in infants, children and adolescents, 2nd edn. Williams and Wilkins, Baltimore, pp 467–481

Cronin W A, Germanson T P, Donowitz L G 1990 Intravascular catheter colonization and related bloodstream infection in critically ill neonates. Infection Control and Hospital Epidemiology 11:301–308

Drew J H, Arroyave C M 1980 The complement system of the newborn infant. Biology of the Neonate 37:209–217

Ducharme F M, Gauthier M, Lacroix J, Lafleur L 1990 Incidence of infection related to arterial catheterisation in children: a prospective study. Critical Care Medicine 16:272–276

duMoulin G C, Paterson D G, Hedley-Whyte J, Lisbon A 1982 Aspiration of gastric bacteria in antacid-treated patients: a frequent cause of post-operative colonization of the airway. Lancet i:242–245

Durandy A, Fischer A, Griscelli C 1979 Active suppression of B lymphocyte maturation by two different newborn T lymphocyte subsets. Journal of Immunology 123:2644–2650

Farley J J, Englander R, Tressler R L, Vink P E 1996 The critically ill child with Human Immunodeficiency Virus infection. In: Rogers M C (ed) Textbook of pediatric intensive care, 3rd edn. Williams and Wilkins, Baltimore, p 945

Filippell M B, Rearick T 1993 Respiratory syncytial virus. Nursing Clinics of North America 28:651–671

Gaur S, Kesarwala H, Gavai M, Gupta M, Whitley-Williams P, Frenkel L D 1994 Clinical immunology and infectious diseases. Pediatric Clinics of North America 41:745–782

Gibb D, Newell M L 1992 HIV infection in children. Archives of Diseases of the Child 67:138–141

Guidet B, Nicola I, Barakett V, Gabillet J M, Snoey E, Petit J C, Offenstadt G 1994 Skin versus hub culture to predict colonization and infection of central venous catheters in intensive care patients. Infection 22:43–48

Hague R A, Rassam S, Morgan G, Cant A J 1994 Early diagnosis of severe combined immunodeficiency syndrome. Archives of Diseases of the Child 70:260–263

Hauger S B 1991 Approach to the pediatric patient with HIV infection and pulmonary symptoms. Journal of Pediatrics 119:S25–S33

Helling T S, Evans L L, Fowler D L, et al 1988 Infectious complications in patients with severe head injury. Journal of Trauma 28:1575–1577

Hughes W T 1994 *Pneumocystis carinii* pneumonia. In: Pizzo P A, Wilfert C M (eds) Pediatric AIDS: the challenge of HIV infection in infants, children and adolescents, 2nd edn. Williams and Wilkins, Baltimore, pp 405–418

Johnson P R, Decker M D, Edwards K M, Schaffner W, Wright P F 1986 Frequency of Broviac catheter infections in pediatric oncology patients. Journal of Infectious Diseases 154:570–578

Kaplan S L 1987 Bacteremia and endotoxin shock. In: Feigin R D, Cherry J D (eds) Textbook of pediatric infectious diseases. Saunders, Philadelphia, pp 910–921

Kasian G F, Elash J H, Tan L K 1988 Bacteriologic surveillance of indwelling urinary catheters in pediatric intensive care unit patients. Critical Care Medicine 16:679–682

Krasinski K 1994 Bacterial infections. In: Pizzo P A, Wilfert C M (eds) Pediatric AIDS: the challenge of HIV infection in infants, children and adolescents, 2nd edn. Williams and Wilkins, Baltimore, pp 241–253

Krensky A M, Clayberger C 1994 Transplantation

immunology. Pediatric Clinics of North America 41:819–837

Kroll J S, Booy R 1996 *Haemophilus influenzae*: capsule vaccine and capsulation genetics. Molecular Medicine Today 4:160–166

Kunin C M, Steele C 1985 Culture of the surfaces of urinary catheters to sample urethral flora and study of the effect of antimicrobial therapy. Journal of Clinical Microbiology 21:902–908

Lennard T W J, Browell D A 1993 The immunological effects of trauma. Proceedings of the Nutritional Society 52:85–90

Lipshultz S E 1994 Cardiovascular problems. In: Pizzo P A, Wilfert C M (eds) Pediatric AIDS: the challenge of HIV infection in infants, children and adolescents, 2nd edn. Williams and Wilkins, Baltimore, pp 483–511

Luskin R L, Weinstein R A, Nathan C, Chamberlin W H, Kabins S A 1986 Extended use of disposable pressure transducers. Journal of the American Medical Association 255:916–920

McCarty J M, Flam M S, Pullen G, Jones R, Kassel S H 1986 Outbreak of primary cutaneous aspergillosis related to intravenous arm boards. Journal of Pediatrics 108:721–724

McGowan J E Jr, Bratton L, Klein J O, Finland M 1973 Bacteremia in febrile children seen in a 'walk-in' pediatric clinic. New England Journal of Medicine 288:1309–1312

Merritt W T, Green M 1996 Nosocomial infections in the pediatric intensive care unit. In: Rogers M C (ed) Textbook of pediatric intensive care, 3rd edn. Williams and Wilkins, Baltimore, p 975

Miller K J, Ackerman A D 1996 Primary and secondary immunodeficiencies. In: Rogers M C (ed) Textbook of pediatric intensive care, 3rd edn. Williams and Wilkins, Baltimore, p 915

Morris J B, Occhionero M E, Gauderer M W, Stern R C, Doershuk C F 1990 Totally implantable vascular access devices in cystic fibrosis: a four-year experience with fifty-eight patients. Journal of Pediatrics 117:82–85

Mueller B U 1994 Haematological problems and their management in children with HIV infection. In: Pizzo P A, Wilfert C M (eds) Pediatric AIDS: the challenge of HIV infection in infants, children and adolescents, 2nd edn. Williams and Wilkins, Baltimore, pp 591–601

Nadel S, Levin M, Habibi P 1995 Treatment of meningococcal disease in childhood. In: Cartwright K (ed) Meningococcal disease. Wiley, Chichester

The National Institute of Child Health and Human Development Intravenous Immunoglobulin Study Group (NICHHDIISG) 1991 Intravenous immune globulin for the prevention of bacterial infections in children with symptomatic Human Immunodeficiency Virus infection. New England Journal of Medicine 325:73–80

Noel G J, O'Loughlin J E, Edelson P J 1988 Neonatal Staphylococcus epidermidis right-sided endocarditis: description of five catheterized infants. Pediatrics 82:234–239

Powell D A, Aungst J, Snedden N, Hansen N, Brady M 1984 Broviac catheter-related *Malessezia furfur* sepsis in five infants receiving intravenous fat emulsions. Journal of Pediatrics 105:987–990

Pruitt B A Jr, McManus W F, Kim S H, Treat R C 1980 Diagnosis and treatment of cannula-related intravenous sepsis in burn patients. Annals of Surgery 191:546–554

Rowley K M, Clubb K S, Smith G J, Cabin H S 1984 Right-sided infective endocarditis as a consequence of flow-directed pulmonary-artery catheterization: a clinicopathological study of 55 autopsied patients. New England Journal of Medicine 311:1152–1156

Stark R P, Maki D G 1984 Bacteriuria in the catheterized patient: what quantitative level of bacteriuria is relevant? New England Journal of Medicine 311:560–564

Tunkel A R, Scheld W M 1995 Acute bacterial meningitis. Lancet 346:1675–1680

Vincent J L 1994 Sepsis and septic shock: update on definitions. In: Reinhart K, Eyrich K, Sprung C (eds) Sepsis: curent perspectives in pathophysiology and therapy. Springer Verlag, Berlin, vol 18, pp 3–15

Wigfall D R 1994 Renal problems. In: Pizzo P A, Wilfert C M (eds) Pediatric AIDS: the challenge of HIV infection in infants, children and adolescents, 2nd edn. Williams and Wilkins, Baltimore, pp 547–557

13

Care of infants and children with multiple injuries

Jenny Walker

INTRODUCTION

Trauma is the most common cause of death in children aged 1 to 15 years. In the 1993 report of the Office of Population Census and Surveys there were 550 recorded deaths in this age group, with a higher incidence in boys than girls. Approximately 90% of all cases of trauma are accidental. However, the causes change with age (Box 13.1). Most commonly the trauma is blunt; it is unusual to see penetrating injuries in the United Kingdom. However, non-accidental injury contributes to a significant number of deaths in infants and children each year.

Box 13.1   Causes of accidents vary with age

- infants and toddlers — falls, vehicle passengers
- preschool children — pedestrians, vehicle passengers
- school children — pedestrians, passengers, cyclists, sporting accidents

---

This chapter will discuss the management of children with multiple injuries affecting the trunk (i.e. chest, abdomen and pelvis) and long bones. Children are smaller than adults, and consequently are more likely to receive multiple injuries when the same force is applied to the smaller area/volume of the patient. The management of children with head injuries is discussed in Ch. 10, but 80% of children who sustain multiple injuries also have a head injury.

The chapter outlines the initial assessment, management and resuscitation of a child with multiple injuries, before describing the specific injuries and their management. The full description of the details of cardiopulmonary resuscitation are found in Ch. 4.

It is essential to remember that children involved in accidents can feel responsible for injuries caused to themselves and others. Guilt and fear may contribute to a variety of psychological reactions which may complicate interpretation of physiological signs. If adults, and in particular their parents, were involved in the accident and the child does not know what has happened to them, this inevitably increases their anxiety. If the child is conscious, it is essential that somebody is designated to reassure him and to explain what is happening.

The child involved in an incident resulting in multiple injuries must arrive on the PICU in the best possible condition. Therefore management before and during transfer must be optimum (Chs 4 and 5). The structured approach to assessment and management will have been followed from the scene of the accident, through treatment in the ambulance, in the receiving Accident and Emergency department and then during the transfer to the PICU. If the child's condition deteriorates at any stage the carers' attention should go back to the beginning of the assessment process to identify the cause of the deterioration and administer appropriate treatment.

This structured approach is described by the following four phases:

- primary survey
- resuscitation
- secondary survey
- definitive care.

If a life-threatening event occurs during the primary survey, it must be dealt with immediately. The primary survey and resuscitation are carried out simultaneously. However, it is identified as a separate phase to enable professionals to adopt a sequential and systematic approach to the primary survey, ensuring that treatment is prioritised and nothing is missed.

PRIMARY SURVEY

The primary survey is conducted using the following sequence:

- *A — Airway with cervical spine control*
- *B — Breathing and ventilation*
- *C — Circulation*
- *D — Disability*
- *E — Exposure.*

A—Airway with cervical spine control

The airway is the most important part of the initial assessment, since, without a clear airway and effective oxygenation, cellular activity is impeded and outcome will be poor. Airway assessment and management with cervical spine control is the first and most important part of the primary survey.

Assessment of the airway involves listening for movement of air throughout the airway and lung fields. Noisy breathing may indicate partial obstruction, whilst minimal sounds could indicate total obstruction. Silence is a serious sign and should not be ignored, as it could suggest complete obstruction. The airway must be cleared of food, saliva, vomit, blood or loose teeth. This should be carried out under direct vision using a yankauer sucker to avoid any foreign body being pushed further into the airway.

If the child cannot maintain his own airway, a jaw thrust manoeuvre is performed until cervical spine injury is excluded. This is performed by lifting the corners of the mandible forward, upwards away from the bed, presuming the child is lying flat on his back. This manoeuvre is painful if the patient is conscious, but is often only required in a semiconscious or unconscious child. The head position needs to be maintained if this manoeuvre is required. A Guedel oropharyngeal airway can be inserted to ensure airway patency. This must be placed in position under direct vision to avoid any further trauma to the airway. If the airway needs to be protected and maintained for a prolonged period, the decision may be made to intubate (Ch. 4).

During assessment and management of the airway, it is essential that the cervical spine is controlled, as any child that has been involved in an accident is presumed to have a cervical (and/or a thoracic or lumbar) spinal injury until it has been excluded. Control of the cervical spine is achieved using a semirigid collar of the correct size. Sandbags, or their equivalent, are placed either side of the head, with tape over the forehead and chin to maintain complete immobilisation in the supine position. If the child is struggling — either because he is frightened, hypoxic, or semiconscious — the sandbags and tape are omitted until the child cooperates. Otherwise the child may produce an injury to the neck in this semirestrained position, by thrashing around, allowing the body to move relative to the neck. Whenever partial or complete removal of immobilisation is required, the cervical spine must be held in position by a trained doctor or nurse using manual in-line traction.

If the child is intubated, the semirigid cervical collar must remain in place until after the patient has been extubated, the X-rays have been assessed and a senior doctor with appropriate training has made a clinical assessment of the child's neck. Two-thirds of cervical spine injuries occur without X-ray change (spinal cord injury without radiological abnormality — SCIWORA), therefore normal X-rays are insufficient to enable the collar and care of the cervical spine to be abandoned. As the child becomes more awake and mobile, the sandbags and tape may be removed as he maintains head alignment relative to the rest of his body. However, the hard collar must not be removed until the child has been clinically assessed.

Key points:

- clear airway — suction
  - — jaw thrust
  - — Guedel airway
  - — intubation
- administer oxygen
- cervical spine control maintained until cervical spine injury excluded both clinically and radiologically.

B — Breathing and ventilation

Once the airway has been cleared and protected, effectiveness of breathing must be assessed and ventilatory support provided as appropriate. The aim of management is oxygenation of both lungs with equal movement of both sides of the chest and bilateral air entry. This may be prevented by the injuries incurred, or by displacement of the endotracheal tube either into the oesophagus or one of the main bronchi.

Key points:

- effective ventilation
- oxygenation of both lungs.

C — Circulation

Assessment of the circulation includes the measurement of pulse, blood pressure, capillary refill time, skin colour and later urine output. Tachycardia may be due to fright, anxiety, pain or hypovolaemia, or any combination of these. Hypotension is a very late sign of hypovolaemia in a child, and other signs should have been detected earlier. Pulse rate, capillary refill time, skin colour and temperature are good early indicators of hypotension in childhood. Changes in these parameters are the most useful signs to assess circulatory status and the response to treatment.

Management will include the insertion of two relatively large cannulae (i.e. large for the size of the child), preferably peripheral, and preferably not in an injured limb or below an abdominal injury. When venous access is obtained (Box 13.2), bloods will be taken for baseline routine investigations including full blood count, urea, electrolytes, sugar, amylase, cross match, and later blood gases. The results of these investigations must be obtained, even if this means contacting the referring hospital following retrieval.

Box 13.2 Venous access

- emergency
  - intraosseous: upper tibia, lower femur, lower humerus
- peripherally
  - percutaneous: any vein on a limb
  - cutdown: long saphenous vein at the ankle
  - cephalic vein in the antecubital fossa
- central access
  - femoral vein in the groin
  - jugular vein in the neck
  - subclavian vein in the chest

If peripheral venous access is impossible, intraosseous access should be considered in the emergency situation, and blood/bone marrow aspirated and sent for crossmatch, blood sugar and blood cultures. The intraosseous needle needs to be replaced by definitive access within 6–8 h, to prevent infection at the insertion site.

This vascular access will be used to resuscitate the child, administer maintenance fluids, replace extra losses and to give colloid or blood as required.

Resuscitation fluid is given as crystalloid and/or colloid at 20 mL/kg body weight. The circulating blood volume in a child is 80 mL/kg. Clinical signs of hypovolaemia are not detectable until 25% of this volume is lost. Fluid resuscitation of 20 mL/kg aims to replace this loss. This volume is given once or twice before whole blood is administered, also at 20 mL/kg if the child is haemodynamically unstable. This regime may need to continue until the point of haemorrhage is located and surgical intervention undertaken to control losses.

After every intervention, the child must be reassessed to ensure that he is making good progress. If there is any sign of deterioration, reassessment of the *Airway*, *Breathing* and *Circulation* must take place to ensure that any life-threatening incidents are dealt with as they are found.

Key points:

- pulse, capillary refill time, skin colour, BP
- venous access × 2
- baseline bloods including crossmatch
- 20 mL/kg fluid bolus
- find and stop continuing haemorrhage.

D — Disability

If all the cardiovascular parameters remain stable, the patient will be assessed for disability. When a head injury is confirmed or suspected, neurological assessment is irrelevant until haemodynamic stability is achieved. Outcome from head injury will be affected if poor oxygenation and hypovolaemia are inadequately corrected. In practice, a brief initial neurologi-

cal assessment will be undertaken simultaneously with assessment of the airway. This assessment is an important indicator of prognosis, since, once the child is intubated, sedated and paralysed, neurological assessment is impossible.

Neurological assessment is quickly undertaken by using AVPU, to assess response:

- *A* — *A*lert
- *V* — responds to *V*oice
- *P* — responds to *P*ain
- *U* — *U*nresponsive.

The pupillary size and reaction are also noted.

Regular neurological observations indicate changes in neurological status. Initially recorded every 15 minutes, they are reduced in frequency as the child's condition stabilises. The open anterior fontanelle in a child under 12–18 months is used to directly assess the presence of increased intracranial pressure, indicated by tension over this area. After exclusion of a local eye injury, unequal pupils and non-reactiveness to light need urgent investigation to identify a serious intracranial problem, which may require neurosurgery.

Key points:

- AVPU
- pupillary size and reaction
- neurosurgical consultation.

E — Exposure

The child must be *fully* exposed to enable a *full* physical examination. Health care professionals must remember that children have a large surface area to weight ratio. The consequent loss of heat can hamper effective resuscitation. Therefore, it is crucial that the child's body temperature is maintained by covering the child as much as possible during examination and investigations. This will also help preserve the child's dignity, as children do not like to be naked in strange surroundings.

Comprehensive physical examination identifies obvious sources of external bleeding and previously unidentified injury.

Key points:

- exposure — remember heat loss and dignity
- full examination.

Other considerations

Radiological investigation

The recommended X-rays in the primary survey are:

- lateral cervical spine
- chest
- pelvis.

Further investigations, including a CT scan of head, chest and abdomen, ± abdominal ultrasound, long-bone X-rays and contrast X-rays depend on the child's injuries.

Key points:

- X-rays
- imaging.

Referrals

The primary survey identifies potential underlying injuries which may require referral to the relevant specialists. These will include Anaesthetists, Paediatric Surgeons, Neurosurgical, Orthopaedic, Plastic, ENT, Ophthalmic and Maxillofacial Surgeons.

Key points:

- specialist referral.

Responsibility

The responsibility for care of this child depends on the local protocols, but it is preferable for a single consultant to have overall management, with the other specialists advising on the care of the child. This arrangement provides continuity of care whilst ensuring all of the child's needs are met.

Key points:

- consultant in overall charge.

History

AMPLE provides a useful mnemonic to obtain a rapid history from the family:

- Allergies
- Medication
- Previous history of illness or injury
- Last meal timing and content
- Events before the accident.

The mechanism of injury is important because it might indicate potential problems which need to be excluded.

The following incidents all increase the risk of cervical spine injury:

- falls from greater than 3 m (10 feet)
- unrestrained passenger in a motor vehicle
- passenger in a motor vehicle where another occupant has been killed
- pedestrian hit by a car
- patient with a significant injury above the clavicle.

Key points:

- AMPLE
- mechanism of injury.

Abdominal distention

Children swallow large amounts of air, especially when they are crying, which increases abdominal distention and tenseness, and may even mimic an acute abdomen in severe cases. Therefore a large-bore nasogastric tube should be passed to enable gastric decompression including removal of food and fluid. An orogastric tube is advised if a basal skull fracture is suspected — to prevent entry of the tube into the intracranial space via the fracture. This tube should be left on free drainage and aspirated regularly. This management will reduce the risk of abdominal injury being confused with gastric dilatation.

Urinary catheterisation may also be necessary, as a full bladder can give the appearance of a distended abdomen, particularly in young children. This also aids the accurate measurement of urinary output.

Key points:

- gastric drainage
- urinary measurement.

Once the primary survey and initial resuscitation

are complete and the child is stable, assessment of the whole child is undertaken with a secondary survey.

SECONDARY SURVEY

The secondary survey will incorporate a complete head-to-toe examination, including:

- head
- neck
- spine
- perineum
- urethral meatus
- scrotum.

This examination must include the front and the back of the child. Experienced personnel can enable full examination by logrolling the child, paying particular attention to the child's airway and protection of the cervical and thoracolumbar spine. This will enable assessment and documentation of all injuries, including:

- lacerations
- bruising and swelling of the skin
- open wounds
- fractures and dislocations of bones and joints.

During the secondary survey a more complete neurological assessment is made if the child is not pharmacologically sedated and paralysed. The Glasgow Coma Score is documented.

Examination of the mouth and external auditory canals is important, to look for signs of injury or presence of blood or cerebrospinal fluid.

Internal examination of the vagina is not performed in children as they are under the age of consent. Rectal examination is rarely helpful, and should only be performed by the senior paediatric surgeon if it is likely to affect the child's management.

Regular monitoring is continued and the secondary survey is interrupted to go back to initial assessment and resuscitation as required.

Key points:

- head-to-toe, front and back examination
- neurological assessment
- regular monitoring.

Once stabilised and appropriately resuscitated, the child will be transported to the PICU (Ch. 5). The precise timing of the transfer in relation to the primary survey/resuscitation/secondary survey depends on the child and his injuries and the interventions since the accident. Observations and results of all investigations must accompany the child.

ARRIVAL ON THE PICU

If possible the child should be weighed on admission to PICU. If this is not possible then the weight is approximated using the formula:

$$\text{weight in kg} = 2 \times (\text{age} + 4)$$

If a Broselow tape is available, the weight can be approximated by measuring the length of the child.

It is important to protect the position of the endotracheal tube during transfer, as this can easily move, causing upper lobe collapse. It could also slip into the right main bronchus, causing collapse of the left lung and mediastinal shift. On arrival in PICU, the airway remains the most important priority. Oxygenation and effectiveness of ventilation can be assessed with an oxygen saturation monitor and regular blood gases.

The endotracheal tube will be fixed according to local practice. If the child continues to require assisted ventilation the oral tube may be changed electively to a nasotracheal tube, as it is easier to manage the child. Prior to tube change, the stomach should be emptied, to prevent aspiration of gastric contents. The stomach contents may be fairly solid, as gastric emptying stops completely for some hours after an accident.

Key points:

- stabilise ABC
- fix or change ET tube
- weigh child
- serial observations.

SPECIFIC INJURIES AND THEIR PRESENTATION AND MANAGEMENT

Health care professionals caring for children following trauma should be aware that multiple injuries are common. They must be able to recognise and interpret the multiple signs and symptoms as they present to ensure effective management and prevention of secondary injury.

Airway

Injuries to the airway are often identified early during resuscitation and primary survey, as airway management is always a priority. If facial injuries exist, a Maxillofacial or Ear Nose and Throat Surgeon may be required, as the need for an emergency tracheostomy is not uncommon.

Breathing (and chest injuries)

Internal chest injuries can occur with very little external bruising or sign of injury. The chest X-ray can be normal, as the ribs in a child are very flexible and bend rather than fracture. The lungs and mediastinum can be crushed, producing severe intrathoracic trauma without external or radiological signs. The presence of a clavicular fracture suggests a severe injury, and underlying chest injuries should be considered.

Chest injuries may lead to respiratory distress. The diaphragm is the major muscle of inspiration in children. Diaphragmatic excursion is hindered by gastric dilatation, necessitating the early placement of the nasogastric or orogastric tube. Hypoxia will lead to irritability, drowsiness, or unconsciousness. The heart rate increases and the skin is pale, but bradycardia and cyanosis are both late signs.

Some injuries are life threatening and will be detected during the primary survey and treated at that time. These injuries include:

- tension pneumothorax
- massive haemothorax
- open pneumothorax
- flail chest
- cardiac tamponade.

Tension pneumothorax

This produces severe respiratory distress and cir-

culatory compromise as air collects outside the lung under tension, the lung collapses and the mediastinum is pushed over to the opposite side of the chest. Venous return to the heart is decreased and cardiac output is reduced, producing signs of severe shock.

A small simple pneumothorax will cause problems for the ventilated child, as the positive pressure applied during ventilation will force air/oxygen out into the pleural cavity. The simple pneumothorax will come under tension and therefore requires a chest drain if ventilation is going to be supported.

Signs.   Signs include:

- hypoxia
- shock
- decreased air entry
- hyperresonance to percussion on the side of the pneumothorax
- distended neck veins
- tracheal deviation away from the side of the pneumothorax.

Emergency treatment.   This comprises:

- administration of high-flow oxygen
- needle drainage of tension pneumothorax via the second intercostal space in the midclavicular line
- definitive chest drain insertion.

An asymptomatic pneumothorax associated with blunt chest trauma may be present and not immediately detected. Respiratory distress and/or chest pain should increase suspicion if unequal chest movement and breath sounds with reduced oxygen saturation are not seen. However, this may not be detected until chest X-ray has been performed.

Massive haemothorax

This prevents adequate oxygenation of the affected lung, because of lung collapse from compression. This presents as a life-threatening respiratory emergency; if excessive blood is lost into the thorax, signs and symptoms of hypovolaemic shock are manifested.

Signs.   Signs include:

- hypoxia
- possible shock
- decreased air entry
- hyporesonance to percussion on the side of the haemothorax.

Emergency treatment. This includes:

- administration of high-flow oxygen
- establishing vascular access and fluid resuscitation
- definitive chest drain insertion
- thoracotomy where rupture of a major vessel is suspected on account of large drain losses.

Open pneumothorax

An open wound into the chest allows air directly through the chest wall into the pleural space surrounding the lung. Collapse of the lung on the affected side occurs, causing an emergency situation.

Signs. Signs include:

- hypoxia
- decreased air entry
- hyperresonance to percussion on the side of the pneumothorax
- sucking noise as air moves in and out of the pleural cavity.

Emergency treatment. This includes:

- administration of high-flow oxygen
- covering of the chest wound on three sides to prevent converting the open pneumothorax to a tension pneumothorax
- definitive chest drain insertion.

Flail chest

Fractured ribs can prevent adequate chest expansion due to pain or a flail segment. When three or more adjacent ribs are fractured in two places, this flail segment moves in the opposite direction to the chest wall during respiration, compromising ventilation and producing hypoxia.

Signs. Signs include:

- pain on breathing
- hypoxia.

Emergency treatment. This includes:

- administration of high-flow oxygen
- analgesia
- possible intubation and ventilation.

When rib fracture occurs in young children, damage to thoracic and abdominal organs must always be suspected.

Cardiac tamponade

This is caused by blood collecting in the fibrous pericardial sac which prevents effective filling of the ventricles, leading to a progressive decrease in cardiac output.

Signs. Signs include:

- shock
- hypotension
- quiet heart sounds
- distended neck veins (if there is not associated hypovolaemia)
- reduced pulse pressure difference in association with fall in systolic blood pressure.

Emergency treatment. This includes:

- administration of high-flow oxygen
- establishing vascular access and fluid resuscitation
- needle drainage of the pericardial collection.

Other chest injuries

Some chest injuries are severe but present later; these include:

- pulmonary contusion
- ruptured major airway
- ruptured great vessel
- ruptured diaphragm.

Pulmonary contusion. This is common in children, as their chest wall is very mobile and the ribs can be compressed to crush the underlying lung, but there might not be any associated rib fractures. Hypoxia is progressive, and often requires ventilation.

Rupture of a major airway (i.e. trachea or main bronchus). This may be fatal but, if not, will present as a persistent air leak into the chest drain. Treatment is oxygen administration and open thoracic surgery.

Rupture of a great vessel (i.e. aorta, pulmonary artery or vein or superior or inferior vena cava). This is usually fatal at the scene of the accident. Occasionally the rupture seals itself and will be suspected from the mechanism of injury (acute deceleration) and from a widened upper mediastinum seen on the chest X-ray. The diagnosis is confirmed with an arch aortogram using contrast medium. Treatment is thoracic surgery.

Rupture of the diaphragm. This results in movement of abdominal contents into the thoracic cavity, causing lung compression and hypoxia. This is diagnosed on the chest X-ray, although positive pressure ventilation may apparently reduce the abdominal contents back into the abdomen. Surgical repair of the diaphragm is required.

The majority of severe chest injuries can be managed with administration of oxygen, establishing vascular access and fluid resuscitation, chest drainage, intubation and ventilation and occasionally pericardial drainage. Only rarely is a cardiothoracic opinion needed.

Circulation

Hypovolaemic shock

All forms of shock occur as a result of failure of the cardiovascular system to supply adequate oxygen and nutrients to the tissues. Lack of intervention causes cellular dysfunction, organ failure and finally death.

Hypovolaemic shock has multiple aetiologies, including a reduction in intravascular volume following trauma to major organs, limbs and large vessels. Reduction in circulating volume causes reduced tissue perfusion and acidosis. Redistribution of blood to vital organs leads to underperfusion and failure of organs such as the kidneys and gut. Figure 13.1 shows the sequence of events which leads to failure of organs and systems.

A reduction in tissue perfusion compromises cellular function. Poor oxygen delivery leads to anaerobic cellular metabolism and pyruvic acid

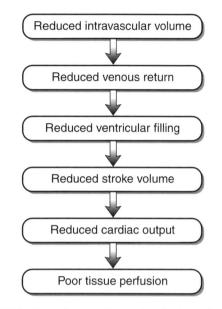

Figure 13.1 An aetiology of hypovolaemic shock. Adapted from Rice (1991).

production. This is converted to lactic acid, which causes changes in cellular pH and eventual destruction of the cell by powerful enzymes released from cell lysosomes (Rice 1991).

Four stages of shock are apparent:

- initial stage
- compensatory stage
- progressive stage
- refractory stage.

Failure to recognise hypovolaemic shock in the early stages can lead to cellular damage and death. There are few clinical symptoms in the initial stage, but shock is evident from reduced cardiac output and tissue perfusion. Decreased oxygen and nutrient delivery produce cellular dysfunction and lactic acidosis, which may be determined from blood gas analysis and blood chemistry results. Poor perfusion is detected by changes in core–peripheral temperature differences, prolonged capillary refill time and cool extremities to the touch.

The compensatory stage is characterised by stimulation of autonomic, hormonal and chemical mechanisms in response to a reduction in cardiac output. These mechanisms stimulate the sympathetic nervous system to increase blood supply to the cardiac and skeletal muscles, whilst reducing circulation to the skin, gastrointestinal tract and kidneys. In addition, heart rate and contractility are improved, pupils dilate, there is increased sweating, and respiration increases in both rate and depth. These responses are associated with the stress response and increased levels of adrenaline and noradrenaline released from the adrenal medulla. Increased corticol levels stimulate the liver to raise blood glucose, and the renin–angiotensin system produces retention of sodium and water. The increased rate and depth of respiration can lead to respiratory alkalosis and a reduction in conscious level. The clinical and biochemical signs associated with this stage can be seen in Box 13.3.

Box 13.3 Signs associated with the compensatory stage of hypovolaemic shock

Clinical signs
- normal blood pressure
- increased heart rate for age
- reduced skin perfusion with pallor, sweating and reduced temperature
- poor peripheral pulses
- urine output < 1 mL/kg/h
- reduced level of consciousness
- reduced bowel sounds
- dilated, reactive pupils

Biochemical signs
- elevated blood glucose, sodium and hydrogen ions
- reduced PaO_2 and $PaCO_2$

The progressive stage of shock is associated with failure of compensatory mechanisms and progression to multiple organ failure. Loss of cardiovascular autoregulatory mechanisms further compromises cardiac output and blood pressure, which leads to further cellular dysfunction (Box 13.4).

Failure of management of previous stages of hypovolaemic shock can lead to irreversible or refractory shock, which will be unresponsive to treatment and lead to death. Early intervention and monitoring of treatment is essential. Early treatment of the cause of hypovolaemia can prevent the cascade of events which leads to irre-

versible shock. Cardiovascular monitoring, using a pulmonary artery thermodilution catheter or Pulsion COLD system (Tibby et al 1997), can provide invaluable information about cardiovascular responses to treatment. If neither of these systems is available, assessment of heart rate, arterial oxygen, oxygen saturation, systemic arterial pressure, right atrial pressure and capillary refill can provide adequate information about cardiovascular function and oxygenation.

Box 13.4 Signs of the progressive stage of hypovolaemic shock

● neurological system	— further reduction in conscious level
● renal system	— acute tubular necrosis and renal failure
● gastrointestinal system	— ischaemia causes ulceration and bleeding — translocation of GI tract organisms
● hepatic function	— jaundice — failure to filter bacteria — reduced metabolism of waste products — increased circulating liver enzymes — reduced clotting mechanisms
● pancreatic function	— pancreatic enzymes increased in blood — myocardial depressant factor further reduces cardiac output
● respiratory system	— impaired gas exchange — raised $PaCO_2$ and reduced PaO_2 — reduction in surfactant production — pulmonary oedema — ARDS

Injuries leading to hypovolaemia are listed in Box 13.5.

Signs. Signs of hypovolaemia include:

- tachycardia
- slow capillary refill time

- poor skin colour and perfusion
- eventual hypotension.

Box 13.5   Injuries leading to hypovolaemia

- chest   — massive haemothorax
           — cardiac tamponade
- abdomen — ruptured liver
           — ruptured spleen
           — disruptured renal vessels
           — disrupted veins draining into the
             inferior vena cava (often
             retroperitoneal and difficult to
             identify, even at laparotomy)
- peripheral — scalp lacerations in a small child
           — pelvic fractures
           — long-bone fractures

Careful examination of all sites where 'invisible' haemorrhage can occur must be undertaken, e.g. gastrointestinal bleeding.

Emergency treatment.   This includes:

- establishing vascular access
- fluid resuscitation
- referral to the appropriate specialist to stop any continuing haemorrhage.

Disability

Head injury (Ch. 10) is common in children because of the disproportionate size of the head in relation to the body. However, spinal injury is rare but has very serious long-term consequences if not detected and appropriately treated. It is important to consider spinal cord injury in any child following major trauma, especially if there is a serious head injury. Therefore spinal injury must be assumed to be present until it has been excluded both clinically and radiologically, although, spinal cord injury without radiographic abnormality (SCIWORA) can occur in the cervical as well as the thoracolumbar region. Protection of the cervical spine is frequently considered but it is also important to protect the thoracolumbar spine. This is best achieved with the child immobilised on a long spinal board. However if this is not available or the child will not tolerate it, they should be nursed flat and log rolled when moved.

Neurological assessment is difficult in young children and impossible in the ventilated, sedated and paralysed child. Management aims to protect the cord, decreasing the possibility of further injury. The careful management of the skin, and bladder and bowel function is important. Early involvement of a consultant in Spinal Injuries assists with diagnosis and management.

Key points:

- immobilisation on a long spine board
- SCIWORA
- neurological assessment
- involvement of appropriate specialist.

Abdominal injuries

In the United Kingdom, the majority of abdominal trauma is associated with blunt rather than penetrating injuries.

Signs and symptoms

Assessment of circulation is essential to detect early signs of hypovolaemia. In addition, frequent observation of the abdomen allows early detection of bruising and assessment of respiratory function. Gastric dilatation from air swallowing must be relieved by passing a nasogastric tube, to avoid confusion relating to symptoms. Careful observations of signs of pain should be made, as tenderness is indicative of peritoneal irritation, suggesting free intra-abdominal blood, urine or bowel content.

Intra-abdominal injuries can involve solid organ rupture, including liver, spleen, pancreas, kidney, bladder or bowel. Bruises on the upper abdomen and lower chest suggest liver and spleen injury. Bruises on the flank and lower chest indicate renal trauma; haematuria increases this suspicion. Seatbelts can produce bruising associated with bowel perforation in the iliac fossa. Bicycle handlebars classically cause injury to the duodenum or pancreas on the posterior abdominal wall as the handlebars crush the child against his own spine.

Investigations

The child's circulation should be monitored to detect signs of hypovolaemia. A double-contrast (intragastric and intravenous contrast) CT scan is the most useful investigation, although this is only performed if the child is haemodynamically stable.

If blood white cell count, liver enzymes or serum amylase are raised, intra-abdominal trauma may be suspected.

Management

Non-operative management of a ruptured liver or spleen is advocated, as the majority of these children will have self-limiting haemorrhage. Emergency laparotomy for internal haemorrhage is only recommended when the child is difficult to stabilise.

Precise fluid management and close monitoring will indicate the need to consult with the paediatric surgeon. Bowel perforation detected either clinically or seen on the CT scan as pneumoperitoneum or leaking of the intragastric contrast requires a laparotomy to locate the injured bowel, and to resect or anastomose as appropriate.

Damage to the pancreas is usually treated non-operatively, similarly to acute pancreatitis, with intravenous fluids, nasogastric aspiration and regular monitoring of serum amylase, calcium, glucose and white cell level. A traumatic pseudocyst may develop some weeks later and be identified on serial ultrasounds. This may require internal drainage.

Signs of haematuria, bruising of the flanks and abdominal pain, may indicate renal damage. However, double-contrast CT scan will identify renal trauma, enabling the function of both kidneys to be assessed. Rupture of the kidney may have occurred. This is usually kept under close non-operative review, as kidneys which have been totally fractured can fully recover as long as the collecting system is intact enough to drain adequately. Temporary percutaneous drainage of urine may allow the damaged kidney to settle and recover. If the CT scan shows an acutely non-functioning kidney, avulsion of the blood supply

to the kidney has occurred. Emergency repair may save that kidney but the time available before the kidney becomes non-viable is very short. In theory, surgery must take place in less than an hour from injury, but it is possible for renal blood flow to be restored up to 6 h after the injury.

In older children and adults, the bladder is protected in the pelvis, but in young children it is an intra-abdominal organ and may be ruptured, especially if full. This may heal on its own if the bladder is continuously drained for a few days, using the smallest silastic urethral catheter. The healing process can be assessed with contrast studies.

Urethral rupture in a boy may be suspected if there is blood at the external urethral meatus and must be excluded, before a urethral catheter is passed, by an ascending contrast urethrogram. The treatment of choice of urethral rupture is by gentle catheterisation by a senior paediatric surgeon to maintain a channel.

Key points:

- resuscitation
- diagnosis
- non-operative management
- surgery, if required, by specialist paediatric surgeon.

Pelvic fractures

Severe fractures of the pelvis can present with hypovolaemia during the assessment of circulation in the primary survey. Urgent venous access is required, with fluid resuscitation and fracture stabilisation by an orthopaedic surgeon using external fixation.

Pelvic fracture without life-threatening haemorrhage will have been diagnosed on the mandatory pelvic X-ray and confirmed clinically during the secondary survey. If external fixation is not required, the management is usually by bedrest. Pelvic fractures are often associated with damage to adjacent organs.

Key points:

- resuscitation
- stabilisation.

Limb injuries

Long-bone fractures

Limb injuries are rarely life threatening except when associated with excessive haemorrhage. This must be treated in the usual manner of urgent vascular access, resuscitation and haemorrhage control. All fractures bleed less when immobilised, with external fixators, splints or backslabs. Control of haemorrhage associated with open bleeding fractures is controlled with direct pressure.

Clinical signs include:

- deformity
- bruising and swelling
- lack of function
- tenderness.

Definitive diagnosis of long-bone fractures is made on X-ray. X-rays are taken to include the joint above and below, and it may be necessary to take bilateral X-rays to compare limbs if diagnosis is difficult.

Despite the fact that the limb injury is rarely life threatening, it is essential to optimise management in order to prevent deformity and disability following recovery. Fracture through a growth plate can affect long-term growth and development of that limb, and a fracture through a joint also has a poor prognosis for later function.

The viability of the limb may be threatened by vascular injury or compartment syndrome. Vascular injury requires urgent surgical attention.

Management of the fracture will include adequate analgesia but this is helped greatly by stabilisation and immobilisation with Thomas splints, back slabs or fixation. Elevation of the limb to decrease swelling is also helpful. Local nerve blocks, e.g. femoral, provide very effective pain relief in the acute situation whilst a fracture is stabilised.

Cleaning and dressing of compound wounds is important, with antibiotic treatment to prevent or treat infection.

Compartment syndrome

This is due to increased pressure within one or more of the muscular compartments of the limb, leading to pain out of proportion to the injury, especially on moving the fingers/toes. The limb will also be swollen. Pallor, paraesthesia and pulselessness are late signs. Regular monitoring of the limb, for presence of distal pulses and signs of swelling, will aid detection of the syndrome and allow early intervention with fasciotomy.

Key points:

- resuscitation
- immobilisation
- analgesia
- compartment syndrome
- neurovascular injury
- infection
- long-term outcome.

Other injuries

These will need referral and management at an appropriate time. They include:

- lacerations
- soft-tissue injury
- severe grazing requiring scrubbing clean to prevent tattooing
- burns and scalds
- eyes — local injury can present as a fixed or dilated pupil
- facial fractures and dental damage.

GENERAL CONSIDERATIONS
Theatre

It is important to remember that if a child is going to the operating theatre, all the relevant surgeons must be present. These may include surgeons specialising in:

- general paediatric surgery
- neurosurgery
- orthopaedic surgery
- ophthalmic surgery
- plastic surgery
- maxillofacial surgery.

It is the responsibility of the child's primary physician/surgeon to ensure that all the relevant teams are present.

Analgesia and sedation

The degree of analgesia and sedation required for each child will vary. However, some children will require complete sedation, analgesia and paralysis whilst others will be breathing and requiring regular oral analgesia.

Analgesia must be regular to be effective. Morphine is often used, as it has a predictable effect. However, morphine can cause respiratory depression, increase constipation and prolong ileus, which must all be anticipated and managed appropriately. However, there are rarely good reasons for discontinuing the drug required.

Codeine produces little respiratory depression and may be used in head-injured patients who are not ventilated. Less severe pain can be controlled with a combination of regular diclofenac and paracetamol.

Non-pharmacological methods to reduce anxiety include the provision of fluids and nutrition to increase comfort and aid healing. It is also helpful for the child to have a dummy/comforter or their favourite toy, and to listen to familiar music. The presence of parents, family and friends is also very important.

Key points:

- intravenous morphine
- enteral analgesia
- fluids and nutrition
- comforters and toys
- familiar music and visitors.

Monitoring

Monitoring of all patients on intensive care is the most important way of assessing improvement or deterioration in the child's condition at a stage when a change in management can be made to improve the situation, or to prevent further deterioration.

The precise monitoring will depend on availability and the child's injuries but can include the following:

- heart rate, BP, CVP, cardiac output
- oxygen saturation, blood gases, oxygen delivery
- temperature (peripheral/core)
- assessment of neurological function
- circulatory observations to affected limbs
- fluid balance:
  — in: crystalloid/medication/colloid/ nutrition
  — out: urine/gastric aspiration/wound/ cavity drainage.

Bladder and bowels

Whilst the child is in the early stages of resuscitation and management, monitoring of urine output is essential, as it is a good guide to the adequacy and stability of the circulation. Hourly urine measurement is often desirable, but the presence of a catheter in the conscious or semiconscious child often causes discomfort and anxiety. These children will often pass urine spontaneously. Nappies can be weighed or the urine collected and measured. Spontaneous micturition can be encouraged with cold wipes over the suprapubic area, or by suprapubic expression if injuries permit.

Catheterisation of the child will be undertaken if precise urine measurement is essential in the management of the child, or if the child does not micturate spontaneously, and occasionally in order to facilitate nursing care. This should be under the direction of the paediatrician/surgeon in charge of the child.

Urethral catheterisation in girls is easily achieved with a fine catheter. However, the urethra of a boy can easily be traumatised or suffer local pressure effects from the catheter, especially at the bend where the penile urethra connects to the bulbar urethra. Urethral strictures can occur years after catheterisation, and can be very difficult to manage. Therefore, urethral catheterisation of a boy is to be avoided unless essential. A suprapubic catheter may be appropriate in some cases. Suspicion of urethral injury must first be ruled out before urethral catheterisation is undertaken. The smallest size pure silicone catheter should be used, as the worst problems of urethral stricture have been seen in boys catheterised with latex catheters. The use of silicone-coated catheters should be discouraged, as the silicone wears off. To decrease further urethral trauma, the catheter must be fixed to the child's abdomen, which does not move relative to the urethral meatus. The child's leg may be a convenient place to secure the catheter, but is potentially very mobile and consequently dangerous and painful.

The child's bowels may not function if there has been gastrointestinal injury leading to an ileus. It is important to know the child's usual bowel habits to assess progress. The use of opiate-derivative analgesia and lack of enteral nutrition slow down gastrointestinal transit and lead to constipation. Delayed bowel activity decreases the child's ability to tolerate enteral nutrition. Therefore, it is important to prevent constipation and encourage bowel action.

If bowel sounds are present, action can be encouraged with a suppository. Dulcolax suppositories are recommended as they have both lubricant and local stimulant activity — unlike the commonly used glycerine suppository, which is often ineffective as it has only a lubricating effect.

Continuing bowel action can be encouraged with lactulose and cisapride.

Key points:

- spontaneous micturition
- non-invasive collecting of urine
- careful catheterisation if necessary
- encouragement of bowel action.

Nutrition

All patients on ICU require nutrition, but children need nutrition both for maintenance and growth as well as tissue healing. Therefore, it is important to commence nutrition early, particularly in children with multiple injuries.

If the child in ICU is nil by mouth, there is an increased incidence of gastric erosions, oesophageal inflammation and even peptic ulceration. It is recommended that the gut be protected by use of intragastric sucralfate or intravenous H_2 antag-

onists. However, there is some evidence that the latter are ineffective.

Initially the child will require intravenous fluids. If there is no contraindication and the gastrointestinal tract is working, enteral nutrition can be started as soon as possible. This could be oral if the child is conscious and cooperative, or via a nasogastric tube. If gastric emptying is found to be a problem, but the rest of the gastrointestinal tract is working, a nasojejunal tube can be used (this is usually inserted under X-ray control). If long-term feeding is anticipated, a gastrostomy feeding tube may be inserted: for example, a percutaneous gastrostomy tube placed endoscopically (PEG).

The precise volume and content of enteral feed will depend on the age, weight and injuries of the patient. Head-injured and ventilated patients are often fluid restricted; burns patients require greatly increased nutrition to counterbalance their catabolism and to enable them to replace lost tissue. The involvement of a paediatric dietician is therefore always recommended. Many children will get diarrhoea if the concentration or volume of feed is increased too quickly. It is advisable to take things cautiously initially, to enable the establishment and tolerance of enteral feeding.

The child's gastrointestinal tract can appear intolerant and be in a state of ileus, when there are no contraindications to enteral feeding. This is especially seen in children who have had a lot of sedation, analgesia and paralysis. The use of cisapride, a prokinetic agent which encourages gastric and small-bowel motility, has been advocated, and is widely used. However, there has been no definite evidence to show that it helps.

If injury or ileus prevent use of the gastrointestinal tract or if intolerance to enteral nutrition occurs, total parenteral nutrition (TPN) should be commenced and gastric acid production buffered with intragastric sucralfate.

A central line will be needed for administration of the TPN. Monitoring of the child's blood and urinary biochemistry will determine the ability of the child to tolerate the carbohydrate load, which may be reduced when he is stressed.

The child can be weaned onto enteral feeds as soon as his condition indicates.

Key points:

- oral
- enteral
- parenteral
- sucralfate/H_2 antagonists/cisapride.

Family

The family must have open access to the child. Staff must be aware of the emotional and legal implications of access when non-accidental injury is suspected, as the injury may have been inflicted by a close family member or friend.

Children on an ICU are usually under the care of more than one consultant/specialist, and it is essential that there is communication between the doctors and nurses in order that everyone who is involved can be clear and honest in their discussions with the family. Parents must be kept informed of their child's management and progress.

Key points:

- open-access visiting
- honest discussions.

Recovery and aftercare

As the child makes progress, monitoring intensity will be reduced. If there is a deterioration, carers must return to the structured approach of assessment identified previously:

- Airway
- Breathing
- Circulation
- Disability
- Treat problems as they are found.

When the child's condition is stable enough for him to leave the ICU, the best site of continuing care needs to be assessed and agreed between all the specialties involved. This may mean that the child goes to a ward where there is particular expertise in the area where the ongoing care lies, rather than the area which gave the major problem on the ICU. For example, a child who has recovered from a ruptured spleen and head injury may be best managed on an orthopaedic ward where the nurses can care for the external fixation on the fractured femur. It is essential that all the specialists continue to review their care of the child to ensure that ongoing management of the various aspects of care continues. The possibility of ear ossicle dislocation following a head injury necessitates a full audiological assessment when the child is well enough to cooperate. Some head-injured children have long-term disability, and the early involvement of a head injury rehabilitation team is invaluable.

The key to successful transfer of the child with multiple specialist involvement from the Intensive Care Unit to the ward for further care is communication, agreement, documentation and discussion with the child's relatives.

Key points:

- select ward for transfer
- all specialists to agree, and to maintain input
- head injury rehabilitation team
- good communication.

REFERENCES AND FURTHER READING

Advanced Life Support Group 1997 Advanced paediatric life support — the practical approach, 2nd edn. BMJ Publishing Group, London

Grosfeld J L, Harris B H 1995 Paediatric trauma and surgical critical care. Seminars in Paediatric Surgery 4 (2).

Rice V 1991 Shock, a clinical syndrome: an update — Part 2: The stages of shock. Critical Care Nurse 11(5): 74–82

Tibby S, Hatherill M, Marsh M, Morrison G, Anderson D, Murdoch I 1997 Clinical validation of cardiac output measurements using femoral artery thermodilution with direct Fick in ventilated children and infants. Intensive Care Medicine 23: 9

14

Care of infants and children with thermal injuries

Tina Sajjanhar

Thermal injuries are a major cause of morbidity and mortality in childhood in the UK. The range of thermal injuries can extend from sunburn to burns sustained from contact with hot water or flames, but should also include the effects of smoke inhalation where there is a primary thermal injury. In 1992–93 over 70 000 accidents involving burns to children under the age of 14 were reported. Half of these occurred in children between 1 and 5 years of age, with a male preponderance (DTI Consumer Safety Unit 1993). About 10% of children presenting to the accident and emergency department with burns will need referral to a burns unit or admission to the local hospital (Grout et al 1993). In 1992 there were 84 deaths of children in the 0–14 year old age group involving thermal injuries at home. The majority of fatalities occur as a result of house fires, often due to smoke inhalation. Older children are more likely to be involved in burns resulting from combustion, whilst the younger age group are more likely to present with scalds. Scalds most commonly occur from spilt hot liquids, but may be due to immersion in bath water or contact with cooking fat.

Mortality from burns has decreased because of improved medical management, public awareness campaigns and stringent legislation regarding flammable materials. However, morbidity remains significant. This chapter outlines the initial resuscitation following thermal injury, the assessment of burns and important aspects relating to fluid management, nutrition, antibiotic use and morbidity.

INITIAL RESUSCITATION

A structured approach is vital, incorporating the basic principles of resuscitation, which should commence at the scene of the incident.

Airway

Airway assessment should include immobilisation of the cervical spine where trauma is suspected, such as a fall from a window at the scene of a house fire. Signs of significant smoke inhalation should be excluded (Box 14.1).

Box 14.1 Clinical features indicating smoke inhalation

- direct burns to the face or oropharynx
- hoarseness or stridor
- soot in the nostrils
- carbonaceous sputum
- mucosal injury
- wheeze
- dysphagia
- drooling or dribbling of saliva

Stridor is a late sign and requires immediate intervention. Full thickness chest or neck burns may lead to physical restriction of the airway, requiring urgent escharotomy. Early endotracheal intubation should be considered when respiratory distress is present, as airway obstruction may progress rapidly. Tracheostomy is required when intubation is not possible.

Breathing

If the child is breathing well spontaneously, 100% humidified oxygen should be given immediately by facemask. Hypoventilation should alert staff to the possibility of carbon monoxide or cyanide poisoning in cases of house fire. The greater affinity of carbon monoxide for haemoglobin leads to a decrease in the presence of oxyhaemoglobin and an increase in carboxyhaemoglobin. The presence of carboxyhaemoglobin does not alter the absorption of selected wavelengths of light used in pulse oximetry to calculate the arterial oxygen saturation. Therefore, whilst pulse oximetry is helpful in determining oxygenation, it will be misleading in carbon monoxide poisoning. Urgent estimation of arterial blood gases and carbon monoxide levels should be made to assess the degree of hypoxia and severity of inhalational injury. Inadequate breathing or cyanosis may require endotracheal intubation with 100% humidified oxygen.

Circulation

If the burn surface area is greater than 10–15%, children are at risk of hypovolaemia due to fluid loss. Intravenous access should be obtained with the largest-bore cannula in the largest vein available. If peripheral access is not available, either because of the position of the burns or as a result of hypovolaemia, venous cutdown or central venous lines may be considered. The intraosseous route can be used temporarily whilst intravenous access is being secured. Blood should be taken for:

- full blood count
- electrolytes and urea
- cross match
- blood glucose
- carboxyhaemoglobin
- carbon monoxide levels
- lactate
- arterial blood gas evaluation.

Intravenous fluids should be commenced as soon as possible. Oral fluids should be withheld in the presence of burns greater than 15%, as secondary ileus may occur.

ADDITIONAL ASSESSMENT

The conscious level should be noted on admission to provide a baseline recording, as changes may be attributable to worsening hypoxia, hypovolaemia or concurrent head injury. A rapid method of assessing a child's conscious level is use of AVPU (see Ch. 13). If a child only responds to pain, this corresponds with a Glasgow Coma Scale score of approximately 8, which may indicate the need for airway intubation. A warm environment is essential, as the burned child is at risk from hypothermia due to loss of heat and fluid from the surface of the burn. Any cold compresses applied prior to admission should be removed to reduce the risk of profound hypothermia, especially in small children. The burn may initially be covered with clingfilm or sterile towels gently laid over the patient whilst the environment is warmed.

Calculation of the child's weight aids estimation of fluid and drug requirements. If the child cannot be placed on scales, the weight may be calculated by the formula:

$$\text{weight in kg} = (\text{age} + 4) \times 2$$

in children over one, or by the use of a Broselow tape. Experienced staff may be able to estimate the weight of the child from observation.

Tetanus prophylaxis should be offered to children who have not been immunised or whose immunisation status is unknown.

ASSESSMENT OF THE BURN

The severity of the burn depends on the following factors:

- time of contact with burn material
- temperature of burn material
- type of burn material
- part of body involved
- age of patient
- surface area of skin involved.

Duration of contact and temperature of the burn material are the most important features. A temperature of 54°C will produce a full thickness burn in 30 s, whilst a temperature of 60°C can produce the same burn in 5 s. A disabled or young, relatively immobile child may be unable to escape from the burn material, making exposure time longer. Scalds from boiling fat and flame burns may lead to more serious injuries because of longer contact times.

The burn surface area (BSA) is best calculated in the child using the Lund and Browder chart (see Fig. 14.1). With increasing age the head contributes less to the surface area and the legs and thighs contribute more. Rapid estimation of BSA is achieved using the child's own palm with extended and adducted fingers, which equal approximately 1% BSA. This is especially useful where burns may be scattered or small. In larger burns it is easier to total the area of unburned skin and deduct from 100.

Over the age of 15 the 'rule of nines' can be used. The head, the front or back of each lower limb or each entire upper limb accounts for 9% of the total body surface, the front or the back of the trunk account for 18% each and the perineal area accounts for the final 1%.

Classification of the depth of burn depends on the layers of skin that are penetrated (Table 14.1 and Fig. 14.2):

- simple erythema
- superficial
- partial thickness
- full thickness.

Simple erythema is not included in the estimation of the total BSA. Frequent assessment of the burn is important, as the burn may progress in depth and extent over time from the initial assessment.

Children with the following burns should be considered for transfer to a specialist burns unit:

- those with 10% or more partial-thickness burns
- 5% or more full-thickness burns
- burns to delicate areas such as eyes, face or hands
- burns involving the airway.

Hospital admission should also be considered for children with burns to the perineal area, to feet, or over joints, or those where non-accidental injury (NAI) is suspected.

FLUID MANAGEMENT

Intravenous fluid resuscitation is the most important factor associated with improved survival after burns. Fluid loss secondary to large burns is a major cause of mortality, making adequate fluid replacement essential for survival. The local and systemic increase in capillary permeability following a burn and subsequent

CHART FOR ESTIMATING SEVERITY OF BURN WOUND

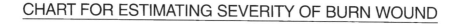

NAME _____ WARD _____ NUMBER _____ DATE _____
AGE _____ ADMISSION WEIGHT _____

LUND AND BROWDER CHARTS

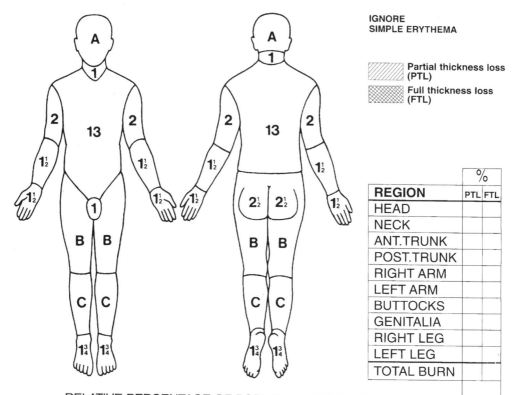

IGNORE
SIMPLE ERYTHEMA

Partial thickness loss (PTL)

Full thickness loss (FTL)

REGION	PTL	FTL
HEAD		
NECK		
ANT.TRUNK		
POST.TRUNK		
RIGHT ARM		
LEFT ARM		
BUTTOCKS		
GENITALIA		
RIGHT LEG		
LEFT LEG		
TOTAL BURN		

RELATIVE PERCENTAGE OF BODY SURFACE AREA
AFFECTED BY GROWTH

AREA	AGE 0	1	5	10	15	ADULT
A=1/2 OF HEAD	$9\frac{1}{2}$	$8\frac{1}{2}$	$6\frac{1}{2}$	$5\frac{1}{2}$	$4\frac{1}{2}$	$3\frac{1}{2}$
B=1/2 OF ONE THIGH	$2\frac{3}{4}$	$3\frac{1}{4}$	4	$4\frac{1}{2}$	$4\frac{1}{2}$	$4\frac{3}{4}$
C=1/2 OF ONE LEG	$2\frac{1}{2}$	$2\frac{1}{2}$	$2\frac{3}{4}$	3	$3\frac{1}{4}$	$3\frac{1}{2}$

For further supplies of this pad or of Flamazine* Cream for the prevention and treatment of infection in burns contact Hull (01482 222200) or your Smith & Nephew Healthcare representative.

Smith+Nephew

Figure 14.1 Lund and Browder chart for estimating severity of burn wound. Reproduced with the permission of Smith & Nephew Healthcare Ltd.

Table 14.1 Classification of burns

Type of burn	Layers involved	Appearance of skin	Healing
Superficial	Epidermis	Red, dry, painful skin Thin-walled blisters No loss of germinal layer	Heals in 3–6 days No scarring
Partial thickness	Epidermis/dermis	White/mottled red (depending on depth) blisters, moist, painful Loss of germinal layer	Heals 10–28 days May lead to contractures May need grafting if deep
Full thickness	Epidermis through to subcutaneous fat	Hard, leathery, waxy white or charred black	Needs grafting Leads to contractures Slow to heal, takes weeks to months

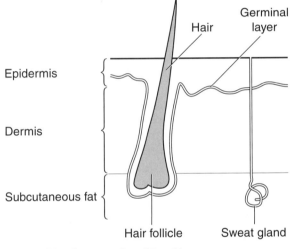

Figure 14.2 Cross-section of the skin.

hypovolaemia, may result in decreased cardiac output.

The choice of resuscitation fluid continues to cause controversy (Derganc 1993, Puffinbarger et al 1994), but hypertonic solutions are not recommended in childhood because of the risk of hypernatraemia, hyperosmolarity and intracellular dehydration. Varied regimes advocate use of both isotonic and colloid solutions, either alone or in combination. Isotonic solutions are currently favoured, with Ringers lactate frequently used in burns units. Colloid solutions may be more effective where the goals are maintenance of serum oncotic pressure, minimising wound oedema and decreasing volume requirements. However, early colloid administration has been reported to be deleterious, as the increased capillary permeability and protein leak cause an increase in lung water and precipitate pulmonary oedema. Some regimes favour the use of colloid solutions, particularly fresh frozen plasma or human albumin solution 4.5%, as fluid replacement, along with isotonic solution for maintenance fluid.

Formulae recommended for calculating fluid replacement for children with burns vary with some specifying the type of fluid to be used. In the UK, the Advanced Life Support Group (ALSG) recommends the Parkland protocol which is taught during the Advanced Paediatric Life Support Course (ALSG 1993). The volume of fluid required for resuscitation can be calculated using the formula:

$$24 \text{ h fluid replacement (mL)} = \text{body weight (kg)} \times 4 \times \text{BSA (\%)}$$

The calculated fluid is commenced after an initial fluid bolus of 20 mL/kg for the treatment of hypovolaemic shock. Half the total amount is given as over the first 8 h commencing from the estimated time of the burn, with the remaining half given over the next 16 h. Maintenance fluid is given in addition to this. This formula tends to underestimate the amount of fluid for small infants and overestimate the amount of fluid for older children, but physiological monitoring can indicate adjustments in volume required.

Other formulae are available, and their use may vary with the set protocols of individual departments.

The goal of fluid therapy is to ensure adequate

resuscitation to stabilise circulation. Indicators of perfusion should be assessed frequently and include:

- capillary refill
- core–peripheral temperature gap
- pulse volume
- heart rate
- pH and lactate levels
- conscious level
- urine output.

Assessment of fluid balance may be assisted by catheterising the child to ensure a minimal urine output of 0.5–1 mL/kg/h. In the intensive care setting, central venous and arterial pressure monitoring aid assessment.

The addition of electrolytes to the maintenance solution can correct imbalances. Infants in particular are at risk of hypoglycaemia, necessitating addition of glucose to the infusion.

Blood transfusions may be required with early and aggressive escharotomy, or when extensive haemolysis leads to a marked drop in haemoglobin. Blood should be reserved for those children who have cardiovascular compromise secondary to anaemia or those who are critically ill, because of the risks associated with transfusion (Mann et al 1994).

ANALGESIA

Children with burns are often distressed and frightened for a variety of reasons, including pain, unfamiliar surroundings and interventions of medical staff. Effective analgesia is a priority and should be administered promptly.

In the acute stage, the ideal analgesia to provide immediate and effective pain relief is intravenous morphine (0.1 mg/kg). Staff should be aware of the risk of respiratory depression and provide appropriate monitoring and supervision. Intramuscular injections are not advocated, as absorption is unreliable and the mode of delivery adds to discomfort. In some cases, a morphine infusion may be required, and in older children the use of patient-controlled analgesia (PCA) should be considered. Older children may be able to use entenox via a mask, although this

may not provide effective analgesia. For dressing changes, oral analgesia including oral morphine and codeine phosphate may be used. Amnesic agents such as midazolam have proved effective in very distressed children and may be used as an adjunct to analgesia.

It is essential that a child is not in pain as this is upsetting to both the child and the parents. A painful experience can be modified by good communication and explanations, especially regarding medical procedures such as inserting intravenous lines. The parents should be allowed to be present wherever possible, as they can help to comfort the child and add reassurance.

SMOKE INHALATION

Improvements in fluid management and a decrease in burn-related sepsis make respiratory failure the most common reason for mortality associated with burn injuries. Smoke inhalation is the most common cause of death in the first 24 h and may occur with little or no visible external burn (Uitvlugt & Ledbetter 1995). Children involved in house fires must be closely observed, as respiratory distress may become apparent in the hours or days following initial exposure (Box 14.1).

When evidence of smoke inhalation is present, the child should either be transferred to a burns unit or observed in an intensive care unit. Bronchospasm and stridor require treatment with bronchodilators and nebulised adrenaline, respectively. Definitive treatment may involve early endotracheal intubation, as oedema can occur rapidly and may necessitate emergency tracheostomy.

The pathophysiology of damage due to smoke inhalation is dependent on the relative effects of:

- direct thermal injury
- asphyxiation
- toxin exposure.

Damage to the lungs by direct heat occurs infrequently, as heat is effectively dissipated by the upper airways before it reaches the lungs. However, direct thermal injury to the tissues surrounding the neck may lead to severe oedema and direct occlusion of the airway, requiring immediate endotracheal intubation.

Up to 80% of deaths involving smoke inhalation are due to asphyxiation and hypoxaemia. Inspired oxygen is reduced by the fire itself and then further because of inhalation of carbon dioxide and carbon monoxide.

Carbon monoxide (CO) has two hundred times the affinity of oxygen for haemoglobin but can be displaced with predictable dissociation kinetics related to the time from exposure and the concentration of inspired oxygen. The half-life of CO is 240 min in air but this is reduced to 40 min in the presence of 100% oxygen. The use of hyperbaric oxygen (oxygen administered in a specialised chamber at three atmospheres of pressure) can reduce the half-life to 25 min. The severity of initial carbon monoxide exposure can be calculated using a nomogram, if the admission carboxyhaemoglobin level and time from exposure are known. Clinical features of carbon monoxide poisoning do not always correlate well with carboxyhaemoglobin levels. However, at CO levels of 20%, features include headaches, confusion and impaired conscious level; the classical appearance of cherry red mucous membranes is not a reliable sign. Levels over 60% are usually fatal. Administration of oxygen should commence at the scene of a house fire and not be delayed until admission to hospital. Administration of 100% oxygen via an endotracheal tube may be adequate treatment in most cases of CO poisoning. In severe cases where there is loss of consciousness due to CO poisoning, in the absence of other injuries, treatment with hyperbaric oxygen may be considered.

Inhaled toxins include tiny carbon particles that can be deposited in the alveoli, and poisonous gases such as hydrogen cyanide that inhibit mitochondrial respiration, leading to cell death. The resultant lung damage is often not apparent for several hours after the exposure. Airway obstruction is gradual, resulting from damage to the respiratory epithelium with impaired ciliary action and mucosal oedema, mucosal necrosis, sloughing and haemorrhage. Chest X-ray is not always helpful in the initial diagnosis of smoke inhalation, as changes may not be present. Whilst in adults bronchoscopy has been found to be a useful adjunct to diagnosis, the procedure is not easy or as reliable in children. Diagnosis should be based on progress and clinical findings in the child.

Treatment of smoke inhalation includes:

- administration of 100% humidified oxygen
- regular pulmonary toilet
- physiotherapy
- nebulized bronchodilators.

These children are at risk of developing acute respiratory distress syndrome (ARDS). Risk factors include ongoing lung damage, an increase in lung water secondary to fluid resuscitation, and the direct effects of mechanical ventilation. The reported incidence of ARDS in the burn population is 4.6%, which is higher than the 0.4–1.1% incidence reported in the general intensive care population, with a comparatively high mortality (Reynolds et al 1993a). In PICU the placement of a pulmonary artery catheter can help in the assessment of volume administration. Secondary lung damage may be avoided by the use of lower ventilation pressures and permissive hypercapnia (Reynolds et al 1993b). Massive thermal injury and burn shock is associated with depressed cardiac function, despite adequate fluid resuscitation, necessitating the use of inotropes to maintain blood pressure. It has been proposed that reduction in cardiac output is caused by myocardial depressant factor released in response to injury.

Although less common, respiratory distress may occur in children secondary to scalds (Hudson et al 1994). The injury is not usually recognised early, and treatment may be delayed, leading to increased morbidity and mortality. Direct thermal injury to the mucosa of the respiratory tract occurs as a result of accidental ingestion of hot fluids or inhalation of steam, with scalds to the face. Stridor is the most common presenting symptom, but may not be immediately apparent, occurring several hours after the initial injury. Mucosal injury may be apparent from oral examination, but the majority of injury is supraglottic and not visible. Children presenting with stridor associated with a scald to the upper body should be suspected of having an associated inhalation injury. The progressive nature of this condition necessitates observation for increasing respiratory distress. Nebulised adrenaline may alleviate distress, but where there is severe obstructive respiratory distress, early intubation is indicated. Bronchoscopy may assist assessment of the extent of the injury. Extubation will depend on the development of a leak around the endotracheal tube, indicating resolution of the mucosal oedema. Secondary bronchopneumonia may occur, delaying extubation.

CIRCUMFERENTIAL BURNS

Circumferential burns of the neck and chest may lead to airway obstruction and respiratory compromise, respectively. Circumferential burns of the chest cause splinting of the chest and difficulty with spontaneous ventilation and are an indication for assisted ventilation. Extremity burns associated with tissue oedema can lead to occlusion of the blood supply, to ischaemia and significant tissue destruction. Doppler monitoring of digital vessels and pulse oximetry are recommended to pick up ischaemia early; regular palpation of the distal pulses is not sensitive enough, as disappearance of the pulse indicates significant injury has already occurred.

If a torniquet-like effect occurs, then urgent escharotomies (longitudinal incisions of the skin) may be required. The incisions should be on both sides of an extremity: e.g. both sides of all affected fingers. If the chest is involved, vertical lines along the anterior and posterior axillary lines are made, with additional midline, midclavicular and transverse incisions if indicated. As the burn is full thickness, no anaesthetic is required. Escharotomies do not lead to additional scarring. Blood transfusion may be required as profuse bleeding can occur.

GASTROINTESTINAL COMPLICATIONS

Gastrointestinal ileus can occur in children even in the presence of 10–15% burns. Insertion of a nasogastric tube will help to decompress the stomach. It is inadvisable to feed children orally until stable. Stress ulcers (Curling's ulcers) in the gastric and duodenal mucosa are a well-recognised complication of burns. The use of enteral feeding even in small amounts raises gastric pH, helping to prevent stress ulcers. In the intensive care setting, the use of H_2 receptor blockers such as ranitidine is associated with an increase in nosocomial infections. Sucralfate is more commonly used for gastric protection.

If gastrointestinal haemorrhage occurs, the reported mortality is high, especially where there is associated sepsis. One study has shown a higher incidence of gastrointestinal haemorrhage occuring within 2 weeks of injury with extensive burns (> 30%), especially where these are full thickness (Zhon et al 1993).

NUTRITION OF THE BURN PATIENT

Burns induce a hypermetabolic state in the child, which occurs soon after injury. It is vital to provide nutrition early to aid host defences and promote successful wound healing (Kien 1987). Hypermetabolism is contributed to by increased evaporation of water and release of stress hormones (catecholamines, corticosteroids). Translocation of bacteria from ischaemic bowel causes a massive release of cytokines and inflammatory mediators which further increase metabolic rate. Early enteral feeding and burn excision have resulted in reduced energy requirements in burned children. Data suggest that provision of twice predicted energy expenditure ensures energy balance in 95% of burned children. Age and underlying nutritional status of the child will affect energy requirements. The resting energy expenditure (REE) is directly related to the size of the burn and the presence of fever. Patients with severe burns (> 60%) benefit from nursing in a warm (33°C) dry environment to decrease the REE.

Burn healing requires increased glucose intake, but fat is the principal substrate for aerobic metabolism, providing energy in the healing phase. Burn patients exhibit relative carbohydrate intolerance, with hyperglycaemia and abnormal glucose tolerance test. This is due to glycogenolysis, increased gluconeogenesis, and high levels of catecholamines causing insulin suppression and peripheral insulin resistance. Blood glucose may not be decreased by insulin administration, but may require reduction in carbohydrate intake. Too much carbohydrate may lead to increased production of carbon dioxide, resulting in acidosis.

Despite the increase in serum free fatty acids caused by catecholamines and glucagon, dietary fat needs to be given in adequate amounts to provide energy. Protein loss results from destruction of tissue, haemorrhage and wound exudate and urinary losses attributed to stress and muscle disuse. Protein needs to provide at least 25% of energy intake. The remaining intake can be divided equally between fat and carbohydrate. Net protein catabolism of zinc-containing enzymes leads to an increased loss of zinc in the urine and hence zinc deficiency. Zinc aids wound healing and should be given with vitamin C, multivitamins and folic acid.

Calorie intake needs to be high, and several formulae are available to determine calorie requirements. These equations include measurement of the child's age, preburn weight and burn surface area; however, local policy will dictate which formula is used in consultation with the nutritional team.

The route of feeding depends on the condition of the child. Where small burns and no facial injuries occur, oral feeding can be encouraged, with high-calorie products used to increase energy intake. Children with moderate burns may initially require intravenous fluids because of the risk of gastrointestinal ileus. When gut function returns, oral feeding can be commenced, although nasogastric feeding may be required, especially where there are accompanying facial injuries. Continued ileus will indicate the need for parenteral nutrition in the interim. Children with severe burns should be tube fed as soon as some gut function returns, as tolerated. This decreases the risk of stress ulceration and bacterial translocation.

Common problems associated with enteral feeding include:

- nausea or vomiting, due to the type of feed, GI disturbance, drugs such as morphine or antibiotics
- anorexia secondary to stress and anxiety, which can be reduced by appropriate timing of procedures and use of analgesic and amnesic drugs
- diarrhoea resulting from secondary lactose intolerance, altered gut flora associated with antibiotic usage, hyperosmolarity of high-calorie feeds; treatment of diarrhoea with anticholinergics should be avoided
- tube discomfort due to nasal irritation or emotional intolerance; tube feeding may be discontinued when it provides < 60 kcal/kg/day
- poor weight gain or wound healing due to inadequate nutrition; high-calorie supplements are not always palatable, therefore supplemental nasogastric or parenteral nutrition should be considered.

Although parenteral nutrition is a useful alternative to enteral feeding when GI problems occur, the placement of a central venous catheter increases the risk of sepsis, thromboembolism, phlebitis and possibly systemic fungal infections. The decision to use parenteral feeding should be made taking this into consideration whilst remembering that the clinical state of the child will dictate the route of feeding.

INFECTION AND USE OF ANTIBIOTICS

Burn patients are at high risk of sepsis because of loss of skin integrity, which allows entry of microorganisms from the skin or the environment. However, the incidence of burn infection and sepsis have been decreased by early excision and grafting of the burn and prompt treatment of suspected sepsis. Routine systemic antibiotic prophylaxis is not recommended, but perioperative antibiotics are thought useful. Selective bowel decontamination with aztreonam has been shown to decrease burn wound colonisation with Gram-negative bacteria. Immunoprotective measures such as the use of immunoglobulin have not been found to be helpful in reducing wound sepsis.

At the time of the burn there is no bacterial infection of the wound. Gram-positive bacteria from hair follicles and sweat glands, and Gram-negative organisms from the intestinal tract, can appear in the wound within 3 days, becoming virulent pathogens. However, the use of early prophylactic systemic antibiotics is associated with early appearance of Pseudomonas in wound and blood cultures. Therefore prophylactic systemic antibiotics are only considered useful when given perioperatively at the time of burn wound excision. Systemic antibiotics may be useful during autografting, as dressings cannot be disturbed for a few days and therefore infection may go unnoticed. A short course of penicillin in the immediate post-burn period may be beneficial, as the incidence of streptococcal colonisation is higher in children than adults. Wound swabs should be sent for microscopy and culture if infection is suspected.

In the diagnosis of septicaemia the use of individual parameters of infection may be misleading. Fever may not be directly related to infection but to the release of inflammatory mediators in the post-burn period. The platelet count often falls because of sequestration within the burn wound. The white cell count may be raised as a result of stimulation of antimicrobial defences rather than infection. The clinician will be guided by the state of the burn and the known history, as well as wound and blood cultures. An upward trend in C-reactive protein and white cell count with a downward trend in platelet count, is more useful than absolute numbers. The parameters used for the diagnosis of sepsis should be used in conjunction with each other and the clinical state of the patient to decide on the relevant management (Housinger et al 1993).

Topical antibiotics are not widely used but may be helpful when the child is too unwell to undergo operative debridement of a burn. Topical neomycin ointment is sometimes used on small areas of burn on the face. Silver sulphadiazine (Flamazine) may be useful on exposed areas such as the cartilage of the ear. Silver sulphadiazine causes discoloration of the tissues, leading to confusion regarding the depth of the burn. It should not be used in the initial stages until the burn has been formally assessed by experienced staff. Antistaphylococcal agents such as Bactroban may be used where there is methicillin-resistant staphylococcal aureus (MRSA).

DRESSINGS

Prior to transfer to the local burns unit, it is advisable to wrap the burn in cling film and not to apply any paraffin to the skin at this stage. The skin is protected and easily visible through this dressing when the child arrives at the burns unit. Fluid from burst blisters is retained, keeping the burn moist.

Burns are debrided early and blisters deroofed before dressings are applied to the underlying tissue. Dressings help to protect the burn and prevent infection. The type of dressings used may vary with local protocols. Low-adherent dressings such as Jelonet, paraffin gauze or Mepitel (plyamide netting coated with silicone gel) are preferred, as these will stick to dry skin and may be used in layers over large burns. The dressings are left in place for 3–5 days and then changed. As the dressings are non-adherent, newly epithelialised skin is not disturbed. A secondary dressing such as cotton wool can be applied over this first layer to absorb the exudate from the burn, and this may need to be changed more frequently. If infection is suspected, the first layer of dressing may need to be disturbed much earlier than anticipated for the wound to be assessed.

Burns on hands and feet can be dressed with liquid paraffin and enclosed in plastic bags to keep them clean and encourage mobility. In the case of full-thickness burns, grafting is advocated, sometimes within 24 h of injury. This provides a more effective barrier to infection and leads to a better cosmetic result. Once the graft has been applied, the area is left undisturbed for 7 days to allow the graft to take.

NON-ACCIDENTAL INJURY

Studies have reported the incidence of non-accidental injury (NAI) in children as varying from 1.7% to 25% (Hobson et al 1994). These studies are not easy to carry out, and injuries will be missed or overdiagnosed depending on the experience of the physician. However, health professionals caring for children need to be aware of the possibility of NAI, as there is up to a 70% chance of further injury from the same environment and up to 40% chance of long-term morbidity.

The most common type of non-accidental burns are scalds. These may follow a particular pattern and are usually deeper than accidental burns as they represent forced exposure.

Particular points in the history to suggest abuse include:

- history does not fit the injury
- child who exhibits 'frozen watchfulness'
- changing/inconsistent story
- carer's story differs from the child's story
- history inconsistent with the motor development of the child
- child already 'at risk'
- delay in seeking medical attention.

On examination the pattern of the burn may suggest abuse:

- discrete burns that have an identifiable pattern such as an iron burn or cigarette burn
- bilateral and circumferential glove and stocking burns involving the extremities
- forced immersion burns involving the buttocks and the perineum, with parallel lines of demarcation laterally
- burn older than history suggests
- evidence of other older injuries such as healed injuries or fractures.

Suspicion of abuse must be reported to the appropriate authorities, usually via the social services. Appropriate action following investigation should be supervised by the local child protection team.

NEUROLOGICAL COMPLICATIONS OF BURNS

The incidence of neurological complications related to burns has decreased because of improved understanding of the pathophysiology and advances in burn management. Seizures are the most common complication, with a reported incidence between 1.5% and 14%. One recent study of burn encephalopathy in children with a mean total burn surface area of 31% reported the incidence of seizures as 1.5% (Mukhdomi et al 1996). Hyponatraemia, known epilepsy, hypoxia, sepsis, drugs and undetermined causes were identified. Hyponatraemia may result from infusion of large volumes of electrolyte-free solution during resuscitation, increased ADH secretion in sick children or administration of glucose infusions to maintain blood sugar without monitoring serum sodium levels. Correction of hyponatraemia should be slow and may involve fluid restriction or infusion of hyperosmolar solutions. A previous history of epilepsy may be related to a lower seizure threshold following a burn; anticonvulsant levels may be affected and must be assessed. Encephalopathy associated with hypoxia is more common, with smoke inhalation leading to acute respiratory distress syndrome. Drug withdrawal from benzodiazepines used for sedation, may also lead to seizures. This study showed a good prognosis following seizures, but other studies have reported a poorer neurological outcome following burn encephalopathy.

OUTCOME OF BURNS

In children, one series has shown that the larger the burn, the greater the risk of mortality (Morrow et al 1996). The majority of burns leading to death are greater than 30% total BSA. Children aged 0–4 years have an increased risk of mortality independent of burn size. In this same series the incidence of inhalation injury in this younger age group was higher and may be related to their immobility and inability to escape the effects of fire.

Very small burns can lead to death in infants and small children without the presence of inhalation injury, probably because of an immature immune system and increased tendency towards hypovolaemic shock. Inhalation injury is a weak predictor of death in children unless associated with a large burn, which in itself has a high prediction for mortality. Flame and scald injuries of similar sizes produce no difference in mortality; however, scalds are more likely to occur in small children and flame burns in older children. Death is commonly due to sepsis, pneumonia and respiratory distress syndrome leading to multisystem organ failure. All children with significant burn injuries are at risk of death and should be transferred to the regional burns unit where possible. In smaller children, toxic shock syndrome can result from the presence of relatively small burns, and any evidence of sepsis should be treated promptly.

PSYCHOLOGICAL ASPECTS

The psychological wellbeing of the child and family must be considered when planning rehabilitation of the burned child. There may be feelings of guilt and helplessness from the other members of the family, especially if there is the chance of permanent physical disfigurement. The child should be incorporated back into the family environment as soon as possible, where normal routine is encouraged. The child may require regular dressing changes and further operations necessitating repeated hospital appointments and admissions. Where possible, these should be kept to a minimum, and this may be achieved in collaboration with the Primary Care Team.

PREVENTION OF THERMAL INJURY

Although the treatment of burns has resulted in an improved mortality, the key lies in the prevention of thermal injuries. Health education programmes highlight dangers facing children, encouraging measures such as installation of smoke detectors in the home. The Primary Care Team is well positioned to advise and support parents regarding dangers in the home. National and local government bodies, fire authorities, the British Standards Association, and volunteer groups are actively involved in fire safety and education supported by government legislation.

REFERENCES

Advanced Life Support Group 1993 Advanced paediatric life support: the practical approach. BMJ Publishing Group, London

Derganc M 1993 Present trends in fluid therapy, metabolic care, and prevention of infection in burned children. Critical Care Medicine 21(9):397–398

DTI Consumer Safety Unit 1993 Home Accident Surveillance System annual report. HMSO, London

Grout P, Horsley M, Touquet R 1993 Epidemiology of burns presenting to an Accident and Emergency department. Archives of Emergency Medicine 10:100–107

Hobson M I, Evans J, Steward I P 1994 An audit of non-accidental injury in burned children. Burns 20(5):442–445

Housinger T A, Brinkerhoff C, Warden G D 1993 The relationship between platelet count, sepsis and survival in pediatric burn patients. Archives of Surgery 128:65–66

Hudson D A, Jones L, Rode H 1994 Respiratory distress syndrome secondary to scalds in children. Burns 20(5):434–437

Kien C L 1987 Nutrition in burn and trauma patients. In: Grand R, Sutphen J, Dietz W (eds) Paediatric nutrition: theory and practice. Butterworths, Boston

Mann R, Heimbach D M, Engrav L H, Foy H 1994 Changes in transfusion practices in burn patients. J Trauma 37(2):220–222

Morrow S E, Smith D L, Cairns, Howell P D, Nakayama D K, Peterson H D 1996 Etiology and outcome of pediatric burns. Journal of Pediatric Surgery 32(3):329–333

Mukhdomi G J, Desai M H, Herndon D N 1996 Seizure disorders in burned children: a retrospective review. Burns 22(4):316–319

Puffinbarger N K, Tuggle D W, Smith E I 1994 Rapid isotonic fluid resuscitation in pediatric thermal injury. Journal of Paediatric Surgery 29(2):339–342

Reynolds E M, Ryan D P, Doody D P 1993a Mortality and respiratory failure in a pediatric burn population. Journal of Paediatric Surgery 28(10):1326–1331

Reynolds A M, Ryan D P, Doody D P 1993b Permissive hypercapnia and pressure-controlled ventilation as treatment of severe adult respiratory distress syndrome in a pediatric burn patient. Critical Care Medicine 21(3):468–471

Uitvlugt N D, Ledbetter D J 1995 Treatment of pediatric burns. In: Arensman R M (ed) Paediatric trauma: initial care of the injured child. Raven Press, New York

Zhon Y P, Zhon Z H, Xue J Z 1993 Burns complicated with gastrointestinal haemorrhage — an analysis of 70 cases. Burns 19(2):150–152

15

Care of children with gastrointestinal disorders

*Heather E. Steele   Elizabeth Gibbons
Karon Dyke*

Children with congenital and acquired gastrointestinal (GI) disorders are frequently seen in PIC. This chapter presents an overview of the management of these children.

ESSENTIAL ANATOMY AND PHYSIOLOGY

From birth, the gastrointestinal tract provides the body with water, electrolytes and nutrients, essential for cell activity. The GI tract also has secretory and barrier functions, is an endocrine organ and is part of the immunological system. Digestive processes are controlled by mechanical, nervous and hormonal mechanisms which may be disrupted during illness.

The GI tract comprises the following organs.

Oesophagus. The distal portion of the oesophagus acts as a sphincter preventing reflux of acidic stomach contents. Immaturity during the first 6 months of life means that approximately 40% of babies demonstrate signs of reflux due to sphincter incompetence (Beasley et al 1991).

Stomach. This has a capacity of aproximately 30 mL at birth, increasing to 1500 mL in adulthood. Gastric secretions are regulated by nervous and hormonal mechanisms. Gastric glands are stimulated by the medulla via the parasympathetic fibres of the vagus nerves and local enteric nervous system reflexes (Fig. 15.1). Stomach emptying is regulated by signals from the stomach and duodenum (Fig. 15.2). The rate of gastric emptying is limited by the amount of chyme processed by the small intestine and by the

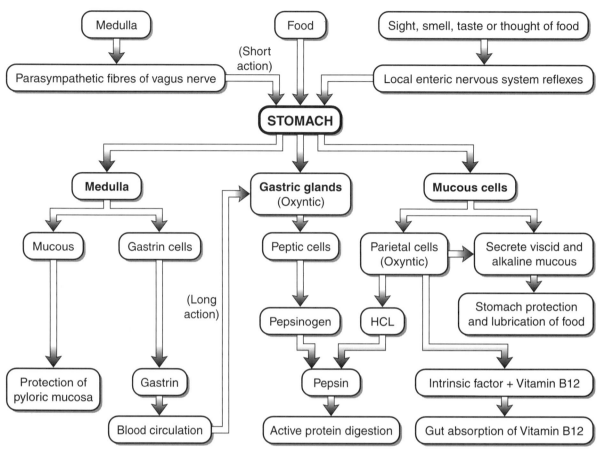

Figure 15.1 Gastric acid secretion.

inhibitory effects of the enterogastric reflex on pyloric activity, including:

- duodenal distention
- irritation of the duodenal mucosa
- acidity and osmolality of chyme
- presence of protein and fat breakdown products in chyme.

Small intestine. This is approximately 275 cm long in neonates, increasing to 5–6 m in adults. The duodenum and jejunum form over half the length of the small intestine and are the primary sites for digestion and absorption of fats, amino acids, sugars and vitamins. The ileum forms the final third and is responsible for the absorption of bile salts and vitamin B_{12}. The ileocaecal valve separates the small intestine from the colon and

prolongs transit time for digestion and absorption to occur. It also reduces contamination of the small intestine by the faecal contents of the colon.

Peristaltic movement is controlled by the myenteric plexus. If the plexus is blocked by drugs or has degenerated due to disease, peristalsis does not occur. Intense irritation of the intestinal mucosa due to infection causes increased peristalsis, thus relieving irritation or excessive distention.

Regeneration capacity of villi is limited in infancy and compromised when malnutrition exists, reducing absorption of nutrients.

Large intestine. This is divided into the caecum, colon, rectum and anal canal, and is approximately 40 cm long in neonates, growing to approximately 150 cm in adults. The principal

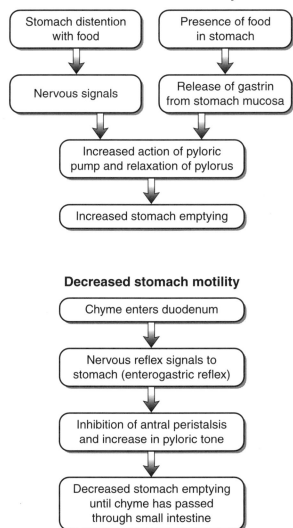

Increased stomach motility

Stomach distention with food

Presence of food in stomach

Nervous signals

Release of gastrin from stomach mucosa

Increased action of pyloric pump and relaxation of pylorus

Increased stomach emptying

Decreased stomach motility

Chyme enters duodenum

Nervous reflex signals to stomach (enterogastric reflex)

Inhibition of antral peristalsis and increase in pyloric tone

Decreased stomach emptying until chyme has passed through small intestine

Figure 15.2 Regulation of stomach emptying (Guyton 1992).

functions of the colon are absorption of water and electrolytes from chyme in the proximal half and storage of faecal matter in the distal portion until it is expelled.

The pancreas. Pancreatic secretions from the acini cells pass into small ducts uniting to form the pancreatic duct. This joins the common bile duct from the liver and gall bladder, entering the duodenum at the ampulla of Vater.

The pancreas is an exocrine and endocrine gland. The exocrine pancreas secretes enzymes responsible for digestion and absorption of fats, carbohydrates and proteins in response to food entering the small intestine. Sodium bicarbonate is also secreted to neutralise acidic stomach contents as they enter the proximal duodenum. The endocrine portion of the pancreas secretes hormones from the islets of Langerhans (Box 15.1).

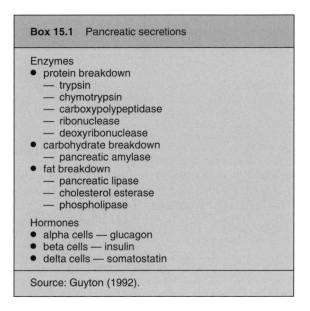

Box 15.1 Pancreatic secretions

Enzymes
● protein breakdown
 — trypsin
 — chymotrypsin
 — carboxypolypeptidase
 — ribonuclease
 — deoxyribonuclease
● carbohydrate breakdown
 — pancreatic amylase
● fat breakdown
 — pancreatic lipase
 — cholesterol esterase
 — phospholipase

Hormones
● alpha cells — glucagon
● beta cells — insulin
● delta cells — somatostatin

Source: Guyton (1992).

The liver. This is located in the right upper quadrant of the abdomen and is attached to the lower surface of the diaphragm. It is covered by peritoneum and a layer of dense connective tissue. The liver is divided into right and left lobes separated by the falciform ligament (Fig. 15.3). The functions of the liver are outlined in Box 15.2. These are immature in neonates leading to:

● deficiency in plasma protein formation
● potential fluid shifts due to changes in oncotic pressure
● deficient gluconeogenesis
● poor conjugation of bilirubin
● lack of blood clotting factors
● reduced ability to break down and excrete drugs.

The lobule, a tiny cylindrical structure, is the functional unit of the liver. It is constructed

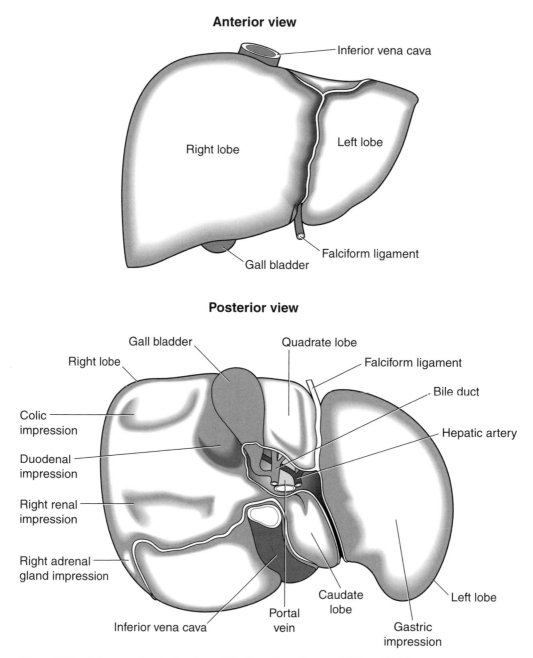

Figure 15.3 Anterior and posterior views of the liver. From Ross and Wilson (1990).

around a central vein and is composed of hepatic cellular plates that radiate outwards from the central vein. Between the adjacent cells of each hepatic plate lie small canaliculi into which the hepatic cells secrete bile. The canaliculi empty into terminal bile ducts in the septa between adjacent liver lobules. Small portal venules that receive their blood supply from the portal veins are also found in the septa. Blood flows from these venules into branching hepatic sinusoids, between the hepatic plates and into the central vein of the lobule. In addition, there are hepatic arterioles in the interlobular septa, which supply arterial blood to the tissues and empty directly into the hepatic sinusoids.

Box 15.2   Functions of the liver

Vascular
1. red cell formation during fetal life
2. formation and destruction of red blood cells
3. synthesis of coagulation factors
4. manufacture of plasma proteins
5. phagocytosis of bacteria, toxins and worn out blood cells by Kupfer cells
6. reservoir for blood

Food
1. carbohydrate metabolism
2. lipid metabolism
3. protein metabolism
4. bile salts synthesis
5. bile production and secretion
6. mineral and vitamin storage
7. vitamin D activation
8. iron storage

Detoxification
1. urea formation
2. degradation of drugs
3. steroid catabolism

Source: Mowat (1994)

The gall bladder and biliary tree. This is a pear-shaped sac located in the fossa of the visceral surface of the liver which stores and concentrates bile until it is required by the small intestine. Bile from the right and left hepatic ducts empties directly into the duodenum via the common bile duct or is diverted into the gall bladder.

CARE OF THE NEONATE WITH CONGENITAL GASTROINTESTINAL DISORDERS

Management of neonatal congenital gastrointestinal abnormalities requires early assessment and diagnosis, preoperative stabilisation, good surgical repair and prevention of postoperative complications.

Oesophageal atresia and tracheoesophageal fistula

Aetiology and physiology

The oesophagus and trachea develop from a common foregut during the 3rd–5th gestational weeks and then separate and lengthen. Oesophageal atresia occurs when the oesophagus fails to develop as a continuous passage. The trachea and oesophagus may fail to separate into distinct structures, forming a tracheoesophageal fistula.

Oesophageal atresia has an incidence of 1:3000–5000. 50% of neonates with this defect are born prematurely, and more than 50% have associated congenital malformations, including chromosomal disorders which influence mortality. The epidemiology and genetics of the defect are unclear. The majority of infants with oesophageal atresia have a blind-ending proximal oesophagus and a fistula between the trachea and distal oesophagus, although there are variations (Fig. 15.4) (Spitz et al 1994, Walker et al 1996).

Clinical signs and symptoms

Maternal hydramnios is an early sign of oesophageal atresia. In newborns the diagnosis should be suspected where there are excessive oral secretions associated with choking or cyanotic attacks. These symptoms will be exaggerated if the defect is not diagnosed prior to feeding. The passage of an oro/nasogastric tube is not possible, and the chest X-ray shows air in the bowel confirming the presence of a distal fistula. Following confirmation of the diagnosis, other abnormalities should be excluded and potential complications prevented.

Surgical management

Prior to surgery the infant will require a nasogastric tube or a Replogle double lumen tube. This is placed in the oesophageal pouch on continuous suction to clear the oropharynx and prevent oral secretions entering the lungs. Nursing in the head-up position is recommended to reduce the risk of gastric reflux through the fistula into

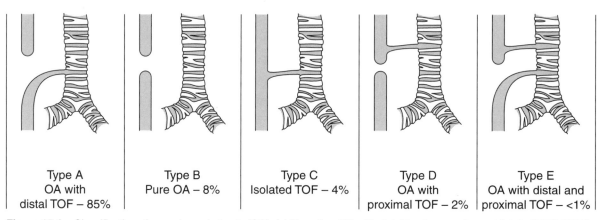

Figure 15.4 Classification of oesophageal atresia (OA): (a) Type A — OA with distal tracheoesophageal fistula (TOF) (85%); (b) Type B — pure OA (8%); (c) Type C — isolated TOF (4%); (d) Type D — OA with proximal TOF (2%); (e) Type E — OA with distal and proximal TOF (< 1%). From Beasley et al (1991).

the lungs, reducing the risk of pneumonitis or atelectasis. The infant may require ventilation if respiratory distress is present. The surgical management of oesophageal atresia depends on the anatomy of the defect. In most cases, primary anastomosis of the oesophagus and division of the fistula is possible via a right thoracotomy and extrapleural approach.

Either a gastrostomy is formed which decompresses the stomach or a silastic transanastomotic nasogastric tube is inserted, providing access for enteral feeding.

Following a difficult primary oesophageal repair, the infant may require several days ventilation with paralysis to allow the anastomosis to heal. Care must be taken when giving the infant suction and also on handling, to avoid hyperextension of the oesophagus and damage to the anastomosis. Contrast studies are performed after 1 week; if no leak is detected, oral feeding is commenced. Some infants do require a chest drain for an anastomotic leak. Parenteral nutrition and prophylactic antibiotics will be required until the leak has resolved. Delayed primary repair may be considered in preterm infants with underlying pulmonary disease, those with associated abnormalities, or where a 'long gap' makes end-to-end anastomosis difficult. The latter may require reconstruction using a colonic or jejunal interposition or mobilisation of the stomach (Rescorla et al 1994).

Outcome

The mortality has decreased, with survival rates of 85–90% irrespective of the type of repair. The main causes of death are associated congenital abnormalities and prematurity with a weight of less than 1500 g (Spitz et al 1994).

Complications in the long-term management of these infants may occur. Infants with oesophageal atresia demonstrate a degree of oesophageal dysmotility, with a high incidence of gastroesophageal reflux requiring medical treatment and occasionally fundoplication. Anastomotic stricture formation is also a common problem which may be aggravated by reflux and require dilatation. A degree of tracheomalacia may be present in a small number of infants, requiring aortopexy. As children grow older, bolus obstruction secondary to oesophageal dysmotility and/or stricture formation may occur.

Despite these complications, studies of adults born with oesophageal atresia show that, following surgical repair, they are likely to enjoy a normal lifestyle (Spitz et al 1994, Engum et al 1995).

Abdominal wall defects

Exomphalos, omphalocele and gastroschisis all describe protrusions of the abdominal contents at or around the umbilicus. Clinical subdivision of these defects is useful for descriptive purposes, although separation cannot be absolute.

These defects are often diagnosed antenatally on ultrasound. This allows time for the parents to receive counselling to consider the severity of the problem and the options for termination or surgery with the need for long-term care. Antenatal diagnosis also enables the mother to be transferred to a regional centre for delivery allowing immediate examination of the baby on delivery, protection of the bowel from further damage and the prospect of arranging early surgery (Nicholls et al 1993).

Exomphalus/omphalocele

Aetiology and pathophysiology. Exomphalos results from incomplete formation of the anterior abdominal wall during fetal development, occurring in 1:2500–5000 births (Yeo 1996). During the third week of development, four somatic folds appear defining the anterior thoracic and abdominal walls. These folds migrate centrally to fuse at the umbilical ring, usually completed by 12 weeks gestation. An arrest in the development of these folds results in an anterior wall defect, forming an exomphalos. The developing loops of intestine are protected by the amniotic membrane and peritoneum, the umbilical cord enters the amniotic sac, and the abdominal muscle wall is normal. Smaller hernias into the umbilical cord usually contain loops of intestine; however, with a larger defect, there may be prolapse of liver as well as bowel into the exomphalos sac. There is a high incidence of other congenital abnormalities accompanying this defect.

Preoperative management. The diagnosis of exomphalus is often made on antenatal ultrasound, allowing careful assessment for associated abnormalities and chromosome screening by chorionic villi sampling or amniocentesis.

If the defect is large, an elective caesarean section can be performed at 36 weeks gestation to optimise preoperative management and prevent haemorrhage from an accidental rupture of the liver during delivery (Yeo 1996). Ventilation may be required if respiration is impaired. A nasogastric tube is inserted and kept on free drainage to decompress the stomach and reduce the risk of the intestines becoming distended as air is swallowed. The gut is protected from infection and heat loss by covering with plastic wrap or inserting the infant's lower body in a specially designed plastic bag. If there are signs of infection or if the gut is compromised, cefuroxime and metronidazole are commenced.

Clinical management. Management is determined by the size of the defect. A small or moderate-sized defect is usually readily closed; attempts at primary closure of larger defects may result in respiratory and haemodynamic instability.

If fascial closure is not tolerated, there are two options for surgery. The most common option is the construction of a temporary silastic pouch/silo to cover the exomphalos. This is reduced over 7–10 days until the silo contents have returned into the abdominal cavity and fascial closure can be performed. The alternative option is to create a large ventral hernia by closing the skin over the defect. This can then be repaired several months later, allowing the baby to grow, but secondary closure is often difficult and the cosmetic result is poor (Yeo 1996).

Postoperative management. Postoperative management is dependent on the surgical technique used to repair the exomphalos. Following closure of a small or moderate defect, the infant should be weaned from ventilation and extubated as tolerated. However, creation of a large ventral hernia may cause respiratory compromise requiring ventilation for a longer period of time. Ventilation often continues while decompression of a silo pouch is achieved. The infant is kept 'nil orally' and receives parenteral nutrition (Dillon & Cilley 1993).

Outcome. 90% survival is estimated, but with underlying congenital abnormalities mortality increases to 40%. In survivors, complications tend to be rare, but can include prolonged intestinal dysfunction, bowel obstruction, sepsis and perforated viscus (Dillon & Cilley 1993).

Gastroschisis

Aetiology and pathophsiology. Gastroschisis

is a rare abdominal wall anomaly that is differentiated by the position of the cord. Classically the umbilical cord is intact, with loops of intestine herniating through a small defect to the right of the cord. There is no sac covering the intestine, and the loops of bowel are thick walled and matted due to exposure to amniotic fluid (Dillon & Cilley 1993).

The exact reason for this defect is unclear, but one widely accepted theory is that the anomaly results from a rupture at the base of the umbilical cord in an area weakened by the involution of the right umbilical vein. Loops of intestine are free to herniate into the amniotic cavity at what appears to be a relatively late stage in fetal development. The reported incidence of the defect varies in the range 1:10 000–20 000; however, there has been an apparent increase in incidence in the last twenty years in Europe and the USA (Stringer et al 1991).

Associated chromosomal or structural defects are rare. All infants have non-rotation and abnormal fixation of the intestine as a result of the defect, and gastrointestinal anomalies such as atresia or stenosis can occur in up to 20% of infants (Dillon & Cilley 1993).

Preoperative management. Following delivery, care must be taken in handling the gut, so that the bowel mesentery is not torn, causing additional intestinal injury. The infant must be kept warm and stabilised prior to surgery.

Surgical management. Options for repair of this defect include:

- primary fascial closure
- primary skin closure
- construction of a silastic pouch with a delayed repair.

Primary closure of the defect enables full enteral feeding to be established and earlier discharge home (Swift et al 1992, Stringel 1993). Large defects with gross visceroabdominal disproportion require a staged repair, usually with the formation of a silo.

Outcome. Infants born with gastroschisis have few associated abnormalities and generally do well postoperatively and long term. Short gut syndrome may develop from prolonged exposure to amniotic fluid in utero, characterised by lactose intolerance and decreased carbohydrate and protein absorption.

Improvements in surgical repair have led to a good prognosis, with survival rates as high as 90–99% (Swift et al 1992, Dillon & Cilley 1993).

Diaphragmatic hernia

Diaphragmatic hernia is a defect occurring in the posterolateral segment of the diaphragm. This varies in size, commonly occurring on the left, with abdominal viscera herniating into the thoracic cavity. Infants born with congenital diaphragmatic hernia have mortality rates of 30–60%, largely due to pulmonary hypoplasia and pulmonary hypertension (Rodriguez et al 1996)

Survival of the infant depends on the presence of sufficient lung tissue and cardiorespiratory and metabolic stability prior to surgery. Recent innovations in the timing of surgery and in intensive care techniques have improved the outlook for some of these infants.

Aetiology

Between 4 and 8 weeks gestation the diaphragm forms, separating the abdominal and thoracic cavities. The defect is essentially a persistence of the pleuroperitoneal canal, resulting in free communication between the two cavities during fetal life. The lungs are in the glandular phase of development as herniation of the bowel into the thoracic cavity occurs, resulting in hypoplasia of the pulmonary structures. Primitive arterial and bronchial branching is usually complete by 16 weeks gestation; therefore, herniation of the bowel at varying times of lung growth results in different degrees of hypoplasia (Weinstein & Stolar 1993). An alternative hypothesis has been suggested on the basis of animal experimentation: that the primary problem is the intrauterine lung hypoplasia, and the diaphragmatic defect and organ displacement occur as a secondary event (Iritani 1984).

The incidence of congenital diaphragmatic hernia is estimated to be in the range 1:2000–5000 births. There appear to be no predisposing factors, although associated congenital anomalies may be present in up to 50% of infants (Rodriguez et al 1996).

85–90% of all congenital diaphragmatic defects are of the posterolateral (Bochdalek) type, 80% are left sided, 15% right sided and 5% bilateral (Weinstein & Stolar 1993). The anterior diaphragmatic defect (of Morgani) arises between the costal and sternal muscular origins of the diaphragm, usually on the right hand side, the infant being asymptomatic and undiagnosed until later in life.

Pathophysiology

Congenital diaphragmatic hernia may be diag-
nosed in utero or immediately after birth. Presenting signs include:

- respiratory distress within 6 hours of life
- asymmetric or distended chest and scaphoid abdomen
- absent breath sounds on affected side
- chest X-ray shows air-filled loops of bowel in the chest.

Failure to make in utero diagnoses results in respiratory distress in 90% of infants, and 10% have insufficient pulmonary function to sustain extrauterine life. The pathophysiological sequence of events explains the potential instability of an infant with diaphragmatic hernia (Fig. 15.5). The

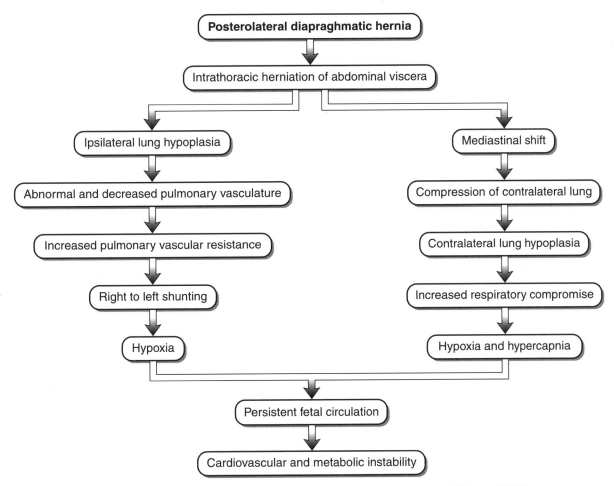

Figure 15.5 Pathophysiology of congenital diaphragmatic hernia. Adapted from Davenport & Holmes (1995).

ipsilateral lung is hypoplastic and has an abnormal pulmonary vasculature that is sensitive and prone to rapid increases in vascular resistance and subsequent pulmonary hypertension. This causes hypoxia resulting in persistent fetal circulation or persistent pulmonary hypertension of the newborn. This is characterised by a right to left shunting of blood across the patent foramen ovale and ductus arteriosus. The contralateral lung is often partially compressed and may be hypoplastic, causing further respiratory compromise (Davenport & Holmes 1995).

Preoperative management

Elective intubation as soon as the defect is suspected is essential to prevent sudden collapse. Management includes:

- avoidance of prolonged bagging via face mask to prevent air entering the abdomen and increasing mediastinal shift
- ventilation using low inspiratory pressures, small tidal volumes and a high rate +/− high frequency oscillation
- nursing with head of cot elevated, reducing pressure of abdominal contents in the thorax
- elective paralysis and sedation to maximise respiratory and cardiovascular function
- prophylactic antibiotics if distended/malrotated bowel could compromise mesenteric perfusion.

If normal blood gases and acid base balance are difficult to maintain then the prognosis is likely to be poor. Oxygen saturation should be monitored on the right hand, reflecting preductal saturation, and on either foot, indicating postductal oxygen saturation. Saturations should be maintained within normal limits running within 5% of each other. If desaturation of both readings suddenly occurs then lung rather than ductal shunting should be considered, including:

- lung collapse and consolidation
- infection
- pneumothorax
- gut distention
- inadequate ventilation.

Careful monitoring is important to detect rapid changes in oxygen saturation. If desaturation occurs with more than a 10% difference between pre- and postductal saturations, urgent treatment is required, including:

- bagging with 100% oxygen
- correction of acidosis
- pulmonary vasodilators
- nitric oxide
- considering ECMO.

Protocols for the management of these infants vary, although no particular regime has been proven superior by controlled trials. The UK ECMO trial suggests an increased survival when used, supporting the American literature (UK Collaborative ECMO Trial Group 1996). For less severe cases, most centres adopt a policy of delayed primary repair and conservative management to minimise the effects of persistent fetal circulation.

Surgery

Surgery is generally delayed until cardiorespiratory stability has been achieved. Some centres suggest that repair of the defect whilst on ECMO can safely be performed, but this is still being explored. Surgical repair is performed through a subcostal or transverse abdominal incision, and the diaphragmatic defect is sutured. If the defect is large, a reinforced silastic or dacron patch may be used. The repair should be taut enough to prevent paradoxical diaphragmatic movement, but not so tight as to deform the chest or raise intra-abdominal pressure.

Postoperative care

Surgical repair of diaphragmatic hernia reduces the compliance of the respiratory system and may exacerbate any preoperative problem. Pneumothoraces can occur on both sides of the chest, requiring a pleural drain. Once the condition of the infant improves, slow weaning from ventilation commences.

Antenatal diagnosis and a greater understanding of persistent fetal circulation have advanced the management of these infants. Research into future treatment has included fetal surgery to reverse intrauterine lung hypoplasia and tracheal ligation to repair the defect (Harrison et al 1990, DiFiore et al 1994). Lung transplantation and liquid ventilation have also been considered but remain experimental and controversial (Weinstein & Stolar 1993, Davenport & Holmes 1995).

Quality of life remains a concern for survivors with borderline pulmonary hypoplasia and/or a neurological insult in the neonatal period (Lund et al 1994). Restrictive airway disease may occur postoperatively, and there is a high incidence of GI motility disorders (Weinstein & Stolar 1993, Norden et al 1994). It is unclear which infants will benefit from the use of ECMO, because of the difficulty in predicting selection criteria. Experience in the USA suggests that ECMO therapy will result in a survival rate of about 40–60%; however, the long-term effects of ECMO are still unclear (Davenport & Holmes 1995, Rodriguez et al 1996).

NECROTISING ENTEROCOLITIS

Aetiology

Necrotising enterocolitis (NEC) is characterised by diffuse or patchy necrosis of the bowel mucosa and submucosa, commonly affecting the terminal ileum and colon. It is an acquired disease of unknown aetiology that develops during the neonatal period (Kliegman 1990, Stringer & Spitz 1993). There is a high mortality rate and delayed morbidity due to the development of short gut syndrome (Kliegman 1990). Although commonly seen in premature or low-birthweight infants, those with congenital heart disease or overwhelming infection are also at risk (Stringer & Spitz 1993).

NEC usually occurs during the first 2 weeks of life, after feeding has commenced (Rushton 1990a). Immaturity of the gastrointestinal tract and introduction of enteral feeding are thought to be associated with the development of NEC (Kliegman 1990). The types of bacteria colonising the gastrointestinal tract are also thought to be related to the occurrence of NEC (Hoy et al 1990,

Millar et al 1992). Other risk factors thought to increase the risk of NEC include:

- **prenatal**
  - fetal distress and hypoxia
  - placental dysfunction
  - prolapsed cord
  - maternal infection
  - premature rupture of membranes
- **perinatal**
  - prematurity < 36 weeks gestation
  - low birthweight
  - traumatic delivery
  - birth asphyxia
  - meconium aspiration
- **postnatal**
  - cold stress
  - respiratory distress syndrome
  - congenital heart disease
  - indwelling umbilical artery catheter
  - sepsis
  - low cardiac output
  - early feeding into a premature gut
  - thromboembolitic states, i.e. polycythaemia.

Signs and symptoms

Initially, infants present with non-specific symptoms, including:

- lethargy
- poor feeding
- temperature instability
- recurrent apnoea
- bradycardias
- hypoglycaemia
- electrolyte imbalance.

The infant's abdomen is distended, blood is passed in the stools, and pneumatosis coli (see below) is present. Advanced NEC can cause cardiovascular and respiratory compromise. If untreated, NEC can lead to gut perforation, sepsis, decompensated shock and death.

Pathophysiology

The early histopathological injury in NEC is

disruption of the intestinal mucosal epithelium. The three factors essential to the pathogenesis of the disease are:

- ischaemic damage to the gut
- bacterial colonisation
- the availability of dietary substrate, usually formula feed

(Roberts 1990, Kliegman 1990).

NEC usually responds to intensive medical treatment, and mild disease can be completely reversible. However, 30–50% of neonates develop complications requiring surgery. Babies with extensive disease have a high mortality (Stringer & Spitz 1993).

When the normal intestinal bacterial flora gains access to the submucosal tissue, hydrolysis of dietary substrate results in the formation of extramural gas, usually in the submucosa. This is called pneumatosis coli, characterising well-established NEC and seen radiographically or at laparotomy. Progressive infiltration of the mucosa and bowel wall with Gram-negative bacteria causes more extensive tissue inflammation, with haemorrhagic necrosis, ulceration and possible perforation of the bowel and sepsis.

Clinical management

Conservative medical treatment is preferable, including:

- commencement of parenteral feeding and nil enterally
- passage of nasogastric tube — replace aspirates with 0.9% KCl saline intravenously
- frequent abdominal girth assessment and measurement
- stools tested for blood and reducing substances
- respiratory and cardiovascular support, including ventilation and inotropes as required
- removal of umbilical arterial lines, to reduce risk of infection
- intravenous antibiotics — benzyl penicillin 60 mg/kg/dose 6–12 hourly, gentamicin 2.5–6 mg/kg daily and metronidazole 7.5 mg/kg/dose 12 hourly (Shann 1996).

Infants requiring surgery usually present with intestinal perforation or persistent metabolic acidosis. Presurgical treatment for haemodynamically unstable, very premature infants can include the insertion of a soft Penrose drain into the iliac fossa to drain air, intestinal contents and peritoneal fluid. This drainage should be sent for laboratory analysis.

Surgery

Surgery is considered for neonates with intestinal perforation where medical treatment has been unsuccessful and for those who are likely to tolerate an anaesthetic. Surgery often involves segmental resection, with ostomy formation and creation of a distal mucus fistula. Following surgery the infant may be nil enterally for up to 10 days, requiring parenteral nutrition.

Reanastomosis of the gut can occur 4 to 6 weeks postoperatively, following contrast studies to demonstrate absence of stricture formation. However, extensive damage to large areas of small bowel and colon may require drastic resection. Short gut syndrome results, affecting gut absorption and dependence on parenteral nutrition, prolonging recovery.

Postoperative management includes assessment and care of the stomas and wound site. Ostomy losses and gastric aspirate need to be replaced intravenously. Parenteral nutrition should continue until the gut has recovered. Enteral feeding may commence slowly after several weeks, with breast milk where possible or hydrolised protein feeds, e.g. Pregestermil.

A further group of rare abnormalities that may require surgery with or without stoma formation and occasionally paediatric intensive care include:

- intestinal atresias
  — duodenal atresia
  — jejuno-ileal atresias
  — complex atresias
- gut malrotation
- Hirschsprung's disease
- meconium ileus.

THE GUT IN MULTIORGAN FAILURE

Protection of the gut

The most important protective agents of the gut are mucin and secretory immunoglobulin A (IgA). Mucin forms a protective layer over the tightly joined cells, maintains selective absorption of nutrients and protects the cell surface from damage from hydrogen and hydrochloric acid. In the intestine, mucin helps prevent toxins and bacteria from translocating into the circulation. Immunoglobulin A secreted from lymphoid tissue in the gut prevents organisms invading and penetrating the mucosa.

The secretion of IgA is initiated by enteral feeding. Administering specific nutrients to preserve the mucosa will help prevent translocation of bacteria into the blood:

- *glutamine* — immunological role, maintaining mucosal barrier and gut-associated lymphoid tissue
- *arginine* — improves cellular immunity and wound healing
- *fatty acids* — promote normal mucosal growth and repair
- *nucleotides* — increase resistance to infection, improving immune function of cells and enhancing T lymphocyte function.

During critical illness, due to the withholding of enteral feeding, the integrity of the gut mucosa and barrier mechanism may be compromised. Some factors encourage bacterial translocation (Box 15.3); therefore, enteral feeding should be considered a priority.

Selective decontamination of the gut

It is suggested that altering gut flora by decontamination may eradicate nosocomial infection. This may be achieved by administering topical non-absorbable antibiotics to the oropharynx and gastric mucosa via a nasogastric tube and administering systemic antibiotics. This is followed by septic screening of the gastrointestinal tract. Studies carried out in adults show a decrease in nosocomial infections following

---

Box 15.3 Specific factors promoting translocation of bacteria

- host immunosuppression or glucocorticoid therapy
- hypovolaemia and septic shock resulting in inadequate perfusion/ischaemia of gut mucosa, and dysfunction of mucosal barrier and increased permeability
- ulceration or local injury to mucosa
- intestinal obstruction, which may cause mucosal injury and bacterial overgrowth
- parenteral nutrition/no enteral feeding, causing hypoplasia of mucosa

Source: Phillips & Olson (1993).

---

selective decontamination, but no significant effect on mortality (Humfreys 1994).

STRESS ULCERATION

The incidence of stress ulceration has declined in critically ill children due to the use of preventative therapies such as antacid therapy, H_2 receptor antagonists and sucralfate (Prevost & Oberle 1993). Some disorders increase the incidence of stress ulceration:

- burns > 35% body surface area = Curling's deep duodenal ulcers
- trauma or central nervous system disease = Cushing's ulcers — deep ulcers throughout the GI tract
- fulminant hepatic failure
- Gram-negative sepsis — stimulates gastric acid production
- respiratory failure
- shock.

Stomach perforation is rare but potentially life threatening if haemorrhage occurs.

Ulcers tend to be superficial, small and multiple, and located in the proximal region of the stomach in non-acid-producing areas. Signs and symptoms include painless GI haemorrhage resulting in melaena and/or coffee ground aspirate.

Management

The primary aim of management is the identi-

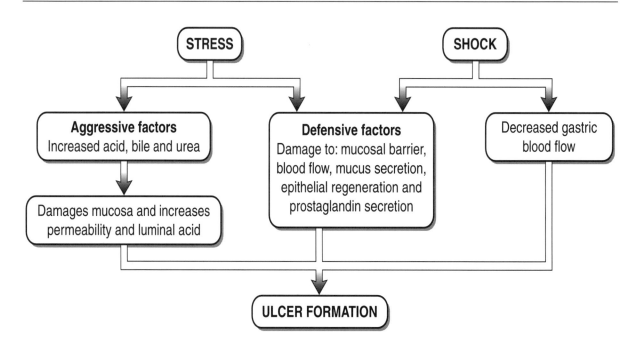

Figure 15.6 Pathophysiology of stress ulceration. Adapted from Prevost & Oberle (1993).

fication of children at risk (Fig. 15.6) and prompt treatment of causative factors, reducing the high mortality associated with haemorrhage. It is suggested that a gastric pH of less than 3.5 increases the incidence of stress ulceration. However, it is now thought that the acidity of mucosal tissue is a more reliable indicator, measured using a specialised nasogastric tube (Tonometer). The liquid gastric pH is assessed and effectiveness of treatment is evaluated by sequential monitoring of gastric pH.

Enteral nutrition is also important in providing protection by improving the gastric mucosal defence and should be considered whenever possible.

PANCREATITIS

This is rarely seen in paediatric intensive care but may be caused by:

- drugs — frusemide, prednisolone, tetracyclines
- infections — coxsackievirus, Epstein–Barr, hepatitis A or B, mumps, mycoplasma
- vascular disorders — systemic lupus erythematosis, thrombotic thrombocytopenia purpura
- metabolic disorders — hyperlipidaemia, hyperparathyriodism, uraemia, malnutrition, cystic fibrosis
- trauma — injury, penetrating peptic ulcer
- obstruction — duodenal obstruction, blockage of papilla of Vater by gallstones, cholelithiasis, tumours.

Signs and symptoms

These include:

- abdominal pain — central, radiating through to back
- nausea, vomiting
- pyrexia
- paralytic ileus
- ARDS or pleural effusions
- haemoconcentration due to fluid shift
- hyperglycaemia due to release of glucagon from damaged cells

- later in disease process, retroperitoneal haemorrhage:
  - grey discoloration of flanks (Grey Turner's sign)
  - grey discoloration of umbilicus (Cullen's sign).

Management

Pancreatic enzymes have vasoactive properties resulting in localised oedema and fluid shifts. Aim of treatment is to rest the pancreas, restore circulating volume and maintain electrolyte balance. Management includes:

- pain relief — avoid morphine and opiate derivatives, which cause increased contraction of sphincter of Oddi and pain
- nil enterally, nasogastric aspiration and fluid replacement
- maintain haemodynamic stability
- maintain electrolyte balance
- maintain fluid balance
- maintain blood sugar levels.

REYE'S SYNDROME

Reye's syndrome is a disease of unknown aetiology characterised by acute toxic encephalopathy and fatty infiltration of the liver. Typically it follows a viral infection such as Influenza A or B, Varicella, RSV, CMV, Rotavirus, or Herpes simplex. These appear to cause mitochondrial injury, specifically in the liver and brain, resulting in cerebral oedema that may cause brain damage or death. The prognosis depends on stage of presentation and extent of encephalopathy. This is most commonly seen between 6 months and 15 years of age. Retrospective studies in 1986 suggested a link between salicyclic acid ingestion and Reye's syndrome. The Committee on the Safety of Medicines in the UK withdrew paediatric aspirin formulations for children aged 12 years or less. Since then there has been a decline in reported cases, possibly linked to aspirin avoidance, but it may also be linked to increased awareness of inborn errors of metabolism as a differential diagnosis (Mowat 1994).

Pathology

Liver pathology shows mitochondrial damage which affects detoxification of waste products. It appears swollen with no evidence of inflammation. Intracellular lipid and fatty infiltration of the kidneys, heart and pancreas are also found (Glasgow & Moore 1993).

Signs and symptoms

The disease appears to start with a viral illness; during the recovery period the child develops vomiting and decreased level of consciousness. This coincides with raised intracranial pressure, characterised by convulsions, coma, or an opisthotonic state.

Clinical management

There are characteristic laboratory findings of Reye's syndrome (Box 15.4); however, inherited metabolic disorders should be considered.

Box 15.4 Laboratory findings of Reye's syndrome

- elevated transaminase (SGOT-aspartate, SGPT-aminotransferase)
- elevated ammonia — disruption in ammonia breakdown urea and excretion
- prolonged prothrombin time — liver function appears to return to normal as disease progresses

---

The overall aim is to protect the brain from irreversible damage secondary to raised intracranial pressure. The collapsed child is dehydrated from excessive vomiting. Rehydration at 50–60% of normal maintenance requirements is a priority. Plasma and/or platelets may be required to correct clotting abnormalities, especially prior to liver biopsy. Anticonvulsants are given to control seizures. The liver should recover spontaneously within 1 month of onset if treatment is successful.

DIABETIC KETOACIDOSIS
Pathophysiology

This is a potentially life-threatening condition

caused by absent or insufficient insulin production.

Insufficient insulin. The transport of glucose across the cell membrane is inhibited, resulting in increased extracellular glucose. Hyperglycemia raises the serum osmolarity, causing osmotic diuresis leading to polyuria, dehydration and polydypsia in an attempt to maintain hydration. If untreated, fluid and electrolyte imbalance leads to haemoconcentration, vascular collapse and shock; serum analysis shows increased potassium levels, which may fall as it is drawn into the cells with glucose. Gluconeogenesis is initiated by the metabolism of free fatty acids and proteins for energy. Fatty acids are metabolised at a greater rate than gluconeogenesis, resulting in ketone formation and accumulation.

Ketoacids and lactic acid production lead to metabolic acidosis. The rising pH and falling bicarbonate stimulates the respiratory centre to increase alveolar ventilation, removing excess acid — manifested by Kussmaul's respirations.

Clinical signs

These include:

- polyuria
- polydypsia
- vomiting and dehydration
- lethargy — impaired level of consciousness (diabetic coma)
- hyperventilation — Kussmaul's respirations
- electrolyte disturbance — dysrhythmias
- shock.

Management

Airway management, monitoring of vital signs, fluid balance and blood glucose levels are essential. Rehydration and electrolyte replacement is achieved using IV isotonic saline and administration of IV glucose according to blood glucose levels. Colloid may be required to restore circulating volume. To manage blood glucose levels, insulin should be administered on a sliding scale, using a continuous infusion according to the blood glucose levels.

Correction of acidosis is essential; this is achieved as gluconeogenesis is inhibited by administration of insulin. Bicarbonate is administered if required when the acidosis is severe.

Potassium supplementation may be required if the child is hypokalaemic in response to the insulin therapy and correction of the acidosis.

GASTROINTESTINAL BLEEDING

Causes include gastrointestinal inflammation or perforation due to stress ulceration, necrotising enterocolitis, oesophageal varices, trauma and poisons. This is also associated with congenital abnormalities such as arteriovenous malformations and pyloric stenosis. Coagulopathies including haemorrhagic disease of the newborn, disseminated coagulopathy and haemolytic uraemic syndrome are also related to GI bleeding.

Clinical signs

These include:

- haematemesis
- melaena
- occult blood in stool
- hypovolaemia.

Management

This is based on treatment of the underlying cause, which may require endoscopic examination and close observation for gastric or intestinal perforation. Supportive management includes:

- airway management
- maintenance of vital signs and haemoglobin
- correction of hypovolaemia.

DISORDERS OF THE BILIARY TRACT
Biliary atresia

Aetiology

This is characterised by absence/obstruction of the biliary tree. The atresia involves isolated segments of the bile duct system or more often the entire biliary tree including the gall bladder. The cause is thought to be the end result of progressive cholangitis caused by inflammation from an infection or toxin in utero or soon after birth.

Signs and symptoms

The infant presents with persistent jaundice beyond the first week of life due to direct (conjugated) hyperbilirubinaemia caused by accumulation of bile in the liver. Pale stools indicate lack of bile drainage, and dark coloured urine is caused by increased bilirubin secretion. Failure to thrive, abdominal distention and pruritis develop later as the liver enlarges and disease progresses. Signs of undiagnosed progressive liver disease are evident between 5 and 12 months.

Management

A modified Kasai portoenterostomy is performed before 60 days of age, using a Roux en Y loop of jejunum (about 40 cm) brought up and anastomosed end-to-side to the porta hepatis and then an end-to-side anastomosis with small bowel. If unsuccessful, liver transplantation is required.

Postoperative management. Routine postoperative laparotomy care is required. Specific complications include:

- ascending cholangitis
- portal hypertension
- progressive liver failure.

CARE OF THE NEONATE WITH UNCONJUGATED HYPERBILIRUBINAEMIA

Erythrocyte destruction results in the production of bilirubin. Two forms of bilirubin exist (Fig. 15.7). Elevated serum bilirubin levels may be due to high levels of either form, so hyperbilirubinaemia is subcategorised into unconjugated and conjugated.

Aetiology

Common in the neonatal period, 50% of newborns develop jaundice from 24 h of age, due to normal physiological processes. This also arises when the mechanisms causing physiological unconjugated hyperbilirubinaemia are aggravated or accentuated by a pathological process (Mowat 1994). Jaundice occurring within the first 24 h of life or persisting for more than 2 weeks should be investigated, as it may be related to haemolysis or liver disease.

Pathophysiology

This is dependent upon the aetiology — excessive production of bilirubin, impaired bilirubin binding/transport, hepatic metabolism or increased recirculation of bilirubin.

Clinical features

Unconjugated hyperbilirubinaemia presents as jaundice and absence of bile in urine (Box 15.5). The concentration of serum bilirubin causing jaundice differs with age.

Box 15.5 Possible causes of neonatal unconjugated hyperbilirubinaemia

- physiological jaundice of the newborn
- displacement of bilirubin by albumin-binding drugs (e.g. sulphonamides, cephalosporins, frusemide)
- decreased binding of bilirubin — e.g. hypoalbinaemia, hypoxia, prematurity, hypoglycaemia
- haemolytic disorders — e.g. ABO incompatibility
- breast milk jaundice
- transient familial hyperbilirubinaemia
- metabolic disorders — e.g. galactosaemia, hypothyroidism
- enteric reabsorption of bilirubin — e.g. meconium retention, high intestinal obstruction

---

If untreated, accumulation of unconjugated bilirubin may result in kernicterus or transient encephalopathy. Kernicterus results from deposition of unconjugated bilirubin in the basal ganglia, corpus striatum and thalamus. Unconjugated bilirubin enters the brain when the serum concentration exceeds the capacity of serum proteins to bind bilirubin. The diffusion of bilirubin into

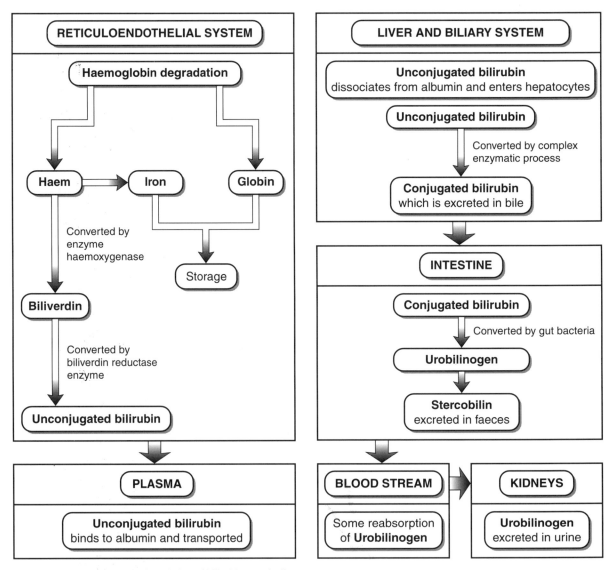

Figure 15.7   A systematic description of bilirubin metabolism.

brain tissue interferes with specific neuronal enzyme activities and may cause necrosis of neurons, resulting in death or permanent neurological damage (Kelnar et al 1995). In the presence of acidosis, hypoxia, hypoalbinaemia, or prematurity, kernicterus may occur when serum bilirubin concentrations are as low as 136 mmol/L. The risk of kernicterus is also increased by the duration of exposure to high serum bilirubin levels, alteration in the blood–brain barrier, and pre-existing brain damage (Mowat 1994).

Management

Critically ill infants have an increased risk of developing unconjugated hyperbilirubinaemia and kernicterus at lower bilirubin levels, because of the many factors interfering with bilirubin metabolism and altering the blood–brain barrier. Early intervention is essential to prevent escalation of bilirubin levels. The initial aim is to prevent kernicterus, but investigation and treatment of the cause is required.

Phototherapy. This reduces levels of unconjugated bilirubin by photochemical reactions. Bilirubin is converted to photobilirubin and lumirubin and excreted into bile without conjugation. Although there are no reported long-term side effects of phototherapy, there are preventable complications such as:

- poor temperature control — infant nursed naked to facilitate maximum exposure
- fluid depletion — increased insensible losses; increased frequency of stools
- increased metabolic rate — increased enzyme activity
- ocular damage — exposure to phototherapy rays
- parental anxiety and reduced stimulation
- increased platelet turnover

(Edwards 1995).

Phototherapy is commonly used when levels of bilirubin reach 250 mmol/L (15 mg/dL) in term infants. In premature infants it should be commenced at lower levels (Mowat 1994).

Exchange transfusion. This is the most rapid and effective method to control unconjugated hyperbilirubinaemia but is only considered if phototherapy has been unsuccessful or the risk of kernicterus is high. It may be necessary in infants with severe haemolytic disorders, to remove antibodies and correct anaemia.

During exchange transfusion, twice the infant's calculated blood volume is progressively replaced with compatible whole blood, thus removing bilirubin. Complications of exchange transfusion may be reduced by using two access sites and the isovolaemic exchange transfusion procedure. This involves simultaneous removal of the infant's blood and administration of the transfused blood, attempting to maintain a more constant blood pressure by reducing the fluctuation in blood flow (Todd 1995). Haemodynamic monitoring is essential for early detection of complications.

CARE OF THE CHILD WITH ACUTE OESOPHAGEAL VARICEAL BLEEDING

Acute oesophageal variceal haemorrhage is one of the complications of chronic liver failure that may cause admission to PICU.

Aetiology

Oesophageal varices result from portal hypertension secondary to disorders of the portal and hepatic venous systems. These may be pre-, intra-, or posthepatic in origin and cause obstruction of normal blood flow (Box 15.6) (Mowat 1994).

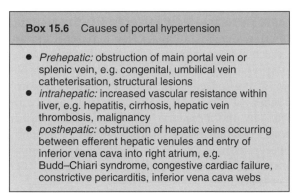

> **Box 15.6** Causes of portal hypertension
>
> - *Prehepatic:* obstruction of main portal vein or splenic vein, e.g. congenital, umbilical vein catheterisation, structural lesions
> - *intrahepatic:* increased vascular resistance within liver, e.g. hepatitis, cirrhosis, hepatic vein thrombosis, malignancy
> - *posthepatic:* obstruction of hepatic veins occurring between efferent hepatic venules and entry of inferior vena cava into right atrium, e.g. Budd–Chiari syndrome, congestive cardiac failure, constrictive pericarditis, inferior vena cava webs

Pathophysiology

Prolonged obstruction of portal blood flow results in increased vascular resistance and hypertension in the portal and splenic circulation. In an attempt to decompress the portal system, collateral vessels develop between the portal and systemic venous system, particularly the submucosal veins of the oesophagus. These oesophageal veins dilate, forming varices which become thin walled, protruding into the oesophagus, and rupture, causing alimentary bleeding (Mowat 1994).

Clinical features

Variceal haemorrhage may be triggered by factors including sepsis and aspirin ingestion or occur without warning. It may present slowly, characterised by melaena or anaemia or suddenly with haematemesis. Slow bleeding may become brisk haemorrhage, requiring emergency treatment. However, both can result in hypovolaemic shock if blood loss is severe.

Liver function may be affected after haemorrhage, due to impaired hepatic perfusion during the period of anaemia and hypotension, resulting in jaundice, ascites and encephalopathy.

Encephalopathy may progress with the presence of blood in the gut, as the high protein content stimulates increased ammonia production (Mowat 1994).

Management

Acute variceal bleeding may be life threatening. Initial management maintains a patent airway, corrects hypovolaemia and arrests bleeding.

Hypovolaemia is treated with fresh whole blood, packed cells, or 4.5% albumin solution/crystalloid fluid until blood products are available. In the presence of coagulopathy, fresh frozen plasma and IV vitamin K may be needed. Overtransfusion must be avoided, as this may cause distention of varices, precipitating further bleeding.

Ventilation may be necessary to provide airway protection until the child's condition has stabilised and further bleeding has not occurred.

Lactulose may be administered to reduce ammonia reabsorption. Control of bleeding includes pharmacological therapy, balloon tamponade and endoscopic sclerotherapy.

Pharmacological therapy. Bleeding may be controlled with continuous administration of vasoactive drugs, including vasopressin (pitressin), glypressin, somatostatin or octreotide. These latter two drugs have not been systematically evaluated in children. Octreotide is similar in nature to somatostatin, but is longer acting and has less effect on systemic circulation than vasopressin (Mowat 1994). These drugs are thought to decrease pressure in the portal venous system by causing vasoconstriction of the splanchnic arterial bed, resulting in decreased blood flow through the varices (Mowat 1994).

Vasopressin has serious side effects related to vasoconstriction of the coronary, mesenteric and peripheral arteries, which may cause myocardial and bowel ischaemia, decreased peripheral circulation and hypertension. Nitroglycerin may reduce systemic vasoconstriction and increase efficiency of vasopressin by reducing portal venous resistance (Mowat 1994).

Balloon tamponade. Persistent bleeding unresponsive to pharmacological intervention may require balloon tamponade with a paediatric Sengstaken-Blakemore tube. This is a three or four lumen tube with two balloons which can be inflated separately inside the oesophagus and fundus of the stomach. The other lumens are for oesophageal and gastric aspiration.

Endotracheal intubation is advisable prior to positioning of the tube, as complications include airway obstruction and aspiration pneumonia. The tube is passed into the stomach either nasally or orally. The gastric port is inflated, and the tube is pulled back until resistance is felt indicating its position at the cardio-oesophageal junction. Application of traction to the fundus of the stomach causes venous compression. Inflation of the gastric balloon alone can arrest bleeding, but the oesophageal balloon may also be inflated to a pressure of 20–30 mmHg. Monitoring of this pressure is important, as oesophageal necrosis secondary to mucosal ischaemia can occur, leading to rupture or erosion. Bleeding often recurs when the balloon(s) are deflated (Mowat 1994). Balloon tamponade should only be used as a temporary measure to allow a period of stability so that preparation can be made for sclerotherapy.

Endoscopy and sclerotherapy. Upper gastrointestinal endoscopy is performed when the child is stabilised, to determine the site of bleeding.

Endoscopic injection therapy thromboses bleeding vessels by injection of a sclerosing agent which causes contraction of the varix. The resulting inflammatory reaction produces thrombosis, eventually forming a fibrous band. Sclerotherapy is difficult with active bleeding and is best performed when bleeding has been controlled using pharmacological agents or balloon tamponade. Repeated sclerotherapy may be needed to completely obliterate the varices.

Complications following sclerotherapy include pleural effusions, transient fever, bacteraemia, ulcers and strictures. Sucralfate minimises the risk of ulceration. New techniques for obliteration of varices include injection of tissue adhesives or thrombin and banding ligation (Mowat 1994, Bornman et al 1994). If frequent bleeding occurs, surgery may be required to decompress the portal system by diverting portal blood to the systemic circulation. The new technique of transjugular intrahepatic portocaval stent shunting (TIPSS) may also become an option in the future (Mowat 1994, Peterson & Laine 1993). Liver transplantation may also be considered but is best delayed until bleeding has stopped.

CARE OF THE CHILD WITH ACUTE LIVER FAILURE

In acute liver failure (ALF) there is severe impairment of function and hepatocellular necrosis resulting in multiorgan failure, including encephalopathy. It may occur in the absence of any recognised underlying chronic liver disease and has a mortality of 30–70% depending upon the aetiology (Mowat 1994, Kelly 1993).

In asymptomatic, undiagnosed chronic liver disorders such as Wilson's disease or autoimmune chronic liver disease, the presenting feature is often hepatic encephalopathy, termed 'acute on chronic' liver failure (Mowat 1994).

Aetiology

There are many causes of ALF (Box 15.7) (Mowat 1994, Kelly 1993). In babies under the age of 1 year, the most likely cause is congenital infection and/or metabolic disease. In older children it is commonly secondary to viral hepatitis, hepatotoxic drugs or chemicals (Kelly 1993).

Pathology

Pathology depends on the aetiology. Liver failure occurs due to hepatic necrosis, hepatocellular degeneration, or cirrhosis (Kelly 1993).

Pathogenesis

The mechanism of ALF is poorly understood. It

is suggested that the process is multifactorial, dependent on the balance between susceptibility of the host, severity and nature of hepatic injury, efficiency of intrahepatic protective mechanisms (i.e. glutathione) and the ability of the liver to regenerate (Kelly 1993). Other factors contributing to liver failure may be altered parenchymal perfusion, endotoxaemia and decreased hepatic reticuloendothelial function (Suchy 1992).

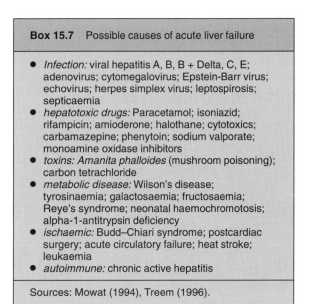

Box 15.7 Possible causes of acute liver failure

- *Infection:* viral hepatitis A, B, B + Delta, C, E; adenovirus; cytomegalovirus; Epstein-Barr virus; echovirus; herpes simplex virus; leptospirosis; septicaemia
- *hepatotoxic drugs:* Paracetamol; isoniazid; rifampicin; amioderone; halothane; cytotoxics; carbamazepine; phenytoin; sodium valporate; monoamine oxidase inhibitors
- *toxins: Amanita phalloides* (mushroom poisoning); carbon tetrachloride
- *metabolic disease:* Wilson's disease; tyrosinaemia; galactosaemia; fructosaemia; Reye's syndrome; neonatal haemochromotosis; alpha-1-antitrypsin deficiency
- *ischaemic:* Budd–Chiari syndrome; postcardiac surgery; acute circulatory failure; heat stroke; leukaemia
- *autoimmune:* chronic active hepatitis

Sources: Mowat (1994), Treem (1996).

Clinical features

ALF can develop within hours or weeks. The clinical presentation varies with aetiology, but generally there is a rapid onset of hepatic dysfunction with coagulopathy, hypoglycaemia and encephalopathy. Liver function biochemistry will be abnormal (Box 15.8). There is progressive or increased jaundice, although it may be absent in the early stages of liver failure (Mowat 1994).

Hepatic encephalopathy. This is an intrinsic part of ALF, causing alteration in neurological function that may progress to coma and death. The underlying pathophysiological mechanisms remain incompletely understood, with several hypotheses existing including the following.

Portal systemic shunting. Blood flow from the

intestine shunts through the liver, causing incomplete removal of potentially toxic metabolites formed by intestinal bacterial degradation of proteins, amino acids and blood.

Box 15.8   Liver function tests

Common biochemical measurements of liver function:

Serum enzymes
- **aminotransferases: alanine aminotransferase (ALT), aspartate aminotransferase (AST)** — intracellular enzymes found in all tissues, particularly liver, heart, skeletal muscle, adipose tissue, brain and kidney. Increased ALT and AST levels indicate hepatocellular necrosis — leakage from damaged tissues. Only hepatocytes have high levels of ALT, therefore liver specific
- **alkaline phosphatase (ALP)** — an iosenzyme contained in liver, bone, intestines and kidney. Hepatic isoenzymes are located mainly in the endothelium of intrahepatic bile ducts. ALP level is increased in liver disease, particularly impaired bile production caused by obstruction/inflammation of hepatobiliary tract.

Bilirubin
Byproduct of haemoglobin breakdown (Fig. 15.7). Measured as total bilirubin — direct (conjugated) and indirect (unconjugated) bilirubin. Increased indirect bilirubin demonstrates decreased ability to conjugate bilirubin. Increased direct bilirubin suggests impaired excretion of bilirubin into bile ducts and biliary tree.

Coagulation studies
Synthesis of coagulation factors (I, II, V, VII, IX, X) occurs within the liver. Decreased plasma concentrations result in prolonged clotting time. Measurement of prothrombin time (PT) evaluates the extrinsic pathway, and partial thromboblastin time (PTT) assesses intrinsic and common pathways of clotting cascade.
   Prolonged PT indicates poor utilisation of vitamin K due to parenchymal liver disease or obstructive jaundice. Improvement in PT after vitamin K administration suggests that vitamin K malabsorption is due to decreased bile secretion. No improvement suggests severe liver disease or disseminated intravascular coagulation. Prolonged PTT indicates hepatic dysfunction or heparin therapy.

Serum albumin
Manufactured by the liver, decreased levels may demonstrate liver synthetic dysfunction or inadequate protein intake. Hypoalbinaemia is found in advanced chronic liver disease; it does not always occur initially in acute liver failure, as albumin has a half life of 20 days.

Source: Mowat (1994).

Accumulation of neuroactive products.   Failure of liver metabolism causes increase in:

- ammonia
- aromatic amino acids — cross the blood–brain barrier, causing changes in brain neurotransmitters by increasing inhibitory and false neurotransmitters and inhibiting synthesis of excitatory neurotransmitters
- synergistic neurotoxins — in combination, ammonia, short chain fatty acids, mercaptans and phenols act as neurotoxins.

Increased gamma-aminobutyric acid (GABA) receptor activity.   GABA is the principal inhibitory neurotransmitter in the brain; accumulation results in neural inhibition.

Alteration in the blood–brain barrier.   Increased permeability allows entry of normally excluded toxic substances.

Hypoglycaemia.   Decreased brain energy metabolism.

Hypoalbinaemia.   Decreased albumin binding of toxins allows free toxins to cross the blood–brain barrier.

Hepatic encephalopathy is thought to be metabolically based, as it is reversible following liver transplantation (Kelly 1993).

It is classified into four grades according to severity (Table 15.1). The development and pro-

Table 15.1   Grades of hepatic encephalopathy

Grade	Signs and symptoms
I	Lethargy Minor disturbance of consciousness or motor function Impaired concentration Day/night sleep reversal
II	Increased drowsiness but responsive to simple verbal commands Disorientation Confusion Agitation and inappropriate behaviour
III	Stuporous but arousable to voice Localisation to pain Incoherent speech Confusion
IV	Coma Unrousable +/– response to pain Decerebrate/decorticate posturing

gression of hepatic encephalopathy to coma depends upon the severity and speed of hepatic damage. It may be precipitated by sepsis, GI bleeding, electrolyte imbalance and sedation (Mowat 1994, Stanley et al 1995).

Coagulopathy. Coagulopathy occurs secondary to dysfunction in the synthesis of coagulation factors, fibrinolytic agents and inhibitors of coagulation (Treem 1996). The coagulation factors that are most commonly decreased are Factors II, V, VII, IX and X, all of which are measured by prothrombin time (PT). PT is the most useful parameter to assess hepatic necrosis (Mowat 1994, Stanley et al 1995),

Other factors contributing to coagulation problems are disseminated intravascular coagulation (DIC) and/or thrombocytopenia (Kelly 1993).

Hypoglycaemia. Hypoglycaemia frequently occurs, due to impaired hepatic gluconeogenesis, decreased hepatic glycogen and elevated levels of plasma insulin caused by altered hepatic metabolism (Kelly 1993, Stanley et al 1995).

Major complications

The child with ALF is at risk of life-threatening complications; therefore, close assessment and monitoring is essential.

Cerebral oedema. Raised intracranial pressure secondary to cerebral oedema, with associated brainstem herniation, is the major cause of death in children with ALF (Treem 1996). The pathogenesis of cerebral oedema in hepatic encephalopathy is unclear but is thought to result from vasogenic and cytotoxic mechanisms. Early detection of increasing cerebral oedema is difficult, as papilloedema rarely occurs. However, signs of spasticity, rigidity, or clinical features of brainstem involvement are indicators (Mowat 1994).

Cardiovascular. Cardiovascular compromise occurs secondary to decreased peripheral resistance and hypotension due to sepsis, endotoxaemia, or increased capillary permeability. Cardiac arrhythmias may occur due to electrolyte imbalance (Kelly 1993, Mowat 1994).

Unexplained hypotension may arise in the late stages, possibly due to central vasomotor depres-

sion. Unexpected cardiac arrest occurs in up to 25% of cases (Mowat 1994).

Respiratory. Respiratory complications arise mainly due to encephalopathy. In the early stages of encephalopathy the child's respiratory rate may increase. Hyperventilation causing respiratory alkalosis leads to decreased cerebral perfusion and oxygen consumption.

As neurological function deteriorates, respiratory effort is reduced, resulting in respiratory acidosis and hypoxia, increasing the risk of atelectasis, aspiration and respiratory infection. Hypoxia also occurs due to intrapulmonary shunting of blood or hypotension (Mowat 1994).

Acid–base and electrolyte imbalance. Deficiencies may occur in sodium, potassium, phosphate and magnesium due to ALF or secondary to supportive therapy. Hypokalaemia may result in metabolic alkalosis which then triggers a compensatory metabolic acidosis. In the presence of metabolic alkalosis, cerebral ammonia uptake may be increased. Metabolic acidosis also occurs due to hepatic necrosis and tissue hypoxia (Mowat 1994).

Renal failure. Prerenal uraemia and/or acute tubular necrosis may occur secondary to dehydration or hypovolaemia. Functional renal failure (hepatorenal failure) is thought to occur due to intrarenal shunting of blood, hypovolaemia, sepsis and electrolyte imbalance (Kelly 1993).

Sepsis. Susceptibility to bacterial and fungal infection is increased in ALF, probably due to loss of macrophage activity in the liver, lowered complement levels and decreased opsonisation (Kelly 1993). The most common bacterial infections are *Staphylococcus aureus*, streptococci and coliforms (Stanley et al 1995).

Gastrointestinal bleeding. GI haemorrhage may occur from gastric erosions and stress ulceration, exacerbated in the presence of coagulopathy.

Management

Management includes supporting hepatic function and prevention or treatment of complications, allowing recovery and regeneration of the liver or survival until a donor is available.

Intensive monitoring of the child's condition is

required. Monitoring of intracranial pressure using an intraventricular device provides the most accurate assessment of cerebral oedema. This may be contraindicated with coagulopathy, due to the risk of haematoma which may increase intracranial pressure (ICP), resulting in medullary coning and death (Kelly 1993).

If the aetiology is unknown, children should be considered infectious until investigations establish a diagnosis. Paracetamol ingestion necessitates specific therapy including gastric lavage, forced diuresis and the administration of n-acetyl-cysteine (Kelly 1993).

Prevention and management of complications includes multiorgan support as follows.

Cardiovascular support

- Maintain perfusion and oxygenation.
- Correct hypovolaemia.
- Administer inotropic support.

Respiratory support

- Progression beyond stage II of hepatic encephalopathy may necessitate elective ventilation and sedation to manage cerebral oedema.
- Oral intubation may be performed due to coagulopathy.

Neurological support

- Hepatic encephalopathy:
  — restrict protein intake to 0.5–1 g/kg/day, reducing production of nitrogenous metabolites
  — enteral lactulose 1–2 mL/kg/4–6 hourly, reducing ammonia reabsorption by producing loose acidic stools
  — avoid sedatives if unintubated, as these exacerbate coma and make neurological observation inaccurate.
- Cerebral oedema:
  — fluid restriction — 50–75% daily maintenance
  — ventilation, paralysis and sedation
  — sedation before stimulation (e.g. lifting, endotracheal suction)
  — nursed with head in midline position; head elevated by 30 degrees, enhancing cerebral venous return

— IV mannitol 0.5 g/kg — monitor serum osmolarity sodium
— maintain CPP in range 50–90 mmHg
— short-term hyperventilation causing hypocapnia reducing cerebral blood volume
— thiopentone coma (0.5 mg/kg IV and maintenance infusion at 0.5–3 mg/kg/h) if increased ICP resistant to mannitol.

- Convulsions:
  — phenytoin, phenobarbitone, or thiopentone infusion if uncontrolled.

Haematological support

- Coagulation support:
  — IV vitamin K
  — fresh frozen plasma/platelets
  — blood transfusion.

Metabolic support

- Hypoglycaemia — maintain blood glucose above 4 mmol/L.
- Correct metabolic acidosis.
- Correct electrolyte imbalance — sodium may aggravate cerebral oedema. Hyponatraemia is usually secondary to dilution.

Renal support

- Prevention and treatment of hypovolaemia.
- IV dopamine to maintain renal perfusion.
- IV frusemide if urine output <0.5 mL/kg/h.
- Haemodialysis or ultrafiltration.

Gastrointestinal support

- Parenteral nutrition if enteral feeds not tolerated.
- H_2 antagonists, supplemented with antacids to maintain gastric pH >5;

Sepsis

- Treat bacterial and fungal infections.

Hepatic support. Currently the only successful intervention for acute liver failure is liver transplantation, despite the trials of other therapies, including charcoal haemoperfusion, exchange transfusion, plasmapheresis, haemodialysis and administration of prostaglandins (Kelly 1993). Research continues, including the development of extracorporeal liver assist devices that contain functioning hepatocytes (Conlin 1995) and hepatocyte transplantation (Asonuma & Vacanti 1992).

Liver transplantation. Liver transplantation is considered for children who develop stage III hepatic encephalopathy to enable early placement on the transplant list (Kelly 1993). Urgent liver transplantation is indicated when the prothrombin time is longer than 90 s after vitamin K administration, irrespective of the grade of encephalopathy (Mowat 1994). The major contraindication is irreversible brain damage (Kelly 1993).

CARE OF THE CHILD FOLLOWING LIVER TRANSPLANTATION

Orthotopic liver transplantation (OLT) is an established treatment for children with acute liver failure and end stage liver disease (Beath et al 1993). By the early 1990s, survival 1 year after transplant exceeds 80% for chronic liver failure or metabolic disorders. In children transplanted for acute liver failure the survival rate is approximately 70%, due to death from cerebral oedema, infection and multiorgan failure. Survival rates continue to increase with improvements in operative techniques, immunosuppression, intensive care and the management of complications (Mowat 1994).

Liver transplantation raises many ethical and moral issues for families and health care professionals. Long-term prognosis is unknown, but the majority of recipients enjoy an improved quality of life with normalisation of growth and development (Stewart et al 1991).

Donor recipient compatibility

The immunological parameter for assessing donor and recipient compatibility is ABO blood typing (Busuttil et al 1988). Cytomegalovirus (CMV) status of the donor is important to establish, as CMV infection after liver transplantation may increase morbidity and mortality (Rubin 1988). If the donor organ is CMV positive the recipient is treated prophylactically with IV ganciclovir or aciclovir and CMV hyperimmune globulin to prevent serum conversion (Mowat 1994).

Organ size compatibility is also considered; however, the donor liver can now be used in differing ways (Box 15.9).

Box 15.9   Types of liver transplants

Reduced size liver transplants (RSLT)
- Developed due to shortage of size-matched donor livers. The divisions used are the right lobe (segments V–VIII), the left lobe (segments II–IV) and the left lateral (segments II–III) (Treacey 1992, Mowat 1994).
- RSLT decreases waiting time and reduces incidence of hepatic artery thrombosis, attributed to the large size of the hepatic artery for anastomosis.
- A major complication is bleeding from the cut surface, minimised using ultrasonic dissection (Mowat 1994).
- Survival rate is equal to that of whole allografts (Slooff 1995).
- The success of reduced size grafts has resulted in split liver transplants, auxiliary transplantation and living related liver donation.

Split liver transplants (SLT)
- SLT is one donor organ surgically divided and transplanted into two recipients.

Auxiliary liver transplantation
- Consists either of transplanting an auxiliary liver into a heterotopic position or removing a lobe of the recipient's liver and placing the graft orthotopically (Mowat 1994).
- Used in fulminant hepatic failure where the native liver may recover and in metabolic disorders where only a mass of adequately functioning hepatocytes is required (Shaw & Wood 1988).

Living related liver transplants (LRLT)
- A living relative of the recipient becomes a donor by undergoing a partial hepatectomy (Lyon 1995).
- Results are comparable to those for cadaveric liver transplants (Kawasaki et al 1992).
- LRLT should improve survival rates, as transplants will be performed earlier before the complications of liver disease become advanced.
- The living donor liver segment is not affected by haemodynamic instability, and cold ischaemia time of the donor organ is reduced (Boone et al 1992).
- Disadvantage — donor risks life-threatening complications.

Postoperative management

Postoperative care of a transplant recipient is

similar to care following any major surgery (Pascucci 1989). It remains a dangerous surgical procedure, with recipients experiencing one or more life-threatening complications in the perioperative or early postoperative period (Mowat 1994).

Postoperative management requires early management of complications (Box 15.10).

Box 15.10 Specific management after liver transplantation

Cardiovascular
- Maintain circulating volume with colloid.
- Fresh frozen plasma (FFP), administered if bleeding is associated with coagulopathy, can mask liver function deterioration.
- Blood is given for haemorrhage or severe anaemia, maintaining packed cell volume (PCV) below 35% (haemoglobin 8–10 g/dL). PCV above 35% is associated with increased risk of hepatic artery thrombosis. Venesection is indicated if PCV is elevated.
- Screen blood products for CMV.
- Assess degree of haemorrhage — observe amount and type of wound drainage.
- Antiplatelet treatment — aspirin and dipyridamole.

Fluid and electrolyte balance
- Accurate fluid balance.
- Abdominal drain loss, high in protein content — replace with 4.5% HAS.
- Initial restriction of crystalloid and sodium intake.
- Electrolyte monitoring and supplements as indicated.
- Blood glucose monitoring.

Respiratory
- Maintain good tissue oxygenation.
- Oral intubation if the child has a coagulopathy, to reduce the risk of traumatic haemorrhage.
- Physiotherapy and postural drainage to reduce risk of atelectasis and consolidation.

Liver function
- Assess graft function — monitor liver function tests, clotting screens, acid base balance and electrolytes
- Abdominal ultrasound and doppler studies assess patency of hepatic vessels.

Immunosuppression
- Combination of cyclosporin, corticosteroids and azathioprine.

Infection
- Routine bacterial cultures of all secretions, discharges and urine at least twice weekly and if clinical signs of sepsis.

Box 15.10 Specific management after liver transplantation (cont'd)

- Removal of abdominal drains, urinary catheter and venous lines as soon as possible to reduce risk of colonisation and tips sent for culture (Mowat 1994).
- Prophylaxis therapy, nystatin and amphotericin for Candida albicans, aciclovir for previous herpes zoster infection, and co-timoxazole for Pneumocystis carinii.

Renal
- Monitor renal function.
- Dopamine to improve renal perfusion, and frusemide to increase diuresis.

Neurological
- Assess neurological function, including electroencephalogram monitoring.

Gastrointestinal function and nutrition
- When nil orally, give H_2 antagonists.
- Maintain gastric pH above 5 with the addition of antacids.
- Parenteral nutrition until enteral feeding commenced when ileus resolved.

Postoperative complications

Cardiovascular. Hypovolaemia may occur if there is:

- inadequate replacement of intraoperative losses
- intra-abdominal bleeding
- vasodilatation as rewarming takes place.

Bleeding occurs from anastomotic suture lines and bleeding points concealed during perioperative hypotension (Baker et al 1992). It also occurs due to an increase in collateral vessels. The risk is increased in the presence of pre-existing coagulopathy or severe portal hypertension.

Hypertension frequently occurs, attributed to cyclosporin and steroids therapy. Up to 50% of children will require short-term antihypertensive treatment (Baker et al 1992).

Bradycardias of unknown aetiology are common but often do not cause cardiovascular compromise (Baker et al 1992).

Fluid and electrolyte balance. Fluid overload may occur due to decreased colloid oncotic pressure secondary to protein deficiency. Fluid shifts from the intravascular compartment to the interstitial space result in oedema and hypovolaemia. Fluid overload may also be attributed to the retention of water and sodium, occurring in response to increased production of antidiuretic hormone as part of the stress response. Electrolyte imbalance is also common, as follows.

- *Hypokalaemia* — revascularisation of the transplanted liver causes rapid uptake of potassium and glucose. To correct hepatocyte potassium deficiency, potassium shifts from the intravascular compartment to the intracellular compartment of the liver.
- *Hyperkalaemia* — early indication that the graft is not functioning well.
- *Hypocalcaemia* — massive blood transfusion may decrease ionised calcium and magnesium serum levels, due to citrate preservative.
- *Magnesium deficiency* — due to cirrhosis or malnutrition. Cyclosporin also causes magnesium wasting (Busuttil et al 1988).

Transient hyperglycaemia may occur as the transplanted liver attempts to regulate glucose metabolism (Baker et al 1992). A persistent hypoglycaemia, unresponsive to increased glucose support, indicates poor liver function, with inability to regulate carbohydrate metabolism.

Respiratory. Respiratory function can be compromised by:

- large abdominal incision
- long operative time
- decreased lung expansion due to elevated diaphragm if the graft is large
- increased intra-abdominal pressure if abdominal complications occur (Baker et al 1992).

Respiratory infections are also common after transplant, and identification of the causative agent is vital to enable prompt treatment (Busuttil et al 1988).

Other pulmonary complications include:

- pulmonary oedema, due to fluid overload or the increase in lung water following major surgery
- right-sided pleural effusions

- phrenic nerve damage (Baker et al 1992). This may occur due to manipulation during surgery. The phrenic nerve is situated close to the suprahepatic vena cava.

Liver function

Liver function is rapidly restored if the graft is successful. This is demonstrated by bile production, normal serum bicarbonate levels, low serum potassium, correction of a coagulopathy within 2 to 3 days after transplant, and return to normal aspartate transaminase levels within a week. Previously high plasma bilirubin levels should also begin to reduce by day 2 (Baker et al 1992).

Liver dysfunction occurs for a number of reasons. Manifestation of poor hepatobiliary function includes coagulopathy, hypoglycaemia, metabolic acidosis, hyperkalaemia, pulmonary and peripheral oedema and decreasing need for sedation. Severe graft failure may require emergency retransplantation (Baker et al 1992).

Causes of graft dysfunction. This can be due to primary non-function, preservation injury, or acute and chronic rejection. Other causes include:

- liver infection due to hepatitis B, C or non- A, B, or C
- sepsis
- bile duct obstruction
- biliary leak
- vascular occlusion of graft — hepatic artery or vein.

Immunosuppression

Lifelong immunosuppressive therapy is essential to prevent and treat acute and chronic graft rejection, as the graft antigens trigger a combined humoral and cellular immune response. Antirejection regimens include a combination of drugs. Maintenance therapy usually includes cyclosporin, corticosteroids and azathioprine. Antilymphocytic/antithymocyte globulins may be given to treat episodes of rejection (Box 15.11 and Table 15.2). The aim is a therapeutic dosage preventing rejection without increasing the risk of infection and toxic side effects (Mowat 1994).

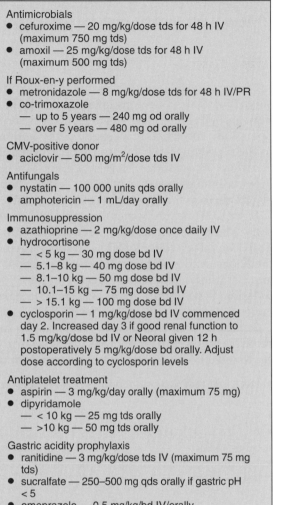

Box 15.11 Medication after liver transplantation

Antimicrobials
- cefuroxime — 20 mg/kg/dose tds for 48 h IV (maximum 750 mg tds)
- amoxil — 25 mg/kg/dose tds for 48 h IV (maximum 500 mg tds)

If Roux-en-y performed
- metronidazole — 8 mg/kg/dose tds for 48 h IV/PR
- co-trimoxazole
  - — up to 5 years — 240 mg od orally
  - — over 5 years — 480 mg od orally

CMV-positive donor
- aciclovir — 500 mg/m^2/dose tds IV

Antifungals
- nystatin — 100 000 units qds orally
- amphotericin — 1 mL/day orally

Immunosuppression
- azathioprine — 2 mg/kg/dose once daily IV
- hydrocortisone
  - — < 5 kg — 30 mg dose bd IV
  - — 5.1–8 kg — 40 mg dose bd IV
  - — 8.1–10 kg — 50 mg dose bd IV
  - — 10.1–15 kg — 75 mg dose bd IV
  - — > 15.1 kg — 100 mg dose bd IV
- cyclosporin — 1 mg/kg/dose bd IV commenced day 2. Increased day 3 if good renal function to 1.5 mg/kg/dose bd IV or Neoral given 12 h postoperatively 5 mg/kg/dose bd orally. Adjust dose according to cyclosporin levels

Antiplatelet treatment
- aspirin — 3 mg/kg/day orally (maximum 75 mg)
- dipyridamole
  - — < 10 kg — 25 mg tds orally
  - — >10 kg — 50 mg tds orally

Gastric acidity prophylaxis
- ranitidine — 3 mg/kg/dose tds IV (maximum 75 mg tds)
- sucralfate — 250–500 mg qds orally if gastric pH < 5
- omeprazole — 0.5 mg/kg/bd IV/orally

Source: The Birmingham Children's Hospital NHS Trust protocol.

Cyclosporin is nephrotoxic. To reduce the incidence of acute renal failure, it is commenced on day two post transplant. Some North American and many European centres also administer it preoperatively. Cyclosporin is given intravenously until intestinal absorption is demonstrated; serum cyclosporin levels need to be closely monitored. The new oral formulation (Neoral) can be given immediately post-

operatively, as it is absorbed in the absence of bile flow.

Rejection

Graft rejection occurs in three forms: hyperacute, acute and chronic. Hyperacute rejection is rare and occurs within 1 to 3 days, probably due to cytotoxic antibodies. The only treatment is retransplantation (Mowat 1994).

Acute rejection occurs in about 70% of recipients within 4–14 days after transplantation and is caused by a cellular immune response mediated by T lymphocytes (Fig. 15.8) (Wahrenberger 1995). Acute rejection is characterised by fever, increased prothrombin time and increased serum levels of bilirubin, transaminase and alkaline phosphatase. Prompt treatment is essential to prevent loss of the graft (Wahrenberger 1995). This is difficult, as systemic or hepatic infection, bile duct obstruction and vascular thrombosis have similar manifestations. Differential diagnosis is made by investigations to exclude the aforementioned complications and by liver biopsy (Mowat 1994).

Pharmacological immunosuppression is used to treat acute rejection, beginning with a 3 day course of methylprednisolone. In 80% of cases intensified therapy reverses rejection. However, the remainder will develop chronic rejection unless immunosuppression is intensified further. This includes discontinuing cyclosporin and commencing tracolimus (FK506) (Mowat 1994).

Chronic rejection usually occurs gradually and is mediated primarily by B lymphocyte antibody reaction, although there is also some T lymphocyte involvement (Fig. 15.9). It is characterised by bile duct loss. The process may be arrested by using FK506 therapy, but generally the only treatment is retransplantation (Wahrenberger 1995).

Infection control

Prevention, early recognition and treatment of infections is vital, as these cause significant morbidity and mortality. The most frequent pathogens seen are *Enterobacteriaceae*, *Candida* or *Aspergillus* species and *Pneumocystis carinii* (Mowat 1994).

Table 15.2 Antirejection drugs

Drug	Action	Side effects
Cyclosporin	Reversible inhibition of T lymphocyte mediated immune responses by suppression of interleukin-2 production	Acute and chronic renal failure Hepatic toxicity Hypertension Fluid retention Convulsions Tremors GI disturbance Thrombocytopenia Haemolysis Gum hyperplasia Hirsutism
Azathioprine	Incorporated into cellular DNA and alters synthesis and function of RNA, preventing cytotoxic T cell proliferation and antibody production	Bone marrow suppression causing leukopenia and thrombocytopenia Hepatic toxicity GI disturbances Alopecia Infection Fever Rash Pancreatitis
Corticosteroids	Inhibit production of interleukins 1 and 2, thereby blocking proliferation of T lymphocytes, and prevent T cell migration to sites of antigen deposits Also decrease lymphocyte, monocyte and basophil counts and have an inflammatory effect	Decreased resistance to infection Fluid retention due to retention of sodium and water Delayed wound healing Hypertension Diabetes Growth impairment Osteoporosis Obesity
Tracolimus (FK506)	Similar action to cyclosporin: blocks secretion of IL-2 and decreases proliferation of cytotoxic T cells	Anaphylaxis Fluid overload Fever Increased susceptibility to infection Lymphoma Neurotoxicity Diabetes
Antilymphocyte/ antithymocyte globulin	Contain lymphocytes from serum of various animals produced in response to injection of human lymphocytes or thrombocytes, and cause marked lymphocytopenia by binding to surface antigens on host T and B cells. This causes opsonisation and removal by the reticuloendothelial system, or lysing of lymphocytes	Severe allergic reactions or anaphylaxis Fever Chills Erythema Pruritis Leucocytopenia Thrombocytopenia Increased susceptibility to infection Lymphoma

Source: Wahrenberger (1995).

Secondary to immunosuppression is the increased risk and effect of opportunistic and community-acquired infections. One of the most hazardous is Epstein-Barr virus (EBV), which can cause lymphoproliferative disease (Chiyende and Mowat 1992). This occurs when there is con-tinual proliferation of B lymphocytes because of failure of the suppressed immune system to respond normally to EBV-infected B lympho-cytes. It is frequently fatal unless immunosup-pression is stopped (Malatack et al 1991). Immunosuppression may also be associated with

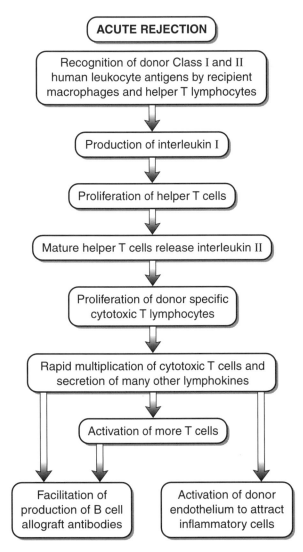

Figure 15.8 Mechanisms of rejection — acute rejection.

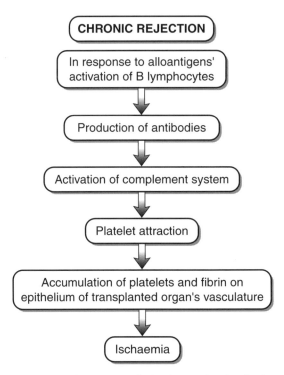

Figure 15.9 Mechanisms of rejection — chronic rejection.

- hypotension
- prolonged cross clamp time of inferior vena cava
- administration of cyclosporin/FK506 and other nephrotoxic drugs
- sepsis
- hepatorenal syndrome.

Neurological function

Alteration in neurological function may occur after transplantation. Electroencephalogram (EEG) monitoring is important, as convulsions are common, associated with encephalopathy, fast administration of cyclosporin, electrolyte and metabolic disturbances and hypertension. Phenytoin is often used and is rarely hepatotoxic, but does enhance cyclosporin clearance, and so the dose of cyclosporin should be increased and levels closely monitored (Baker et al 1992). Children transplanted for acute liver failure and those who suffer severe graft dysfunction may develop acute hepatic encephalopa-

an increased incidence of lymphoma and other malignant diseases.

Renal function

Renal failure may occur, requiring treatment with haemodiafiltration/haemofiltration until renal function improves. Causes include:

- pre-existing nephropathy
- abdominal tamponade secondary to haemorrhage

thy and are at risk of raised intracranial pressure (Mowat 1994).

Gastrointestinal function and nutrition

GI complications include paralytic ileus, stress ulceration, gastritis, and small and large bowel perforations caused by trauma during transplantation (Baker et al 1992).

CARE OF THE CHILD FOLLOWING INTESTINAL TRANSPLANTATION

Significant progress has been made in intestinal transplantation due to advances in surgical techniques and immunosuppression with tracolimus (FK506); however, only a few transplant centres worldwide are currently performing intestinal transplants (Kelly & Buckels 1995).

Permanent intestinal failure occurs in children with extreme intestinal loss due to surgical removal or congenital abnormalities causing inadequate absorptive function (Kocoshis 1994, Kelly & Buckels 1995) (Box 15.12). These children are dependent on parenteral nutrition for survival. This is not feasible, because of the life-threatening complications of septicaemia secondary to line contamination, loss of vascular access and irreversible liver disease (Reyes et al 1993). The aim of transplantation is to restore intestinal function, enabling the discontinuation of parenteral feeding.

Box 15.12   Causes of intestinal failure

- short gut syndrome as a result of neonatal surgery
- microvillus inclusion disease
- mucosal abnormalities
- autoimmune enteropathy
- aganglionosis

Source: Kelly & Buckels (1995).

Complications include infection, rejection and lymphoproliferative disease. Behavioural problems with feeding may also occur, and the emotional demands upon the child and family are immense (Kelly & Buckels 1995).

Intestinal transplantation may take the form of:

- isolated small bowel transplants
- combined liver and small bowel transplants
- multivisceral transplants: liver, small bowel, stomach and pancreas.

The type of transplant depends on the remaining function of the gastrointestinal tract and the presence of abnormalities in other organs.

Specific postoperative management

Intestinal transplantation is technically equivalent to liver transplantation but has significant postoperative complications related to rejection, infection and nutrition (Buckels et al 1993). The postoperative course may be more complex and protracted, with the recipient requiring an extended period in intensive care, especially after combined organ transplants. Initial postoperative pharmacological management following intestinal transplantation is similar to that for major abdominal surgery and liver transplantation (Box 15.13).

Postoperative complications

Fluid and electrolyte balance.   Fluid overload secondary to postoperative fluid shifts into the extracellular compartment and peritoneum is common, although dehydration can occur in the initial postoperative period due to large stoma losses. Fluids are restricted to 60% of maintenance requirements and stoma losses replaced with intravenous 0.9% saline. Sepsis, hepatic dysfunction, or increased stoma bicarbonate excretion may result in metabolic acidosis requiring intravenous bicarbonate and replacement of gastrointestinal losses with Hartman's solution (Beath et al 1994).

Immunosuppression.   Greater immunological problems are experienced in intestinal transplants than in other transplanted organs due to the large number of the mesenteric lymph nodes and Peyer's patches of the small bowel graft which provide an antigenic stimulus to the recipient (Gunning 1994). A combination therapy of

Box 15.13 Medication after liver and small bowel transplantation

Antimicrobials
- ciprofloxacin — 5 mg/kg/dose bd for 14 days IV
- amoxil — 25 mg/kg/dose tds for 14 days IV (maximum 500 mg tds)
- metronidazole — 8 mg/kg/dose tds for 14 days IV
- co-trimoxazole — up to 5 years—240 mg od orally
  — over 5 years—480 mg od orally
- ganciclovir — 5 mg/kg/dose bd IV for 14 days then oral acyclovir
- aciclovir — <5 years 200 mg/kg/dose qds orally
  — >5 years 400 mg/kg/dose qds orally

If CMV positive donor to CMV negative recipient:
- anti-CMV IgG — 500 mg/kg IV on days 1, 2, 7 postoperatively
  — 250 mg/kg IV on days 14, 21, 28 postoperatively

Antifungals
- nystatin — 100 000 units qds orally
- amphotericin — 1 mL/day orally

Selective decontamination of digestive system
- fluconazole — 3 mg/kg od IV for 5 days postop
- colistin — 1.5 mega units/dose tds orally
- gentamicin — 2.5 mg/kg/dose tds orally

Immunosuppression
- azathioprine — 2 mg/kg/dose once daily IV
- hydrocortisone
  — <5 kg — 30 mg dose bd IV
  — 5.1–8 kg — 40 mg dose bd IV
  — 8.1–10 kg — 50 mg dose bd IV
  — 10.1–15 kg — 75 mg dose bd IV
  — >15.1 kg — 100 mg dose bd IV
- tacrolimus (FK 506) — commenced immediately postop 0.075 mg/kg/dose bd via nasojejunal/nasogastric tube

Dose adjusted to maintain tacrolimus levels 15–20 ng/mL (whole blood essay) for first 14 days then 10–15 ng/mL until 3 months postop.

Box 15.13 Medication after liver and small bowel transplantation (*cont'd*)

Antiplatelet treatment
- aspirin — 3 mg/kg/day orally (maximum 75 mg)
- dipyridamole — < 10 kg — 25 mg tds orally
  — > 10 kg — 50 mg tds orally

Gastric acidity prophylaxis
- ranitidine — 3 mg/kg/dose tds IV (maximum 75 mg tds)
- sucralfate — 250–500 mg qds orally if gastric pH < 5.
- omeprazole — 0.5 mg/kg/bd IV or orally

Source: Birmingham Children's Hospital NHS Trust

steroids, azathioprine and tracolimus (FK506) is given. Tracolimus levels are monitored and maintained at 20–40 ng/mL.

Intestinal function and rejection. Hypermotility secondary to disruption in the enteric nervous system may occur but can be controlled with medication such as loperamide (Reyes et al 1993, Kelly & Buckels 1995). The incidence of rejection after small bowel transplantation is high, with the greatest risk in the first 7–14 days. It may, however, occur at any time if immunosuppression is inadequate (Beath et al 1994).

Assessment of intestinal rejection by clinical observation includes:

- measurement of stoma losses (10–15 mL/kg/day)
- measurement of reducing substances and steatocrit in stomal fluid
- observation of stoma colour to assess graft perfusion.

Endoscopic examination through ileostomy and bowel histology may also be required (Kocoshis 1994). In acute rejection, endoscopic examination shows a dusky mucosa with focal ulceration, and in severe rejection there will be mucosal sloughing and graft necrosis (Gunning 1994). Episodes of acute rejection are treated with increased dosage of tacrolimus, a single dose of methylprednisolone and, if rejection persists, increasing maintenance steroids (Beath et al 1994, Gunning 1994).

During episodes of rejection, bacterial translocation may occur due to increased intestinal mucosal permeability. Until the episode of rejection is resolved, additional antibiotics are required (Gunning 1994, Kelly & Buckels 1995).

In chronic rejection, villous atrophy, muscular

fibrosis and subintimal thickening may occur, causing ischaemia and fibrosis of the intestine and mesentery. This is not normally diagnosed until the graft is removed and may result in late graft loss (Kelly & Buckels 1995).

Nutrition. During the process of weaning from parenteral nutrition and episodes of rejection, dehydration may occur secondary to high stoma losses. A high fluid intake is required, including intravenous fluid replacement and enteral dioralyte. Enteral feeding via jejunostomy is commenced when paralytic ileus has resolved. Iso-osmolar feeds are initially introduced, gradually increasing concentration and volume. Oral/intravenous essential fatty acid and fat-soluble vitamin supplements may be required.

Infection. The risk of infection is high, especially from cytomegalovirus enteritis, Epstein-Barr virus, *Pneumocystis carinii*, atypical mycobacteria and fungal infections. Prophylaxis is given against *Pneumocystis carinii* using co-trimoxazole and against CMV using ganciclovir and CMV hyperimmune globulin. Selective decontamination of the bowel with Colomycin, amphotericin and gentamicin is given to reduce bacterial translocation which can occur following harvesting and implantation (Beath et al 1994, Gunning 1994).

Renal function. The risk of renal impairment is high postoperatively, especially as the therapeutic dose of tacrolimus required may cause nephrotoxicity.

REFERENCES

Asonuma K, Vacanti J P 1992 Cell transplantation as replacement therapy for the future. Critical Care Nursing Clinics of North America 4(2):249–254

Baker A, Ross-Russell R, Mowat A P 1992 Intensive care management of children following orthotopic liver transplantation. British Journal of Intensive Care (July/August): 229–240

Beasley S W, Myers N A, Auldist A W 1991 Oesophageal atresia. Chapman and Hall Medical, London

Beath S V, Brook G D, Kelly D A et al 1993 Successful liver transplantation in babies under 1 year. British Medical Journal 307:825–828

Beath S V, Kelly D A, Booth I W, Freeman J, Buckels J A C, Mayer A D 1994 Post operative care of children undergoing small bowel and liver transplantation. British Journal of Intensive Care 4(9):302–306

Boone P, Kelly S, Smith C S 1992 Liver transplantation: living related donations. Critical Care Nursing Clinics of North America 4(2):243–248

Bornman P C, Krige J E J, Terblanche 1994 Management of oesophageal varices. Lancet 343:1079–1084

Buckels J A C, Mayer A D, Beath S V, Kelly D A, Booth I W 1993 Birmingham protocol for liver and small bowel transplantation.

Busuttil R W, Brems J J, Hiatt J R 1988 Pediatric liver transplantation. In: Maddrey W C (ed) Transplantation of the liver. Current Topics in Gastroenterology. Elsevier, New York, pp 309–330

Chiyende J, Mowat A P 1992 Liver transplantation. Archives of Disease in Childhood 67:1124–1127

Conlin C 1995 Extracorporeal liver assist device: hope for the future. Critical Care Nurse Quarterly 17(4):73–78

Davenport M, Holmes K 1995 Current management of congenital diaphragmatic hernia. British Journal of Hospital Medicine 53(3): 95–101

DiFiore D P, Mitchell J, Kharaasch V, Quigley S, Kuehn M, Wilson J M 1994 Experimental fetal tracheal ligation reverses the structural and physiological effects of pulmonary hypoplasia in CDH. Journal of Pediatric Surgery 29(2):248–257

Dillon P W, Cilley R E 1993 Newborn surgical emergencies. Pediatric Surgery 40(6):1289–1313

Edwards S 1995 Phototherapy and the neonate: providing safe and effective nursing care for jaundiced infants. Journal of Neonatal Nursing (October):9–12

Engum S A, Grosfield J L, West W, Rescorla F J, Scherer L B 3rd 1995 Analysis of morbidity and mortality of 227 cases of oesophageal atresia and/or tracheoesophageal fistula over two decades. Archives of Surgery 130(5):502–508

Glasgow J F T, Moore R 1993 Current concepts in Reyes syndrome. British Journal of Hospital Medicine 50:10

Gruppi L A, Killen A R, Rodriguez 1990 Liver transplantation: key nursing diagnoses. Dimensions of Critical Care Nursing 9(5):273–279

Gunning K E J 1994 Intensive care management of small bowel transplantations. British Journal of Intensive Care 4(7):242–245

Guyton A C 1992 Human physiology and mechanisms of disease, 5th edn. WB Saunders, Philadelphia

Harrison M R, Langer J C, Scott Adzick N, Golbus M S, Filly R A, Anderson R L, Rosen M A, Callen P W, Goldstein R B, deLorimer A M 1990 Correction of CDH in utero v. critical clinical experience. Journal of Pediatric Surgery 25(1):47–57

Hoy C, Millar M R, MacKay P, Godwin P G R, Langdale V, Levene M I 1990 Quantative changes in faecal microflora preceding NEC in preterm neonates. Archives of Disease in Childhood 65:1057–1059

Humfreys H 1994 The future of selective decontamination of the digestive tract in trauma. Care of the Critically Ill 10(5):228–230

Iritani I 1984 Experimental study of pathogenesis and embryogenesis of CDH. Anatomical Embryology 169:133–139

Kawasaki S, Makuuchi M, Ishizone S 1992 Partial liver transplantation from living donors. Transplant Proceedings 24(1):470–472

Kelly D A 1993 Fulminant hepatitis and acute liver failure. In: Buts J P, Sokal E M (eds) Management of digestive and liver disorders in infants and children. Elsevier Science, Amsterdam, pp 577–594

Kelly D A, Buckels J A C 1995 The future of small bowel transplantation. Archives of Disease in Childhood 72:447–451

Kelnar C J H, Harvey D, Simpson C 1995 The sick newborn baby, 3rd edn. Baillière Tindall, London, pp 277–306

Kliegman R M 1990 Models of the pathogenesis of necrotizing enterocolitis. Journal of Pediatrics 117 (suppl): 52

Kocoshis S A 1994 Small bowel transplantation in infants and children. Gastroenterology Clinics of North America 23(4):727–742

Lund D P, Mitchell J, Kharasch V, Quigley S, Kuehn M, Wilson J M 1994 Congenital diaphragmatic hernia: the hidden mortality. Journal of Pediatric Surgery 29(2):258–264

Lyon H D 1995 Living related liver transplants: an option for pediatric patients. Critical Care Nursing Quarterly 17(4):37–47

Malatack J J, Gartner C J, Urbach A H, Zitelli B J 1991 Orthotopic liver transplantation, Epstein-Barr virus, cyclosporin and lymphoproliferative disease: a growing concern. The Journal of Pediatrics 118(5):667–674

Millar M R, MacKay P, Levene M, Langdale V, Martin C 1992 Enterobacteriaceae and neonatal necrotising enterocolitis. Archives of Disease in Childhood 67:53–56

Mowat A P 1994 Liver disorders in childhood, 3rd edn. Butterworth-Heinemann, Oxford

Nicholls G, Upadhyaya V, Gornall P, Buick RG, Corkery J J 1993 Is specialist centre delivery of gastroschisis beneficial? Archives of Disease in Childhood 69:71–73

Norden M A, Butt W, McDougall P 1994 Predictors of survival for infants with CDH. Journal of Pediatric Surgery 28(5):650–652

Pascucci R C 1989 Pediatric intensive care. In: Gregory G A (ed) Pediatric anesthesia. Churchill Livingstone, New York, pp 1289–1388

Peterson W L, Laine L 1993 Bleeding as a consequence of portal hypertension. In: Sleisenger M H, Fordtran J S (eds) Gastrointestinal disease: pathophysiology/diagnosis/management, vol 1, 5th edn. WB Saunders, Philadelphia, pp 172–177

Phillips M C, Olson L R 1993 The immunological role of the gastrointestinal tract. Critical Care Clinics of North America 5:1

Prevost S S, Oberle A 1993 Stress ulceration in the critically ill. Critical Care Clinics of North America 15(1):163–169

Rescorla F J, West K W, Scherer L R 3rd, Grosfeld J L 1994 The complex nature of Type A (long-gap) oesophageal atresia. Surgery 116(4):658–664

Reyes J, Tzakis A G, Todo S, Abu-Elmagd K, Starzl T E 1993 Post operative care of small bowel transplant recipients. Care of the Critically Ill 9(5):193–198

Roberts P M 1990 NEC: etiology, treatment, prevention and nursing care. Critical Care Nurse 10(4):38–53

Rodriguez M, Kanto W P Jr, Howell C G, Hatley R B,

Bhatia J 1996 Early diagnosis of diaphragmatic hernia and survival: a time for appraisal? Neonatal Intensive Care 9(2):42–46

Rubin R H 1988 Infectious disease problems. In: Maddrey W C (ed) Transplantation of the liver. Current Topics in Gastroenterology. Elsevier, New York, pp 279–308

Rushton C H 1990a Necrotising enterocolitis — Part 1: Pathogenesis and diagnosis. American Journal of Maternal Child Nursing 15:296–300

Rushton C H 1990b Necrotising enterocolitis — Part 2: Treatment and nursing care. American Journal of Maternal Child Nursing 15:309–313

Shann F 1996 Drug doses, 9th edn. ICU, Royal Children's Hospital, Melbourne, Australia

Shaw B W, Wood R P 1988 The operative procedures. In: Maddrey W C (ed) Transplantation of the liver. Current Topics in Gastroenterology. Elsevier, New York, pp 87–110

Slooff M J 1995 Reduced size liver transplantation, split liver transplantation and living related transplantation in relation to the donor organ shortage. Transplant International 8(1):65–68

Spitz L, Kiely E M, Morecroft J A, Drake D P 1994 Oesophageal atresia: at risk groups for the 1990s. Journal of Pediatric Surgery 29(6):723–725

Stanley A J, Lee A, Hayes P C 1995 Management of acute liver failure: aetiology, complications and management. British Journal of Intensive Care (January):8–15

Stewart S M, Hiltebeitel C, Nici J, Waller D A, Uauy R, Andrews W S 1991 Neuropsychological outcome of pediatric liver transplantaton. Pediatrics 87:367–376

Stringel G 1993 Large gastroschisis: primary repair with a Goretex patch. Journal of Pediatric Surgery 28(5):653–655

Stringer M D, Spitz L 1993 Surgical management of neonatal necrotising enterocolitis. Archives of Disease in Childhood 69:269–275

Stringer M D, Brereton R J, Wright V M 1991 Controversies in the management of gastroschisis: a study of 40 patients. Archives of Disease in Childhood 66:34–36

Suchy F J 1992 Fulminant hepatic failure. In: Behrman R E (ed) Nelson's textbook of paediatrics. W B Saunders, Philadelphia, pp 1024–1025

Swift R I, Singh M P, Ziderman D A, Silverman M, Elder M A, Elder M G 1992 A new regime in the management of gastroschisis. Journal of Pediatric Surgery 27(1):62–63

Todd N V 1995 Isovolemic exchange transfusion of the neonate. Neonatal Network 14(6):75–77

Treacey S 1992 Reduced-size liver transplantation for infants and children. Critical Care Nursing Clinics of North America 4(2):235–242

Treem W R 1996 Hepatic failure. In: Walker A W, Durie P R, Hamilton R J, Walker-Smith J A, Watkins J B (eds) Pediatric gastrointestinal disease: pathophysiology, diagnosis, management, vol 1, 2nd edn. Mosby, St Louis, pp 343–393

UK Collaborative ECMO Trial Group 1996 The Lancet 348:75–82

Walker W A, Durie P R, Hamilton J R, Walker-Smith J A, Watkins J B 1996 Pediatric gastrointestinal disease, 2nd edn. Mosby, St Louis

Wahrenberger A 1995 Pharmacologic immunosuppression: cure or curse? Critical Care Nursing Quarterly 17(4):27–36

Weinstein S, Stolar C J H 1993 Newborn surgical emergencies. Pediatric Clinics of North America 40(6):1315–1333

Wilson K J W 1990 Ross and Wilson Anatomy and physiology in health and disease. Churchill Livingstone, Edinburgh pp 184–185

Yeo H M 1996 Surgical intervention for the repair of exomphalus. Professional Nurse 11(4):226–227

16

Haematological and oncological problems in paediatric intensive care

S. P. Attard-Montalto

INTRODUCTION

Malignant disease presents once in every 1–10 000 children and, as shown in Table 16.1, up to one third have acute leukaemia, while the rest have solid tumours. Approximately 50% of these children will survive long term, though this figure improves with individual cancers: e.g. up to 70% of children with acute lymphoblastic leukaemia are now cured. Nevertheless, the dramatic improvement in prognosis for childhood cancer over the past three decades has been achieved by an escalation in the intensity of therapy at the price of increased acute and chronic morbidity. Although current trends in oncological practice are geared toward reducing this morbidity, the continuing escalation in intensive therapy will inevitably lead to an increased admission rate to PICU. Therefore, it is important that PICUs are set up to accommodate these children with potentially curable malignant disease if they are to survive the

Table 16.1 Malignant disease in childhood

Disease	% of all cancer
Acute leukaemia[a]	30
Central nervous system tumours	20
Lymphoma[b]	12
Soft tissue sarcoma	8
Neuroblastoma	6
Nephroblastoma (Wilms')	5
Bone tumour	4
Others	15

[a] ratio 6:1 acute lymphoblastic to acute myeloblastic leukaemia
[b] 7% non-Hodgkin's; 5% Hodgkin's lymphoma

acute emergencies and ultimately continue to survive long term.

Despite the life-threatening nature of severe haematological and malignant disease, the need for intensive care treatment for this group of patients is relatively uncommon. In children with an underlying haematological condition, admission to PICU usually follows severe infection or a haemolytic or haemorrhagic crisis. In those with malignant disease, although emergencies may result from direct pressure effects or obstruction by the tumour, they are usually caused indirectly by complications of the malignant disease and its treatment, including pancytopenia leading to infection, and metabolic derangement. This chapter will review the more common haematological and oncological conditions presenting in PICU and limit the discussion to the *intensive* aspects of treatment alone.

HAEMATOLOGICAL PROBLEMS

Anaemia and haemolysis

Anaemia

The haemoglobin level varies with age, and anaemia is defined as a haemoglobin below the normal range for the age of the child (see Table 16.2). Anaemia is extremely common in patients on PICU. It may be present on admission but often develops later due to reduced bone marrow function as a result of the ongoing debilitating condition or infection (Bagby 1987). It is exacerbated by repeated venesection and procedures associated with blood loss. Routine assessment of the blood count is therefore mandatory on all intensive patients, and anaemia should be corrected at regular intervals.

Table 16.2 Haemoglobin range with age

Age	Normal range of Hb (g/dL)
Newborn	13–22
Infancy	9–13
1–6 years	10–14
6–12 years	11–15
>12 years (female)	12–16
>12 years (male)	13–16

Sickle cell anaemia

Haemolytic disorders rarely necessitate admission to PICU unless they complicate some other severe insult such as infection or poisoning. However, sickle cell anaemia can result in acute crises which require intensive care. This disease is caused by the presence of an abnormal haemoglobin chain (HbS) which crystallises when exposed to low concentrations of oxygen in the bloodstream. As a result, the red cells assume a sickle shape and block the microcirculation, leading to infarcts. Severely affected children present with 'crises' usually triggered by an intercurrent infection, dehydration, acidosis and deoxygenation. Haemolytic crises occur when red cell breakdown is markedly increased, and an acute on chronic anaemia develops with jaundice. Infection, often with parvovirus, may trigger an aplastic crisis with bone marrow shutdown and a pancytopenia on the peripheral blood count. Painful crises are common and usually due to infarction of the bones, lung or spleen. The latter usually results in functional 'asplenia' by early childhood and increases the risk of pneumococcal septicaemia. Vasculo-occlusive crises involving the central nervous system may result in devastating neurological sequelae. Sickling within visceral organs, with concomitant pooling of blood, results in a sequestration crisis which, when affecting the lung, has a high mortality in the acute phase. Children present with shortness of breath, hypoxia, severe anaemia (< 6 g/dL) and pulmonary infiltrates on the chest X-ray.

A rapid screening test for HbS will confirm the diagnosis. Treatment involves the administration of oxygen, rehydration, correction of acidosis and aggressive antibacterial therapy, particularly against pneumococcal disease. Opiates are usually required for adequate analgesia. Cerebrovascular accidents and lung sequestration crises are indications for an emergency exchange transfusion, which should not be performed outside the PICU setting. The aim of this treatment is to reduce the amount of circulating HbS to 20–30% of the total haemoglobin. Patients with lung sequestration and persistent hypoxia, despite increased ambient oxygenation, may require full ventilatory support.

Bleeding disorders

Homeostasis is maintained by an intact vascular system together with normal coagulation. Therefore, bleeding may result from rupture of blood vessels and major organs associated with trauma and surgical procedures, or is the result of an abnormality in blood clotting. The latter is normally maintained by platelets clumping together and the production of an overlying fibrin mesh, thereby consolidating the platelet clot.

Haemorrhage

This is usually due to accidental or operative trauma. Management essentially involves stemming the blood loss at source and replacement of the amount lost. Hence, a surgical opinion must be sought and the blood pressure restored using plasma substitutes and whole blood as soon as this is available. When recurrent transfusions are required over a relatively short period of time, platelets and clotting factors must be replaced, since these are also lost in the haemorrhage and their residual circulating levels diluted by the transfusions.

Thrombocytopenia

Thrombocytopenia, defined as an absolute platelet count less than $100 \times 10^9/L$ in children, may follow decreased platelet production and increased platelet degradation (Box 16.1). Bone marrow dysfunction is a common complication of severe, debilitating illnesses and may result in thrombocytopenia even in those who do not have a primary abnormality of the bone marrow (e.g. leukaemia) and who have not received cytotoxics or radiotherapy. Therapeutic drugs are a common cause of thrombocytopenia, and all medications should be reviewed in patients with a low platelet count.

Normal or increased platelet production may still be associated with thrombocytopenia when platelet consumption is increased. This occurs with severe sepsis, disseminated intravascular coagulation (DIC) and autoimmune disease, e.g. systemic lupus erythematosis (SLE). In isoimmune disease, e.g. immune thrombocytopenic purpura (ITP), antiplatelet antibodies develop, usually after a preceding viral infection. These attach to platelets which are then identified as 'abnormal' and removed by the spleen.

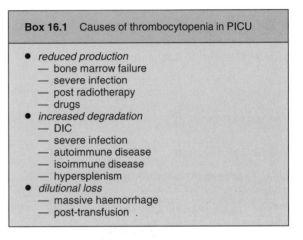

Box 16.1 Causes of thrombocytopenia in PICU

- *reduced production*
  - bone marrow failure
  - severe infection
  - post radiotherapy
  - drugs
- *increased degradation*
  - DIC
  - severe infection
  - autoimmune disease
  - isoimmune disease
  - hypersplenism
- *dilutional loss*
  - massive haemorrhage
  - post-transfusion .

A platelet count less than $15 \times 10^9/L$ is likely to result in spontaneous haemorrhages, usually manifest as small pinprick petechiae on the skin, mucosal surfaces and fundi. These are easy to miss and should be looked for in all those at risk. Below a count of $10 \times 10^9/L$ the risk of severe, sometimes fatal, haemorrhage involving the brain, lungs and gastrointestinal tract increases as the platelet count falls.

Coagulopathies

Congenital coagulopathy. Formation of the fibrin web is dependent on several clotting factors involved in two clotting cascades. Congenital abnormalities in factor production such as haemophilia A (factor VIII), Christmas disease (factor IX) and Von Willebrand's disease (low factor VIII and abnormal platelet adhesion) lead to bleeding disorders.

Acquired coagulopathy. Disseminated intravascular coagulation (DIC) is associated with a severe, acquired coagulation defect. As shown in Box 16.2, DIC is triggered by the release of procoagulant material which 'sets off' the clotting cascade, and may follow extensive endothelial damage commonplace in severe septicaemic states. Widespread activation of the clotting mechanism with extensive deposition of fibrin and platelet aggregation ultimately leads to consumption of clotting factors and platelets with fulminant haemorrhagic consequences. Furthermore, the problem is compounded by an increase in fibrinolysis, with breakdown products being released into the circulation, where they interfere with further clot formation.

Box 16.2   Causes of disseminated intravascular coagulation

Endothelial damage
- infection
  - — Gram-negative septicaemia
  - — meningococcal disease
  - — falciparum malaria
  - — severe viraemia
- severe burns, trauma
- hypothermia, heat stroke

Release of procoagulants
- acute myeloid leukaemia (M3 type)
- anaphylactic reactions
- severe transfusion reactions
- snake bites
- liver failure

Coagulopathy is also a feature of hepatic diseases, since the liver is the main source of clotting factors. Vitamin K is involved in the production of factors II, VII, IX and X. Its deficiency, due to immaturity, biliary obstruction, malabsorption, cancer-malnutrition and drugs such as warfarin and cephalosporin, leads to prolonged bleeding. Finally, normal function of the clotting factors may be disrupted by antibodies found in autoimmune diseases, e.g. SLE.

Management of the coagulopathies.   Treatment involves the control of the underlying condition, e.g. SLE, infection and correction of the coagulopathy (Lee 1992). The latter may require a single factor substitute, e.g. factor VIII concentrate in haemophilia A, or several clotting factors

using fresh frozen plasma (FFP). In DIC, platelet transfusions are necessary in addition to FFP and fibrinogen concentrates. Vitamin K is useful in augmenting vitamin K-dependent coagulation factors, whereas nasal desmopressin (DDAVP) and adrenaline increase levels of factor VIII and Von Willebrand factor (VWF).

Fibrinolytic inhibitors, e.g. tranexamic acid, prevent the breakdown of clots once these have formed, helping to 'contain' a coagulopathy in cases of persisting haemorrhage. Protamine sulphate has antiheparin properties and is mostly used postoperatively to revert the coagulopathy induced by heparin during bypass surgery.

Blood products

Blood products are associated with serious side effects, including fatal anaphylactic reactions, and should be treated with the greatest of respect. All blood products should be checked by two qualified members of staff who should ensure that every unit administered corresponds to the appropriate child. If in doubt, all products should be returned to the blood transfusion centre for reassessment. Major adverse reactions usually develop during the infusion (but even up to 2 h later) and present with a raised temperature, rigors, breathlessness, pain in the chest, back or limbs, headache, tachycardia and hypotension. A rise in temperature and fall in blood pressure may be the only signs in sedated, ventilated children. The infusion should be stopped immediately, the child resuscitated with volume if hypotensive and given intravenous hydrocortisone (25–100 mg) and chlorpheniramine (2.5–10.0 mg). Mannitol diuresis in order to maintain a high urine flow is indicated with severe haemolysis. Shocked patients require intravenous adrenaline (1 in 10 000) and occasionally renal dialysis. The blood product should be returned to the laboratory for further analysis together with a fresh sample of the patient's serum and urine. The majority of serious transfusion reactions occur as a result of clerical, medical and nursing errors and can be avoided by obsessive checking of all transfusion details. Minor reactions due to patient alloantibodies against the transfusion product are common especially during platelet transfusions and manifest as a fever, rigors and an urticarial rash. They are usually controlled by temporarily stopping the infusion and by the administration of intravenous hydrocortisone and chlorpheniramine.

Red cells. It is important to maximise the oxygen-carrying capacity in compromised patients on PICU. Hence, anaemia should be corrected, ideally by the administration of packed cells which comprise the centrifuged erythrocytes from a unit of single donor whole blood. Whole blood can be used in the emergency situation of acute blood loss. 'Standard' units of red cells/whole blood contain large numbers of white cells which carry histocompatibility (HLA) antigens and may result in HLA-immunisation. This creates problems with subsequent cross-matching of red cell and platelets so that, in children destined to receive multiple transfusions, it is prudent to use leucocyte-depleted red cells. Blood should be administered over a period of 3–4 h (except with acute haemorrhage), and covered with a diuretic midway through the transfusion in order to avoid circulatory overload. Patients with severe anaemia (Hb < 5 g/dL) should be given smaller volume transfusions over 5–6 h to avoid pulmonary oedema (Jayabose et al 1991). The volume of packed cells required can be calculated using the formula:

$$\text{volume red cells (mL)} = \text{desired increase in Hb (g/dL)} \times \text{patient weight (kg)} \times 4$$

Platelets. Platelets express A and B antigens only to a small extent and it is not essential for platelet transfusions to be ABO and Rhesus compatible. Platelet transfusions are extracted from voluntary donors (British Committee for Standards in Haematology 1992) and, unless stated otherwise, each transfusion bag is the product of several pooled donor platelets. Impurities include white cell degradation products which commonly lead to minor 'platelet reactions'. Therefore, many haematology units routinely cover every platelet transfusion with intravenous chlorpheniramine (2.5–10.0 mg) and hydrocortisone (25–100 mg) (Schiffer 1991). Those children likely to require multiple platelet transfusions, e.g. bone marrow recipients or children with acute myeloid leukaemia, should be treated with single donor platelets (British Committee for Standards in Haematology 1992). An increment in the peripheral platelet count of less than $10 \times 10^9/L$ one hour after the transfusion indicates the presence of antiplatelet antibodies, and these children require HLA-matched, single donor platelets (British Committee for Standards in Haematology 1992).

Platelets are indicated in cases of thrombocytopenia with signs of bleeding, with or without an associated coagulopathy. If the patient has no skin, mucosal or fundal petechiae and is not actively bleeding (including microscopic haematuria), platelets are given 'routinely' if the platelet count falls below the following levels (Schiffer 1992):

- $< 20 \times 10^9/L$ — to avoid the risk of spontaneous haemorrhage
- $< 50 \times 10^9/L$ — for invasive procedures, e.g. insertion of central line, lumbar puncture.

However, acidosis, sepsis, hypo- and hyperthermia all result in platelet dysfunction, and a lower threshold for platelet transfusion should be maintained if these complications prevail. Platelets are supplied in units of variable volume. In general, neonates require 10 mL/kg, children aged 1–5 years require 2–3 units, those aged 5–10 need 3–4 units, and adolescents require 5–8 units. They should be infused over a period of about 30 min.

Plasma. Plasma and plasma substitutes (e.g. 4.5% human albumin solution) are used as first line volume expanders to treat hypovolaemia and hypotensive situations. Initially 20 mL/kg is given, though it is often necessary to repeat this dose several times, especially during severe shock.

Fresh frozen plasma (FFP). FFP consists of human plasma, freshly collected and stored at –30°C, in order to preserve coagulation factors. It is given in aliquots of 10 mL/kg (10–15 mg/kg) over 1–2 h in situations where clotting is significantly deranged: e.g. DIC, following cardiopulmonary bypass, liver dysfunction, or warfarin overdose.

Cryoprecipitate. This product is rich in factor VIII and fibrinogen and is used to replace these factors in children with haemophilia A and Von Willebrand's disease. It is supplied in units of about 50 mL and should be given in a dose of 10 mL/kg.

Irradiated blood products. These should be requested for children at risk of developing antibodies, e.g. bone marrow transplant recipients, and those with significant immunoparesis involving T-cell function, e.g. children with Di George syndrome and absent thymus gland.

Cytomegalovirus (CMV)-negative blood products. Transmission of CMV may cause problems in the newborn and immunosuppressed children. Hence, CMV-negative products should be given prior to and after bone marrow and renal transplantation, and in CMV-negative patients infected with the human immunosuppression virus (HIV).

Blood filters. These can be used to reduce white cell contaminants in transfusions, thereby reducing the number of antibody reactions in those who require regular red cell transfusions, e.g. thalassaemia major. By reducing the number of infused leucocytes, filters also reduce the risk of CMV contamination and HLA sensitisation. Most are not effective as an antibacterial barrier.

ONCOLOGICAL PROBLEMS

Cancer patients are at risk of life-threatening complications as a result of the tumour itself or its treatment. PICU management will involve direct control of these complications, specific anticancer therapy and general support of the debilitated, often septicaemic, child. The latter includes careful attention to the nutritional state, a problem that is easily overlooked in children with cancer who may be 'expected' to lose weight and develop cancer-cachexia.

Pressure effects

Mediastinal mass and airway obstruction

Rarely, children present with increasing respiratory distress due to upper airway obstruction caused by an enlarging mediastinal mass (Spain & Whittlesley 1989). This superior mediastinal syndrome is usually associated with superior vena caval obstruction, so that progressive stridor and cough is accompanied by facial suffusion, oedema and collateral venous congestion (Issa et al 1983). Most cases are due to enlarged mediastinal lymph nodes involved with T-cell leukaemia and non-Hodgkin's lymphoma. Pleural effusions may accompany these lesions, further aggravating the respiratory distress.

If the clinical condition permits radiographs, computerised tomography scanning of the chest and echocardiography will define the extent of the lesion and help plan for a diagnostic biopsy. However, the aim of primary treatment should be to safeguard the airway. Intubation can be extremely difficult and must be performed by experienced personnel. Extubation may not be possible until the tumour bulk has been significantly reduced. In the case of lymphoma, this is normally achieved following initial chemotherapy including steroids. However, in those where a biopsy and therefore histological confirmation of the tumour type is not possible, empiric radiotherapy can be given to shrink the tumour mass. These measures may, however, result in a temporary deterioration in respiratory status as a result of postirradiation oedema. When significant effusions are also present, pleurocentesis and pericardiocentesis may alleviate a degree of the respiratory embarrassment.

Cardiac involvement

Tamponade may be caused acutely by a rapidly developing malignant pericardial effusion and, in the long term, by postirradiation fibrosis. Intracardiac obstruction is a feature of tumour-thrombus extension into the right side of the heart, usually due to a Wilms' tumour extending from the kidney, through the renal vein, into the inferior vena cava. Children present with shortness of breath, cough and cardiomegaly on the chest radiograph. Treatment involves cardiorespiratory support and pericardiocentesis under echocardiographic guidance when tamponade is present. Extension of tumour-thrombus requires preoperative chemotherapy and open heart surgery.

Raised intracranial pressure

Raised intracranial pressure (ICP) is characterised by an altered level of consciousness, headaches and vomiting which are usually worse in the morning. Raised ICP, clumsiness, ataxia and focal neurological signs are common features in children presenting with a brain tumour. Emergency measures to reduce the ICP include high dose dexamethasone (1–2 mg/kg), 20% mannitol (0.5–2 g/kg), and hyperventilation to maintain a PCO_2 of 3.5–4.5 kPa. Therapeutic neurosurgery and, in some cases, a suitable ventricular shunt procedure will be required, preferably once the condition has stabilised. Seizures should be treated with benzodiazepines in the first instance, followed by phenytoin which should be continued for several months after neurosurgery.

Spinal cord compression

Spinal cord compression is a medical emergency usually caused by metastatic destruction of the vertebral bodies or intraspinal tumour extension with sarcoma, neuroblastoma, leukaemia or lymphoma (Packer et al 1985). Dexamethasone, 1–2 mg/kg, should be commenced immediately. If appropriate, tumour shrinkage should be achieved with chemotherapy. Otherwise, emergency surgical decompression or localised radiotherapy is required.

Metabolic derangement

Tumour lysis

Several tumours are exquisitely sensitive to chemotherapy and undergo rapid lysis when exposed to even small doses of cytotoxics. These include T-cell leukaemia and B-cell lymphoma (Burkitt type), which may present with significantly bulky disease. Shortly after the commencement of chemotherapy, these bulky tumours lyse 'en masse', thereby releasing intracellular break-down products into the circulation (Silverman & Distelhorst 1989). The sudden surge in plasma potassium, phosphate and uric acid results in severe metabolic derangement, acidosis and secondary hypocalcaemia, sometimes with seizures and acute renal failure as a result of uric acid nephropathy (Silverman & Distelhorst 1989). Serum pH and electrolyes, including potassium, calcium, phosphate and urate, must be monitored at least twice daily. Children should be hydrated with 2–3 L/m^2 intravenous fluids without potassium additives prior to and after commencing chemotherapy. Hyperuricaemia can be controlled with the use of allopurinol, which blocks uric acid synthesis, and uricozyme, which converts uric acid to a more soluble metabolite. However, allopurinol also increases the xanthine level which, in turn, is poorly excreted in the presence of alkalosis. For this reason alkalinisation is no longer recommended for the treatment of tumour lysis syndrome. Hyperkalaemia must be corrected if fatal arrhythmias are to be avoided. A potassium-binding resin should be started, whilst intracellular influx of potassium is encouraged by intravenous calcium gluconate (100–200 mg/kg) and an insulin-dextrose infusion. Renal dialysis, preferably by haemodialysis which is more efficient at removing uric acid, is occasionally required to control the acidosis, hyperkalaemia and hyperphosphataemia.

Hyperviscosity syndrome

Hyperviscosity can arise when the presenting leukaemic white cell count in the peripheral blood exceeds $100 \times 10^9/L$ (Ablin 1984). Patients may be agitated, confused with blurred vision, breathless and hypoxic. Hyperviscosity predisposes to tumour lysis, pulmonary vascular sludging, alveolar damage, thromboses and haemorrhages which, when they occur in the CNS, may be fatal (Ablin 1984). Therapy includes measures to counteract tumour lysis and platelets to reduce the risk of bleeding. The latter do not significantly increase blood viscosity unlike red cells. However, a partial exchange transfusion using fresh red cells may be given to those in heart failure. Leukapheresis is indicated in those with marked symptoms of hyperviscosity and with metabolic derangement.

Syndrome of inappropriate antidiuretic hormone (SIADH)

SIADH may occur in those with severe pulmonary sepsis, brain tumours, lymphoma and following cytotoxic drugs, especially vincristine and cyclophosphamide. Excessive release of antidiuretic hormone (ADH) leads to water retention, plasma hyposmolality and hyponatraemia (Silverman & Distelhorst 1989). The latter, if severe, result in seizures and coma and may be fatal. Fluid restriction is usually sufficient in less severely affected cases, whereas frusemide (1 mg/kg) and sodium supplementation at a rate of 2 mmol Na^+/h is necessary in comatose patients and when the plasma sodium is less than 120 mmol/L.

Treatment-related problems

Bone marrow failure

Many cytotoxic agents are active against rapidly dividing cells. These include malignant cells as well as normal bone marrow cells. Hence, profound myelosuppression is a common side effect of chemotherapy and is a requisite for successful bone marrow transplantation. The resulting pancytopenia requires supportive therapy in the form of regular red cell and platelet transfusions (Jayabose et al 1991, British Committee for Standards in Haematology 1992). White cell infusions are neither a practical nor an effective measure. Whenever myelosuppressed patients, particularly those with a peripheral neutrophil count of less than 1×10^9/L, develop a significant temperature ($>38.5\,°C$), septicaemia must be assumed (Young 1986). A thorough examination should be followed by a chest radiograph, swabs of clinically suspect sites, urine and blood cultures. Blood cultures should be taken from peripheral and central catheters, and broad spectrum intravenous antibiotics commenced (Young 1986). Recovery of the peripheral blood count may take 7–14 days following a single course of

chemotherapy, but may be considerably prolonged in patients on PICU, especially following bone marrow transplantation (BMT) and in those with overwhelming sepsis. For those patients, bone marrow recovery can be encouraged with the use of growth factors, e.g. granulocyte colony stimulating factor (G-CSF) (Lieschke & Burgess 1992a,b). These drugs must be commenced soon after the administration of chemotherapy or BMT. The duration of treatment is titrated against the rise in neutrophil count but, in general, G-CSF is continued for 14 days. Although expensive and not without side effects, these drugs reduce the duration of neutropenia, but have no beneficial effect on the platelet count.

Immunosuppression and septicaemia

Cancer patients are often immunosuppressed as a result of the malignant process and its treatment, and are at particular risk of infection (Table 16.3). Infections are often not localised but manifest as septicaemia. Causative organisms often originate from the patient's oral and gastrointestinal flora, including *Pseudomonas aeruginosa*, *E. coli* and *Klebsiella* species (Table 16.4). Therefore, combination antibiotics with Gram-positive and negative cover are required, and ceftazidime, 50 mg/kg/dose intravenously three times daily, and gentamicin, 2.5 mg/kg/dose intravenously three times daily, are effective first

Table 16.3 Immunosuppression and sepsis in the cancer patient

Immune defect	Causes	Infecting organisms
Altered defence barriers	Mucosal ulceration, skin trauma Tumour infiltration, indwelling catheters	Bacteria
Decreased cellular immunity	Decreased neutrophil numbers	Bacteria, fungi
	Decreased neutrophil function	Bacteria, fungi
	Altered T-cell function	Bacteria, fungi, viruses
Decreased humoral immunity	Decreased B-cell function	Encapsulated bacteria

Table 16.4 Common infecting organisms in children with cancer

Bacteria		Viruses	Fungi	Others
Gram-positive	*Gram-negative*			
Staphylococci	Escherischia coli	Herpes simplex	Candida	Pneumocystis
Streptococci	Klebsiella	Varicella zoster	Aspergillus	
Corynebacteria	Enterobacteriacae	Cytomegalovirus		
Clostridia	Pseudomonas	Adenovirus		
Listeria	Anaerobes			

line agents (Young 1986). They should be given for at least 48 h in those where blood cultures are negative and continued for longer if the temperature does not settle and/or the clinical condition remains poor. The choice of first line antibiotics will depend on the customary flora for each individual unit. If cultures are positive, antibiotics must be tailored to the sensitivity of the organism(s), and continued for at least 10 days.

Graft versus host disease (GVHD)

GVHD results from the toxic effects of donor lymphocytes on the immunocompromised host. It is usually manifest as cutaneous reactions, liver dysfunction, diarrhoea and pancytopenia. If severe, the prognosis is extremely poor, and for this reason some workers advocate routine pre-irradiation of all blood products with the aim of killing any donor lymphocytes (Greenbaum 1991). However, the true benefit of this practice is unclear.

OPPORTUNISTIC INFECTIONS

These infections are due to organisms which do not normally cause significant problems in non-immunocompromised individuals.

Bacterial infections

Bacteraemias are common in the immunocompromised host, usually involving commensal organisms normally found in the respiratory tract, oral mucosa, perianal region, gastrointestinal and genitourinary tracts. For this reason, empirical treatment with broad spectrum antibiotics must be started with the earliest signs of infection (usually fever).

Fungal infections

Fungaemia should be suspected in an immunosuppressed patient with signs of sepsis who does not respond to intravenous antibiotics. Candida may be grown from blood and urine cultures, although a liver biopsy is necessary to confirm hepatic candidiasis. In this condition a persistent fever is accompanied by right upper quadrant pain and multiple deposits in the liver on ultrasonography. Treatment involves a prolonged course of intravenous amphotericin B or fluconazole. Aspergillus tends to present with focal, later widespread and confluent pulmonary infiltrates. Respiratory embarrassment and deterioration in the radiological appearance progresses despite antibiotics, and 30% of patients with aspergillus pneumonia will go on to develop disseminated aspergillosis. Many will require ventilatory support, and bronchoalveolar lavage is often necessary to confirm the diagnosis. Amphotericin B, although highly nephrotoxic, is the treatment of choice. Liposomal amphotericin is less toxic, possibly more effective, but considerably more expensive.

Viral infections

Viral pneumonitis is potentially extremely serious in the immunocompromised cancer patient, especially following bone marrow transplantation. Specific antiviral treatment is only available against a few viruses: high dose intravenous acyclovir against herpes viruses, e.g. herpes simplex or varicella-zoster; ganciclovir and immune globulin against cytomegalovirus; and ribavirin against respiratory syncitial virus (RSV). Nevertheless, patients who develop a pneumonitis due to these agents, or to adeno- or measles viruses, often require ventilatory support. PICU management is complicated by severe problems in maintaining satisfactory oxygenation, and the mortality associated with viral pneumonitis remains high.

Immunocompromised patients on PICU who have had contact with chickenpox, i.e. within 24 h before and any time after the index case develops varicella vesicles, should be given zoster immune globulin (ZIG) if their varicella antibody status is negative (if known). In addition, any clinical signs of emerging chickenpox in the patient should prompt the commencement of high-dose intravenous acyclovir.

Protozoal infections

Pneumocystis carinii is probably the commonest cause of opportunistic pneumonia in the immunocompromised host. It is a ubiquitous organism present in most children but is reactivated in those whose immune function is deficient. Fever and cough precede progressive breathlessness and hypoxaemia. Severe cases will require ventilation when the diagnosis can be confirmed by induced sputum cultures, bronchoalveolar lavage, or lung biospy. High-dose co-trimoxazole can result in an improvement in oxygenation within 3–4 days and has considerably reduced the mortality associated with pneumocystis pneumonia. Pentamidine should be reserved for those patients who fail to respond to co-trimoxazole. Prednisolone in a dose of 2 mg/kg for 5 days

(and reducing over the next 2 weeks) confers an added advantage with regard to morbidity and mortality, and its use is currently accepted practice in this condition.

INTENSIVE CARE NURSING OF THE PAEDIATRIC CANCER PATIENT

Due care should be taken if cytotoxic agents have to be given to the patient on PICU. Gloves, goggles and aprons are used to handle these drugs, and spillage, or contact with the eyes or mucosal surfaces, must be avoided. Any contact should be treated immediately with thorough washing using soap and water. In order to minimise the incidence of cytotoxic 'burns', extra care must be taken to ensure correct function of all access cannulae, catheters and ports, and the cytotoxics injected or infused in accordance with the prescribed/documented instructions. Adequate hydration and anti-emetics are important adjuncts to chemotherapy and should be provided as a routine.

Immunosuppressed patients should ideally be nursed in a single cubicle. General nursing hygiene should apply in accordance with good nursing standards. In addition, strict hand washing with soap or an alcohol-based antiseptic before and after attending to the patient is essential. The use of single-use aprons, gowns and gloves may help reduce the risk of contamination of the patient with foreign organisms. Routine regular use of a mouth wash and an oral antifungal agent such as nystatin should be encouraged in the neutropenic patient. Per rectal examinations and suppositories may result in a bacteraemia and should be avoided if at all possible.

REFERENCES

Ablin A R 1984 Managing the problem of hyperleukocytosis in acute leukaemia. American Journal of Pediatric Hematology and Oncology 6:287–291

Bagby G C 1987 Haematological aspects of systemic disease. Hematology/Oncology Clinics of North America 1:167–350

British Committee for Standards in Haematology 1992 Guidelines for platelet transfusions — British Committee for Standards in Haematology, Working Party of Blood

Transfusion Task Force. Transfusion Medicine 2:1777–1780

Greenbaum B H 1991 Transfusion-associated graft-versus host disease: historical perspectives, incidence and current use of irradiated blood products. Journal of Clinical Oncology 9:1889–1902

Issa P Y, Brinhi E R, Janin Y, Slim M S 1983 Superior vena cava syndrome in childhood. Pediatrics 71:337–341

Jayabose S, Tugal O, Ruddy R 1991 Transfusion therapy for

severe anaemia. American Journal of Pediatric Hematology and Oncology 13:114

Lee C A 1992 Coagulation factor replacement therapy. In: Hoffbrand A V, Brenner M K (eds) Recent advances in haematology, 6th edn. Churchill Livingstone, Edinburgh, pp 73–88

Lieschke G J, Burgess A W 1992a Granulocyte colony-stimulating factor and granulocyte-macrophage colony-stimulating factor (Part I). New England Journal of Medicine 327:28–35

Lieschke G J, Burgess A W 1992b Granulocyte colony-stimulating factor and granulocyte-macrophage colony-stimulating factor (Part II). New England Journal of Medicine 327:99–106

Packer R J, Rorke L B, Lange B L 1985 Cerebrovascular accidents in children with cancer. Pediatrics 76:194–201

Schiffer C A 1991 Prevention of alloimmunisation against platelets. Blood 77:1–4

Schiffer C A 1992 Prophylactic platelet transfusion. Transfusion 32:295–298

Silverman P, Distelhorst C W 1989 Metabolic emergencies in clinical oncology. Seminars in Oncology 16:504–515.

Spain R C, Whittlesley D 1989 Respiratory emergencies in patients with cancer. Seminars in Oncology 16:471–489

Young L 1986 Empirical antimicrobial therapy in the neutropenic host. New England Journal of Medicine 81:237–242

FURTHER READING

Freifeld A G, Hathorn J W, Pizzo P A 1993 Infectious complications in the pediatric cancer patient. In: Pizzo P A, Poplack D G (eds) Principles and practice of pediatric oncology, 2nd edn. JB Lippincott, Philadelphia, pp 987–1019

Hoffbrand A V, Pettit J E (eds) 1993 Blood transfusion. In: Essential haematology, 3rd edn. Blackwell Scientific, London, pp 392–407

Lange B, D'Angio G, Ross A J, O'Neill J A, Packer R 1993 Oncologic emergencies. In: Pizzo P A, Poplack D G (eds) Principles and practice of pediatric oncology, 2nd edn. JB Lippincott, Philadelphia, pp 951–972

Sergeant G R 1992 Sickle cell anaemia, 2nd edn. Oxford University Press, Oxford

Psychosocial, Nutritional and Pharmacological Issues

SECTION CONTENTS

Section 3 has been written by UK experts to provide an overview of common issues relevant to the management of infants and children in intensive care. The physiological needs of critically-ill children often form the highest priority for practitioners, but the importance of nutrition and pharmacokinetics may not be considered early in the child's management. The psychosocial issues affecting the child and family will need to be addressed to assist the family to cope with their stay and prepare for the future. Therefore, this section of the book provides information important for the ongoing management of infants and children requiring intensive care.

17

Family support in paediatric intensive care

Caroline Haines
Michelle Wolstenholme

The reasons for admission of a child to the Paediatric Intensive Care Unit (PICU) are diverse. Each child exhibits unique physical, psychological, emotional and developmental characteristics, each of which needs to be addressed. Disruption in normal family routine can lead to signs of stress in both the child and her family. The promotion of Family Centred Care within paediatric nursing can help to reduce family stress. It not only recognises the importance of the family to the wellbeing of the child (Jay & Youngblut 1991), but also recommends that nurses and parents work together in mutual participation, to enhance quality of care for the child (Rushton 1990).

Being aware of the differing definitions and interpretations of 'family' within our changing society is vitally important. Traditionally, the family was seen as a heterosexual married couple with children; however, today a much broader concept of a group of people who love and care for each other may be more appropriate. Stressed families may not be able to comfort their child in the normal way. The ability to identify the predominant sources of family stress can assist PIC staff to implement strategies to help them manage these difficult situations in the most constructive way.

This chapter will address the theories of stress. Following this the sources of stress for parents and siblings will be discussed with application to clinical practice in paediatric intensive care.

STRESS

The general concept of stress is familiar to lay

people and professionals alike; however, its complex nature has made it difficult to reach agreement over a specific definition. Despite this, three essentially different, but integrated, approaches to the definition and the study of stress have been developed (Cox 1978):

- 'engineering approach'
- 'physiological approach'
- 'interactional approach'.

By considering these approaches to stress and applying them to the behaviours exhibited by all family members involved following the admission of a child to PIC, it is hoped that staff will gain a greater insight into the process. With this insight, they will then be able to offer each individual more support during this particularly stressful period in their lives.

Engineering approach

This approach identifies influences from the environment which give rise to a stress reaction (Cox 1978). On entering a PICU, parents can potentially experience stress from the sights and sounds of the alien environment. This approach can be likened to a piece of elastic. Slight pulling of the elastic will have no detrimental effect; however, when the elastic is overstretched it snaps. Hence, when stress is no longer tolerable, physical and psychological damage may occur (Cox 1978). However, this model only identifies what causes stress and not how the person reacts to it.

Physiological approach

This approach to stress was influenced by the work of Selye (1974), who as a medical student noted changes in the human body when a person was ill, regardless of the nature of the complaint. He explained the stress response as the body's non-specific reaction to demands placed upon it (Selye 1974). This response to stress is referred to as the General Adaptation Syndrome (GAS) and consists of three stages.

1. The first stage, or alarm reaction, involves physiological changes caused by the sympathetic nervous system (SNS). The SNS is activated whenever the body needs to use energy, often referred to as the fight or flight response. The hypothalamus acts as the orchestrator of the SNS; the anterior lobe of the pituitary gland is stimulated to release adrenocorticotrophic hormones which stimulate the adrenal glands and adrenal medulla to secrete catecholamines prepared by the body for flight or fight (Table 17.1). If this stage is prolonged then physical symptoms of a loss of appetite, weight and strength loss, a lack of ambition, and facial expressions associated with general malaise can be evident.

2. The second stage or resistance reaction refers to the body's reduction in sympathetic

Table 17.1 Reactions to activation of the sympathetic and parasympathetic nervous systems

System	Function/ organ	Sympathetic reaction	Parasympathetic reaction
Cardiovascular	Heart rate	↑	↓
	Blood pressure	↑	↓
	Limbs (trunk)	Dilation of blood vessels to voluntary muscles	Voluntary muscle contraction
Respiratory	Respiratory rate	↑	↓
Neurological	Pupils	Dilate	Constrict
Gastrointestinal tract	Saliva secretion	Suppressed	Stimulated
Urinary	Bladder muscle	Relaxed	Contracted
Endocrine	Adrenal glands	Stimulated to secrete ↑ adrenaline and noradrenaline	↓secretion
	Liver	Glucose released from glycogen	Sugar stored
	Emotion	Experience strong emotion	↓experience of strong emotion

activity. If the stressor is not removed from the body, the adrenal cortex is stimulated to increase secretion of glucocorticoid hormones which control blood glucose levels, and there is additional shrinkage of the thymus, spleen and lymphatics. These physiological changes affect the body's general immune system and response to illness.

3. The third or final stage is exhaustion. The body's resources become depleted, blood sugar levels drop and death may occur due to hypoglycaemia.

The GAS refers only to the physical effects of stress on the body, whereas a holistic approach takes into account the physical, environmental and psychological effects of stress. Awareness of the physical effects of stress, such as alertness, agitation, nervousness and sweating, can, however, be useful in the initial assessment of parents on the admission of their child to PICU, and their potential ability to cope with the situation.

Interactional approach

This approach refers to the relationship between individuals and their environment and is therefore a more psychologically based approach to stress. It combines elements of the two previous models (Cox 1978) and recognises that stress can be an individual perceptual phenomenon influenced by prior psychological processes (Cox 1978). It highlights the importance of feedback mechanisms, thus ensuring the approach becomes cyclical rather than linear (Fig. 17.1).

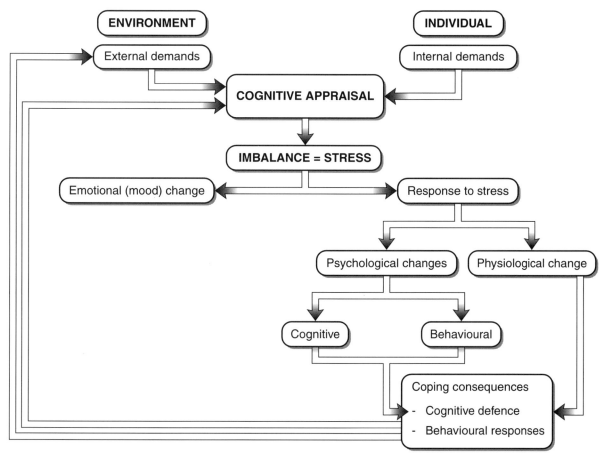

Figure 17.1   The interactional model of stress (Cox T 1978 Stress. Macmillan, London, with permission).

PARENTAL STRESS

The admission of any child to PIC not only exposes families to inordinate amounts of stress from environmental factors, but it also causes an abrupt alteration to their role as a parent (Jay 1977). Parents enter hospital as the primary carers, but have to relinquish the major part of this role to the nursing and medical staff when their child's needs can no longer be met by themselves (Farrell & Frost 1992). The role of a parent to a healthy child changes to that of a parent to a critically ill child (Miles & Carter 1983, La Montagne & Pawlack 1990), which causes immense grief and feelings of helplessness.

Additional stressors such as financial constraints, work commitments, marital problems or personal injury in individuals' lives can also have dramatic effects on how they cope with particular stressful events. Identification of these parental stressors is therefore necessary in order to develop nursing interventions that can help facilitate the adaptation of families.

Specific parental stressors and differing coping mechanisms have been investigated by several researchers in recent years; however, since 1982, Miles & Carter appear to have led the research into parental stress. Miles & Carter (1982) developed the Parental Stressor Scale: Paediatric Intensive Care Unit (PSS:PICU), a tool which identified seven main dimensions of stress experienced by parents in PIC (Table 17.2).

Within this framework, parents tend to find the child's behaviour and emotions particularly difficult to accept. They become distressed by seeing their child cry, being in pain, unable to communicate, sad and frightened. It is at these times that the child is at its most vulnerable and turns to his parents for support, guidance and love. However, the parents themselves also feel vulnerable. Their parental role has significantly altered and they may be grieving for their healthy child, whilst adapting to the needs of their critically ill child. Therefore, parents are often unable to provide totally for their child's needs. This may improve as the child's stay in PIC progresses and they become more familiar with the situation and environment. Initially,

Table 17.2 Dimensions of stress experienced by parents of children in PIC, according to the PSS: PICU[a]

DIMENSION	EXAMPLES
1. Child's behavioural and responses.	Crying, demanding, emotional, frightened, restless, rebellious.
2. Alteration to parenting role.	Not being able to see, visit, hold or care for child.
3. Staff behaviour.	Laughing, joking, talking too much or not enough.
4. Staff communication.	Use of jargon, giving inconsistent, unintelligible or insufficient information to parents.
5. PICU sights & sounds.	Alarms, equipment, other sick children.
6. Painful or distressing procedures conducted on the child.	Cannulation, suctioning, physiotherapy.
7. Child's appearance.	Puffiness or change in skin colour.

[a]Miles & Carter (1982).
It is this tool that has continued to be used in recent years in replica studies investigating parental stress in PIC (Miles et al 1989, La Montagne & Pawlack 1990, Jay & Youngblut 1991, Haines et al 1995).

parents may be unable to hold their child because of the critical nature of her condition; they may be frightened or even afraid to touch him. Patience, understanding and consideration for the family's needs must therefore be considered and be addressed by staff in a very individual manner. The child himself may be linked to electronic monitoring equipment, a ventilator plus several intravenous infusion lines, and thus may have an inordinate amount of equipment attached to him which may significantly alter his physical appearance. Additionally, the constant intervention required by nursing, medical and allied health staff to ensure the child's stability can not only be overwhelming, but may add to the tremendous anxiety and stress experienced by the family (Kasper & Nyamathi 1988, Carnevale 1990, Haines et al 1995).

Communication between staff and parents can fluctuate greatly depending on individuals and circumstances. Parents should be well informed of their child's progress and have regular meetings with medical and nursing staff (Kirschbaum 1990). Ensuring the information given to parents is consistent, understandable, relevant and honest is essential for the establishment of a good rapport and trust. Assessing each parent individually and discussing with them their understanding of the situation and their ability to comprehend the information, is vital if the needs of each are to be met. This could be achieved by the appropriate implementation of a framework or model of nursing care which enables a comprehensive assessment of the child and parents, to identify actual or potential communication problems. Primary Nursing, which not only strengthens the partnership and continuity in care concept of nursing, but also minimises the number of nurses caring for any one child and family, could be beneficial (Rogers et al 1992). This reduces the amount of adapting the child and family have to do, thus not only allowing fostering of good nurse-to-nurse communication links, but more importantly of good communication links between the nurse, child and parents (Manley 1989).

Explaining to parents the potential variety and fluctuation in the degree of dependency of the children in PIC is extremely valuable, if they are to understand why their child may receive more intense nursing and medical input on some days in comparison to others (Haines et al 1995). Restricting information to parents and poor communication links can increase stress levels for families, and these in turn can be easily relayed to the child. This additional worry, fear and potential agitation in the child can then cause a further delay in their recovery (Jay & Youngblut 1991).

The variety and fluctuation in staff behaviour can have significant impact on parental stress levels (Miles & Carter 1982). Some parents may interpret the relaxed, joking behaviour of staff in a critical care environment as being particularly inappropriate, whilst others may appreciate the informality. Some may see the rushed, distant and concerned manner of staff as a deterioration in their child's condition, whilst other parents may be oblivious or unaffected by their manner. Interpretation of any behaviour is very individual; however, staff in a critical care environment need to be particularly receptive to the stressors experienced by parents and act in a professional manner at all times.

The physical aspects of the PIC environment can add additional stressors to these factors. The high degree of technology, intensity of the work, constant light, sights of other sick children and urgency of the environment can magnify these issues further.

Coping mechanisms exhibited by parents to deal with these stressful situations may be broad and varied. They are seen as conscious ways of trying to adapt to both stress and anxiety in a positive and constructive way. They may be achieved by using both thoughts and behaviours directed towards searching for information, problem-solving, seeking help from others, recognising individual feelings and establishing personal goals and objectives (Gross 1992) (Table 17.3).

Unconscious reactions such as defence mechanisms of denial, hostility, isolation and distortion of facts are not uncommon, and PIC nursing staff are in an ideal position to recognise these and to promote more appropriate coping strategies in parents.

Coping styles and mechanisms do not tend to be conscious behaviours. Parents may initially be unable to proceed straight to their child on entering the PICU for the first time; however, once a parent acclimatises to the environment, progression towards the child may occur more naturally. Parents may become very withdrawn, either being reluctant to leave the child or alternatively being unable to visit for long periods. These parents obviously require support, understanding and time to adjust to the situation. Mothers and fathers may react very differently and individually at times of stress. It is important to remember that the role of the primary carer is changing (Baker & Lane 1994), as fathers and child minders may provide the day-to-day care for children of mothers who are working. Family structure may be complicated by divorce or death of a parent. The stressors for single parents may be more complex (Baker & Lane 1994). PIC nursing staff must assess individual needs and intervene appropriately to assist with parental coping.

Problem-and emotional-focused coping behav-

Table 17.3 Some coping mechanisms and their corresponding defence mechanisms

Coping mechanism	Description	Corresponding defence mechanism
Objectivity	Separating one thought from another, or our feelings from our thoughts, which allows us to obtain a better understanding of how we think and feel and an objective evaluation of our actions.	Isolation
Logical analysis	Carefully and systematically analysing our problems in order to find explanations and to make plans to solve them, based on the realities of the situation.	Rationalisation
Concentration	The ability to set aside disturbing thoughts and feelings in order to concentrate on the task in hand.	Denial
Empathy	The ability to sense how others are feeling in emotionally-arousing situations so that our interactions take account of their feelings.	Projection
Playfulness	The ability to use past feelings, ideas and behaviour appropriately so as to enrich the solution of problems and to otherwise add some enjoyment to life.	Regression
Tolerance of ambiguity	The ability to function in situations where we or others cannot make clear choices – because the situation is so complicated.	–
Suppression	The ability consciously to forget about or hold back thoughts and feelings until an appropriate time and place to express them arises.	Repression
Substitution of thoughts and emotions	The ability consciously to substitute other thoughts or feelings for how we really think or feel in order to meet the demands of the situation.	Reaction formation

Sublimation can be thought of as a coping mechanism *and* a defence mechanism, because it involves chanelling anxiety in socially desirable ways and so is positive and constructive.

Adapted from Gross (1992).

iours may emerge in some parents (La Montagne & Pawlack 1990). Problem-focused behaviour may include seeking social support from the nurse involved in the child's care, or from social groups. Emotional-focused behaviours include guilt, anger, sadness and despair. Parents may feel guilty and seek reassurance that what they did was correct, or blame someone else for not detecting the seriousness of their child's condition (Kasper & Nyamathi 1988, Kirschbaum 1990).

PIC nurses who are not only aware of parental stressors but also coping styles can be effective mediators in helping to reduce these stressors, thus enabling parents to develop their own coping styles. However, nurses do perceive the needs of parents very differently, and an accurate assessment of them is therefore essential.

SIBLINGS

Recognition of the needs and coping strategies of siblings of critically ill children is an area of immense significance to the maintenance of the family.

Parents are responsible for providing support to the siblings of the affected child, however they themselves may already be suffering from great stress, and it is therefore often difficult for them to know what to tell the child.

Parental perception of how well the child may cope with a critically ill sibling may be influenced by their own defence mechanisms of denial, anger, intellectualisation, worry or fear. Research has shown that parents do tend to restrict the information given to siblings of critically ill children (Titler et al 1991, Kleiber et al 1995). Some wish to protect the well child from painful information; others doubt their ability to communicate effectively with the child when discussing their critically ill sibling, or feel they are not old enough to understand (Kleiber et al 1995).

Dependent upon physical and developmental

age, withholding information from siblings of critically ill children, provision of too detailed information, prevention or significant encouragement of visiting to the critical care environment and the ill child, can often lead to added stress within the family. A reduction of communication between parents and non-hospitalised children can leave siblings wondering what is wrong and what the outcome will be, an unrealistic sense of responsibility and guilt for the child's problems or a fear of the same illness affecting them (Titler et al 1991). Behavioural problems, deterioration in school work, regression and anger may also be evident in their attitude.

Children generally tend to be curious, concerned and perceptive about the medical treatment of an ill sibling and about the expectations for the future.

The pre-school child, although restricted in ability to verbally express feelings and needs regarding her sibling's illness, displays concerns through altered behaviour and play. Her comprehension of illness severity, the PIC environment and its implications are limited; however, this should not necessarily restrict parental explanations or visitations to their sibling.

Some school-aged children may ask numerous questions requiring significant in-depth information about the ill child's condition, the environment and the equipment being used, and may even ask directly whether the ill child is going to die.

Adolescents' comprehension of the situation is similar to that of their parents. Questions and concerns regarding their sibling's reason for admission, equipment and likely survival, need to be answered with honesty and sincerity. Discussion about the situation and any subsequent alteration in their behavioural characteristics must be addressed individually and with understanding.

Providing comprehensive, honest and direct information for all siblings is vitally important if they are to remain part of the family and able to cope with their sibling's illness. Attempts to shelter siblings from unpleasant information can increase their fears and fantasies. They know when something is wrong, and without further explanation they only have their own imagination to draw on.

Despite the whole family being affected by the admission of a child to PIC, parents may be unaware of the effect of this experience on their well child and may not have the knowledge or skills to assist in the understanding of the situation. Health care professionals need to provide support, guidance and help to parents to enable them to support their well child. Explaining to parents that school-aged children have a need for knowledge and have the ability to understand complex issues, may enable them to encourage their well children to ask questions about their sibling's illness. Once provided with this information, parents can then be assisted in formulating a plan to include the school-aged siblings in the information tree (Kleiber et al 1995). Parental comfort or discomfort with information-giving to the siblings should be assessed and the appropriate guidance and help given.

Developmental age of siblings will influence how much information may be given and by which method. Discussing the situation and circumstances with siblings can often enlighten families and health professionals as to how they perceive the situation to be and how much information can be tolerated. The expertise of play specialists, counsellors and support workers and the use of role-play and information booklets are just a few of the options available. Whichever is chosen, practising what the parents want to say to the siblings can be invaluable.

If the admission to PIC is planned, then siblings can be involved in preadmission visits which may assist them to continue their family role during the hospital admission. The need for time alone with their critically ill sibling, or with their parents, is often overlooked because of the increased stressors on all family members in this situation. Ensuring their daily routine continues in some form can be extremely difficult; however, siblings tend to need this reassurance in order for them to cope with the situation (Titler et al 1991, Kleiber et al 1995). Although it may seem inappropriate for siblings to want to go and play with friends, attend parties, go shopping or alternatively stay constantly with their critically ill sibling, these needs should be accepted and considered as they tend to be the coping mechanisms of each individual.

By considering many of these issues, the information and coping needs of the siblings of critically ill children will begin to be addressed, with the hope that disruption to the family during a particularly stressful period will be minimised.

CHILD

Children are less able than adults to cope with an altered environment, because of their age, development and limited life experiences. Their ability to cope is further reduced when they are admitted to PIC, where the child may be separated from his family, exposed to unusual sights and sounds and painful treatment. Child development proceeds at a relatively rapid rate, and therefore even a short period of hospitalisation can produce stress, interfere with development and, in some cases, cause regression (Wilson & Broome 1989). Consideration of the age range and thus stage of development, assists identification of appropriate strategies that may be used to help the child cope.

Infants are the most vulnerable of children in terms of development, as they are unable to comprehend information given to them, they need food, rest, stimulation, warmth and love. In PIC, they may not receive sufficient rest because of the noisy environment and required interventions. They are unable to understand why they cannot have food or regular contact with people. Developmental delay may occur as a result of a lack of opportunity for stimulation because of their illness and medications. Immunisations may be delayed, making the infant more susceptible to infectious diseases.

Toddlers have very similar needs to infants but may experience more anxiety from separation and the strange environment (Wilson & Broome 1989). They have developed relationships with their family, being able to recognise individuals, and may fear separation more than the infant. Any routine that is significantly interrupted can be confusing and frightening for the toddler. Bowlby (1985) describes this concept as separa-

tion anxiety, where a profound disturbance to the child's development can occur as a result of separation from his/her parents. These issues can have a detrimental effect on the self esteem and coping ability of the parents (Bowlby 1985) and should be considered as part of the ongoing assessment of the child and family.

The child is able to comprehend more information, both verbally and non-verbally, and may determine parental feelings from facial expressions, tone of voice and actions. They may not want to upset their parents further by disclosing their fears. Behavioural regression often occurs as a coping method of the child's experience. This may be due to loss of independence and control over choice of clothing and play or sleep periods.

Adolescence is often confusing, as it is a time of rebellion, in which the adolescent seeks more independence and development of self. It can also be a very bewildering time during which puberty occurs, privacy is vitally important and fears for the future become more prevalent.

Healthcare professionals need to work in partnership with families and the adolescent, negotiating care whilst ensuring that a good quality of life is maintained. A major aspect of this is effective communication between all parties. To promote a trusting relationship, honesty is essential. Interventions directed at the individual needs of adolescents will encourage trust and assist her to cope during admission to intensive care. The need for independence and privacy from parents usually sought by the adolescent often becomes unimportant when faced with the additional stress of being in intensive care. Inclusion of significant friends and encouragement of normal routine may reduce additional stress caused by interference with normal lifestyle.

Adolescents may be embarrassed by their parents assisting in their personal hygiene needs; this needs to be handled with great care. The adolescent and the parents need to be happy with the situation to ensure that stress relieved for one party is not inadvertently transferred to another.

Consistency on the part of the caregivers, by practising a 'primary nursing' or 'named nurse' concept, is important (Rogers et al 1992) not only for the development of trust, but also to provide stability for the child and the family.

Young children often find the presence of their family comforting, enhancing their ability to cope. Allowing '24 hour' visiting and encouraging parents not only to participate in their child's care but allowing them to stay near the unit in a comfortable waiting area or parental accommodation, is valuable (Jansen et al 1989).

Holistic needs of the family must be considered. For those parents who are unable to be resident, effective communication and support mechanisms must be considered.

Humanising strategies to assist the child to cope with the alien environment include:

- displaying family photographs and favourite posters
- providing favourite toys and comforters
- enabling children to listen to favourite music
- enabling them to watch videos and television
- facilitating visits from friends and siblings.

Provision of the above can assist individual growth and development, as can the expertise of play specialists (Jansen et al 1989, Bossert 1994, Wilson & Broome 1989).

Intubation, assisted ventilation and drug therapies such as sedation and muscle relaxation can interfere with the child's ability to communicate normally and may cause frustration. Involvement of speech therapists can provide support and suggestions for alternative communication methods. Nasotracheal intubation is preferred in children, and one advantage of this is that it does allow the children to mouth words, facilitating communication with their family and others.

TRANSITIONAL CARE

Transition from the PICU to a ward area can be a stressful experience for children and families. They will have become familiar with the environment, routines, staff and equipment within the PICU, and the move to the ward will engender additional stresses for which families have to adapt their behaviour in order to cope. Early planning of the transfer of a child to the ward

area is vital to reduce this stress (Braun & St Clair 1994). PIC nurses are in the ideal position to coordinate this activity and ensure families cope with the transition. Additional strategies that facilitate coping include:

- discussion with the child and family prior to the transfer
- de-intensifying the child by removing monitoring equipment and lines
- meeting ward nursing staff
- providing written information about the ward philosophy and facilities
- discussion with other families previously with a child in PIC
- comprehensive nursing handover involving parents where appropriate
- providing detailed written information regarding the transfer, to assist communication
- transfer during normal working hours to optimise healthcare follow up.

Particular concerns identified by families include the loss of the 1:1 nurse:patient relationship and reduced presence of medical staff. The emphasis on transfer to the ward environment needs to be on the promotion of independence and rehabilitation.

By ensuring the child and family have been adequately prepared for transition to the ward, and by guaranteeing new staff are comfortable with the care and treatment required, transfer of the child and family will be made less stressful.

IMPLICATIONS FOR CLINICAL PRACTICE

A significant number of stressors and coping strategies affecting families admitted to PIC have been identified. Parents need to be able to dictate the pace of their involvement in their child's care to feel comfortable in the PIC environment. This should be reflected in the unit philosophy, which also may provide parents with insight into the aims of treatment for their child. Support for parents from individuals not directly involved in the child's care can be invaluable. The type of support involved is dependent on their knowledge and experience but will incorporate both practical and psychological help. These people include:

- social workers
- other parents
- psychologists
- counsellors
- religious/cultural representatives
- healthcare assistants.

All PIC staff must ensure that families' cultural beliefs are respected, irrespective of whether they differ from their own. Care should be taken not to place pressure on parents to conform to what may be considered right for one culture but taboo for another. In British society there is an increasing number of ethnic groups. Use of translators may be required to ensure effective communication. For convenience, there may be a tendency to involve a family member as interpreter. However, this can place added stress on an individual at a particularly difficult time and could lead to inaccurate or selective provision of information to other family members. Careful consideration should be given to choice of translator, for this reason.

In conclusion, recognising parental stress and assisting family coping is an important aspect of the work of PIC staff, which should be included in educational programmes. Early recognition and introduction of strategies to reduce parental stress will assist with stress reduction in the child. Recent research into and understanding of these issues has lead to changes in practice such as visiting policy and parental participation (Etzler 1984, Cunliffe 1987, Miles et al 1989, La Montagne & Pawlack 1990, Farrell & Frost 1992, Haines et al 1995). However, further relevant research into cultural and religious differences is required to ensure that the needs of all children and families are met appropriately.

REFERENCES

Baker S, Lane M 1994 The good father: How is the role of the father in child care changing? Child Health June/July:28–31

Bossert E 1994 Factors influencing the coping of hospitalised school-age children. Journal of Pediatric Nursing. 9(5):299–306

Bowlby J 1985 Separation, anxiety and anger. Volume 2 of Attachment and loss. Hogarth Press, London

Braun R, St Clair C 1994 Transitional family care; PICU to pediatrics. Critical Care Nurse 8:65–68

Carnevale F M 1990 A description of stressors and coping strategies among parents of critically ill children: a preliminary study. Intensive Care Nursing 6:4–11

Cox T 1978 Stress. Macmillan, London

Cunliffe P H 1987 Communicating with children in the intensive care unit. Intensive Care Nursing 3(2):71–77

Etzler C A 1984 Parents' reaction to paediatric critical care settings: a review of the literature. Issues in Comprehensive Paediatric Nursing 7:319–331

Farrell M F, Frost C 1992 The most important needs of parents of critically ill children: parents' perceptions. Intensive and Critical Care Nursing 8:130–139

Gross R D 1992 Psychology — the science of mind and behaviour. Hodder & Stoughton, London

Haines C, Perger C, Nagy S 1995 A comparison of the stressors experienced by parents of intubated and non-intubated children. Journal of Advanced Nursing 21(2):350–355

Hazinski M F 1992 Nursing care of the critically ill child. Mosby Year Book, St Louis

Jansen M T, DeWitt P K, Meshul R J, Krasnoff J B, Lau A M,

Keens T G 1989 Meeting psychosocial and developmental needs of children during prolonged intensive care unit hospitalization. Child Health Care 18(2):91–95

Jay S S 1977 Pediatric intensive care: involving parents in the care of their child. Maternal–Child Nursing Journal 6(3):195–204

Jay S S, Youngblut J M 1991 Parent stress associated with paediatric critical care nursing: linking research and practice. AACN Clinical issues 2(2):276–284

Kasper J W, Nyamathi A M 1988 Parents of children in the paediatric intensive care unit: what are their needs? Heart and Lung 17(5):574–581

Kirschbaum M S 1990 Needs of parents of critically ill children. Dimensions of Critical Care Nursing. 9(6):344–352

Kleiber C, Montgomery L A, Craft-Rosenberg M 1995 Information needs of the siblings of critically ill children. Children's Health Care 24(1):47–60

La Montagne L L, Pawlack R 1990 Stress and coping of parents of children in a paediatric intensive care unit. Heart and Lung 19(4):416–421

Manley K 1989 Primary nursing in intensive care. Scutari Press, England

Miles M S, Carter M C 1982 Sources of parental stress in pediatric intensive care units. Child Health Care 11(2):65–69

Miles M S, Carter M C 1983 Assessing parental stress in the intensive care unit. Maternal–Child Nursing Journal 8(5):345–359

Miles M S, Carter M C, Riddle I, Hennessey J, Eberly T W 1989 The paediatric intensive care unit environment as a source of stress for parents. Maternal–Child Nursing Journal 18(3):199–219

Monat A, Lazarus R S 1977 Stress and coping — an anthology. Columbia University Press, New York

Rogers M B, Cole S, Goode M 1992 Looking forward. Paediatric Nursing 4(2):23–25

Rushton C H 1990 Strategies for family centered care in the critical care setting. Pediatric Nursing 16(2):195–199

Selye H 1974 Stress without distress. Hodder & Stoughton, London

Titler M, Cohen M, Craft M 1991 Impact of critical illness on the family: perceptions of patients, spouses, children and nurses. Heart & Lung 20:174–182

Wilson T, Broome M E 1989 Promoting the young child's development in the intensive care unit. Heart & Lung 18(3):274–279

18

Care of the dying child

Mollie Cook

The death of a child is a tragic life event that is particularly hard to accept, the loss leading to grief that can be the most painful, enduring and difficult to survive. Harriet Sharnoff Schiff (1978) called it the ultimate tragedy, where the parents violate natural law by outliving their child.

The pain of losing a child, whether a baby or older, cannot be measured. However, experience suggests that those losing a baby yearn for the positive memories gained from building a relationship with an older child, whilst parents having such memories state that feelings of loss are actually increased. In all cases, there is the sense of an unfulfilled life script.

Death of a child in the Intensive Care Unit is particularly stressful for both family members and staff. Everyone involved can experience a sense of failure or helplessness through their inability to prevent the child's death.

Caring for the dying child and her family is both a privilege and a challenge. The staff involved participate in the construction of a memory which will remain with the family. The management of the death will have significant implications for the parents' adjustment to life without their child. This chapter will therefore consider the physical, emotional and psychological needs of the dying child and her family within the Intensive Care setting.

Causes of death in intensive care

Technological advances have reduced childhood mortality, but approximately 1:10 children requiring intensive care do not survive. Where the

319

cause of death is a traumatic event, the resulting shock, disbelief and anger expressed is often a difficult challenge for those caring for the child and family. The needs of the family are the most important consideration at this time.

Overwhelming acute illness often leads to rapid deterioration of the child's condition and to sudden death, which leaves parents stunned and disbelieving. The parents often blame themselves for not detecting signs of serious illness sooner. Rationalisation is often evident from questions such as 'could a playmate have infected my child'? Fear for the safety of siblings often comes from such a death, resulting in overprotection and excessive concern for their health. Anxiety relating to infectious illnesses can lead to avoidance by other families within the community, causing parents further grief.

Sudden death can also result from congenital abnormalities which require surgery, in the first few years of life. Risks of surgery, although discussed, are often disregarded because of the parents' faith in the surgeon's expertise. The shock and disbelief associated with such a death are often exacerbated by the child having appeared well preoperatively, and the parents equating giving consent with signing a death warrant. The question 'what if' is often provoked by the child's dying in theatre, without her parents present. Despite thorough preoperative preparation, death is still a huge shock.

Death of a neonate is particularly hard if mother and child have no contact at the birth. Supported participation in her baby's care must be encouraged, especially where anticipatory loss causes emotional and physical withdrawal which may lead to future feelings of guilt. The death of a twin is particularly stressful, with parents experiencing divided loyalties and needing reassurance of the dying baby's life, no matter how short.

Caring for the dying child

Admission to Intensive Care often necessitates urgent resuscitation and intubation, giving little time for decision making or discussion with the child and parents. Staff must support the parents to enable them to support their child through this frightening experience.

Case note 1

A dying child in her teens, frightened by her deteriorating condition which required elective intubation and ventilation, asked if she was going to die. Unsure of the likely outcome, both staff and parents experienced much anxiety while supporting one another to respond to her question.

The urgency of such situations allows little time for exploration of the child's anxieties and feelings about dying. This is particularly relevant to the older child who is more aware of the significance of serious life-threatening illness and death.

Intubated children who remain conscious or semiconscious require considerable reassurance and explanation, regarding the equipment, environment and required interventions. Although more comforting when delivered by the parents, such explanations may be better articulated by experienced nursing staff. The child needs assurance that she will not be left alone. An unconscious state should not exclude appropriate reassurance, as the child may be aware of what is happening to her.

Strategies for communicating with the conscious/intubated child include:

- picture or word boards appropriate to the child's age
- aids for writing and drawing
- use of computers
- use of closed questions with identified responses for 'yes' and 'no'
- art therapy
- play therapy
- story creation and telling.

The child's world and experience of death

A child's understanding of death develops through different experiences into a complete concept at around the age of 8 years (Lansdowne

& Benjamin 1985). Younger children may have some understanding of the meaning of 'dead', although this will be limited by the child's experience, stage of thinking, linguistic ability and stories she has heard. In contrast, it is accepted that an adolescent perceives death as the inevitable, permanent cessation of life, which can happen to herself as well as others. However, whilst aware of the severity of her condition, she may deny the possibility of death. Whilst persisting in a degree of 'magical' thinking, school age children are developing the concept of the permanence of death.

Dying children seem to experience more fear and anxiety of clinical procedures, mutilation and death than those with chronic non-terminal illness. It is possible that a child may be aware of the likelihood of death despite not being informed of her prognosis. Despite their incomplete concept of death, younger children should be prepared for death to allay their fears.

Sensitive assessment of the child's understanding and parents' feelings and beliefs about death will determine the information given to the child. Children pick up environmental cues, such as hushed bedside tones, tearful parents and unexpected visits from friends/family, suggesting that something is wrong. Talking with the child may enable her to explore her feelings, reducing fear and the sense of isolation and vulnerability. The child's behaviour — for instance, withdrawal, regression and anger towards parents or hospital staff — may suggest the child's need to talk about death but inability to do so because of fear of family reactions.

Case note 2

Children do not always ask directly about their condition and may require help in self-expression. A 14-year-old girl who expressed the wish to die was in fact very scared and needed to talk about her fears.

When a dying child asks about death, although painful, it is important that parents and staff respond with truthful answers appropriate to the child's level of understanding. Staff need to explore their own fears regarding illness and death, as these have the potential to form barriers to communication and can be sensed by the child.

One of the greatest fears of dying children is separation. The presence of parents and siblings is vital to reduce feelings of abandonment and to detect behavioural cues indicating the child's distress. Special consideration is required when considering the emotional needs of the sedated and paralysed child. The family should be informed that conversations held at the bedside may be heard by the child, despite her apparent lack of response to noise.

Another important fear of the dying child is pain; therefore, effective pain relief is essential to relieve anxiety in both the child and parents. Elimination of pain must be a priority where death is inevitable, despite possible professional concerns over potentially hastening the child's death. A pain-free, dignified death is not only the right of the child, but can contribute to a positive grieving process for the parents.

Comfort is provided by attending to the physical and hygiene needs of the child, enabling parental and sibling involvement in decisions regarding times for washing, toiletries used, clothes for the child and rest pattern. Such involvement reduces siblings' feelings of isolation and maintains their inclusion within the family.

Involvement of the family provides for the individual needs of the child, such as adolescent boys who like to wear aftershave and girls wearing their favourite hairstyle or nail polish. For the older child, privacy is important and must be considered at all times.

Individual comfort-needs may also be met through consideration of the following:

- positioning of the child
- effects of drug therapies, e.g vasoconstrictors on skin integrity
- physiotherapy to prevent stiffness and contractures
- pressure-relieving aids, including special mattresses and beds
- massage oils and lotions, e.g. aromatherapy oils such as lavender to induce relaxation

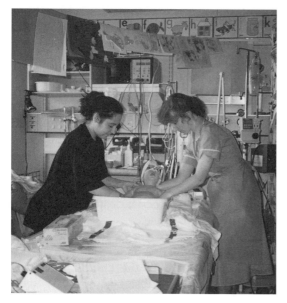

Figure 18.1 Family-centred care.

- toys, clothes and bedding from home
- posters and special photographs
- audio and video tapes.

Preparing and supporting parents

It is important that parents are given the opportunity to hold their child. At times this requires encouragement and support from nursing staff to ensure that parents feel confident and safe while surrounded by equipment and invasive monitoring. This facilitates the gradual process of saying 'goodbye'. Ongoing, unrestricted contact with family and friends will also facilitate this valuable process, but may not always be possible when life-saving interventions are required.

Case note 3

The mother of a dying neonate being nursed in Intensive Care, who herself required intensive nursing, gained great comfort knowing that her baby was lying on her nightdress and could therefore smell her — the only contact they would have.

Support of the family is essential. Grief and anxieties, beliefs and fears about death, may affect their ability to deal with difficult and stressful communications with their child whilst trying to provide optimum care and support. Knowledge of and relationship with the parents gives insight into the support strategies useful in helping the parents care for their child. As parents experience increasing difficulties, a supportive team of professionals is essential to ensure that feelings of parental inadequacy are acknowledged and minimalised. Consistency of honest communication, whilst not removing all hope, is paramount throughout the multidisciplinary team. Team Nursing will promote a supportive, trusting relationship, reducing the possibility of inconsistent or conflicting information. When death is acute and sudden, it is particularly difficult for professionals involved, as relationships with the family are limited. In this situation, parents are often concerned about involving siblings, wishing to protect them and anxious about their reactions. They must be supported and encouraged to be open and honest to enable the siblings to grieve.

Unexpected death of a child

Parents whose children are admitted to Intensive Care often feel that this is where their critically ill child will be cured, because it is a 'centre of excellence'. Sudden and unexpected death is a huge shock, the child having been swiftly transferred from A & E or another hospital. Such parents are psychologically unprepared, often disbelieving and denying the situation, and experiencing severe feelings of guilt, trying to make sense of what led to the admission, while adapting to the reality of the situation. Optimum communication is essential, as is providing every opportunity for contact with their child. Their involvement and consultation is both crucial and empowering in helping them work through their reactions to the death. They will be emotionally vulnerable, maybe hostile and intensely angry toward those caring for them and their child. Although difficult, it is important that staff support them through these feelings. Heightened sensitivity accompanying grief will also mean positive experiences will be treasured, while negative encounters and thoughtless comments will add to their pain (Miles & Perry 1985). Professionals feel they need to 'get it right' for these parents, but each situation is unique, and parental reactions are unpredictable. It is sensitive response to their cues which is important.

Death of a child with chronic illness

Parents of chronically sick dying children pose different challenges. They find it extremely hard to accept that no more can be done. This feeling is sometimes shared by staff, and long-term relationships can haze professional boundaries.

Information on the parents' experiences with their child's illness, previous coping strategies, and their cultural and religious needs, together with the relationship formed, will help to identify potential problems that may influence their ability to deal with their child's death. Again, this information must be shared within the multidisciplinary team to ensure optimal support.

Breaking bad news

Informing parents of the terminal nature of their child's illness or even of their death is one of the hardest tasks facing the professional. What matters most to parents is that the news is delivered in a sincere, sensitive manner. Celia Hindmarch (1993) quotes an outraged mother being told of her daughter's death by a yawning doctor, and conversely a bereaved father who appreciated the distress shown by his son's doctor.

The person imparting such news should be known and trusted by the parents, and possess good communication skills. A comfortable, private room should be chosen to ensure freedom from interruptions. Whenever possible, parents should be seen together; if this is not possible a close relative or friend should be present to give support and to listen to the facts that distraught parents may not hear. Eye contact is very important. Information should be given in a clear, calm manner, avoiding ambiguity and thereby preventing misunderstandings. Questions require

honest answers; withholding information will ultimately lead to greater distress and anger.

Time is required for assimilation of information and expression of response. Parents' understanding should be checked, and those points that appear confusing and difficult to assimilate should be repeated. An empathetic, comforting manner can facilitate talk of past loss and grief, and the need to express this should be respected. Continuing parent support must be assured.

Some parents, aware of their child's imminent death, may utilise the anticipatory grieving mechanism. They start grieving when prognosis is known. Such grieving may be evident in the way parents start talking about the seriousness of their child's condition and the probability of death. They may share fond memories and speak of the future without their child, including asking about procedures when children die and how these will be enacted. If prognosis of death is not definite but likely, parents often comment that it is safer to assume the worst and plan for it to avoid the possible turmoil of emotions if given hope for their child's survival. Parents may feel it appropriate to take their child home to die. Preparation may commence during this period with the help of available community services.

Supporting parents through this period of acceptance and preparation for their loss is an important part of the nursing role, which involves providing unconditional respect for all the emotions that parents express. If parents deny the severity of their child's condition, it is necessary to avoid reinforcement of such denial, by gently and consistently confirming the severity and terminal nature of their child's illness. This may be achieved by sensitively verbalising deteriorating observations of the child and not reinforcing positive parental statements, whilst maintaining parental confidence in the quality of the care given to the child.

Withdrawing from the environment is also a pain-avoidance mechanism. It may seem that there are fewer visits and less contact. This may be difficult for nursing staff to accept, but the reason for withdrawal must be recognised. Contact with local community support should be made to communicate the reality of the child's condition.

Making decisions

The time may come when decisions have to be made regarding the continuance or possible withdrawal of treatment. These decisions require serious consideration of the needs of both child and family. During this time it is helpful for nursing staff, with whom a relationship has been formed, to act as advocates encouraging parents to share their feelings and concerns. Broaching this subject is difficult for the professional, who may see it as a failure, when their prime aim is to save life. Continuation may offer only futile resuscitation attempts and recurrent, possibly painful treatments, while withdrawal may highlight many issues — emotional, religious, cultural and legal — all deserving respect and full discussion. The decision may be particularly difficult for parents whose children have survived many acute setbacks during a chronic illness or who remain conscious and alert despite the serious, terminal nature of their condition. Parents must be given the time needed to ensure full understanding of their child's condition, and have the opportunity to seek opinions from other members of the medical profession. Many parents in this painful situation experience tremendous guilt over 'giving up' on their child, and should not be allowed to feel that they have made the withdrawal decision alone. The consultant must take responsibility for the final decision if parents are unable to face this reality.

If brain death has been established and the implications explained, assimiliation of this information may take some time. The concept of brain death is hard to grasp, especially when parents observe their child's monitored heartbeat, and chest movements delivered by the ventilator. When parents deny brain death, it can be helpful for nursing staff to cease referring to the child as living, when carrying out care. This helps reinforce the child's death, and if consistent, will gradually help parents come to terms with it.

Organ donation

The subject of organ donation is very sensitive, and staff can find it difficult to raise, especially if death is sudden and parents are shocked and disbelieving. Although it may seem insensitive to broach the subject, many parents express regret if they have been unable to donate, due to their inability to think clearly at the time or to staff feelings regarding the request. It may be appropriate for a close friend or relative to open discussions with the parents, prior to discussion with nursing or medical staff. Often, older children have previously discussed their desire to donate organs if the opportunity arose; if so, it is important for the parents to carry out their child's wishes. Many parents gain great comfort and meaning in their loss, knowing someone is benefiting from what seems to be a pointless death. They will need time to discuss options with the Transplant Coordinator, who may be helpful in providing consistency and clarity of terminology. Some parents find agreement difficult and a final decision impossible, which must be respected and accepted.

Prior to donation, time should be given for the parents to hold and to say goodbye to their child. They may wish to organise accompanying toys, and clothes for their child to wear following last offices in theatre. Sometimes parents may wish to see their child again on the ICU following donation; they should be made aware that the body will be cold and will weigh less following major organ harvesting.

Organ donation is often possible in cases involving the coroner. Heart valves and corneas may be harvested up to 24 h after circulatory arrest where the parents wish to donate, but there is no time prior to the child's death. The Transplant Coordinator will maintain ongoing contact with the family following donation, informing them of the wellbeing of the anonymous recipients. This is an important service which can provide comfort during a sad and painful grieving process. If the donated organ fails, parents can feel devastated, experiencing further feelings of bereavement.

Caring for the family at time of death

Death may occur because of cardiopulmonary arrest, and in this instance it is particularly important to keep parents fully informed of events during the resuscitation attempt. In this situation, parents lose any sense of control, and failure to keep them fully informed at this time may lead to extreme anxiety and anger. A member of staff should be available to provide timely information and support, either within view of the resuscitation or, if parents do not wish to be present, in a private room nearby. The language used must be carefully chosen and medical jargon avoided. It is necessary to reinforce the seriousness of the situation and possibility of death, while maintaining some hope.

Many professionals express misgivings regarding the presence of parents at a resuscitation. While these should be considered, the rights of the parents to see what is being done for their child must be respected. Assumptions are made that extremely-upset parents require protection or that they may try to interfere with the treatment. Members of the medical and nursing team often feel inhibited and vulnerable. Exposure to the parents' acute emotions may interfere with professional defences used to cope with one's own feelings. It is likely that parents attending resuscitation attempts are more concerned with their child than with the treatment (Hindmarch 1993). Indeed, parents have stated that their own feelings of guilt and shame have been reduced having seen efforts taken to save their child and knowing everything possible was done.

During resuscitation, parents should be informed of any deterioration, while being aware that treatment continues. When drug therapy fails to gain a positive response, concerns of the team should be made known. At this time parents often begin to question the futility of the resuscitation and may ask about the effects of oxygen deficit on the brain and other organs. An awareness of their child's impending death may prompt parents to ask for treatment to stop so they may hold their child. If baptism has not previously been performed, they may request it, and should there be insufficient time for the hospital Chaplain to attend, this responsibility may fall on the nursing staff.

When the child's death is anticipated, time is available to help prepare the parents and for their involvement in the decision making.

Parents are often concerned about the way their child will die; assurance that adequate sedation and pain relief will be given is essential. Parents should be informed that their child may continue to breathe, albeit abnormally, for a period of time. In addition, changes in colour and body temperature should be explained. Adequate time should be given to discuss these issues, as they often concern parents, particularly those that have never experienced death. Preparation proves more beneficial than withholding information to protect parents from what may be shocking or distressing. The timing and process of treatment withdrawal should be planned with the parents, helping them to choose what feels right for both themselves and their child. If parents wish, facilities should be provided giving privacy for family and friends to be present. Assurance must be given that their nurse will be available throughout this time.

When death is imminent the maximum amount of monitoring equipment and invasive lines should be removed, if coagulation is normal. The parents should be encouraged and supported to hold their child to say goodbye. This may be too difficult for them. Only one parent may wish to stay with their child, or they may ask the nurse to do so, but their decisions must be respected and supported. Some parents find it too hard and frightening to be left alone with their dying child, whereas others need privacy to experience this important time.

Unfortunately, it is not always possible for parents to be present, and the news may be given by phone or on their arrival at the hospital. In the former, it is important that they be prepared for the news, ideally not being alone when receiving it, and advised not to drive when travelling to the hospital. When talking of the death, it is helpful to assure parents that everything possible was done for their child, that they died pain free, and they were not alone — a photograph of a staff member holding their child can be important and comforting to the parents.

The family visiting the child after death

Members of the family and friends may also

wish to say goodbye. This final visit is important, proving the reality of the child's death, especially for those not present at the time of death. This will assist grieving. Where the child is disfigured due to cause of death and/or treatment given to maintain life, special consideration and preparation should be given when encouraging parents to be with their child. Memories of their child's appearance can stay with them, possibly exacerbating suffering experienced (Miles & Perry 1985). Irrespective of appearance, it is usually important for parents to be present after their child's death, and the reality of the mutilation may be less than they would otherwise fantasise. However, parents may choose to remember their child as they looked before, in happier times. Should one parent not wish to see their child, that decision should be respected and supported. It may be that a visit to the Chapel or Funeral Director is more appropriate, and this can be suggested if a hospital visit feels too difficult. Particular sensitivity is required for parents of a neonate who has died, as they may be saying hello and goodbye to their baby at the same time, experiencing very complex emotions.

Case note 4

A mother whose baby had died aged 12 days, following cardiac surgery, gained great comfort from being able to hold him next to her skin — something she had been unable to do, even at his birth.

Siblings are often called the 'forgotten mourners'. They also experience grief, and what they are told of the death is of great importance. Their understanding depends on their age and development, with older children showing more distress, on account of their greater understanding of the reality of death. Involvement rather than isolation helps siblings deal with their grief.

Throughout this time, the parents should be aware of the availability of the hospital chaplaincy and offered their services. Some parents have no religious faith but gain comfort from their child's receiving a blessing. Religious and cultural needs must be taken into account when caring for the dying child and her family, adhering to traditional rituals where orthodox practice exists. It is prudent to note these religious and cultural tenets, including names of the appropriate religious ministers, preventing confusion which can cause anxiety and difficulty for staff caring for the family.

When the family feel the time is right, last offices can be performed, including any specific religious practices relevant to the individual child. The child should be washed and wounds covered with clean dressings. Parents should be encouraged to help with this, as it is their last opportunity to physically care for their child. However, if it is too difficult for them, they should not be pressurised. They may have a special outfit for their child to wear; if not, it is comforting if suitable clothing can be provided by the Unit in the short term.

This is also the time when mementoes may be obtained for the parents. These include photographs of the child and family, hand and/or foot prints and a lock of hair. When a twin has died, a photograph of the babies together can be of great importance in the future, especially to the surviving twin. Some parents do not want a photograph of their dead child at this time, but often change their minds. A photograph should be kept safe should they later request it. Instant photographs may be copied if the quality is poor. When a neonate has died, there will be few mementoes available, so baby's wrist band, birth card and ultrasound scan may be very important to those parents experiencing birth and death so closely together.

Caring for the bereaved family

Time taken prior to leaving the hospital is very individual. Parents often need someone to listen; *being there* is more important than *doing*. Staff should feel able to express their own feelings, enabling parents to recognise that staff also cared for their child, whilst maintaining a professional supportive manner. Many staff feel unsure and insecure when caring for parents in such pain and distress.

Case note 5

A father whose son had died, wrote 'You know as well as I do that there is no good way to give bad news. Gentle words don't humanise brutal facts. A newly bereaved parent is inconsolable, and no amount of cups of tea or soft furnishings can cushion the unacceptable.

Treat us like lost children! We are stunned by the enormity of the loss and can't think of anything else. Leave us for a little while, maybe, but be around. We are in an unfamiliar world. This is your domain. You know about the systems and practices and you are thinking more clearly than we are.

Please don't expect yourselves to soften the blow. No-one can! ... Being there, giving practical help, however basic, is enough. Don't take anything we say personally and accept that we are grateful for your help even though we appear to ignore it' (Shawe 1992).

Anger, often expressed by a bereaved parent at this time, is a particularly difficult emotion for staff members to experience, possibly generating feelings of professional failure. It is important to stay with such parents, enabling them to express these emotions in a safe place. Worried relatives sometimes suggest the use of tranquillisers for distraught parents, often because of their own anxieties in caring for them, and careful thought should be given before taking this option.

Case note 6

'Robby was dead and I was being given a pill to make it go away. Impossible' (Sharnoff Schiff 1978).

Conversely, some parents especially following unexpected death, appear shocked and numb, later stating the feeling to be trance-like, remembering only certain details. Whichever emotions are experienced, certain aspects will be recalled in the finest detail — often the way they were told of their child's death, and the treatment given by the staff caring for them at that time.

It is necessary to provide the parents with information needed to deal with the procedures to be carried out during the following days. These include details of death certificate collec-

tion, registration of death, coroner involvement, if applicable, funeral arrangements and, most importantly, ways of being supported through the grieving period. Although this is given verbally, possibly in the presence of a family member or friend, a package of such information together with a contact name and telephone number of a staff member is beneficial, so parents can read it when they are better able to assimilate the details (Miles & Perry 1985).

It is essential that recognition is given of the time and patience required by the grieving family from the staff. The Department of Health guidelines, 'Care of the dying in hospital' suggest that a designated person be made responsible for the follow-up support of these parents who are made aware of the help and support that will be available to them. Communication with other departments and agencies is imperative – a routine clinic appointment card arriving weeks following the child's death, can produce profound distress for the newly grieving parents.

Continuing care of the family

Invitation to a 6 week follow-up meeting with the consultant who treated their child, together with social worker, bereavement counsellor or genetic counsellor as appropriate, is vital. This fulfils the need of grieving parents to re-explore the course of their child's illness. This is particularly important in the case of a postmortem, where previous questions may now be answered. Equally, it is around this time that the parents' support network seems to fall below the normal level; therefore such a follow-up meeting often has greater importance (Koocher 1994).

Parental grief and mourning

The features of grief and mourning have been studied in depth, but the death of a child is still at times underestimated, the natural order of life is changed. Sumner et al (1991) suggest that psychiatric disturbances are three times more likely in parents whose children have died in PICU. However, a study at the Alder Centre in 1991 suggested that these disturbances are in fact normal for grieving parents, the loss of a child being unlike other bereavements. The grief process for a parent is, by its nature, complicated, perhaps without resolution. Peppers and Knapp (1980) suggest there may be 'shadow-grief' in grieving mothers and 'enduring sorrow', the loss of a child being the loss of a future and security. Life is disorganised by grief, but can gradually be reorganised in a new way by helping parents on their personal journeys. It is important that needs are met on an individual basis. The intensive care unit may be unable to provide such ongoing support, but it is important that close liaison is maintained with community professionals, referring on to appropriate helping agencies or voluntary support networks, all of which

may prevent an unhealthy outcome from incomplete mourning.

Continuing contact with the intensive care unit can, however, provide comfort for many parents, thereby acknowledging the importance of their dead child. Receipt of a letter from a particular nurse, or a card on the anniversary of the death can give much comfort.

Case note 7

A mother invited to a bereaved parents support group stated that 'suddenly the hospital was not a place full of professional strangers but a place of caring people who had really cared for my son.'

REFERENCES

Hindmarch C 1993 On the death of a child. Radcliffe, Oxford
Koocher G P 1994 Preventative intervention following a child's death. Psychotherapy 31(3):377–382
Lansdowne R, Benjamin G 1985 The development of the concept of death in children aged 5 years to 9 years. Child Care, Health and Development 11:13–20
Miles M Y S, Perry K 1985 Parental responses to sudden accidental death of a child. Critical Care Quarterly 8(1):73–84

Peppers L G, Knapp R J 1980 Motherhood and mourning. Praeger, New York
Sharnoff Schiff H 1978 The bereaved parent. Penguin, Harmondsworth, p 3
Shawe M (ed) 1992 Enduring, sharing, loving. Darton, Longman and Todd, London, p 83
Sumner M, Dinwiddie R, Matthew D J, Skuse D H 1991 Loss on a paediatric intensive care unit: parental reactions. Care of the Critically Ill 7(2):64–66

19

Managing pain in critically ill children

Jayne Fisher   Dawn Harrison

Critically ill children experience pain for a variety of reasons. These include:

- trauma
- surgical intervention
- intubation
- invasive procedures, e.g chest drain insertion, central line placement and suctioning.

Exposure to the paediatric intensive care (PIC) environment, with its unfamiliar sights and multiple sounds, can contribute to the child's experience of pain. Previous painful experiences also contribute by increasing anxiety. The age at which a child can recall a painful experience remains open to debate, but Johnston (1993) suggests that there is no clear evidence that a child under 6 months of age retains a memory for past painful experiences.

Pain is a complex, personal and multidimensional phenomenon incorporating both physiological and psychological components (Carter 1994) which often transcend conventional medical and nursing interventions. Therefore, no single profession assumes responsibility for pain control. Consequently, enormous disparity exists between the management of paediatric and adult pain. Multiple misconceptions surround the neonate's response to pain. The complexities of assessment deter many, and the difficulty in attaining accurate information about medications results all too frequently in ineffective management of paediatric pain. There is a vital role to play in the ongoing assessment and provision of optimal pain relief, as there is insufficient research to guide the practitioner (Brill 1992).

This chapter provides an overview of the physiology of pain, assessment tools appropriate for use in the PIC environment, current pharmacological management, and non-pharmacological approaches to pain management.

PHYSIOLOGY OF PAIN

Perception of pain is complex and varies greatly from one individual and from one occasion to another, because of factors such as personality, mood, environment and the duration of the pain. However, we have some understanding of the pathways involved in the transmission of acute pain signals and how they are modified (Fig. 19.1).

Acute pain is frequently caused by tissue damage. The resulting inflammatory reaction causes local release of mediators such as prostaglandins, histamine, bradykinin, substance P and noradrenaline. Pain sensation is detected by free nerve endings or nociceptors and transmitted along unmyelinated slow C fibres (dull, diffuse pain) or small myelinated fast A fibres (sharp, well-localised pain), to cell bodies in the dorsal root ganglia. Fibres from these cells synapse in the substantia gelatinosa, Rexed laminae II and III, and the nucleus proprius, laminae IV to VI, of the dorsal horn of the spinal cord, causing activation of interneurons, resulting in the release of substance P, an 11 amino acid neuropeptide.

Subsequent activation of neurons in laminae VII and VIII of the anterolateral cord results in transmission of ascending signals via the spinothalamic and spinoreticular tracts. This is an oligosynaptic system which sends signals to various areas of the central nervous system including the posteroventral thalamic nucleus and brainstem reticular formation (Fig. 19.2). These nuclei project somatotopically to the somatosensory area of the postcentral gyrus of the cerebral cortex and diffusely to the whole non-primary cortex, respectively; the former mediates pinprick sensation while the latter is responsible for a range of sensations from irritating to excruciating. A multisynaptic system ascends from the posterior cord, including Lissauer's tracts which carry axons from neurons of the substantia gelatinosa to the posteromedial

ventral nucleus of the thalamus. This system has no facility for somatotopic localisation, but allows the full appreciation of diffuse persistent pain. These pathways develop early in fetal life and are essentially complete by the time of birth (Rogers & Helfaer 1995, Thorpe 1996).

Descending control originates in the cerebral cortex, diencephalon and brainstem, accounting for the emotional responses and previous experiences of pain. Descending inhibition of pain pathways at the level of the dorsal horn neurons is mediated by various nuclei such as the mesencephalic periaqueductal grey, some of the raphe nuclei and the locus caeruleus. Endogenous opioid peptides, serotonin and noradrenaline are the likely neurotransmitters involved. These descending pathways develop late in fetal life and continue to mature over the first year of life.

The Gate Control Theory of pain (Fig. 19.3) assists the understanding of the interaction of pain pathways. The 'gate' resides in the substantia gelatinosa, where the transmission of pain signals is either blocked or enhanced. Inhibitory signals are mediated by thick myelinated AB fibres which respond to light touch, vibration, scratching and rubbing, resulting in closure of the gate by preventing activation of T (target) cells. Central control can alter the sensitivity of the gate. Cognitive processes such as fear and anxiety can enhance pain by opening the gate mechanism, whereas behavioural interventions, for instance relaxation or distraction techniques, may reduce the perception of pain by closing the gate.

Treatment of pain can be targeted at various points in the pathway. The synthesis of prostaglandins at the site of injury can be effectively blocked by non-steroidal antiinflammatory drugs (NSAIDs) such as diclofenac. Local anaesthetics may be used to block the transmission of impulses along nerve fibres, the non-myelinated C fibres being most readily affected; these drugs may also be used by the extradural and intrathecal routes to block transmission in spinal nerve roots and the spinal cord itself. The opiates act at sites within the central nervous system, increasing centrally-mediated inhibition from the mesencephalic periaqueductal grey or blocking afferent impulses at the level of the substantia

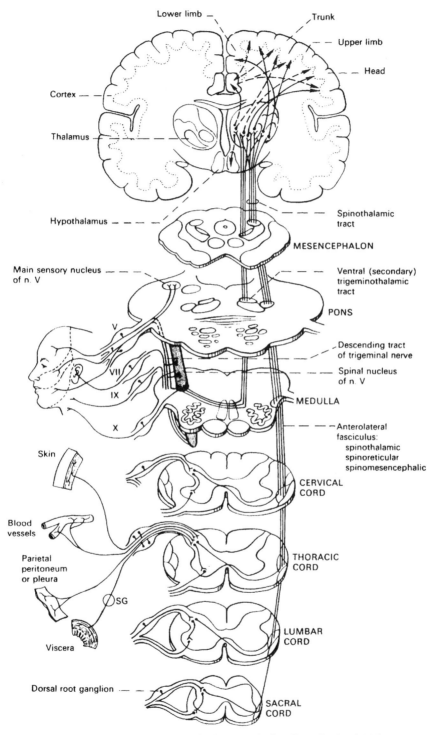

Figure 19.1 Primary neural pathways of pain transmission. From Bonica (1990).

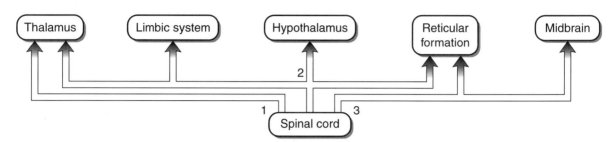

Figure 19.2 Projection tracts from spinal cord to brain centres. Final pathways will be to cortex where pain perception occurs. 1, spinothalamic tract system; 2, spinoreticular tract system; 3, spinomesencephalic tract system. Adapted from Puntillo (1991).

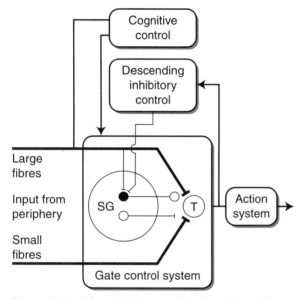

Figure 19.3 Schematic diagram of the Gate Control Theory of pain. SG, substantia gelatinosa; T, transmission cells. From Thorpe (1996).

gelatinosa. The latter site of action explains the effectiveness of extradural and intrathecal opiates. Tramadol is thought to act by enhancing descending serotoninergic and noradrenergic inhibitory pathways. At present the manufacturer does not recommend use of this drug in children, but experience has shown that it can be effective in the child over 25 kg, where a dose of 2 mg/kg intravenously every 4–6 h has controlled pain effectively (Mikhelson & Ciplin 1993).

ASSESSMENT OF PAIN

Successful pain management is based on assess-ment relevant to the child's developmental and cognitive level. The Royal College of Surgeons and Royal College of Anaesthetists Report (1990) concluded that accurate assessment is essential if intervention is to be effective.

Within the paediatric critical care environ-ment, pain assessment is exceptionally challeng-ing. The child's ability to communicate pain is affected by altered level of consciousness, intuba-tion, paralysis and/or sedation, developmental level, cultural background and parental presence or absence. Physiological responses to hypoxia, pyrexia, reduced cardiac output and raised intracranial pressure can mimic pain symptoms, including tachycardia, tachypnoea, pallor and agitation. The foundations of good pain manage-ment rest on the accurate and timely recognition of pain experienced by children.

The preverbal and preschool child presents particular challenges because of their limited vocabulary and inability to communicate pres-ence and intensities of pain. Older children may also present difficulties because of their limited vocabulary and inexperience (Schechter 1989, Eland 1990). The underlying principle to an accurate pain assessment appears to be the ability of the practitioner to classify the child's level of cognitive development, as this can prove to be one of the most influential factors in selecting a tool that can be utilised effectively. The nurse should discuss the child's previous experience and developmental level with the parents, as these will influence how the child reacts to pain.

Pain assessment tools used in clinical practice can be divided into three major categories:

- behavioural
- physiological
- self report.

Behavioural assessment

This is subdivided into infant and child assessment.

Infant assessment

The infant's facial expression is used as a baseline for assessment in the *Neonatal Facial Coding System* (NFCS) developed by Grunau and Craig (1990). Studies performed by the authors elicited various responses to pain, notably open lips, mouth stretch, taut tongue, brow bulge and eye squeeze.

Facial expression is documented as the most reliable behavioural assessment tool in the neonate's response to pain (Craig et al 1992, Dale 1986, 1989, Marvin & Pomietto 1991). Crying is a universally accepted sign of distress in the infant. The experienced assessor is able to recognise and differentiate types of cry such as pain, hunger or other discomfort. Wolff (1974) described the cry of the infant in pain as displaying an urgent need for a response. On suffering pain, infants will display a loud cry which ceases when the painful stimulus is withdrawn. Infants of 6 months and older have been proven to associate objects and individuals with pain and will begin to cry before the stimulus has occurred. Although various studies have been performed on the infant's physical response to pain no data can be elicited to show any specific motor activity in response to the experience (Craig et al 1992).

Child assessment

Young children have difficulty in accurately using self-report assessment tools. To overcome this problem and to reliably document pain behaviour in 1–5 year olds, a variety of assessment criteria have been developed.

Tarbell et al (1992) developed the *Toddler–Preschooler Postoperative Pain Scale* (TPPS) from

evaluation of previous studies. The scale uses three observational categories (Box 19.1)

Box 19.1 Observational categories of the Toddler–Preschooler Postoperative Pain Scale

- verbal pain expression: verbal pain, complaint cry, scream, groan, moan, grunt
- facial pain expression: open mouth, lips pulled back at corners, closed eyes, furrowed forehead
- bodily pain expression: rubbing area, touching painful area.

The preschool child has limited ability to communicate the intensity, duration and quality of pain, necessitating the use of behavioural assessment tools. Assessment based on behaviour alone creates the danger of inappropriate assumptions being made. The principal behavioural tool used is the *Children's Hospital of Eastern Ontario Pain Scale* (CHEOPS) (McGrath et al 1985), which was developed for use in assessment of postoperative pain in under-5s.

Six behaviours are observed which are indicative of pain. Potential total scores from all categories are: 4, indicating an absence of pain, to 13, suggesting severe pain. Carter (1994) supports CHEOPS as a valid measurement tool when compared with observational pain scales. This scale can be utilised effectively in PIC, although practitioners should remember that other factors can influence a child's behaviour, including parental presence and perception of stress.

Physiological assessment

The reliability of physiological responses to pain is often questioned. Activation of the adrenergic nervous system may only be observed during the initial pain stimulus; therefore, tachycardia, hypertension, pupil dilation and diaphoresis could be attributed to other stimuli. Chronic pain can cause a rebound effect of vagal stimulation, including a fall in heart rate, respiratory rate and blood pressure.

Physiological responses to pain appear more

obvious in infants. Neonatal responses to short periods of pain have been extensively researched, utilising heel prick or circumcision as a source of acute pain. However, critics of physiological assessment suggest that neither of these can reproduce the pain a sick neonate is likely to undergo whilst receiving intensive care (Carter 1994).

Self-report techniques

Self report tools rely on the child's capacity to communicate her level of pain. Children under the age of 6 rarely understand the concept of pain, and are unable to communicate its severity (Eland & Anderson 1977); therefore, self-assessment tools are inaccurate in preschool children. However, it has also been suggested that children of 5 years can accurately communicate their pain on a rating scale relevant to their cognitive development. Despite the proliferation of paediatric pain assessment tools, research regarding the appropriateness of these instruments within the paediatric critical care environment is limited.

Faces scales (Fig. 19.4)

Wong & Wilson's (1995) faces scale uses a range of six faces in cartoon form, ranging from a smiling face that is free of pain to a face which displays the maximum amount of pain that one could feel. The child then chooses the face relevant to how he feels. Further scales have evolved based on similar principles, notably Douhit's (1990) faces scale, which uses slightly more detail, and Beyer's Oucher scale. Faces scales in use have been clinically validated; however, their use in the critical care environment is limited to the assessment of the conscious postoperative child.

Hester poker chip pain assessment tool

With this tool (Hester 1979) the child is given five 'poker chips' and informed that each 'chip' represents a 'piece of pain': one chip equates to a 'little pain', whereas all chips represent a 'big pain'. The child is then asked to display the intensity by selecting the relevant number of chips. A score of 0–5 provides information on the effectiveness of analgesia. Although the tool has been validated for use with children receiving immunisation, it could be adapted for use in PIC in the assessment of the awake postoperative child when used in conjunction with play therapy. Ross & Ross (1988) question its validity on the grounds that young children may not possess adequate numeracy skills. They suggest that chips of differing sizes could be a suitable adaptation.

Eland color tool

Using a body outline (front and back view) and eight crayons, the child is asked to point to the crayon which represents her biggest pain. She then chooses three more crayons representing pain which is a 'little less pain', 'little pain' and 'no pain'. The crayons selected are then arranged in order of pain representation. The child is asked to show on the body outlines where it hurts and to colour that area using the relevant crayon colour. This enables the professional to identify the site and intensity of pain, resulting in effective evaluation of analgesia. Impaired motor strength and coordination in the critically ill child may hinder use of this tool.

Oucher scale

This scale was developed to assist clinicians in measuring pain in 3–12-year-olds, facilitating intervention and ongoing evaluation. Photographs of the face of a 3 year old boy, ranging from no pain to a photograph of the same child suffering a painful experience, are displayed on a vertical scale. The tool can be utilised in two ways: preschool children can identify the face which represents how they feel (or how the pain makes them feel); the older child who has adequate numeracy skills may utilise the numbers to rank pain on the scale from 0 to 100.

The visual analogue scale

This scale uses the mother's perception of her children's pain. It comprises a 10 cm line with 'no

Pain Rating Scales for Children

PAIN SCALE/DESCRIPTION	INSTRUCTIONS	RECOMMENDED AGE
FACES Pain Rating Scale* (Nix, Clutter, and Wong, 1994; Wong and Baker, 1988): Consists of six cartoon faces ranging from smiling face for "no pain" to tearful face for "worst pain"	Explain to child that each face is for a person who feels happy because there is no pain (hurt) or sad because there is some or a lot of pain. Face 0 is very happy because there is no hurt. Face 1 hurts just a little bit. Face 2 hurts a little more. Face 3 hurts even more. Face 4 hurts a whole lot, but Face 5 hurts as much as you can imagine, although you don't have to be crying to feel this bad. Ask child to choose face that best describes own pain. Record the number under chosen face on pain assessment record.	Children as young as 3 years

0	1	2	3	4	5

| Oucher[†] (Beyer, 1989): Consists of six photographs of child's face representing "no hurt" to "biggest hurt you could ever have"; also includes a vertical scale with numbers from 0 to 100; scales for African-American and Hispanic children have been developed (Villarruel and Denyes, 1991) and validated (Beyer, Denyes, and Villarruel, 1992) | *Photographs:* Explain to child that face at bottom has "no hurt"; second picture, "just a little bit of hurt"; third picture, a "little bit more"; fourth picture, "even more hurt"; fifth picture, "*pretty* much hurt'; and last picture, "biggest hurt you could ever have." Ask child to choose face that best describes own pain.
Numbers: Explain to child that 0 means you have "no hurt"; 0 to 29, "little hurts"; 30 to 69, "middle hurts"; 70 to 99, "big hurts"; and 100, "biggest hurt you could ever have." Ask child to choose any number between 0 and 100, not just numbers pictured on Oucher, that best describes own pain. | Children 3–13 years; use numeric scale if child can count to 100 by 1s and identify larger of any two numbers (as in original instructions), or by 10s (Jordan-Marsh and others, 1994); otherwise use photographic scale |
| Numeric Scale: Uses straight line with end points identified as "no pain" and "worst pain"; divisions along line are maked in units from 0 to 10 (high number may vary) | Explain to child that at one end of the line is a 0, which means that a person feels no pain (hurt). At the other end is a 10, which means the person feels the worst pain imaginable. The numbers 1 to 9 are for a very little pain to a whole lot of pain. Ask child to choose number that best describes own pain. | Children as young as 5 years, provided they can count and have some concept of numbers and their values of more or less |

No pain   Worst pain

0	1	2	3	4	5	6	7	8	9	10

| Poker chip tool[‡]: Uses four red poker chips placed horizontally in front of child | Tell child, "These are pieces of hurt." Beginning at the chip nearest child's left side and ending at the one nearest child's right side, point to chips and say, "This [the first chip] is a little bit of hurt and this [the fourth chip] is the most hurt you could ever have." For a young child or for any child who does not comprehend the instructions, clarify by saying, "That means this [the first chip] is just a little hurt; this [the second chip] is a little more hurt; this [the third chip] is more hurt; and this [the fourth chip] is the most hurt you could ever have." Ask child, "How many pieces of hurt do you have right now?" Children without pain will say they don't have any. Clarify child's answer by words such as "Oh, you have a little hurt? Tell me about the hurt." Elicit descriptors, location, and cause. Ask the child, "What would you like me to do for you?" Record number of chips selected. | Children as young as 4 to $4\frac{1}{2}$ years, provided they can count and have some concept of numbers |

*Several variations of faces scales exist. Complimentary copies of Wong/Baker FACES Scale are available from Purdue Frederick Co., 100 Connecticut Ave., Norwalk, CT 06856; (203) 853-0123, ext. 4010. For translations of FACES, see Appendix F.
[†]Oucher is available for a fee from Judith E. Beyer, PhD, RN, P.O. Box 47004, Aurora, CO 80047-0004.
[‡]Instructions for Poker Chip Tool and Word Graphic Rating Scale from Acute Pain Management Guideline Panel: *Acute pain management in infants, children, and adolescents: operative and medical procedures; quick reference guide for clinicians*, AHCPR Pub No 92-0020, Rockville, MD, 1992, Agency for Health Care Policy and Research, Public Health Service, US Department of Health and Human Services. Poker Chip Tool developed in 1975 by Nancy O. Hester, University of Colorado Health Sciences Center, Denver, CO. Spanish instructions from Jordan-Marsh M and others: *The Harbor-UCLA Medical Center Humor Project for Children*, Los Angeles 1990, Harbor-UCLA Medical Center.

Figure 19.4   Pain rating scales for children. From Wong & Wilson (1995), with permission.

pain' at one end and 'as painful as it could possibly be' at the other. Mothers are asked to plot their perception of the intensity of pain, giving a score between 0 and 10. Eland (1990) found that a parent's perception of pain correlates closely with the child's perception.

Linear scales

There are a number of linear scales in use, ranging from the well-known pain thermometer to simple descriptive scales. They can be adapted for use in the critical-care setting, although impaired motor coordination and altered visual perception may affect reliability.

The majority of the above tools can be implemented for use in the conscious child. Accurate assessment is difficult in the paralysed and sedated child. There is little documented evidence of assessment tools relevant to the ventilated and sedated child. Many critical care areas use sedation scoring as an alternative (see Box 19.2).

Box 19.2 Sedation score

1. unresponsive
2. moving with suction or handling only
3. moving spontaneously
4. awake but settled
5. irritable and unmanageable.

PHARMACOLOGICAL MANAGEMENT OF PAIN

There are many effective analgesics available (Table 19.1) but there is limited research into their use within paediatric intensive care, the majority of information being extrapolated from adult studies (Berde 1989). Analgesic agents currently used in PIC include opioids, non-opioids and local anaesthetics. The type of analgesia utilised is determined by assessment or whether systemic or local therapy is indicated. A multiplicity of adjunctive medications, including sedatives, anticonvulsants, anxiolytics and neuroleptics, are also used. There has also been an increase in the use of regional analgesia, particularly in postoperative patients.

Table 19.1 Commonly used analgesics in the PICU

Drug	Dose	Route/method
Fentanyl	4–8 µg/kg/h	Intravenous infusion
Morphine sulphate	10–30 µg/kg/h	Intravenous infusion
Alfentanil	30 µg/kg/h	Intravenous infusion
Diclofenac	1–3 mg/kg/24 h	Oral/rectal
Paracetamol	10–15 mg/kg/dose	Oral/rectal

Table 19.2 The four main opioid receptor sites

Receptor	Location	Action
mu (µ) receptors	Thalamus Substania gelatinosa of the spinal cord	Respiratory depression Euphoria Supraspinal analgesia Physical dependence
Delta (δ) receptors	Deep cortex of the brain Amygdala	Respiratory depression Euphoria Supraspinal analgesia Physical dependence Morphine less effective at these receptors than endogenous encephalins
Kappa (κ) receptors	Spinal cord Hypothalamus	Spinal analgesia Miosis Sedation Hypothermia Secretion of ADH
Sigma (σ) receptors		Dysphoria Hallucinations Respiratory stimulation Vasomotor stimulation

Opioids

Opioid analgesics continue to be the single most important group of drugs in the management of pain within paediatric intensive care. Opioids, whether naturally occurring or synthetic, are drugs with a morphine-like effect, producing analgesia by acting as either complete or partial agonists at opioid receptor sites throughout the central nervous system (CNS), imitating the effects of endogenous opioids.

There are four main opioid receptor sites (Table 19.2). Dysphoria and hallucinations occur particularly with mixed agonist–antagonist drugs (Snyder 1984). The variance in action and side effects of differing opioids may relate to the disparate receptor sites. The most commonly used opioids, morphine and fentanyl are agonists. Pure agonists essentially have no ceiling effects, increased doses provide increased intensity of analgesia and sedation (Brill 1992).

Effects of opioids are shown in Box 19.3. (see also Table 19.3.) Respiratory depression is of particular concern in infants because of immaturity of hepatic conjugation and difference in the number of receptor sites dependent on age (Brill 1992).

Box 19.3 Effects of opioids

- suppression of the autonomic responses to noxious stimuli, such as tachycardia, hypertension and sweating
- dose-dependent respiratory and CNS depression
- diminished response of the respiratory centre to hypercapnia and hypoxaemia
- decreased respiratory rate and tidal volumes
- dysphoria and euphoria
- cough suppression
- nausea and vomiting
- reduced gut motility
- increased sphincter tone
- urinary retention
- histamine release
- vasodilatation
- pruritis.

Morphine

Morphine remains the most commonly used opiod, as it is inexpensive, extensively researched and flexible in administration. Morphine usage results in histamine release, particularly following rapid intravenous administration, resulting in hypotension and/or bronchospasm.

Fentanyl

Fentanyl is a potent, synthetically derived opioid structurally related to pethidine. It is approximately 80–100 times more potent than morphine (Paice & Buck 1993). Fentanyl's profound lipid solubility results in rapid onset of 90–180 s, although its duration of action is up to 40 min, which is shorter than morphine. It has few adverse effects on haemodynamics and generates much less histamine release than morphine. Adverse effects include muscular rigidity, particularly after rapid intravenous administration and spontaneous respiration, necessitating muscle relaxants or naloxone if ventilation is sufficiently compromised.

Alfentanil

Alfentanil is a short-acting analogue of fentanyl which differs from fentanyl in its distribution and elimination from the body. It has approximately one-third the potency of fentanyl. When administered in low doses it does not appear to have any advantage over fentanyl, exerting very similar cardiorespiratory effects.

Table 19.3 Cardiovascular effects of common analgesics and sedatives

Drug	Heart rate	Blood pressure (arterial)	Cardiac index	Systemic vascular resistance	Central venous pressure	Pulmonary artery pressure
Morphine	↓	mild ↓	no change	↓	↓	minimal ↓
Fentanyl	↓	no change	no change	no change	no change	no change
Midazolam	minimal change	mild ↓	mild ↓	minimal change	mild ↓	no change
Chloral hydrate	no change to mild ↓	no change	no change to mild ↓	no change	no change	unknown
Opioid and midazolam	↓	↓↓	↓–↓↓	↑	↓	↓

Adapted from Kaplan (1983).

Antagonists, tolerance and cessation

With all opioids it is important to appreciate that the duration of the respiratory depression exceeds the duration of the analgesic or sedative effect. Opioid antagonists such as naloxone must be administered with caution on account of the side effects of dysphoria, nausea and vomiting, anxiety and potentially severe pain. Naloxone is a mu and kappa antagonist, competitively inhibiting kappa and mu antagonists. More severe side effects can occur, including tachypnoea, tachycardia, hypertension, pulmonary oedema and even sudden death.

Prolonged administration of opioids may result in tolerance, necessitating increased drug dosage. Physical dependence can occur, and therefore abrupt cessation of opioids should be avoided to prevent withdrawal syndrome. Gradual weaning prevents the child experiencing uncomfortable symptoms that can also mimic the onset of sepsis.

Non-steroidal antiinflammatory drugs (NSAIDs)

NSAIDs have analgesic, antiinflammatory and antipyretic properties due to interference with prostaglandin production. They include ibuprofen, diclofenac and aspirin. Aspirin is not recommended for use in children less than 12 years, because of its possible association with Reye's syndrome. Prostaglandins are naturally occurring fatty acids responsible for sensitising the nerve endings to pain transmission and enhancing oedema formation and leukocyte infiltration. The pain cycle is interrupted by interference with arachidonic acid metabolism preventing prostaglandin release in response to cell damage (Fig. 19.5). NSAIDs are very effective when used in combination with opioids for acute pain and singular use for chronic pain. The most significant side effect is gastrointestinal bleeding, which also commonly occurs in critically ill children as a result of stress.

Paracetamol

Paracetamol is extremely useful for mild to moderate pain. It has no antiinflammatory properties but is effective as an antipyretic. Although not as effective as ibuprofen, administration does not result in the potential problems of gastric irritation or platelet aggregation.

Adjunctive medications for pain control

Sedatives and hypnotics consitute an important adjunct to pain management; they should not be administered in place of analgesia but used in conjunction with other agents to provide effective analgesia. Sedatives can eliminate the emotional aspects of pain by inducing sleep, anxiolysis and amnesia. Benzodiazepines and chloral hydrate are the mainstay of sedative therapy.

Benzodiazepines

Benzodiazepines facilitate the inhibitory effect of gamma aminobutyric acid (GABA) on neural transmission at limbic, thalamic, hypothalamic

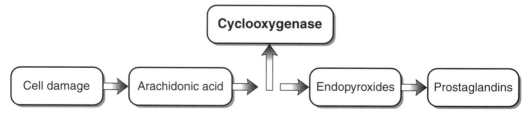

Figure 19.5 Mechanism of NSAIDs in interrupting the pain cycle: NSAIDs interfere with the cyclooxygenase system, inhibiting the formation of prostaglandins.

and spinal receptors in the CNS, preventing overstimulation of the brain. Benzodiazepines cause sedation, anxiolysis and amnesia for the duration of the infusion. Differences between benzodiazepines are the duration of action and the degree of amnesia attained. Administration also results in skeletal muscle relaxation through the inhibition of afferent spinal pathways. This effect is potentiated when used in combination with neuromuscular blocking agents. Lorazepam and diazepam are not recommended for use as sedation for children (Rogers & Helfaer 1995).

Midazolam is the most commonly used benzodiazepine in the PICU because of its compatibility with most intravenous solutions and lack of cardiovascular side effects, providing the patient is not hypovolaemic (Park & Navapurkar 1994).

Tolerance to midazolam is well documented but is easily overcome by increasing the doses during administration. This can become problematic if the sedation is abruptly discontinued but can be overcome by gradual weaning. Abrupt withdrawal can result in abnormal movements, fitting, a hyperaware state and cardiovascular instability. There is little research exploring benzodiazepine withdrawal in paediatric intensive care; that available looks at the use of midazolam in combination with fentanyl or morphine (Marsh et al 1994). A gradual reduction in the infused dose, and/or substitution with an oral benzodiazepine, appears to avert withdrawal symptoms.

Chloral hydrate

Chloral hydrate is frequently administered during weaning from mechanical ventilation because it is well tolerated haemodynamically, although the belief that it does not cause respiratory depression remains disputed (Eland & Banner 1992). It also has potentially significant side effects, including depressing sleep patterns and irritating the gastric mucosa.

Propofol

Propofol has a recognised role for the sedation of ventilated adults, since it enables rapid weaning and extubation compared with other agents. Neither the manufacturers nor the Committee on the Safety of Medicines (CSM) recommend the use of propofol for continuous sedation in PIC or for the induction of anaesthesia in children less than 3 years of age; therefore it is not licensed in the UK. The CSM (1992) cited 66 worldwide reports of serious adverse effects and some fatalities in children continuously sedated with propofol. Parke et al (1992) detailed 5 deaths in the UK, all associated with the requirement for doses in excess of those suggested for adults.

Modes of administration

Effective analgesia within intensive care is dependent upon the selection of an appropriate drug and dose given via the appropriate route. The route is determined by the type of analgesic, access, duration of effect and desired action.

Intramuscular administration of medication is avoided in children because of inconsistent variables in absorption rate, due to altered tissue perfusion. Oral administration may be inappropriate because of trauma, surgical interventions and the inability to initiate the profound analgesic effect required, due to delayed absorption (Llewellyn 1996).

Intravenous administration offers the advantage of complete bioavailability, immediate effect and painless administration. Proponents of intermittent intravenous bolus medication assert that it enables assessment of the efficacy of both the drug and route of administration. However, given the pharmacokinetic profile of most drugs, and technological advances in infusion pumps, continuous infusion achieves the desired effect with lower doses. A continuous therapeutic level of analgesia can be achieved without the potential adverse effects of intermittent bolus and fluctuating serum levels (Fig. 19.6). Careful titration using an appropriate pain and/or sedation scoring tool minimises the risk of overdosage.

Patient-controlled analgesia

Patient-controlled analgesia (PCA) may be used

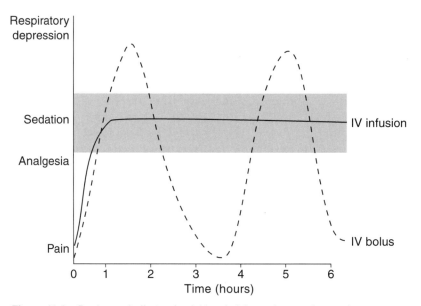

Figure 19.6 Dosing and effects of opioids administered as continuous intravenous infusion, compared with those for intravenous bolus.

within PIC with the post-operative child, non-ventilated child or long-term ventilated child. PCA is delivered via a computerised infusion pump programmed to deliver medication as a continuous infusion, as interval doses, as a bolus dose or a combination of the three. Comprehensive education of both the child and parents prior to use is important if it is to be used effectively. Favourable outcomes with PCAs have been noted in children as young as 5 years (Gillespie & Morton 1992, Gaukroger 1993).

Regional blockades/anaesthesia

Advances in paediatric anaesthesia have resulted in the increased use of regional blockades, epidural, caudal and spinal analgesics. Regional anaesthesia works by modulating or blocking the sodium transmission of afferent nociceptors (Berde 1989). The most commonly used local anaesthetics are bupivicaine and lignocaine, used either singly or in combination with morphine or fentanyl (Lloyd Thomas 1990).

Peripheral nerve blockade and wound infiltration are extremely effective adjuncts for providing postoperative analgesia. Local infiltration is of particular relevance in PIC when painful procedures are undertaken. Care must be taken to prevent intravenous administration, as dysrhythmias, myocardial depression and fitting can result. Epidural, caudal and spinal analgesia are extremely convenient, safe and effective modes of administration for children, producing few of the systemic side effects of opioid administration (Berde 1989, Brill 1992). Administration results in the opioids' binding predominantly with the kappa receptor sites in the spinal cord. This enables restricted CNS blockade and prolonged duration of analgesia. As with all opioid administration the risk of respiratory depression must be considered and can occur up to 24 h after opioid administration (Lloyd Thomas 1990). The use of segmental thoracic epidural in trauma patients with flail chests or rib fractures is documented (Brill 1992). Intrapleural administration after thoracotomy or major unilateral abdominal or retroperitoneal surgery has being explored in the USA.

Nitrous oxide analgesia: entonox

Nitrous oxide mixture has limited use within

PIC, being restricted to the non-intubated child undergoing painful procedures. It has a rapid onset of approximately four minutes and a short duration of action that produces sedation, amnesia and dissociation. When combined with oxygen in a 50:50 concentration, analgesia and not anaesthesia is produced, respiratory depression being avoided.

NON-PHARMACOLOGICAL INTERVENTIONS

Non-pharmacological interventions encompass a wide variety of strategies. These can be used independently or, more commonly in PIC, in combination with pharmacological interventions for pain management. Vessey et al (1994) classify the non-pharmacological interventions into direct and intrapsychic approaches. Direct approaches are primarily sensory, including touch, massage, aromatherapy, acupuncture and transcutaneous nerve stimulation. Touch is one of the most effective means of communication which nurses can encourage between the family and child. The use of acupuncture, aromatherapy and transcutaneous nerve stimulation in PIC is in its infancy, with little known about their effective outcomes. Reduction of environmental stimuli is important in stress reduction, incorporating day and night regimes by turning down lights and reducing noise and coordinating care to prevent unnecessary disruption to the child. The regular changing of position has also been demonstrated to be effective in reducing pain (Berde 1989).

Intrapsychic approaches incorporate distraction techniques, imagery and hypnosis. Distraction is a means of diverting attention onto something other than the pain, such as television, videos, music, books and toys and is potentially effective for short procedural pain (Carter 1994). Intrapsychic approaches are restricted by the child's chronological age, developmental age and previous experiences. Ideally they should be introduced by a skilled practitioner and practised with the child and family prior to the pain experience.

REFERENCES

Berde C B 1989 Paediatric post operative pain management. Paediatric Clinics of North America 36(4):921
Bonica J J 1990 The management of pain, vol 1. Lea & Febiger, Philadelphia
Brill J E 1992 Control of pain. Critical Care Clinics of North America 8(4):203–217
Carter B 1994 Child and infant pain: principles of nursing care and management. Chapman and Hall, London
Committee on the Safety of Medicines 1992 Serious adverse effects and fatalities in children associated with the use of propofol (diprivan) for sedation. Current Problems 34
Craig K D, Prkachin K M, Grunall R V E 1992 Cited in: Turk D C and Meback R (eds) The handbook of pain assessment. Guilford, New York, pp 256–276
Dale J C 1986 A multidimensional study of infants' responses to painful stimuli. Pediatric Nursing 12:27–31
Dale J C 1989 A multidimensional study of infant behaviour associated with assumed painful stimuli: phase II. Journal of Pediatric Health Care 3:34–38
Douhit J L 1990 Psychosocial assessment and management of paediatric pain. Journal of Emergency Nursing 16(3, part 1):168–170
Eland J 1990 Pain in children. Nursing Clinics of North America 25(4):871–882
Eland J M, Anderson J E 1977 The experience of pain in children. Pain: a source book for nurses and other health care professionals. Little Brown, Boston, pp 453–473

Eland J M, Banner W 1992 Assessment and management of pain in children. Cited in: Hazinski M F, Nursing care of the critically ill child, 2nd edn. Mosby, St Louis
Gaukroger P B 1993 Patient controlled analgesia in children. Cited in: Schechter N L, Berole C B, Yaster M (eds) Pain in infants, children and adolescents. Williams & Wilkins, Baltimore, pp. 203–211
Gillespie J, Morton N 1992 Patient controlled analgesia for children: a review: Paediatric Anaesthesia 2:51–59
Grunau R V E, Craig K D 1990 Facial activity as a measure of neonatal pain expression. Cited in: Tyler D C, Krane E J (eds) Advances in pain research and therapy, vol 15: Paediatric pain. Raven Press, New York
Hester N K 1979 The pre-operational child's reaction to immunisation. Nurse Research 28(4):250
Johnston C 1993 Development of psychological responses to pain in infants and toddlers. In: Schecter N L, Berde C B, Yaster M (eds) Pain in infants, children and adolescents. Williams & Wilkins, Baltimore, pp 65–74
Kaplan J 1983 Cardiac anaesthesia. In: Cardiovascular pharmacology, vol 2. Grune & Stratton, New York
Llewellyn N 1996 Pain assessment and the use of morphine. Paediatric Nursing 8(3):32–35
Lloyd Thomas A R 1990 Pain management in paediatric patients. British Journal of Anaesthesia 64:85–104
Marsh D F, Cronin S, Munro H M, Taylor B L, Smith G B 1994

Acute withdrawal syndrome in children recovering from sedation with midazolam and morphine. Care of the Critically Ill 10(42):42

Marvin J A, Pomietto M 1991 Pain assessment in infants (0–12 months) using Neonatal Facial Action Coding System. Journal of Pain and Symptom Management 6:193

McGrath P J, Johnson G, Goodman J T, Schillinger J, Dunn J, Chapman J 1985 The CHEOPS: a behavioural scale to measure post operative pain in children. Advances in Pain Research and Therapy. Raven Press, New York, pp 395–402

Mikhelson V A, Ciplin L E 1993 The use of Tramadol following surgery and in the PICU. 7th World Congress of Pain, Aug 22–27, Paris

Paice J A, Buck M M 1993 Intraspinal devices for pain management. Nursing Clinics of North America 28(4):921–935

Parke T J et al 1992 Metabolic acidosis and fatal myocardial failure after propofol infusion in children: five case reports. British Journal of Anaesthesia 305:613–616

Park G R, Navapurkar V 1994 Sedation in the critically ill patient: the place of midazolam. Care of the Critically Ill 10(1):5–9

Puntillo K A 1991 Pain in the critically ill: assessment and management. Aspen, Maryland

Rogers M C, Helfaer M A 1995 Handbook of paediatric intensive care, 2nd edn. Williams & Wilkins, USA

Ross D, Ross S 1988 Assessment of paediatric pain. Paediatric Nursing 11:73–91

Royal Colleges of Surgeons and of Anaesthetists 1990 Commission on the provision of surgical services. Report of the Working Party on Pain after Surgery. RCS/RCA, London

Shechter N 1989 The undertreatment of pain in children: an overview. Paediatric Clinics of North America 36(4):781–794

Synder S H 1984 Drug and neurotransmitter receptors in the brain. Science 224:22

Tarbell S E, Cohen I T, Marsh J L 1992 The toddler–preschool post-operative pain scale: an observation scale for measuring post-operative pain in children age 1–5, preliminary report. Pain 50:273–280

Thorpe D M 1996 Pain management in the critically ill. Cited in: Ruppert S D, Kernicki J G, Dolan J T (eds) Dolan's critical care nursing, 2nd edn. Davis, Philadelphia

Vessey J A, Carlson K L, McGill J. 1994 Use of distraction with children during acute pain experience. Nursing Research 43(6):369–372

Wolff P H 1974 Active language: the natural history of crying and other vocalisations in early infancy. Cited in: Stone L J, Smith H T, Murphy L B (eds). The competent infant. Tavistock Publications, London

Wong D L, Baker C M 1988 Pain in children: comparison of assessment. Paediatric Nursing 14(1):9–17

Wong D L, Wilson D 1995 Whaley and Wong's nursing care of infants and children. Mosby-Year Book, Inc., St Louis

FURTHER READING

Beider L H, Weaver K, Edwards W 1990 Post-up patient controlled analgesia in children. Paediatric Nursing 16(6):549–554

Bergman et al 1991 Reversible neurological abnormalities associated with prolonged midazolam and fentanyl administration. Journal of Paediatrics 4:644–648

Carpenter P J 1990 New method of measuring young children's self report of fear and pain. Journal of Pain and Symptom Management 5(4):233–240

Koren G et al 1985 Post-operative morphine infusion in newborns: assessment of disposition characteristics and safety. Journal of Paediatrics 107(6):963–967

McIlvane W B et al 1988 Continuous infusion of bupivicaine via intrapleural catheters for analgesia after thoractomy in children. Anaesthesiology 69:261

Schechter N L, Berde C B, Yaster M 1993 Pain in infants, children and adolescents. Williams & Wilkins, Baltimore

Shelly M C et al 1991 Midazolam infusions in critically ill patients. European Journal of Anaesthesiology 8:21–27

Szyfelbein S K, Osgood P F, Carr D B 1985 The assessment of pain and plasma B endorphin immuno activity in burned children. Pain 22:173

Yaster M, Deshpande J K 1988 Management of paediatric pain with opioid analgesics. Journal of Paediatrics 113(3):421

20

Care of the child requiring long-term ventilation

Trudy A. Ward

Advances in health care have enabled many more children with chronic respiratory insufficiency to survive and live ordinary lives. The numbers of children with assisted ventilation in the United Kingdom alone increased five fold between 1990 and 1998 (Robinson 1990, Ward unpublished data, Jardine, Wallis & UK Working Party 1999). These children have very different needs in comparison with critically ill children, although they may well present initially in the Paediatric Intensive Care Unit (PICU) during the acute phase of their condition.

This chapter aims to discuss the complex health needs related to these children and their families, and the multidisciplinary process which is required to ensure a child-focused, family-centred approach.

DEFINITIONS AND TERMS

Previously a child requiring mechanical ventilation for 1 month or more was accepted as the arbitrary definition of 'long-term ventilation'

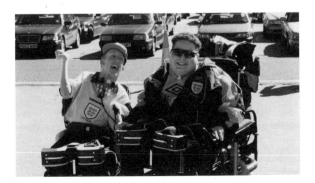

(Goldberg 1984, Newton-John 1989). In 1990 Robinson proposed a definition of long-term ventilation as any child with assisted ventilation for 6 months or more.

The UK Working Party on Paediatric Ventilation defines long-term ventilation as 'any child who, when medically stable, continues to require a mechanical aid for breathing, after an acknowledged failure to wean, or slow wean, three months after the institution of ventilation' (Jardine, Wallis & UK Working Party 1999).

The long-term ventilated child has been described in a number of ways from the 1970s to the present day; examples include: technology-dependent children, ventilator-dependent children, ventilator-assisted children and children with assisted ventilation. These may all have the same meaning but they present us with different images. In former terms the image is of equipment dependency, whereas the last term, children with assisted ventilation, presents us first with a positive image of a child requiring assistance and secondly a piece of equipment. It is important for health care professionals to consider images presented by medical and/or health terms, particularly when the image is likely to be presented throughout the child's life. Positive images promote value and positive self esteem which is of paramount importance to those growing up with a disability. We will therefore use the term 'child with assisted ventilation' throughout the rest of this chapter to describe any child requiring long-term ventilation / respiratory support. The author's definition of 'long-term ventilation' is when, over a period of time (which may be variable but usually between 1 and 6 months), in the absence of acute respiratory disease, and following a ventilation weaning programme for a minimum period of 1 month, the child is unable to sustain adequate spontaneous ventilation and requires mechanical ventilation.

In the 1980s, the USA and Australia were debating children with assisted ventilation and designing home care programmes (Ad Hoc Task Force 1984, Schreiner et al 1987, Davidson-Ward and Keene 1988). The Australian literature provides us with much debate on the issue, reflecting a world-wide interest in home care. The home care industry was growing, largely because of escalating hospital costs and because the number of individuals with assisted ventilation at home was increasing rapidly (Gillis et al 1989, Newton-John 1989). In the USA in the 1980s one PICU alone had 80% of its beds occupied by children receiving long-term ventilatory support (Gillis et al 1989).

In the late 1980s Europe also began designing home care programmes, particularly in France, Holland and Switzerland, and the United Kingdom has also been implementing home care programmes for many years (Robinson et al 1992).

In the 1990s, however, there has been a developing debate in the UK on the issues of service provision, including home care programmes, particularly as the number of children has increased from 35 in 1990 to in excess of 80 in 1996 (Robinson & RCN Working Group unpublished data). In 1996 a Working Party on Paediatric Long-term Ventilation was formed to raise awareness of the current issues and to be involved in research. A research study was undertaken which had two main outcomes:

1. data on the epidemiology of children with assisted ventilation in the UK
2. core guidelines for the discharge home of the child on long-term assisted ventilation in the UK.

There were 136 children (0–16 years) registered on the database in 1997 (Jardine, Wallis & UK Working Party 1999).

Children with assisted ventilation in the United Kingdom

Children with assisted ventilation in the UK have presented with the following:

- congenital central alveolar hypoventilation ('Ondine's Curse')
- spinal cord trauma, e.g. high cervical injury following a road traffic accident or non-accidental injury
- neuromuscular conditions, e.g. myopathy, spinal muscular atrophy, muscular dystrophy

- neuropathy, e.g. poliomyelitis, Guillain Barré syndrome
- metabolic conditions, e.g. glycogen storage disease (Pompes)
- lung disease: bronchopulmonary dysplasia
- infection, e.g. meningitis, poliomyelitis
- thoracic abnormality, e.g. scoliosis, Larsen's syndrome, cerebral palsy.

(Robinson 1990, Robinson et al 1992, Robinson & RCN Working Group unpublished data, Jardine, Wallis and UK Working Party 1999).

PROCESS OF LONG-TERM MECHANICAL VENTILATION

Wherever possible the decision on long-term ventilation should be through informed choice for the child and family. Where a child is known to have a pre-existing health condition, e.g. a neuromuscular disorder, the child and family can have the opportunity to sit down with the health care team and access information and knowledge about the condition and its possible long-term implications for that child and family — e.g. that the child will eventually require assisted ventilation. The appropriate information for each child needs to be up to date, reviewed regularly and presented in an unbiased manner. Some health care professionals, for example, may not be aware of existing children with assisted ventilation living at home and attending mainstream school.

Children who have been given appropriate knowledge about their condition, including the eventual need for assisted ventilation, often decide to go ahead and try out the various options available to them. The adaptation to a life with assisted ventilation is less stressful if the child and family are better prepared.

Unfortunately, there remain situations where a child presents in acute respiratory failure and mechanical ventilatory support is commenced as a means to maintain the child's life without prior warning. It is an acute event which requires immediate intervention, and it is only once the child is stabilised that the full extent of his condition is realised. With children, for example, who have sustained a spinal injury, it is difficult to know the full extent of the injury at the outset.

With children who have a neuromuscular condition, the diagnosis may be made late or health care professionals may have been reluctant to discuss the issue of respiratory failure. When the underlying condition is not known at the time of the acute event or where it is known but the family and child have not had the opportunity to discuss all the options available to them, the child presents in the ICU with the acute event requiring ventilatory support. This is the phenomenon of entrapment, first described by Gillis et al (1989): the child and the family have had no control or choice in the process, and withdrawal of treatment becomes ethically, legally and emotionally complex (Farrell & Fost 1989). It is important for health care professionals to be aware of the phenomenon in order that a balanced debate on the ethical dilemma can ensue, and that the consequences, both positive and negative, of modern advances in critical care on the lives of people are discussed. It is equally important that as many children as possible are not entrapped into assisted ventilation but given the opportunity to choose the options available to them, promoting respect for the child as an individual and as a person who needs to be able to make an informed decision about her life.

MODES OF ASSISTED VENTILATION IN CHILDREN

There are a variety of modes of ventilation suitable for children. A full assessment of the child's physical, psychological, developmental, social and biological needs, together with the family needs, is necessary in choosing the most suitable mode of ventilation.

Factors influencing the choice of mode of ventilation in children include:

- the time, per 24 h, which ventilatory support is needed
- the child's ability to protect his airway
- the child's ability to cough
- the likelihood of upper airway obstruction with external negative pressure ventilation (ENPV)

- whether the child has a thoracic abnormality
- the age and weight of the child
- whether the child has any nasal and/or facial problems
- the psychological profile of the child, e.g. preferences, whether frightened of being placed in a box (Cabinet ENPV), whether unable to tolerate facial appliances
- the psychosocial profile of the family, e.g. available support
- the degree of mobility the child has or is likely to have
- local expertise and resources.

Commonly used modes of assisted ventilation in children are listed in Box 20.1.

Box 20.1 Commonly used modes of ventilation in children

- intermittent positive pressure ventilation (IPPV)
  — t IPPV: IPPV through a tracheostomy
  — n IPPV: IPPV through a nasal or facial mask
- external negative pressure ventilation (ENPV)
  — chest cuirass
  — poncho/jacket/pneumowrap/raincoat
  — cabinet/tank
- diaphragm pacing / phrenic nerve stimulation.

Intermittent positive pressure ventilation

Positive pressure ventilation is the most commonly used method of assisted ventilation, particularly as there have been advances in the development of more user-friendly domicilliary appliances. There are two modes:

- t IPPV: intermittent positive pressure ventilation via a tracheostomy. A proportion of children will have had formation of a tracheostomy during the acute phase and will therefore continue to use this site for ventilation. Many children prefer to have objects away from their face. This mode is used particularly where the child has lost the ability to cough and protect their airway.
- n IPPV: intermittent positive pressure via a nasal or facial mask. With this mode the child can receive continuous positive airway pressure

(CPAP) or bilateral positive airway pressure (BiPAP). Face masks are not usually used in young children, although comfortable quality facial masks for small children are being developed. This is because they are not usually tolerated in children aged 5 or under, and also the continuous use of high-pressure facial masks can increase the development of facial distortions over time.

There are a growing number of lightweight, portable positive pressure ventilators for home use.

External negative pressure ventilation

This is where negative pressure is applied to the chest wall by creating a vacuum within a rigid structure around the thorax, enabling airflow into the lungs via the child's mouth/nose.

Advantages to using ENPV are:

- It avoids intubation or formation of a tracheostomy.
- The child has a reduced susceptibility to infection because she is using her own airway to breathe.
- The child's airway can be aspirated without any disturbance in ventilation.

Disadvantages are:

- There is a risk of aspiration in children with impaired consciousness or neuromuscular conditions, who are unable to protect their airway.
- Upper airway obstruction may occur — for example, during REM sleep.
- The cabinet or tank is bulky and heavy. It has a frightening appearance; although, this can be reduced by decorating the tank e.g. Thomas the Tank Engine.
- There is limited access to the child.
- A major disadvantage, particularly if ENPV is needed during the day also, is the immobility of the child, which has a negative effect on his long-term development.
- In addition the child needs someone to put on and take off the equipment, whereas, with positive pressure ventilation, often very young children can manage their ventilation independently.
- In a child with a severe kyphoscoliosis or a

severe anatomical distortion the cuirass and poncho are difficult to apply. Skin integrity around the child's neck, arms, hips and legs needs to be checked regularly as pressure is increased around these areas. Equally, the child's circulation around these areas needs to be observed regularly, as there is a risk of the appliances being fitted too tightly.

Diaphragm pacing

Diaphragm pacing by electrical stimulation of the phrenic nerves was first developed by William Glenn in 1972 (Glenn et al 1984, Bauer et al 1992). The diaphragm pacer is made up of external and internal parts. Externally, there is a transmitter which controls the impulse to the phrenic nerves and antennae. This is taped to the child's skin at the distal end over each receiver. Internally there are two receivers, surgically placed subcutaneously, and the electrodes connected to each phrenic nerve. The transmitter radio frequency signal is emitted from the antennae. The receivers convert the radio frequency signal to an electrical impulse, which is carried by a wire from the receiver to the stimulating electrode on the phrenic nerve. The phrenic nerve is electrically stimulated and the diaphragm contracts.

Indications for the use of diaphragm pacing in children

Diaphragm pacing may be considered in the child who presents with the following:

- assisted ventilation required 12–24 h per day
- intact cervical roots 3–5 (phrenic nerve)
- normal diaphragm muscle and absence of clinical signs of neuropathic or myopathic processes
- absence of any significant lung disease
- absence of supplemental oxygen requirement during activity, if awake pacing is contemplated
- absence of a severe chestwall abnormality
- absence of airflow obstruction.

Children most likely to benefit from diaphragm pacing are those with congenital, central alveolar hypoventilation or those with high cervical cord transection (Weese-Mayer et al 1994). One issue to consider, when deciding whether diaphragm pacing is an option for a particular child, is that continous stimulation of one phrenic nerve for long periods can damage the nerve and diaphragm. Also, diaphragm pacing is usually alternated with another mode of assisted ventilation, for example IPPV via a tracheostomy, particularly if assisted ventilation is needed 24 h per day. Finally, there is a risk that upper airway obstruction may occur, particularly during sleep. This is because, although vocal cords in children tend to be in the mid position, they can be drawn together, causing obstruction on inspiration, due to the child's small larynx and the greater negative pressure caused by the forceful diaphragmatic contractions. In addition, the upper airway muscle contraction is not coordinated during non-centrally mediated phrenic nerve stimulation. Formation of a tracheostomy or CPAP is therefore needed during periods of sleep.

The current view on the most effective mode of diaphragm pacing is continuous simultaneous pacing of both hemidiaphragms with low-frequency stimulation and a slow respiratory rate (Glenn et al 1984). Weese-Mayer et al 1994 confirm that bilateral continuous low-frequency pacing is the optimum mode for children for more than 15–20 h per day, up to the age of 10–12 years.

The advantages of diaphragm pacing centre on increased mobility and improved self esteem. With regard to the child's mobility, the transmitter appliance is small, lightweight and portable, easily fitting into a 'waistbag'. The child is able to move around more freely than if she were attached to a ventilator, and is able to participate in most sports. The child does, however, have to take care not to take part in excessive exercise, as the pacer has a fixed respiratory rate. Children with both high cervical cord transection and central alveolar hypotension, perceive themselves to be more 'normal' when they use pacers as opposed to ventilators. This may be an important factor when considering the child's perceived benefit and increased self esteem.

HEALTH MANAGEMENT AND INTERVENTION

There are essentially three phases of multidisciplinary management and intervention regarding children with assisted ventilation:

1. the acute phase
2. the transitional/rehabilitation phase
3. the home, review and respite phase.

The acute phase

It is not the purpose of this chapter to discuss the detailed management of acute respiratory failure in children. The management of a child with assisted ventilation in the acute phase does, however, require a consistent holistic approach.

Respiratory function is a fine balance between muscle power, central respiratory drive, and the respiratory load placed upon the child. Ventilatory muscle power and central respiratory drive must be sufficient to overcome the respiratory load, otherwise respiratory failure occurs. Assisted ventilation will be needed if the cause of the imbalance is not reversible. The aim initially, therefore, is to reduce the respiratory load, increase the central respiratory drive and improve ventilatory muscle power.

Management of reducing the respiratory load includes:

- treating infections aggressively with antibiotics and reducing the risk of further infections through effective infection control measures.
- improving the physiological state of the airways through the use of nebulised bronchodilators, particularly when attempting to reduce bronchospasm
- aggressive physiotherapy, particularly percussion, vibrations and postural drainage to reduce pulmonary resistance, assist mucoidary activity and the removal of secretions, and reduce atelectasis. Diuretics are usually prescribed to reduce interstitial and alveolar oedema where present.

Management to improve the child's ventilatory muscle power includes the commencement of balanced enteral feeding and then, as soon as it is tolerated, allowing the child to have an ordinary oral diet, thus improving his nutritional state and avoiding metabolic imbalances. Serum electrolytes are monitored regularly to promote optimum muscle activity through electrolyte stability.

Each child's fatigue threshold has an effect on her muscle power, which in turn will affect her ability to wean from assisted ventilation. The fatigue threshold is the limit by which the child is able to perform the work of breathing in relation to the respiratory load. Following acute respiratory failure, weaning is usually focused on enabling the child to take on an increasing proportion of the work of breathing. All the child's available energy is used to breathe in order to wean from assisted ventilation which leaves little reserve for other activities. In chronic respiratory failure, a child initially has an acute respiratory event that requires him to perform the work of breathing above his fatigue threshold. Reduction in the work of breathing can be achieved, but it often remains above the child's fatigue threshold.

Ventilator weaning techniques are designed to improve ventilatory muscle power in an attempt to raise the child's fatigue threshold (Keens et al 1990). Sprint weaning has the desired effect whereby the child's muscles are trained with periods of muscle activity, followed by rest periods. The child has a period of time when the ventilator takes over the work of breathing completely, ensuring total ventilatory muscle rest. The child then has short periods of time during the day whilst fully awake when she is disconnected from the ventilator for approximately four times per day. These initial sprint periods may last for a few minutes, increasing gradually as tolerated by the child. Non-invasive monitoring using pulse oximetry and end tidal CO_2 monitoring is used to aid assessment of the child in addition to observing for signs of respiratory distress: tachypnea, recession, hypoxia or hypercapnia. The sprint is stopped if respiratory distress occurs. Sprint weaning is particularly effective where ventilatory muscle fatigue is thought to be a component.

With chronic respiratory failure weaning, the child is weaned off ventilation completely during the day prior to attempting to reduce sleeping ventilatory support. The child also needs complete ventilatory support during rests.

Psychosocial and developmental needs

The child's psychological state should be assessed and his needs addressed by the nurse in collaboration with the child and adolescent mental health team (CAMHS) providing specialist advice and support to the child, family and health care professionals. Interventions which enable the child and family's psychosocial and developmental needs to be met are:

- the child's having unlimited contact with her parents, primary caregivers and siblings
- the allocation of a team of nurses with a primary nurse coordinator, which promotes a consistent, individualised approach to care
- the provision of play therapy.

Indications for assisted ventilation at home

Indications for considering assisted ventilation at home following the acute phase are primarily to prolong the child's life and to improve his quality of life. In some instances, assisted ventilation may be used to provide symptom control for a child with a life-limiting condition. Children with neuromuscular conditions, for example, who are at the end stage of their illness may require assisted ventilation as a palliative measure to reduce the unpleasant sensations of choking on excessive secretions.

The child may only require assisted ventilation for part of the 24 h, e.g. nocturnal ventilation or whenever they fall asleep. Factors which influence the decision to commence assisted ventilation with home ventilation as a goal are:

- the presence of risk factors for developing respiratory failure
- the child's current respiratory status
- the rate of deterioration of respiratory function
- the likely effect of assisted ventilation on the child's survival
- the likely effect of assisted ventilation on the symptoms of the underlying condition

- the child's likely quality of life in relation to other disability/illness
- the child's wishes
- the child and family's abilities and the support available

(adapted from Kinnear 1994). All these factors are considered together where there is the opportunity to decide to commence assisted ventilation.

The risk factors for developing respiratory failure include the clinical condition of the child, e.g. a child with a progressive degenerative condition such as muscular dystrophy. Treatment with nasal ventilation is effective in reversing the nocturnal respiratory failure without significant disturbance to lifestyle (Khan et al 1996).

In assessing the child's current respiratory status with a view to determining the presence of chronic respiratory failure, consideration should be given to the evidence of the following:

- a child with poor or absent respiratory effort during sleep, suggesting congenital or acquired alveolar hyperventilation syndrome
- paradoxical abdominal movement which may suggest poor phrenic nerve or diaphragmatic function
- poor oxygen delivery and increasing carbon dioxide retention as evidenced through pulse oximetry trends
- suprasternal tug and snoring or stridor, suggesting upper airway obstruction.

Lung function studies, ultrasound, X-ray screening, nerve conduction studies, central nervous system imagery and muscle biopsy all provide information about the child's current respiratory status which often confirms the immediate assessment of the child in chronic respiratory failure showing signs of increased effort to breathe, cyanosis, a pained expression, and sitting upright with head partially extended for maximum airway effect.

The rate of deterioration of the child's respiratory function is usually determined through regular assessment of her respiratory function where lung function studies indicate progressive deterioration over increasingly short periods of time.

How assisted ventilation will affect the child's survival rate in the long term does raise quality of life issues, but it is an important consideration within the overall assessment of the appropriateness of a child's living long term at home with assisted ventilation. For example, long-term ventilation at home may not be appropriate for a child with degenerative brain disease or persistent vegetative state.

Assisted ventilation should be considered along with other symptoms the child is experiencing and other disabilities or other health problems the child has and an assessment made of the positive or negative effects of commencing it. As mentioned previously, the child should be given the opportunity to discuss his health and be enabled to make an informed choice as to whether he would like to commence assisted ventilation. Health care professionals can gain much insight into this issue from children and young adults with muscular dystrophy.

Discharging a child home with assisted ventilation can be a complex process. However, this should not compromise the goal of getting the child home as soon as possible. Living with a child with assisted ventilation is challenging as well as rewarding. Each family needs to be assessed as to their understanding of the reality of taking their child home. Parents or primary carers need to be committed to taking their child home, and health care professionals need to ensure that appropriate support will be available for the child and family once the child is at home.

The transitional/reHabilitation phase

Once the child is over the acute phase of the life-threatening event, and her health has been optimised, she is usually ready to be transferred to a transitional service. The term 'transitional' implies moving on with change. Transition is defined as 'a passing from one condition or place to another', also 'a passage from an earlier to a later stage of development' (Shorter Oxford Dictionary 1975). It is during this phase away from an acute PICU environment that the child and family begin to take control over their lives, with the health care professionals' providing

specialist knowledge, training, intervention, advice and support to enable the family to reHabilitate and adapt to their new lifestyle.

A concept inherent in paediatric reHabilitation is Habilitation, which is the 'activities and interactions that enable an individual with a disability to develop *new* abilities and skills and to achieve his or her maximum potential' (Bramadat & Melvin 1987). The child will be relearning previous skills and also developing new skills and abilities. It is a process of active change on the part of the child. ReHabilitation is a different process for the child as opposed to the adult, as the former is a growing individual, approaching different physical, psychological and cognitive developmental stages, hence the author's use of the highlighted spelling reHabilitation throughout the remainder of this chapter.

The appropriate setting for the coordination and reHabilitation of the child with assisted ventilation and her family is a centre able to provide a multidisciplinary team consisting of medical, nursing, therapy, social work and reHabilitation engineering professionals. Some Transitional Services are based in the hospital setting, usually but not always, next to the Intensive Care Unit. Others are based in the community and are designed more as a home environment.

There are advantages and disadvantages to both settings. Hospital-based services have ready access to all acute services and staff; however, they tend to be very clinical and not conducive to promoting new and adaptive strategies and skills for going home and meeting the child and family's ordinary needs. Other disadvantages are that the environment, with its hospital routine, is too protective to provide learning in real life situations, and it continues to cushion the child and family against home-based problems.

Community-based services have to be more self sufficient, particularly regarding staff teams. The child may have to travel to hospital for specialist investigations. However, the less clinical 'home' environment enables adaptation to the realities of going home for the child and family, and enables the developmental, ordinary needs of the child and family to be met more effectively

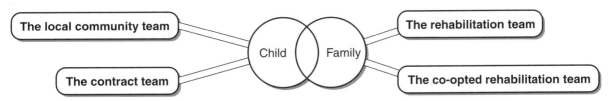

Figure 20.1 An integrated multidisciplinary approach in the transitional/rehabilitation phase. Each child should have a coordinator or case manager. This is often the role of the paediatric nurse.

Box 20.2   The reHabilitation team

- paediatric rehabilitation consultant / consultants in neurodisability
- respiratory paediatrician
- paediatric nurses and child care workers
- physiotherapist
- occupational therapist
- rehabilitation engineers / clinical engineers
- educational psychologist
- speech and language therapists
- child and adolescent mental health team.

Box 20.3   Co-opted reHabilitation team members

- paediatric ear, nose and throat consultant
- orthotic specialist
- orthopaedic / spinal injury consultant
- neurophysiology specialist
- dietician
- liaison worker / teacher
- others, e.g. ophthalmologist.

Box 20.4 Local community team

- general practitioner and community paediatrician
- paediatric community nurses and child care workers
- social worker
- educational officer
- voluntary support services
- health visitor and school nurse.

Box 20.5   The contract team

- service, business/contracts manager
- health commissioner
- social service officer
- educational officer
- specialist interagency commissioning team.

---

because the transition and integration to home has already begun. Another advantage to a community model is effective and appropriate risk management in that community environments are better able to organise and implement 'pilot' outings within an ordinary community and give a clearer picture of the child and family's ability to manage when at home.

The transitional service provides:

- assessment of the child's and family's needs by the multidisciplinary team
- reHabilitation for the child and family in preparation for going home
- regular review and respite care.

During the transitional phase, there need to be effective communication links with the child's local community teams. The reHabilitation team is also in an ideal position to assist families and their advocates, for example, solicitors, to gain the necessary compensation for the child's growing needs. Figure 20.1 and Boxes 20.2–5 show the teams of professionals involved.

The *aims*, therefore, of a transitional service are:

- to provide effective transition to home and school
- to provide a co-ordinated, holistic and integrative multidisciplinary service
- to provide assessment, reHabilitation and review for children with assisted ventilation and their families, to enable them to live at home and re-integrate into their own community

- to restore, as far as possible, the child's original quality of life or to establish an alternative life plan
- to promote the child's developmental needs, in balance with their complex health needs. There is the risk of them becoming institutionalised and living a highly clinical existence. It is, therefore, important to recognise and meet the child's ordinary developmental needs
- to promote long-term family health and wellbeing through establishing support and communication networks and providing respite care where needed.

The challenge which the child and family are taking on is long term, probably for life, and families need to be enabled and empowered to take control of their lives and adapt positively to having a child with assisted ventilation at home.

Multidisciplinary assessment

Multidisciplinary assessment of the child. A multidisciplinary referral assessment is usually carried out before transfer to the transitional service, followed by a comprehensive assessment during the first month of admission. The assessment should be an integrated approach involving as many disciplines as appropriate to the child's needs. Multidisciplinary assessment is used to develop reHabilitation and health maintenance programmes for the child. Adopting an interdisciplinary approach will enable the child's needs to be assessed holistically. Assessment also enables the child to maximise his potential whatever level of ability he has. Assessment, together with the next phase, reHabilitation, focuses on the child's long-term health maintenance, reducing complications associated with the child's health condition and the development of abilities.

Assessment includes the child's health, development, social, emotional, family and cultural needs, as well as assessment of her communication, functional and cognitive abilities (see Fig. 20.2)

Individual personal profile. A personal profile of the child's personality and health history prior to either the acute episode or admission to the transitional service is compiled by the team. The personal profile also enables the child to contribute

by expressing his wishes and concerns. It may be appropriate for a member of the child and adolescent mental health team to access the child and family, as adaptation to life with assisted ventilation can present many emotional challenges.

Health. Assessment of the child's health needs is usually carried out by the appropriate medical and nursing professionals depending on the child's health diagnosis, e.g. Respiratory Paediatrician, Neurodevelopmental Paediatrician, Consultant in Spinal Injury or Paediatric Rehabilitation, Paediatric Nurse. Health assessment is documented in detail in the literature and is beyond the scope of this chapter; however, an important consideration is that the child should be assessed globally; this includes their acute health intervention, the child's neurological and respiratory status, the child's growth trend and stage of development, vision, hearing and nutritional intake. Also the child should have access to a variety of health care professionals such as Specialist Paediatricians, an Orthotist, a Dentist, a Podiatrist, as well as Health Visitors and Paediatric Community Nurses, as part of the child's ongoing health maintenance programme. It is at this stage that the feasibility that the child with assisted ventilation can live at home is fully assessed.

Mobility. The child's fine and gross motor abilities are usually assessed by the Physiotherapist and Occupational Therapist. The Physiotherapist, Occupational Therapists, Paediatric Rehabilitation Consultant and Specialist ReHabilitation Engineers, who include Clinical Engineers, assess the child's postural abilities, including their sitting, lying and standing posture, for the provision of positioning equipment and switches (where appropriate) to enable the child to improve their functional ability and take part in usual activities of life.

Social, emotional, family and culture. Members from the CAHMS team, Social Worker and Paediatric Nurse assess the child's social, emotional, family and cultural needs and include the child's coping strategies, response to change and adaptation to their altered self and abilities. This is usually carried out through in-depth interviewing with the child and family together with the use of formal psychological tests.

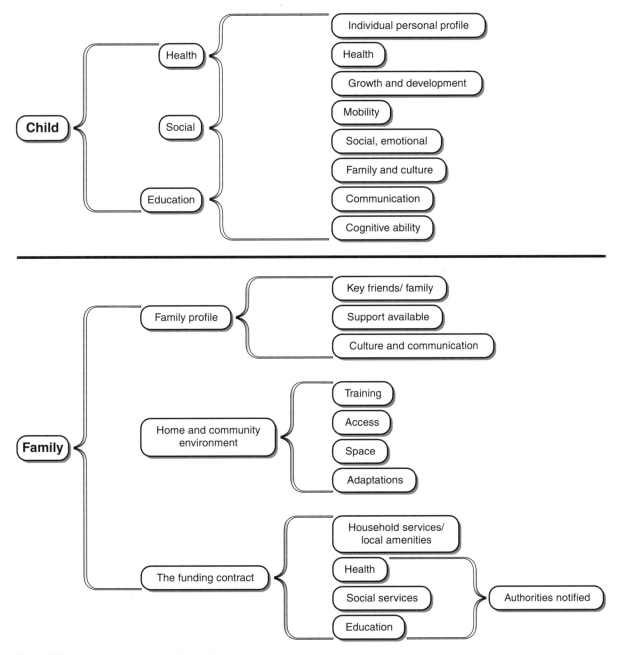

Figure 20.2   Components of multidisciplinary assessment.

Activities of daily living.   Assessment of the child's activities of daily living skills include: their oral skills, their ability to eat and drink, their ability to dress and undress themselves, their ability to wash themselves and meet their own personal hygiene needs. Activities of daily living skills are usually assessed by the Paediatric Nurse, the Occupational Therapist and the Speech and Language Therapist.

Cognitive ability.   The child may need an educational statement of need. The whole team will be involved in providing input into the child's educational statement following a period of reHabilitation and will liaise with the child's local Education Authority, and Educational Psychologist prior to the completion of their educational statement of need.

The child's cognitive ability and educational attainments, as appropriate, are assessed by the Educational Psychologist, Occupational Therapist and/or Teacher, and include assessment of their attention and concentration span, perception, memory recall, reading and writing skills. In the preschool child, development and play is assessed by the Educational Psychologist, Play Specialist and/or Paediatric Nurse.

Communication. The child's ability to communicate is assessed by the Speech and Language Therapist. This includes assessment of the child's expressive and receptive language comprehension and alternative means of communication. The Speech and Language Therapists, Occupational Therapists and ReHabilitation Engineers can also assess the child for switch and communication provision. The Paediatric Nurse along with the Speech and Language Therapist provide advice on appropriate speaking tubes where appropriate.

It should be noted that key professionals may take a lead in the above areas of assessment, but the whole reHabilitation team, child and family are involved in the process.

Multidisciplinary assessment of the family. Assessment of the family focuses on the individual family profile, the home and community environment, and the funding contract.

The family profile. A family profile is compiled by the whole team with considerable input from the family members themselves. Compiling the family profile involves:

1. gathering information on the family members and friends
2. establishing the current level and type of support available either from friends, extended family, voluntary or statutory agencies
3. obtaining relevant cultural information
4. defining the family's communication

network: for example, establishing who is the lead member of the family, how they prefer to be kept informed, and whether English is their first language. Culture and communication are often interlinked.

The family's training needs. This will be an initial assessment of training needs which may alter considerably once the family has built up confidence in their own ability to meet their child's complex health needs. Assessment includes finding out how much each family member is able to take on. A flexible time plan is developed.

Home and community environment. The family home, including access to the space available for equipment, and initial adaptations likely to be needed, are assessed primarily by the Occupational Therapist. The Social Worker, Educational Psychologist and Paediatric Nurse assess the local health, social and educational services and agencies which may be appropriate for the child and family once they are in the community.

The funding contract. At the assessment stage, information regarding the present funding arrangement, the child's health authority, social services and education authorities are recorded. The relevant Health Commissioner, GP, Social Service and Educational Officers are informed of the child's admission.

The purpose of an integrated multidisciplinary assessment which includes a variety of medical, nursing, therapy and reHabilitation engineering professionals with the child and family, is that there is, at the end of the assessment period, a clear, holistic, integrated assessment of the child and family rather than a collection of mini reports.

Multidisciplinary reHabilitation

The next stage is the reHabilitation itself (see Fig. 20.3).

ReHabilitation—the child. To enable the child with assisted ventilation to go home with her family and attend playgroup, nursery or school, requires a period of reHabilitation. ReHabilitation is defined as 'the *relearning* of previous skills,

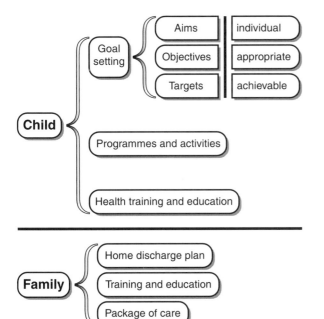

Figure 20.3   Components of reHabilitation.

which often requires adjustment to altered functional abilities and altered lifestyle' (Bramadat & Melvin 1987).

Multidisciplinary assessment is used to develop the interdisciplinary reHabilitation programme. At the start of the reHabilitation programme the focus may well be on the child's health needs; however, a flexible integrated approach ensures that the child's global needs begin to be met in tandem with his complex health needs.

Goals.   Following on from the initial multidisciplinary assessment is the process of planning and goal setting. Planning focuses on organising interventions and draws upon the following:

- information from the assessment
- knowledge about the child's condition
- knowledge about potential interventions
- knowledge about local resources
- parental knowledge of the child
- the child's level of self-awareness
- negotiations (and compromise) with all relevant people.

Planning usually occurs weekly or fortnightly and involves members of the reHabilitation team, parents and the child where appropriate.

The key to successful goal planning and achievement is involving the child and maintaining their motivation.

Aims, objectives and targets are set in the planning phase. The aims are the goals set at the level of handicap at the limits of foreseeability. Objectives are the goals set at the levels of the child's disability, focusing on change over a medium time span. The targets are the goals set at the level of the child's disability or impairment, defining the performance to be reached within a defined time or actions to be undertaken (Rivermead Annual Report 1995). Any number of goals are set, which need to be individual to that child, appropriate and achievable.

The level and degree of change that the child and family are experiencing are acknowledged in the planning phase. Some goals may, for example, have to be postponed and reset at a later date. Priority goals for children with assisted ventilation going home are:

- to ensure the safety of the child: normalisation of respiratory function and growth
- to ensure the child's ability to use respiratory equipment safely and appropriately
- to prevent or minimise problems
- to enable the child to interact and develop in the world around her, however complex her disability.

Programmes and activities.   From the goals; programmes and activities are developed by the team and reviewed weekly. Programmes can be individual discipline led but are always interdisciplinary in process: for example a Physiotherapist may develop a mobility and posture programme and then all members of the team and family carry the programme through, each evaluating the child's progress.

Activities have a recreational focus, promoting the child's developmental and ordinary needs whilst also having a reHabilitative goal: e.g. singing — promotes voice projection and fluency and also experimentation with lung volumes.

Children benefit from a reHabilitation programme that is designed as near to their everyday life as possible, e.g. within a school or nursery context or afterschool activities.

Health training and education for the child. A major role of the reHabilitation team is to ensure that the child has the required knowledge to make informed choices of health care and lifestyle options, appropriate to their level of understanding, and to assist them to develop strategies to enable them in the acquisition of knowledge and new life skills.

Much of the knowledge shared may centre on appropriate information-giving; however, teaching skills related to the programme are also encouraged. The training cycle may consist of:

- information-giving from the team member
- the child's observing
- the child's carrying out the skill
- evaluation — does the child fully understand what he is doing?

Positive encouragement and feedback are of paramount importance in assisting the child to develop new skills and adapt to change. Certificates of achievement and star charts can be used. Additional team members are co-opted where they have specialist knowledge and skills: for example, the Tissue Trauma Nurse.

The Paediatric Nurse is often the primary link with the child during the reHabilitation phase. The reHabilitation programme needs to be carried out throughout a 24 h period. The nurse and child care team are accessible to the child 24 h per day, providing assessment, planning, intervention and evaluation, and the child receives ongoing feedback, enabling a consistent approach. Over time, as their confidence increases, the parents gradually take on the reHabilitation role, with the nurse and child care workers supporting and advising when required.

Rehabilitation for the family. Enabling and empowering the child with assisted ventilation and her family to return home requires a commitment, both with attitude and approach, to the philosophy of family-centred care (Box 20.6). Key elements within the philosophy of family-centred care include: recognition that the family is central in the child's life; that the family is consistent whereas health care professionals fluctuate. Recognition that families have strengths, individuality, choices and needs. Recognition of cul-

tural diversity and respect for different methods of coping, which includes the promotion of family-to-family support and networking amongst families going through similar experiences.

Box 20.6 The philosophy of family-centred care

- recognising that the family is central to the child's life
  - the family is consistent
  - the health care team fluctuates
- recognising that families have strengths
- recognising each family's individuality
- recognising that families have choices and needs
- recognising that families have different methods of coping, which should be respected
- recognising that family-to-family support and networking is promoted
- recognising that health care professionals understand and incorporate the developmental needs of children and young people
- recognising that accessible health care services are developed which are flexible and responsive to family identified needs
- enabling child/parent/professional collaboration at all levels of health care
  - e.g. care of the individual child
  - service development, implementation and evaluation
  - policy development
- recognising and respecting the racial and cultural diversity of families.

Fundamental to family-centred care is the understanding and incorporation of the developmental needs of children and young people into health care services and also the promotion of accessible health care services which are flexible and responsive to family-identified needs.

Another key element to family-centred care is partnership. Family-centred care facilitates child/parent, professional collaboration. Within this philosophy of care there is a shift from a professional-centred approach to a collaborative approach. Collaboration is about working together, an equal partnership based on mutual respect and trust, with shared knowledge, problem solving, goal setting and decision making.

The role of the paediatric nurse, within this philosophy of care, is to enable, empower and strengthen families as well as to promote the acquisition of the skills and competencies necessary to meet their needs. This philosophy enables and empowers the child and family through involvement and facilitates shared responsibility and accountability.

The family's rehabilitation programme focuses on the home discharge process and consists of:

- the home discharge plan
- training and education for the family
- the child and family's package of care.

The home discharge plan.   The home discharge plan begins as soon as the child is admitted to the acute unit; however, the assessment in the transitional phase usually provides more detailed and appropriate information from the family on which to develop a more realistic time scale and action plan. Box 20.7 shows an example of a discharge plan.

Training and education for the family.   The paediatric nurses' role in sharing knowledge and enabling the acquisition of skills with regard to home ventilation is fundamental to empowering and strengthening families. The more the family understand their child's condition and health needs the better they are able to adapt to their child's disability and new lifestyle, and develop more effective coping strategies. The development of skills appropriate to their child's needs also promotes independence and integration towards an ordinary life for the child and family. Training and education consists of theory, skills, equipment, protocols and guidelines, with timescales developed for each topic area.

The child and family's package of care

The package of care is a negotiated document consisting of:

- the multiagency funding contract. All appropriate agencies such as, health, social services and education explore the allocation of funding for the child. The multidisciplinary assessment, together with knowledge, is used to establish appropriate costings according to the child and family's individual needs
- the confidentiality, responsibility and accountability contract. This is a contract developed with the family which clearly sets out confidentiality, responsibility and accountability issues. The home care team, for example, has access to sensitive, private information through working in a private home
- the agreed level and type of support given to the family, which includes the skill mix and establishment of the home care team and that the skill mix will be reviewed as the child's needs change.

The skill mix and establishment of the home care team will be individual to each child and family situation.

Consideration is given to the child's health, social, developmental and educational needs, and the family's ability to contribute to the care of their child without excessive burden being placed upon them.

Regarding Registered Nurse skill mix, consideration should be given to the following:

- the period of time that the child receives ventilation, e.g. nocturnal or 24 h ventilation
- the mode of ventilation that the child uses
- the health stability of the child
- the mobility of the child, e.g. whether the child is fully mobile or immobile due to paralysis.

A multidisciplinary, multiagency needs assessment should be compiled.

In establishing the level and type of support given to the family the contract should consider including the following:

- 24 h telephone access to a Specialist Paediatric Nurse for advice and support
- designation of a primary nurse responsible for assessing, planning, implementing and evaluating the child's care, taking into account the views of the family
- recruitment of trained child care workers who are appointed with input from the family during the selection process. The child care workers could include people with Nursery Nurse, Play Specialist, Child Development, National Vocational Qualification (NVQ) and disability training.

Time in months	1/12	2/12	3/12	4/12	5/12	6/12

- Multidisciplinary assessment
- The child's health status maintained, e.g.
  - mode of ventilation stabilised
- List of agreed goals with a time scale: e.g.
  - child will be on full oral diet
  - child will have range of seating aids (posture and mobility assessment)
  - child will be able to use her voice effectively
- Funding agreement
  - health/social services/education
- Contracts
  - commissioners/family
- Training and education
  - family/child
- Home environment
  - assessment/adaptations/access
- Recruitment and training of home care team
- Equipment
  - costing/trial/purchase
- Transport
- Review
- Respite agreement

Figure 20.4   Home discharge plan.

Living at home: review and respite phase

Multidisciplinary review of the child and family is necessary for the following reasons:

- to enable the child to continue to live at home and integrate fully into her community
- to evaluate the life plan developed in the rehabilitation phase
- to maintain the child's health, promote continued developmental and ordinary needs in balance with complex health needs
- to promote continued long-term family health and wellbeing.

The family and child will undergo change through growth and development as individuals and as a family. The child's needs will change over time, as will those of the family. The child, for example, may not initially attend school or nursery but eventually his life plan programme will need to develop with him to incorporate his educational need, including the support needed to enable him to attend school.

The child's health will need to be maintained to prevent or reduce the long-term effects of disability. Examples include preventing and/or reducing ventilation complications, altered mobil-ity and posture problems, and adapting to developmental changes.

The family's health and wellbeing needs to be maintained to enable the family to develop the ability to cope with the long-term effects of living with a child with assisted ventilation, and to allow family members, including siblings, to grow and develop positively with the experience.

Family members who assume primary responsibility for managing the care of children with a disability experience many stressful feelings and frustrations. These include the financial difficulties related to the complex adaptations to the new environment, the variety of health-related appointments, the fatigue associated with the ongoing care needs of the child, the restrictions to everyday life placed upon them, and role conflict: for example, am I a mother or a nurse? Family members who are caring for individuals with assisted ventilation at home have reported a moderate level of both the burden and the negative impact of caregiving but also a positive sense of mastery of the caregiving role and satisfaction with caregiving (Findeis et al 1994). Noyes' (1999) research, which sought the views of young people using assisted ventilation, offers much insight into their experiences and those of the family.

Family support is a vital component to family

adaptation and survival. In reviewing the family, the multidisciplinary team will be evaluating with the family how they are managing, whether the level of support they have is sufficient, and what strategies will enable the family to cope more effectively. Family networks, such as Contact a Family, informal networks, and the provision of respite care, as well as appropriate levels of information sharing from health care professionals, enable families to adapt in the long term with their alternative life plan.

The review interval varies from child to child. It may initially be monthly, progressing to 3 monthly, then 6 monthly to yearly depending on the health stability of the child. It is beneficial for the family and child to stay as a family whilst in the review phase of the programme. Some transitional services provide bungalow accommodation for families during the multidisciplinary review. The length of stay is dependent on the child and family's needs.

Respite care for children with assisted ventilation is not readily available in the UK, although a couple of centres are developing in this area. An important factor in the development of respite facilities for these children would be that the environment should be as near a home as possible, with activities which would benefit the child as well as the respite benefiting the other family members.

Evaluation of all children with assisted ventilation involved in home care programmes should be carried out by the multidisciplinary team on an ongoing basis. Information for the evaluation should be obtained from as many sources as possible, e.g. family, child, multidisciplinary team, local health care team and school. The sharing of experiences enables more effective programmes to be developed for further children going home.

Health outcomes for these children in evaluating the effectiveness of reHabilitation and home care programmes, have been identified as:

- improved health
- successful transfer to the community
- maintenance of the family unit and

independent living
- sustained school attendance
- hospital readmission rates (Noyes 1999).

SUMMARY

- Children with assisted ventilation have very different needs in comparison with the critically ill child in the paediatric intensive care environment.
- Advances in health care and the move towards home-based living for people with complex health needs, have contributed to an increase in the numbers of children with assisted ventilation living at home.
- Despite this growing trend in children and young people requiring assisted ventilation, there remain few providers of health care who have developed services for the three phases of health care management and intervention for these children and families.
- The role of the nurse as a case manager, coordinator, health educator and trainer, who works collaboratively with the child, family and other professionals, is fundamental to the three-phase health care management and intervention. These children need a multidisciplinary approach which incorporates a child-focused, family-centred and reHabilitative philosophy.
- The UK is moving towards a nationally consistent approach for children with assisted ventilation through the UK Working Group and collaboration with national initiatives for adults with assisted ventilation. For example, a transitional reHabilitation service is being developed at Chailey Heritage which incorporates a clinical pathway of assessment, reHabilitation, reintegration home and review, in an environment where children are able to meet their clinical needs in ways that least disrupt their ordinary needs.
- Finally, health care professionals working with these children need to evaluate home care programmes to ensure that the services are appropriate and effective in meeting their complex health needs and to ensure an optimum quality of life for these children and their families.

REFERENCES

Ad Hoc Task Force on Home Care of Chronically Ill Infants and Children 1984 Guidelines for home care of infants, children and adolescents with chronic disease. Paediatrics 74(3):434–436

Bauer G A et al 1992 Mechanism of unexpected death in a patient with (2 quadriplegia ventilated by a phrenic nerve stimulator. American Journal of Physical Medicine and Rehabilitation 39–40

Bramadat I J, Melvin C L 1987 Habilitation: application of a concept. Clinical Nurse Specialist 1(2):76–79

Davidson-Ward S L, Keene T G 1988 Ventilatory management at home. In: Ballard R A (ed) Paediatric care of the ICN graduate ventilatory management at home. Saunders, Philadelphia, pp 166–176

Farrell P M, Fost N C 1989 Long term mechanical ventilation in paediatric respiratory failure: mechanical and ethical considerations. American Review of Respiratory Disease 140:S36–S40

Findeis A, Liaison J L, Gallo A, Skekleton M 1984 Caring for individuals using home ventilators: an appraisal by family caregivers. Rehabilitation Nursing 19(1):6–11

Gillis J, Tibballs J McEniery J et al 1989 Ventilator dependent children. Medical Journal of Australia 150 2 Jan:10–14

Glenn W W L et al 1984 Ventilatory support by pacing of the conditioned diaphragm in quadriplegia. New England Journal of Medicine 1050–1055

Goldberg A I 1984 Home care for ventilator dependent children: a regional approach to a solution. The Child's Doctor 1(2):28–31

Jardine, Wallis and UK Working Party on Paediatric Ventilation 1998

Khan Y, Heckmatt J, Dubowitz V 1996 Sleep studies and supportive ventilatory treatment in patients with congenital muscle disorders. Archives of Disease in Childhood 74:195–200

Keens T G, Jansen M T, Dewitt P K, Davidson Ward S L 1990 Home care for children with chronic respiratory failure. Seminars in Respiratory Medicine 11(3):269–281

Kinnear W J M 1994 Assisted ventilation at home. A practical guide. Oxford University Press, Oxford

Newton-John H F 1989 Long term mechanical ventilation of patients in Australia. The Medical Journal of Australia 150 2 Jan:3–6

Noyes J 1999 Voices and choices: the health, social care and eduction of young people who use assisted ventilation. The Stationery Office, London

Rivermead Annual Report 1995 Rivermead Rehabilitation Centre, Oxford

Robinson R O 1990 Ventilator dependancy in the UK. Archives of Disease in Childhood 65:1235–1236

Robinson R O, Cartwright R, Fuller W, Jones M, Samuels M 1992 The ventilator dependent child. In: McCarthy G (ed) Physical disability in childhood — an interdisciplinary approach to management. Churchill Livingstone, Edinburgh

Schreiner M S, Donar M E, Kettrick R G 1987 Home mechanical ventilation. Pediatric Clinics of North America 34(1):47–60

The Shorter Oxford Dictionary vol 11, 1975. Oxford University Press, Oxford

Weese-Mayer D E, Hunt C E, Brouvillette R T 1994 Diaphragm pacing in infants and children, ch 26. Williams & Wilkins, Baltimore, pp 389–399

21

Legal and ethical issues in paediatric intensive care

Stephanie Wheeler   Kate Hall

Clinical situations presented to PIC practitioners demand use of scientific, pharmacological and technological developments. In consequence, many issues arise which require legal and ethical consideration. This chapter provides an overview of these issues for PIC practitioners. Specific areas of the legal and ethical framework are examined, with illustrating vignettes assisting this process, in the following sequence:

- basic legal and ethical framework for clinical practice
- principle of Justice and resource allocation
- consent
  — proxy consent and children's rights
  — consent and refusal to treatment/research
  — competency and the Gillick case
- life support and brainstem death
  — ordinary/extraordinary means
  — sustenance technologies versus medical technologies
- child protection and the Children Act 1989
  — issues and philosophy
- legal and ethical indicators for role expansion in PIC.

THE BASIC LEGAL AND ETHICAL FRAMEWORK FOR PRACTICE

The current health service requires new skills, placing greater responsibility on health care practitioners. Responsibility delineates legal accountability, which concerns how much a nurse or any health care practitioner can be held to account in law for her/his actions (Dimond

1995). Dimond frames accountability in four arenas which facilitate an understanding of what can be loosely termed the basic legal framework in:

- civil law
- criminal law
- contract law
- accountability to the profession.

Civil and criminal law represent a person's responsibility to society: criminal law involves the sanctions of the state resulting in punishment; civil law involves the actions of an individual for, primarily, compensation. Contract law (whilst being part of the civil law) is identified separately because it governs agreements between parties.

Vignette 1 illustrates the four arenas of accountability in a case of drug error in PIC.

Vignette 1

Lydia, a neonate with severe tetralogy of Fallot needs to have a patent ductus arteriosus maintained requiring prostaglandin E2, 0.005 µg/kg/min as an IV infusion. The prescription reads 0.05 µg/kg/min. The PIC nurse, Jane, prepares the infusion as per prescription and gives the medication.

Idea taken from Dimond (1995) with permission of the publisher, Prentice Hall Europe, Hemel Hempstead.

Jane is fully qualified and there is an obvious expectation of her duty and standard of care. The duty of care arises from her professional and contractual relationship with the patient and her employers. Her standard of care is currently measured by the Bolam Test, an earlier case (Bolam v Friern Barnet HMC, 1957) which asserts that 'professionals are to be judged against the standards of their peers' (Montgomery 1992, p 83). In addition Dimond (1995, p 30) refers to Whitehouse v Jordan 1981:

'When you get a situation which involves the use of some special skill or competence, then the test as to whether there has been negligence or not is … the standard of the ordinary skilled man exercising or professing to have that special skill. If a surgeon failed to measure up to that in any respect (clinical judgement or otherwise) he had been negligent and should be so adjudged'.

Dimond (1995) points out that any professional group can take the place of the word surgeon. In consequence, Jane's actions are considered in the light of this test. In giving the medication, Jane is negligent and accountable in all four arenas. The standard of care expected is clearly set out in *Standards for the administration of medicines* (UKCC 1992a). This specifically requires that nurses verify drug dosages on prescriptions. It is evident in this vignette that the nurse did not confirm the dosage of prostaglandin.

Accountability related to moral/ethical issues is reflected in consumer expectations that health care professionals act ethically in the best interests of those in their care. A nurse/doctor is legally and morally accountable for his/her actions and should be able to provide a rationale for these (Fletcher et al 1995). Ethics is the branch of philosophy concerning values. Professionals often make statements concerning values and make them explicit in codes of conduct. Nurses are guided by their *Code of professional conduct* (UKCC 1992b) and governed by the United Kingdom Central Council which deals with allegations of misconduct through a Professional Conduct Committee. The Medical Act 1983 gives similar power to the General Medical Council (GMC) to deal with misconduct of Doctors. Doctors are guided ethically by values inherent in their *Duties of a doctor* (GMC 1995) and the 'Blue book' (GMC 1993). The British Medical Association (BMA) has made a particular contribution to the medical ethics arena. Similarly, the Royal College of Nursing (RCN) provides guidance on ethical matters such as research, advanced directives ('living wills') and resuscitation. The RCN and BMA are increasingly working together, recently producing the booklet concerning advanced statements (BMA 1995).

Ethical theories, principles and rules provide a framework for value consideration and ethical decision making. Beauchamp & Childress (1994) encapsulate the basic ethical framework, arguing that knowledge of this will improve judgements and actions. The framework consists of two theories, four principles and four rules. It has been popularised in this country by Gillon (1985) and used by many ethicists (Tschudin 1992, Rumbold 1993, Thompson et al 1994).

The framework itself will not provide a panacea to all problems but it does serve as a background and guide to ethical issues. Certainly, it raises awareness of the issues surrounding paternalism and offers other approaches. Cribb (1995) suggests that this four-principle approach is a valuable tool for individuals with differing philosophies to communicate within the same framework.

In Beauchamp & Childress' (1994) linear model, two major ethical theories are examined: deontology (non-consequential) and utilitarianism (consequential). Briefly summarised, the secondary terms indicates the emphasis. The deontological approach emphasises the process of an action independent of outcome, hence the term non-consequential. In this approach, ethical rules are applied: for example, the rule of veracity. By contrast, the utilitarian approach emphasises the consequences or outcome of actions independent of the process. It could be defensible using this theory to be somewhat 'economical' with the truth if this were thought to be beneficial to the patient. There are distinctions, however, in the consequential perspective, which can be divided into act and rule utilitarian. The act utilitarian appeals purely to the principle of utility. In other words, what action would maximise benefits and produce best outcomes for patients, independent of the process. The rule utilitarian considers both process and outcome; therefore, ethical rules are applied. So truth-telling, for example, would be an important feature. This is an interesting dimension because nurses and doctors do want to consider both process and outcome in patient care — the features of their actions as well as the outcomes in individual cases.

The four principles in the ethical framework are:

- non-maleficence
- beneficence
- respect for autonomy
- justice.

Simply, non-maleficence is fundamental to health care practice. Florence Nightingale commanded that her nurses should 'first, do the patient no harm'. In fact the maxim 'primum non nocere'. (above all, or first, do no harm) is embedded in the Hippocratic Oath and all professional codes and guidance.

The principle of beneficence is to do good, and the Health Service was set up with this aim. Of course health care practice, in attempting to do good, can cause harm. The two principles need to be continually balanced. High-technology intervention involves risk, and clinical practice requires skilled, competent cost–benefit analysis.

The word autonomy is derived from the Greek — *autos*, self, and *nomos*, rule — simply meaning self rule. Respect for autonomy is currently of interest in health care practice, as recognition of paternalistic attitudes is leading professionals to work in partnership with patients. The public are more informed and rightly expect consultation about health care choices. Informed consent is set within the principle of respect for autonomy and is considered in more detail below.

The principle of justice in health care is related to the allocation of resources involving notions of fairness, equity and desert. The deontological ethical theory serves the principle of justice as a key feature in moral reasoning. The principle of justice, in terms of allocation of resources in PIC, is examined in Vignette 2, using the linear model. It is also necessary to examine the rule layer. There are four ethical rules:

- veracity
- fidelity
- confidentiality
- privacy.

Veracity involves free and open communication between professionals, children and families. It could be argued, for example, that non-disclosure of information is as deceitful as lying. Beauchamp & Childress (1994) give three arguments for professional obligations of veracity:

- respecting autonomy
- the ethical rule of fidelity
- the importance of truth-telling.

Without truth there cannot be a trusting relationship, and lying demonstrates disrespect for persons.

The ethical rule of fidelity is linked with truth-telling, promise-keeping and faithfulness. Beauchamp & Childress (1994) state that the relationship between doctor and patient is based on trust and confidence. The doctor therefore becomes a trustee of the patient's medical welfare. This shows the importance of fidelity in the doctor–patient relationship. However, nurses may have a conflict between loyalty to the physician and to the patient. In consequence, this may cause nurses to choose between obligations of fidelity.

Confidentiality and privacy rules are closely connected in professional and patient relationships. Clause 10 of the Code of Professional Conduct (UKCC 1992b) requires that nurses 'protect all confidential information concerning patients and clients obtained in the course of professional practice and make disclosures only with consent, where required by the order of a court or where you can justify disclosure in the wider public interest'. They suggest that public interest involves individuals, groups or society as a whole and covers matters which place others at serious risk, such as serious crime, child abuse and drug smuggling (UKCC 1996).

Doctors as well are bound under the Hippocratic Oath to respect patient confidentiality in almost every circumstance. There are certain situations, however, that require disclosure of confidential information. Non-accidental injury and suspected child abuse require nurses and doctors in the interest of the child and the public to report their concerns. The law gives powers for the police to have information made available in their investigations under the following legislation (Dimond 1995):

- Road Traffic Act 1972
- Prevention of Terrorism (Temporary Provision) Act 1984
- Police and Criminal Evidence Act 1984.

In addition to these, Kennedy and Grubb (1994) refer to the GMC's *Professional conduct and discipline* (1993) where the obligation of confidence is stated, and they highlight where statutory provisions create exceptions:

- The Abortion Regulations 1991
- Public Health (Control of Diseases) Act 1984
- National Health Service (Venereal Disease) 1974
- NHS (Notification of Births and Deaths) Regulations 1982
- Misuse of Drugs (Notification of, and Supply to Addicts) Regulations 1973
- Data Protection Act 1984
- Rights and Responsibilities of Doctors 1992.

PRINCIPLE OF JUSTICE AND RESOURCE ALLOCATION

The Principle of Justice can be a difficult concept to enact when considering equity in relation to the distribution of health care resources. Vignette 2 indicates a contemporary issue arising from the health service reforms legislated with the NHS and Community Care Act 1990. The apparent lack of resources in the local area puts Katie at further risk in transferring to the PICU. If she is not adequately stabilised or the transfer team is not specifically trained, the risks increase. Recent research by Barry & Ralston (1994) showed that adverse events occurred during transport in 42 of 56 children studied. They further found that inexperienced staff incapable of performing basic resuscitative measures may have contributed to morbidity. The research also highlighted inadequate and in some cases malfunctioning equipment in the transfer process. The rationale for providing dedicated PIC facilities is advanced in *Care of the critically ill child* (British Paediatric Association 1993) and outlined by de Courcy-Golder (1996). Wright (1996) highlights three issues concerning the distribution of resources in health care:

- that public expectations are increased with advances in technology
- resources are finite
- nursing practice is influenced by resource decisions.

> **Vignette 2**
>
> Katie, a 7-year-old is brought into A & E department following an RTA, and the medical team diagnose a brain haemorrhage. The District Hospital has no PIC provision, and attempts to secure an IC bed elsewhere are proving difficult. Finally, a bed is found two hundred miles away. Katie and the transfer team begin a hazardous journey.

According to Wright (1996), estimations of health-care expenditure in 1992–1993 were 29.3 billion pounds. However, he points out that the UK's spending on health is 6.6% Gross Domestic Product (GDP) — less than the European average of 8%. The issue is not how much money is available but how it is distributed.

Justice is present whenever a person is due something which may be a benefit or a burden. Distributive justice refers to equal and fair distribution of all benefits and burdens in society, such as taxes, property, opportunities and resources: for example, health care and privileges. There are theories of justice which emphasise certain material principles such as giving to each person according to

- an equal share
- need
- effort
- contribution
- merit
- free-market exchanges

(Beauchamp & Childress 1994). Some theories of justice accept more than one of these, and Beauchamp & Childress argue that sometimes all six are present. These are recognised as important aspects of justice. Currently there is much debate concerning access to resources based on the individual's effort, contribution and ability to pay rather than on clinical need.

Four theories of justice are put forward by Beauchamp & Childress (1994):

- utilitarian
- libertarian
- communitarian
- egalitarian.

Utilitarian and libertarian theories are recognisable in the UK and the USA, respectively. The former attempts to maximise benefits — the NHS tries to provide the 'greatest good for the greatest number' — and the latter involves the free market, where most health care is based on a private system and the ability-to-pay principle. Communitarian theories do not stress rights and obligations in individual human relationships but regard the shared values of groups and communities and the common good to be most important. Egalitarian theories, the main exponent of which is John Rawls (1971), possibly present the greatest challenge to utilitarian and libertarian theories. In Rawls' theory, justice as fairness involves cooperation between people who are equal and free. In this respect society has an obligation to reduce or eliminate inequalities or at least those aspects that hinder 'fair equality of opportunity'. So having a disease or disability is seen as causing 'undeserved restrictions' on a person's potential. For health care, a system based on this theory endeavours to balance opportunity fairly through equal access and allocation of resources. Priorities in allocation should concern preventing and compensating any limits in human function and potential. Beauchamp & Childress (1994) argue that Rawls' theory involves egalitarian implications in that every member of society, despite position, status or wealth, should have equal access to health care. Health care in this approach is an adequate level not a maximum, so anything above this involves personal cost. This is interesting, as better services are then provided in the private sector. This situation can be seen developing alongside the NHS in this country.

It could be argued that the UK has an egalitarian tradition, although Seedhouse (1994) claims the NHS historically lacks design and has missed opportunities to clearly define health. In attempting to characterise principles guiding the NHS, Seedhouse (1994) found a lack of consensus but has extracted and consolidated four:

- it should meet all health needs
- everyone should receive the best care
- it should be egalitarian

- health care costs should be kept to a minimum.

Currently, there are many debates concerning the first principle; resources are finite and demand is potentially infinite. Many would not argue with the second principle, but there are questions concerning notions of 'best care'. What is best and what constitutes care? The third principle is highlighted in this section in attempting to review the theories of justice. The fourth principle is easily recognisable and more pressing in the market-oriented health service.

Provision of regional services disadvantages emergency admissions such as Katie (Powell & Rushforth 1996). Utilitarian concerns for justice, however, would seek to maximise benefits; hence, regional PICUs might give the 'greatest good for the greatest number'. Libertarian theories would allow the private sector to provide the appropriate services. Any treatment Katie required, emergency and long stay, would be a free-market enterprise and choice exercised on the basis of ability to pay. Justice in this situation, in egalitarian terms, requires equal access to service provision, fair opportunity to be admitted and a social obligation to deal with the undeserved clinical need. If the service is regionalised, it could be argued that immediate access is dependent on where the individual lives, questioning issues of fair opportunity and equality. There may be alternative solutions: for example, nursing Katie in an adult Intensive Care Unit with appropriate resources, but this raises issues of equity. De Courcy-Golder (1996) highlights the poor organisation and fragmentation of PIC in this country, leading her to support the case for developing a national system for tertiary PICUs which are properly accredited. This involves a considerable investment, but she argues that medium to long-term benefits would outweigh the disruption and that the costs would be offset by savings in improved clinical outcomes and better quality. Equity in this argument would seem to be addressed, and there is a strong likelihood that this proposed development in PICUs would correspond with egalitarian theories of justice.

CONSENT

This subject is at the heart of most ethical and legal considerations, particularly in relation to children. Elliston (1996) questions the arbitrary age limit of 16 years to make decisions about medical interventions. Regardless of physiological and psychological development, the rights of the child and the role of the parents/guardian constitute a keenly debated area of consent to / refusal of treatment.

The mentally competent person who has reached the age of 18 years will be considered able to make all decisions about his/her health care and participate in research. Dimond (1995) points out, however, that Section 8 of the Family Law Reform Act (1969) provides for a minor of 16 or 17 years to give valid consent to treatment.

The Children Act (1989), for the first time, gives some recognition to the child's wishes and involvement in health care decisions. The Act also highlights that children may express personal preferences which do not always concur with those of their parents. The overriding principle is recognition of children as individuals. This legislation would lead one to believe that decisions made by children in the main are respected. Sadly, this is not the situation. Elliston (1996) traces the case law in England and Wales in the medical context, where apparently two standards are set to determine competence of a child to make a decision: the presumptive test and an evidential test.

The presumptive standard relates to Section 8 of The Family Law Reform Act 1969. There is no provision for a different standard of assessment of competence of the 16 year old. In consequence, as Elliston (1996, p 30) argues, 'the statute appears to intend that the consent of a 16 year old should be as valid in law as if they were an adult, that is that they are to be regarded as self-governing for this purpose'.

The evidential standard is highlighted by Elliston (1996) regarding the famous case of Gillick v West Norfolk and Wisbech Area Health Authority 1985. Apparently, Lord Fraser and Lord Scarman put forward two judgements in terms of the child's competence: in the former.

'sufficient discretion to be able to make as wise a choice in their best interests'

and in the latter,

'attainment of intelligence and understanding of the medical issues'.

Elliston (1996) argues that English law appears to favour Lord Fraser's judgement, and in any event the child must satisfy the evidential test rather than a presumptive test. However, these tests for determining competence to consent to medical treatment do not allow for the child to refuse. Elliston suggests that the courts have created additional requirements for assessment when a child refuses treatment.

In considering the ethical dimension the health care practitioner should focus on the principle of respect for autonomy. Observing self rule would necessitate ultimate right to consent and refusal of treatment to be located with the child. The assumption here is that the child is conscious. The possibility of advanced directives has emerged regarding children but as yet has not been fiercely debated.

Current health care ethicists place great emphasis on respect for autonomous choices. Gillon (1985) points out that the principle of respect for autonomy is central in both deontological and utilitarian ethical perspectives.

The British Medical Association summarises autonomy as 'the capacity to think and decide independently (competence), the capacity to act on the basis of that decision, and the ability to communicate in some way with other people' (BMA 1993, pp 73–74).

Informed consent involves respecting autonomy, incorporating ethical rules of truth-telling and confidentiality. It is argued that, in any theory of autonomy, *liberty* and *agency* are essential features. Liberty requires *independence from controlling influences*, and agency is the *capacity for intentional action* (Beauchamp & Childress 1994). However, where choice is exercised, judgements about so-called competence are involved. Controversy surrounds the concept of competence, with recent discussions focusing on standards. Generally, it is about the ability to understand the treatment or research procedure, to weigh up risks and benefits and make a decision (Beauchamp & Childress 1994). In English law Kennedy & Grubb (1994) outline five categories for competency:

1. evidencing a choice
2. reasonable outcome of choice
3. choice based on 'rational' reasons
4. ability to understand
5. actual understanding.

Respecting autonomy must be exercised in relationship to informed consent. Gillon (1985, p 113) provides a widely accepted definition for medical intervention: 'that consent means a voluntary, uncoerced decision, made by a sufficiently competent or autonomous person on the basis of adequate information and deliberation, to accept rather than reject some proposed course of action that will affect him or her'.

In the case of children the BMA (1993) argues that where there is sufficient intelligence and understanding it should be presumed that decision-making for or against treatment is valid.

In reality, refusal to consent is hugely problematic. It has already been indicated by Elliston (1996) that, in the case of children where refusal of treatment occurs, a much more rigorous test of competence is applied than in adults. She argues that there is no justification for using a more stringent test to determine competence and that it is illogical to distinguish between consent and refusal. Elliston suggests that current ethical perspectives should give individuals equal right to consent or refuse treatment. Vignette 3 illustrates a familiar issue involving consent. Jehovah's Witnesses are bound by their religious beliefs to refuse blood products in the management of their care. The salient point for clinical practice involves safeguarding the interests of the child. In this case the staff have no indication of Susan's beliefs and it cannot be assumed that she shares her parents convictions. Even if she did, because she is unconscious, there is no way of satisfying her competence in the decision-making process. There is a dilemma regarding the duty of care to act in Susan's best interests, respect her autonomy but take account of her parents' wishes.

Vignette 3

A 10-year-old girl (Susan) has had a farm accident in which she sustained a head injury. She is on a ventilator in PIC. 12 hours post admission, neurological observations suggest raised intracranial pressure and surgical intervention is necessary. Her parents are Jehovah's Witnesses.

There are a number of issues for consideration: the tradition of paternalistic practice invites immediate action to do whatever is necessary to safeguard Susan's life, beneficence is a compelling principle. Principles need to be weighed, however: beneficence needs to be balanced with non-maleficence; a cost–benefit analysis is necessary. Practitioners need to consider first if there is a way around this situation that respects both clinical need and religious preference. What are the risks in not giving blood to Susan? Are there alternatives to blood products? If the risks of not giving blood are too great, practitioners are faced with overriding the parents' wishes. The legal way forward is detailed in the Children Act 1989, which provides for application for an order under section 8:

- specific issue order — requiring certain action be taken.
- prohibited steps order — prohibiting a particular procedure.

Parents as well have a right to apply to the court under section 8. Professionals liaise with social services to apply to the court. If the core of the dispute is whether or not the child should receive a transfusion, the professionals will be asking for a 'specific issue order' authorising the administration of blood. The parents will want a 'prohibited steps order' banning treatment contrary to their faith. The courts in England to-date have ordered that blood transfusions can take place in such situations. Fletcher et al (1995) suggest that the courts are more sensitive to parental conviction and urge practitioners to consider the psychological effects of children returning to families following such intervention.

Elliston (1996) reviews an alternative approach found in Scottish law which does not emphasise parental power to consent and allows for full consent at age 16 years without assessment of competence. The position under the new Children (Scotland) Act 1995 allows for refusal of treatment by a competent child under 16 years (Norrie 1995). Equally, they can give consent, unless the same reasons for overriding their decision are used as with an adult, e.g. public health.

An even more radical approach is offered by Alderson & Montgomery (1996), who argue that children should be presumed to be competent from compulsory school age. This means that parents would have to consider children's participation in the decision-making process. They recommend a code of practice be established under an Act of Parliament for children's health care rights to raise standards, provide information and clarity on legal issues.

Consent and research

Research involving human subjects or participants must be assessed by an ethics committee who are particularly concerned that researchers obtain informed consent. The term participant, used with qualitative methodologies, implies involvement in the study but does not ensure informed consent. Dimond (1996) argues that ethical principles in the research process are not always enforceable by law. However, she points out that there are parallel laws. She also makes the important point that anything illegal, such as research on embryos after 14 days' gestation, is not made legal by having consent. The case of children's consent to research is governed by the law and notions of competent decision-making. The age of 18 confers the right to decide about any medical care and to agree, or not, to take part in 'therapeutic' or 'non-therapeutic' research. Therapeutic research primarily aims to benefit the individual involved, whilst non-therapeutic research may or may not benefit the individual but focuses on gathering information (BMA 1993). It is important to point out the limits of research. In the question of therapeutic research the law measures this in terms of a risk–benefit ratio. For non-therapeutic research or research involving those who are incompetent to consent, this ratio is of concern in the regulation of the research (Kennedy & Grubb 1994).

The Medical Research Council (MRC 1991) considers live-born children, including those with mental handicap or illness, up to the age of 18 years. It makes some important points which concur with the ethical framework that respecting self rule is fundamental, that there are rights 'to be free from bodily interference whether physical or psychological' and that these principles are recognised in English law. Interestingly, however, the MRC states only three elements to consent: 'the information, the capacity to understand it and the voluntariness of any decision taken' (MRC 1991, p 6). Beauchamp & Childress (1994) detail informed consent, dividing it into three stages involving seven elements:

- threshold elements (preconditions)
  1. competence (to understand and decide)
  2. voluntariness (in deciding)
- information elements
  3. disclosure (of material information)
  4. recommendation (of a plan)
  5. understanding (of 3 & 4)
- consent elements
  6. decision (in favour of a plan)
  7. authorisation (of the chosen plan)

(Beauchamp & Childress, 1994, p 146).

Consideration of these important and sequential elements delineates the serious nature of the process of consent and the right to refuse treatment, intervention or participation in research. The American experience of health care which is dependent on libertarian theories of justice is more litigious. Yet it is a pertinent reminder that market-oriented health systems in the UK will naturally emphasise rights and responsibilities and in consequence set the stage for civil action if these are not achieved. Correspondingly, the public are far more informed about matters regarding their own health care and the legal process.

Gillick competence

The Gillick case (1985), which involved a mother pleading on behalf of her child, is recognised as a milestone in cases involving child consent. She brought to court an argument against providing contraception to children under 16. Her contention was based on two points: that, as it is illegal to have sex with an under-age person, medical practitioners would be colluding in a crime; and that any unauthorised treatment of a child under 16 constituted battery. The House of Lords ruling did not concur that either an illegal act in providing contraception was performed or that it constituted battery. The Law Lords pointed out that the chief characteristic in the case of children was the achievement of intelligence to facilitate understanding of what is proposed in order to give valid consent (Fletcher et al 1995). Following this case 'Gillick competence' has been widely used to elucidate the child's ability to give consent.

The notion of 'Gillick competent' can be applied to therapeutic research where benefits are anticipated. It is much more difficult to attempt to obtain consent for non-therapeutic research, where there is no direct benefit to the child. In either situation, however, if the under 16 year old is judged able to consent, parental approval must be sought as well (MRC 1991). This is reflected in the current nursing and medical emphasis on partnership. Essential to any good practice is involvement of parents and significant others in the planning and delivery of care. Dimond (1996) reminds us that, since the Gillick case, the ability of those under 16 years to give valid consent has received more consideration. In terms of the child's rights, however, Fletcher et al (1995) point out that in two recent Court of Appeal rulings, individuals under 18 years of age have been unable to refuse treatment when this is considered to be in their best interests.

LIFE SUPPORT AND BRAINSTEM DEATH

PIC practice incorporates extremes of the ethical and legal framework, which can have profound psychological effects on parents, children and staff. Brainstem death is perhaps the worst scenario, because hope and rehabilitation are no longer possible. There is the potential for organ donation, which entails sensitive communication to gain possible consent, but this too involves a whole subset of ethical and legal issues. Watkinson (1995) showed that experienced critical care nurses are in favour of organ donation but, in the case of young adults and children, they were more profoundly affected. Importantly, his findings also demonstrated a strong correlation between nurses' knowledge of brainstem death and having this positive attitude.

Brainstem death and organ donation are discrete and should be considered as unrelated. The person who has been diagnosed as brainstem dead is not automatically a potential organ donor. The preservation of the life for the harvesting of organs is not permitted, where there is little chance of reasonable recovery (New et al 1994).

Organ transplantation is now an acceptable form of treatment, but there are few deaths from brainstem damage that meet the strict criteria for brainstem death. This limits the potential number of organs available. Approaches to the next of kin need to be sensitive and informed. Legislation governing organ donation includes the Human Tissue Act 1961 and the Human Organ Transplant Act 1989. Dimond (1995) suggests that consent is necessary and briefly outlines the debate to increase the availability of organs for transplantation. The opt-out system requires individuals to carry a card if they do not wish their organs to be donated. This would mean that if no card was found, all organs could be harvested. The major concern about this system is the permanent possession of such a card. The implication in this approach is that a person's body is available for donation unless otherwise stated and would cause the individual a 'burden of proof'. The ethical and legal aspects of respect for autonomy, consent, human rights and dignity are involved. The public are mainly in favour of organ donation but find brainstem death incongruous (Gibson 1996). In 1995 Gibson highlighted the key role of critical care nurses in identifying potential donors. Following diagnosis of brainstem death the monitoring of vital signs to maintain function of organs for donation causes nurses distress and problems with patient dignity. In order to understand and support organ

donation and transplantation, Sque and Payne (1994) suggest a framework provided in the notion of Gift Exchange Theory. This theory illuminates the giving and receiving of gifts and simply involves the giver, the gift, the receiver and the object of reciprocity. In applying this to cadaveric organ transplantation, there is the donor, the organ and the recipient.

It may be useful to postulate some possible scenarios in PICU. A child may wish to donate his/her organs and indeed carry a card, and the parents may agree or disagree with this. In the presence of agreement, there is no problem provided of course the donation is suitable. If the parents disagree, all aspects of consent should be considered. If the child dies, it is unlikely that the health care team would pursue organ donation if the parents refused, despite the child's wishes to the contrary. The best evidence appears in the case of adults, where, although there is no right of veto by relatives to donor consent, hospitals do not pursue relative's objections (Gibson 1996). Another possibility is that the child refuses and the parents consent. This would again involve ethical and legal considerations and may be an example where a nurse acts as advocate for the child.

Vignette 4 crystallises the sharp edges of ethical and legal reasoning and accountability in end-of-life decisions. Advances in medical technologies have raised the public expectation of prolongation of life and return to health following disease and injury. In David's situation, however, his parents actively seek not to have his life prolonged. There are particular justice, equity and fairness issues about not prolonging life and withdrawal of treatment in the presence of handicap and disability. Campbell & McHaffie (1995) cite a case heard by the court of appeal in 1981 which authorised a child with Down's syndrome to have surgery for intestinal obstruction against parental wishes. Contrary to this position, however, they cite a case in 1989 where a High Court judge allowed no further attempts to prolong life in a 4-month-old infant with hydrocephalus, severe cerebral palsy and blindness. These cases illustrate that clinicians and the courts seem to both consider and estimate notions of so-called 'quality of life'. Health economists and clinicians have for some time been using the measurement of Quality Adjusted Life Years (QUALYs) (Williams 1985). This system involves scoring life expectancy in relation to health, ill health and death. A score below 0 suggests poor quality of life (Fletcher et al 1995). These scores are used in two ways: to decide which treatments are most beneficial, producing a positive QUALY, and to calculate which patient can be treated and which patient is denied treatment. As one might expect, there is criticism concerning equity and justice. Seedhouse (1994) criticises QUALY because it is arbitrary, conceptions vary and it is really a mechanism for managerial and economic control of health care resources.

Vignette 4

David, an 18-month-old severely physically and mentally handicapped child, is admitted to PIC with respiratory failure secondary to a pneumococcal chest infection. The parents do not wish the nursing and medical team to strive to prolong David's life unnecessarily.

Where withdrawal of life-support in infants born with major congenital abnormalities is concerned, Campbell & McHaffie (1995) suggest these are most likely to be considered in the public arena. They specify that disorders of the central nervous system are the largest subgroup within the infant category. In older children, brain damage related to infection, haemorrhage and hypoxic ischaemia are conditions where withdrawal of life support may be considered. Recent publicity around the 'Child B' case also raises the issue of children suffering from a terminal disease, such as cancer. Further, it illustrates health care rationing and concerns of equity (New 1996).

It is important to clarify what is meant by life-prolonging treatments. Beauchamp & Childress (1994) make certain distinctions concerning treatment and non-treatment decisions. These are set within the principle of non-maleficence but will, of course, necessarily involve balancing

beneficence and other possible competing principles. The distinctions are as follows:

- withholding and withdrawing life-sustaining treatment
- extraordinary and ordinary treatment
- artificial feeding and life-sustaining technologies
- intended effects and merely foreseen effects.

Withholding treatment means not to start something, and withdrawing treatment means stopping treatment. Whilst health care practitioners and family members feel some justification in not starting treatment, they do not feel this regarding withdrawing treatment that has already begun. This is interesting in David's case, since implicit in the parents' request is a plea for withholding treatment. Yet Beauchamp & Childress (1994) argue that distinctions between withholding and withdrawing treatment are ethically irrelevant. This is because decisions about these should be based on benefits and burdens of treatment understood by the patient or surrogate, and consideration of patients' rights. So where does this now position David's parents' request? In order to attempt to answer this, it is necessary to work through the other distinctions above.

Notions of extraordinary and ordinary treatment are in themselves open to misinterpretation. *Ordinary* has often been taken to mean usual or customary, whereas *extraordinary* has often been taken to mean unusual or uncustomary (Beauchamp & Childress 1994). However, there are problems with this because ordinary treatment has simply been viewed as routine, inexpensive, natural and somehow non-invasive and therefore obligatory; whilst extraordinary treatment is often seen as expensive, invasive, complex, artificial and therefore optional. The point here is that whatever treatment is available and concurs with patient wishes is ethically indistinguishable. Another salient point is that, in the vignette, David's consent is not possible but, if optional and obligatory distinctions are used, a cost–benefit analysis of treatment must take place.

Sustenance and medical technologies can be significantly different. The former involves nutrition and hydration given enterally and parenterally. The latter involves advanced technological interventions including artificial ventilation. Arguments rest on the balance of perceived benefits and burdens. For David, it would be necessary to discuss this balance with his parents when the situation of sustenance technologies arises. The case of Airedale NHS Trust v Bland 1993 is familiar to most practitioners. Brahams (1995) points out that successive courts clarified that the discussion about Tony Bland was not about euthanasia. In the event the health care team was permitted to withdraw sustenance technologies. The Royal College of Nursing supported the House of Lords decision but with some reservations. Their argument was that hydration and nutrition are basic fundamental needs involving administration and management of care (Friend 1993).

Intended effects versus merely foreseen effects contains a well-known principle or doctrine known as 'the rule of double effect' (RDE). There are particular subtleties involved in this principle which prohibits the intentional use of harm. Familiar to this is, for example, providing pain control and management in extreme suffering or terminal situations. The administration of analgesia should primarily be to alleviate pain and suffering, not intentionally to cause death. Yet death may be hastened as a foreseen but unintentional consequence of administering analgesia. Campbell (1995) explains this in relation to Dr Nigel Cox, who unfortunately intended his patient's death as the only means of preventing further suffering and pain. Dr Cox's behaviour was against the rule of double effect.

In David's situation the parents have a clear intention not to prolong his life, and the obvious foreseen effects of non-intervention would be death. This conclusion does not necessarily justify or allow for this decision.

Beauchamp & Childress (1994) advanced the argument using notions of optional and obligatory treatments. However, they include several categories to develop these notions. These are quite intricate and involve close examination in the primary text. In brief, quality of life considerations that are particularly controlled and linked for competent patients with the principle of respect for autonomy are invoked. In the case of children in circumstances such as David's, Beauchamp & Childress (1994, p 218) state 'Such quality of life judgements need to be restricted by justifiable criteria of benefits and burdens, so that quality is not reduced to arbitrary and partial judgements of personal preference or of the social worth of a child'. Sadly, David is neither autonomous nor competent. If, in his case, the health care team and parents cannot agree on intervention or non-intervention, application to the court will be necessary for the appropriate order.

CHILD PROTECTION AND THE CHILDREN ACT 1989

Staff involved in child protection issues have a primary aim of prevention. Current trends in nursing are promoting health and healing and providing holistic and therapeutic care in partnership with patients and other professionals. Child protection involves current legislation, the Children Act 1989, and a legal and ethical framework. Roberts et al (1996, p 32) highlight prevention of childhood injury as a national priority in the *Health of the nation* document. Their recent research involving a review of 11 randomised controlled trials of home-visiting programmes demonstrated that these can reduce childhood injury. It is unlikely that Paediatric Intensive Care nurses and doctors will be involved with primary prevention; the nature of the service means that the child abuse issues faced are likely to be of the gravest nature. It is important to have a sense of perspective and review the epidemiology of child abuse. Yet Parton (1985) warns that viewing child abuse from a dominant disease model only ignores the wider legal and socially deviant aspects. Incidence and prevalence rates establish the type of injury and indicate the likelihood of the need for PIC. Hallett (1995), in analysing prevalence and incidence, reviews three main data sources: sample surveys and prevalence estimates based on clinical samples, and data from child protection registers. She argues, however, that there are 'definitional ambiguities' concerning child abuse which cause problems in these estimates. The register data only reflects those cases that have come to the attention of practitioners. Hallett (1995), primarily reviewing the work of Creighton (1992), estimates from the NSPCC register data, where three main clusters of abuse are determined: moderate, serious and fatal. From these it would appear that the moderate category involves the largest percentage of cases. Creighton (1992) defines these categories as:

- moderate — all soft tissue injuries of a superficial nature
- serious — all fractures, head injuries, internal injuries, severe burns and ingestion of toxic substances
- fatal — all cases resulting in death.

It is extremely difficult to establish precise indicators of the likelihood of children receiving PIC from the present statistics. Yet, it would appear from Creighton's (1992) work, from figures compiled from 1988 to 1990 of a sample of 2786 abused children, 61 had skull fractures (2%), 20 had subdural haematomas (1%), and 12 children had brain damage. These are the most likely forms of injury requiring PIC; the vast majority of cases in this sample, however, involved bruising to the head and face or to the body and limbs — 41% and 43%, respectively — which is less likely to require PIC. This last statement should not imply that PIC nurses and doctors by virtue of their specialist role are not involved in early detection and prevention of child abuse. The current emphasis is on working together in a multidisciplinary context (DoH 1991, Murphy 1995).

Vignette 5

4-year-old Hannah is brought into accident and emergency unconscious. She is intubated and is taken to PIC. Her injuries include facial bruising and bilateral retinal haemorrhages; there is also bruising to her back. Her mother and cohabitee arrive later to the unit, pleading ignorance to any of her injuries.

Vignette 5 suggests a possible serious injury requiring PIC. The first considerations in practitioners' duty of care are to respond to Hannah's clinical needs. Hannah is in a place of safety by virtue of being in hospital, and because she is unconscious it is unlikely that her mother would try to remove her. Assessment would indicate that these injuries are non-accidental, and Hannah's mother and her cohabitee are not prepared to give any explanation. Clearly an investigation needs to take place. Health care practitioners and other professionals have a duty to report any suspected or actual child abuse. Referral to Social Services is necessary in the first instance. Any practitioner involved with the family, such as the Health Visitor and General Practitioner, will need to be informed. The legal framework is provided in the Children Act 1989. Stainton Rogers & Roche (1992) point out that, in terms of changes in child protection, a major emphasis in the Act is for courts not to intervene unnecessarily. Two main recommendations are given:

- resources should be available to support families with stress in child care
- practitioners should work in partnership with parents to achieve voluntary agreements in protecting children.

Whyte (1997) makes a case for family nursing and reviews the work of Casey (1993) and Nethercott (1993), who identifies the particular knowledge and skills necessary in family-centred care. Parents should be accepted as partners in care, and nursing should not be used as a source of power. Particular skill is required to work with parents and carers who are under suspicion of abuse. Where no cooperation occurs, this obviously frustrates the investigation and requires greater patience on the part of practitioners. If Hannah's mother attempts to remove her, an Emergency Protection Order will need to be sought. Application for this is to the court, who must be satisfied that there is reasonable cause to believe that the child has suffered or is likely to suffer significant harm. In any event, there needs to be a case conference for professionals and family to share information and recommendations for plans of action and possible registration on the Child Protection Register. The police are responsible for collecting evidence to decide if a case should be put before the criminal court. *Working together* (DoH 1991) encourages parental attendance at case conferences. Professionals' attitudes and views have been shown to differ in relation to this practice. Macaskill & Ashworth (1995) found that social workers were largely supportive of parental attendance but were aware of potential problems. However, Cooper & Pennington (1995) found that there were differences between the attitudes of nurses and social workers to parental attendance. These included:

- resistance to parental involvement
- effects of parents upon conference dynamics
- management of parental involvement.

Practitioners need to apply ethical principles and rules in child protection. The principle of respect for autonomy in the case of Hannah's mother who refuses to cooperate must be overridden in the best interest of her child. Clearly, beneficence and non-maleficence need priority, and justice would require that all situations where abuse is suspected are properly investigated and children are made safe. This does not mean that the ethical rules of confidentiality and veracity are not considered, as the duty to disclose suspected child abuse takes precedent (Wheeler 1995). There are tensions surrounding confidentiality and child protection for Health Visitors, as trust needs to be maintained to gain access for ongoing visiting. Veracity is a key component of professional and patient–client relationships and can be seriously undermined when investigation of suspected and actual child abuse occurs. The ethical and legal framework cannot be applied as a mathematical equation. Cribb (1995) argues that one of the benefits of philosophical ethics is that it allows for reflection and acknowledging uncertainties.

PROFESSIONAL AND LEGAL ISSUES REGARDING ROLE EXPANSION IN PAEDIATRIC INTENSIVE CARE

The dynamic nature of health policy and the changing pattern of health care delivery since the inception of the NHS in 1948 has influenced the role of the nurse. This is particularly apparent following the Griffiths Report (Griffiths 1983) and NHS and Community Care Act (DoH 1990). Public expectation has similarly shifted, with greater interest in and criticism of health care delivery. Practitioners are redefining their roles to incorporate characteristics of clinical activities which were previously undertaken by doctors and other health care professionals. Greenhalgh (NHS Executive 1994) paved the way for role changes amongst junior doctors and nurses. In the USA and UK, specialist nurse practitioners are taking over the management of care for specific groups of patients. Specific legal and professional issues must be addressed to ensure appropriate accountability if this care has traditionally been provided by a doctor.

Both the nursing and medical professions acknowledge the need for practitioners to work in partnership with each other (UKCC 1992c, GMC 1995). *The scope of professional practice* (UKCC 1992c) outlined the principles for expanding nursing practice, and Dimond (1994) traces this development and the current emphasis on skill, knowledge and competence. The UKCC has underlined the need to use the Code of Professional Conduct as the foundation for clinical practice and that practice must meet the changing needs of patients. The UKCC's most recent document, *Guidelines for professional practice* (1996), reflects the motto 'protect and honour' which sums up the principles for professional judgement. Equally the GMC (1995) supports the delegation of care to other practitioners competent in the relevant therapies or procedures. However, it warns against delegating tasks which require medical knowledge and skills. There is considerable freedom for nursing practitioners to develop their skills across traditional professional boundaries, and this is the rationale of *The scope of professional practice*. What governs the extent of skills development are the fundamental principles that underpin the notion of accountability in professional practice, and these are endorsed explicitly by the UKCC in the *Code of professional conduct* (1992b), *The scope of professional practice* (1992c) and are in evidence in the GMC's *Duties of a doctor* (1995).

There are no clear definitions of accountability (Watson 1995), yet it is a central theme in any discussion about the changing role of the nurse. The arenas of accountability have already been discussed earlier in this chapter. Accountability is the hallmark of professionalism and applies to all professionals in the context of their area of work. It can be characterised by responsibility, authority and autonomy, although it is argued that nursing has limited authority and therefore is unable to exercise autonomy (Watson 1995). Accountability demands knowledge, and, as nursing is in essence a practice discipline, there is a level of competence and mastery whereby decisions about clinical interventions are based on a sound body of knowledge. There is a need for practitioners to keep their knowledge and skills up-to-date through continuing education and training. This is supported by the UKCC through PREP (UKCC 1990). Currently, there is no mandatory requirement for doctors to undertake continuing professional education, although it is considered to be an element of good practice by the Royal Colleges.

Standards for practice are essential, as practitioners accused of negligence will be assessed against these. Negligence is defined as an act or omission for which one is liable, where: a duty of care is owed by the defendant to the plaintiff, there is a breach in the standard of that duty, and the breach has caused reasonably foreseeable harm. The measure of the standard is currently that set out in the Bolam Test. Regardless of whether a nurse or doctor carries out a task, the courts will assess the activity based on acceptable standards outlined by a perceived expert in the practice (Dimond 1994). The standard of care should be set and monitored by the profession itself. One approach to standard setting is the development of evidence-based multidisciplinary protocols or clinical guidelines outlining practice. Due to the increasingly complex nature of the decisions that practitioners have to make about interventions and treatment options, protocols can provide useful guidance.

Therefore, the development of specialist skills in PIC should be based on sound education and training. Research evidence should be used to guide practice in order that this can be justified when required by patients and their families or by the profession.

CONCLUSION

The section above concerning the expanding role in PIC indicates that there are always going to be changes in practice, skill standards and expectations and corresponding legal and ethical considerations. It is difficult in this sense to draw conclusions that would not mislead practitioners into a belief that there is always a prescribed course of action. Attempts have been made both to raise awareness and stimulate colleagues to challenge their own value bases and, in turn, their practice. This chapter has outlined the basic legal framework that currently exists and offered an ethical counterpart and applied these to various situations illustrated in vignettes. Whilst these refer to PIC, the general ethical and legal principles can be consistent and therefore applicable in all health care settings.

REFERENCES

Alderson P, Montgomery J 1996 Health care choice: making decisions with children. Institute for Public Policy Research, London

Barry P W, Ralston C 1994 Adverse events occurring during interhospital transfer of the critically ill. Archives of Disease in Childhood 71:8–11

Beauchamp T, Childress J F 1994 Principles of biomedical ethics, 4th edn. Oxford University Press, New York

Brahams D 1995 The critically ill patient: the legal perspective. In: Tingle J, Cribb A (eds) Nursing, law and ethics. Blackwell Science, Oxford

British Medical Association 1993 Medical ethics today: its practice and philosophy. BMJ, London

British Medical Association 1995 Advanced statements about medical treatment. BMJ, London

British Paediatric Association 1993 Report of a working party on paediatric intensive care. BPA, London

Campbell A G M, McHaffie H E 1995 Prolonging life and allowing deaths: infants. Journal of Medical Ethics 21:339–344

Campbell R 1995 The critically ill patient: an ethical perspective — declining and withdrawing treatment. In:

Tingle J, Cribb A (eds) Nursing, law and ethics. Blackwell Science, Oxford

Casey A 1993 Development and use of the partnership model of nursing care. In: Glasper E A, Tucker A (eds) Advances in child health nursing. Scutari, London

Cooper N, Pennington D 1995 The attitudes of social workers, health visitors and school nurses to parental involvement in child protection case conferences. British Journal of Social Work 25:599–613

Creighton S 1992 Child abuse trends in England and Wales, 1988–1990. NSPCC, London

Cribb A 1995 The ethical dimension. In: Tingle J, Cribb A. Nursing, law and ethics. Blackwell Science, Oxford, ch 2, p 21

de Courcy-Goulder K 1996 A strategy for development of paediatric intensive care within the United Kingdom. Intensive and Critical Care Nursing 12:84–89

Department of Health 1990 The NHS and Community Care Act. HMSO, London

Department of Health 1991 Working together under the Children Act 1989: a guide to arrangements for inter-agency cooperation for the protection of children from abuse. HMSO, London

Dimond B 1994 Legal aspects of role expansion. In: Hunt G, Wainwright P (eds) Expanding the role of the nurse: the scope of professional practice. Blackwell Science, Oxford

Dimond B 1995 Legal aspects of nursing, 2nd edn. Prentice Hall, London

Dimond B 1996 Legal issues. In: De Raeve L (ed) Nursing research: an ethical and legal appraisal. Baillière Tindall, London, ch 9, p 118

Elliston S 1996 If you know what's good for you: refusal of consent to medical treatment by children. In: McLean S (ed) Contemporary issues in law, medicine and ethics. Dartmouth, Aldershot

Fletcher N, Holt J, Brazier M, Harris J 1995 Ethics, law and nursing. Manchester University Press, Manchester

Friend B 1993 RCN favours stopping active care for Bland. Nursing Times 89(6):7

General Medical Council 1993 Professional conduct and discipline: fitness to practise. GMC, London

General Medical Council 1995 Duties of a doctor: guidance from the General Medical Council. GMC, London

Gibson V 1995 Nurses' experiences of organ donation. Care of the Critically Ill 11(5):176

Gibson V 1996 The factors influencing organ donation: a review of the research. Journal of Advanced Nursing 23:353–356

Gillon R 1985 Philosophical medical ethics. Wiley, Chichester

Griffiths R 1983 NHS Management Enquiry Report (The Griffiths report). DHSS, London.

Hallett C 1995 Child abuse: an academic overview. In: Kingston P, Penhale B (eds) Family violence and the caring professions. Macmillan, Basingstoke, ch 1, p 21

Hunt G, Wainwright P 1994 Expanding the role of the nurse: the scope of professional practice. Blackwell Science, Oxford

Kennedy I, Grubb A 1994 Medical law: text with materials, 2nd edn. Butterworths, London

Macaskill A, Ashworth P 1995 Parental participation in child protection case conferences: the social worker's view. British Journal of Social Work 25:581–597

Medical Research Council 1991 The ethical conduct of research on children. MRC Ethics Series, MRC, London

Montgomery J 1992 Doctors' handmaidens: the legal contribution. In: McVeigh S, Wheeler S (eds) Law, health and medical regulation. Dartmouth, Aldershot

Murphy M 1995 Working together in child protection. Arena, Aldershot

Nethercott S 1993 A concept for all the family: family centred care — a concept analysis. Professional Nurse 8(12):794–797

New B 1996 The rationing agenda in the NHS. British Medical Journal 312:1593–1601

New B, Solomon M, Dingwall R, McHale J 1994 A question of give and take: improving the supply of donor organs for transplantation. Research report No 18. King's Fund Institute, London

NHS Executive 1994 The Greenhalgh Report: the interface between junior doctors and nurses (executive summary). Greenhalgh and Company Ltd, Leeds

Norrie McK K 1995 Children (Scotland) Act 1995. W Green/Sweet and Maxwell, Edinburgh

Parton N 1985 The politics of child abuse. Macmillan, London

Powell C, Rushforth H 1996 Paediatric intensive care: what is the solution? British Journal of Nursing 5(11):652

Rawls J 1971 A theory of justice. Harvard University Press, Cambridge, MA

Roberts I, Kramer M, Samy S 1996 Does home visiting prevent childhood injury? A systematic review of randomised controlled trials. British Medical Journal 312:29–33

Rumbold G 1993 Ethics in nursing practice, 2nd edn. Baillière Tindall, London

Seedhouse D 1988 Ethics: the heart of health care. Wiley, Chichester

Seedhouse D 1994 Fortress NHS: a philosophical review of the National Health Service. Wiley, Chichester

Sque M, Payne S 1994 Gift exchange theory: a critique in relation to organ transplantation. Journal of Advanced Nursing 19:45–51

Stainton Rogers W, Roche J 1992 Putting it all together: the Children Act 1989. In: Cloke C, Naish J (eds) Key issues in child protection for health visitors and nurses. Longman, Essex, ch 9, p 102

Tschudin V 1992 Ethics in nursing: the caring relationship, 2nd edn. Butterworth Heinemann, London

Thompson I E, Melia K M, Boyd K M 1994 Nursing ethics, 3rd edn. Churchill Livingstone, Edinburgh

United Kingdom Central Council for Nursing, Midwifery and Health Visiting 1990 The Report of the post-registration and practice project. UKCC, London

United Kingdom Central Council for Nursing, Midwifery and Health Visiting 1992a Standards for the administration of medicines. UKCC, London

United Kingdom Central Council for Nursing, Midwifery and Health Visiting 1992b Code of professional conduct, 3rd edn. UKCC, London

United Kingdom Central Council for Nursing, Midwifery and Health Visiting 1992c The scope of professional practice. UKCC, London

United Kingdom Central Council for Nursing, Midwifery and Health Visiting 1996 Guidelines for professional practice. UKCC, London

Watkinson G E 1995 A study of the perception and experiences of critical care nurses in caring for potential and actual organ donors: implications for nurse education. Journal of Advanced Nursing 22:929–940

Watson R 1995 Introduction: accountability in nursing. In: Watson R (ed) Accountability in nursing practice. Chapman and Hall, London, ch 1, p 1

Wheeler S 1995 Child abuse: the health perspective. In: Kingston P, Penhale B (eds) Family violence and the caring professions. Macmillan, Basingstoke, ch 2, p 50

Whyte D A 1997 Family nursing: a systemic approach to nursing work with families. In: Whyte DA (ed) Explorations in family nursing. Routledge, London

Williams A 1985 Economics of coronary artery by-pass grafting. British Medical Journal 291:326–329

Wright S G 1996 The distribution of resources in health care. Professional Nurse 11(9):583–586

22

Nutritional needs of the critically ill child

Alison French   Anne-Marie England

IMPORTANCE OF NUTRITIONAL SUPPORT FOR THE CRITICALLY ILL CHILD

Nutrition is the provision of daily amounts of macro and micro nutrients to meet an individual's requirement for growth and repair. Nutrition is vital for life. During childhood, nutrient requirements per kilogram of body weight are proportionally higher than in adults, because of the demands of growth and development (Taylor and Goodinson-McLaren 1992, Huddleston et al 1993). For critically ill children, the added metabolic stress caused by disease, sepsis or trauma results in an even greater requirement for all nutrients. This is often not seen as a clinical priority when the focus of treatment for critically ill children is on the life-saving measures.

Provision of adequate nutrition is essential to promote healing and maintain muscle mass. Consequently, adequate and appropriate nutritional support influences the length of time for which a child requires supportive ventilation, and it should result in a shorter stay in PIC.

However, the overall metabolic and physical problems associated with admission to PIC can make the provision of adequate nutrition difficult (Box 22.1). A multidisciplinary Nutritional Care Team (NCT) can overcome many of these problems, ensuring that nutrition is optimised via enteral or parenteral routes.

Nutritional substrates

These are essential to maintain health and facilitate growth and development. Energy is provided by the macro nutrients: fat, carbohydrate and protein. The proportions of these required in the diet varies with age, but a balanced feed will provide the correct proportions.

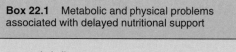

Box 22.1 Metabolic and physical problems associated with delayed nutritional support

- paralytic ileus
- poor gastric emptying
- fluid restriction and high requirement for IV drugs
- hyperkalaemia
- acute renal failure
- multiple surgery over consecutive days
- haemodynamic instability
- metabolic instability
- multisystem organ failure.

Protein

Protein is required for growth and repair and for the production of certain hormones and enzymes: for example, digestive enzymes. It can also be used as an energy source if there is insufficient glucose or fat. Protein consists of twenty amino acids, ten of which are considered essential for normal growth in children (see Box 22.2). Protein may be supplied as whole protein, peptides (short chains of up to five amino acids), or amino acids.

Box 22.2 Ten essential amino acids

- cystine
- histidine
- isoleucine
- leucine
- lysine
- methionine
- phenylalanine
- threonine
- tryptophan
- valine.

Arginine is probably essential too! From Francis (1987).

Carbohydrate

Carbohydrate can be split into two groups: starches and sugars. Both are digested to glucose, which is essential as the fuel for adenosine triphosphate (ATP) production via the Krebs Citric Acid Cycle. Glucose, a simple sugar or polymer, tends to provide the carbohydrate in many feeds. However, disaccharides such as sucrose and lactose may also be used.

Fat

Fat, in the form of lipids, is essential for growth. It is energy dense — providing 9 kcal/g, compared with 3.75 kcal/g for carbohydrate and 4 kcal/g for protein — making it an important source of calories. Essential fatty acids are necessary for cell wall formation and are increasingly recognised as vital for neurological development in neonates (Crawford 1993).

Vitamins

Vitamins are divided into water- and fat-soluble types, both being essential for normal physiological processes. Vitamin C is necessary for healing and formation of new tissue. B group vitamins are vital to metabolism, being present in many of the enzymes involved in energy production. They have small stores in the body and are depleted in a few days, making provision in adequate amounts essential. Fat-soluble vitamins A, D, E and K have larger stores, and are drawn on during starvation. They have important roles in the immune system, clotting mechanisms, bone development and tissue integrity. Stores are proportional to the size and age of the child; therefore smaller and younger children require earlier intervention to prevent deficiencies.

Minerals and trace elements

Minerals and trace elements have vastly different reserves: iron reserves are relatively low, whilst calcium reserves in the form of bone are large. It is still vital to provide adequate amounts of all these nutrients to enable growth to catch up after discharge from PICU and hospital.

'New' nutrients

Certain nutrients may be considered essential during metabolic stress. For example, glutamine, normally a non-essential amino acid, is released in quantity from the muscles and appears to be part of the normal response to trauma and sepsis. It helps to maintain the integrity of the gut and may improve immune function (Wilmore et al 1988). Glutamine is present in most enteral feeds as part of the protein, although supplements may be required. It is not found in parenteral nutrition (PN) solutions.

The presence of medium-chain triglycerides in enteral feeds improves protein synthesis and maintains body, mucosal and liver mass. The mechanism for this is not fully understood (Schwartz et al 1987).

Polyunsaturated fatty acids (PUFA) help to decrease the immune response by having an anti-inflammatory function (Alexander et al 1986). Food itself helps to maintain gut integrity, preventing translocation of microorganisms and possibly preventing multiorgan failure (Inoue et al 1988).

METABOLIC RESPONSE TO STRESS AND INFECTION

The metabolic response to injury or trauma can be divided into three phases, allowing the tissues to mobilise for defence and repair:

- ebb phase
- flow or catabolic phase
- anabolic phase

(Thomas 1994).

The ebb phase lasts for a few hours and is characterised by activation of the sympathetic neural and humoral factors, general depression of metabolic function and a reduction of energy expenditure.

The flow phase is characterised by increased basal metabolic rate and an increase in core temperature. Protein catabolism and increased lipolysis provide a pool of amino and fatty acids. Gluconeogenesis and glycogenolysis take place in the liver, causing the circulating levels of glucose to rise. Glycogen from muscle and liver is consumed within 24 h before fat stores are mobilised. As these primary energy stores are exhausted, body protein will also be utilised. The depletion of muscle mass and resulting debility is a severe consequence of progressive catabolism. All of these responses are mediated by 'stress' hormones, with raised levels of cortisol, glucagon and catecholamines. The result of their combined action is to produce glucose, which is essential for brain cell activity. Peripheral insulin resistance, which makes utilisation of glucose in the muscle more difficult than in brain cells, is due to the antagonistic effects of glucocorticoids and other polypeptides, causing mild hyperglycaemia. Nutritional therapy during this time cannot match all losses, but the aim is to minimise the effects of catabolism. It is impossible to replace all proteins lost; therefore a negative nitrogen balance is expected.

The anabolic phase is unlikely to occur in the acutely critically ill child. Appetite improves, making it possible to maintain a positive nitrogen balance and increase protein synthesis and rebuild muscle mass. Fat stores and reserves of protein are very different with age in childhood. Inadequate intake of nutrients in the absence of metabolic stress may lead to death through inanition (starvation) within a short period of time. A premature infant weighing 1 kg has minimal reserves, sufficient for 4 days only, and nutritional support must be started urgently. In contrast, a toddler has sufficient stores to last about 40 days and a teenage girl stores enough to survive about 50 days without food (Lennard-Jones 1992). These times are all curtailed when metabolic rate rises because of stress.

Hypercatabolism

Stress factors for different types of trauma have been calculated (Elia 1992). Burns and major fractures have the greatest effect on the metabolic rate, increasing energy requirements up to 180% of normal. A very high energy requirement can be impossible to meet artificially; therefore, early commencement of nutritional support is essential.

Consequences of nutritional deficiency

A deficit of nutrients has significant consequences for the child:

- poor healing of wounds and traumatised tissue, e.g. bone, muscle and skin
- depletion of muscle mass and power
- poor immune function and poor resistance to infection
- altered structure and function of the gut
- depression of mood, and apathy

(Booth 1994).

Poor wound healing

Wound healing is a complex process that has precise requirements. It occurs in three phases: inflammation, proliferation and maturation, all requiring specific nutrients. Some of these are needed in all three phases and some in only one. Daily provision of adequate nutrition is vital to the formation of a strong scar. All of the nutrients listed in Box 22.3 are required in larger than normal amounts during illness (Meyer et al 1994).

Box 22.3 Nutrients required for wound healing

- energy (calories)
- protein
- fatty acids (omega 3 series)
- vitamin C (ascorbic acid)
- vitamin A
- vitamin B2 (riboflavin)
- vitamin B5 (pantothenic acid)
- vitamin B6 (pyridoxine)
- vitamin E
- zinc
- iron
- manganese
- copper
- selenium
- silicon — not normally considered a nutrient

From Meyer et al (1994).

Muscle weakness

Muscle weakness results from inadequate provi-

sion of energy and protein but may be a consequence of atrophy from long-term sedation with or without pharmacological paralysis. Muscle loses power before it loses mass, and, without power, muscle cannot work. This has particular relevance in PIC, as loss of power and mass of the respiratory muscles can increase the length of time for which assisted ventilation is required. Similarly, cardiac muscle depletion will lead to impaired cardiac output and possible heart failure. The effects of muscle weakness caused by poor nutrition can be seen fairly soon after the child's admission and can result in an increased overall length of stay.

Poor immune function

The immune system cannot function properly with inadequate nutrition (Keithley & Eisenberg 1993). The normal production and maturation of white cells is inhibited by insufficient substrates to make new cells, resulting in increased susceptibility to infections; this in turn increases metabolic stress and places further demands on energy stores.

Altered structure and function of the gut

Starvation causes gut mucosal atrophy, increasing gut permeability. This can result in gut barrier failure and translocation of bacteria, contributing to sepsis and multiple organ failure (Mainous et al 1994). A starved gut takes longer to accept enteral nutrition when re-introduced, delaying eventual recovery.

Depression of mood and apathy

A period of semistarvation can result in mental state changes including apathy, depression and decreased attention span (Lennard-Jones 1992). These manifestations can be multifactoral for the child requiring a prolonged stay in PIC. Whatever the cause, the lethargic child with decreased interest and motivation can be difficult to engage in any activity, resulting in a longer rehabilitation and delayed discharge.

Nutritional requirements of the critically ill child

Children of varying ages have different nutritional requirements due to the contrasting rates of growth of the body systems. Trauma, sepsis and disease all have an effect on the requirement for nutrients. Other factors to be considered include the mode of ventilation, degree of sedation, pharmacological paralysis, mobility, pyrexia and pre-existing nutritional status.

Estimation of nutritional requirement is best done by the dietitian in discussion with the Nutritional Care Team (NCT). It is impossible to calculate an absolute requirement for each child, because the degree of illness and/or injury suffered is unique. Any estimation is a starting point, altering as the child's condition changes. Regular monitoring of nutritional requirements is vital to provide effective nutritional support. Specific stress factors are taken into account when formulating a regimen for feeding. The NCT will recommend the best enteral feed or parenteral regimen to meet these requirements.

NUTRITIONAL ASSESSMENT OF THE CRITICALLY ILL CHILD

A comprehensive nutritional assessment determines pre-existing nutritional status and establishes a baseline for the measurement of the effectiveness of nutritional support. Nutritional assessment involves a complex series of anthropometric, biochemical and observational measurements. It is unlikely that any one professional will have all the skills necessary to do this accurately, so a multidisciplinary nutritional team can be advantageous.

The Nutritional Care Team

A team approach represents the most effective and efficient way of clinical nutrition management, saving time, improving outcome and cost-effectiveness (Lennard-Jones 1992).

Members of a Nutritional Care Team

The composition of the Nutritional Care Team varies according to local needs. A team which meets regularly, understands the contribution made by all the individual members, undertaking a daily ward round and controlling the budget for enteral and parenteral feeds, will be the most effective (Lennard-Jones 1992). Ideally the team comprises of a Clinician, Dietitian, Pharmacist, Nurse Specialist, PIC Nurse, Clinical Chemist and Microbiologist.

The clinician. A doctor with an interest in nutrition liaises with the relevant medical or surgical team and accepts overall responsibility for the Nutritional Care Team. This role may be assumed by a Gastroenterologist or a Paediatric Intensivist. The doctor is responsible for ensuring that a full history is taken, regular detailed clinical assessments are made and that Parenteral Nutrition (PN) is prescribed appropriately.

The dietitian. The Dietitian is responsible for assessing the ideal feed intake for children referred to the team, calculating nutritional requirements, and designing the feed and administration regimen. The choice of route does not alter the calculation of requirements. The Dietitian also provides advice and guidance regarding the administration and the constituents of parenteral nutrition.

The pharmacist. The Pharmacist is responsible for the preparation of parenteral feeds and advises clinicians of available constituents, ensuring individual nutritional requirements are met. The pharmacist will advise on the compatibility of the constituents, anticipate any drug and nutrient interreactions and give guidance on PN administration.

Nurse specialist in nutritional care. A Nutritional Care Nurse is responsible for the assessment of the child's nutritional status. The role also involves advising on the care of intravenous lines, management of enteral feeding tubes and training of carers. In some units this may be the role of an Intensive Care Nurse.

The Clinical Chemist provides advice on metabolic monitoring, and the Microbiologist will advise on treatment of sepsis.

The role of the PIC nurse in nutritional care

The child requiring intensive care is usually intubated, ventilated and sedated and may be pharmacologically paralysed. This reduces or removes the child's ability to convey hunger and thirst through verbalising or facial expression. Adequate nutrition is achieved in partnership with the parents and NCT by establishing the normal dietary habits of the child and devising a plan to meet these. Parents of the child with a long-term or chronic illness may normally be responsible for their child's enteral or parenteral feeding. Use of collaborative care planning will assist in reinforcing the parental role and facilitating involvement in their child's care.

Aims of nutritional assessment

A full nutritional assessment provides information on existing nutritional status, current diagnosis and requirements, enabling formulation of a feeding regimen. Regular monitoring of nutritional status identifies whether the current regimen is adequate or needs modifying (Richardson 1995).

Anthropometry

All children admitted to hospital should be weighed where possible, for the calculation of drugs, fluid and nutrient requirements. For the critically ill child this may require specialist equipment. In children under 2 it is likely that the parents may know a recent weight. Where weighing is impossible, estimated weight can be calculated by plotting the child's length onto a centile chart. Measurement of head circumference (in the absence of head trauma or swelling) gives further information about the child's growth. Additional measurements of arm anthropometry indicate whether the weight should be at the top or bottom of the centile.

Arm anthropometry is non-invasive and takes little time or equipment. This should be carried out on a free-hanging, non-dominant arm. A mid-upper arm circumference (MUAC) is measured using a tape measure. This is repeated twice a week and will indicate if fat and muscle stores are being depleted or maintained.

Triceps skinfold thickness (TSF) is easily measured with a skinfold calliper by an experienced practitioner to reduce error and improve reproducibility. Triceps skinfold thickness and upper-arm muscle measurements estimate mid-arm muscle mass (MAMM) using the formula:

$$MAMM = MUAC \text{ (cm)} - [0.3142 \times TSF \text{ (mm)}]$$

By comparing these figures with standard tables the skeletal muscle mass and degree of malnutrition can be estimated.

Biochemical markers of nutritional status

Sick or postoperative children are likely to have abnormal electrolytes levels and haematological markers. Serum albumin is an inaccurate guide to nutritional status. C-reactive protein is slightly more sensitive, but must be interpreted as part of the overall picture.

Observational assessment

This is dependent upon accurate recording of fluid intake and output. It is important to record when and why feeds were discontinued, so that the total volume of feed delivered in a 24 h period can be reviewed by the Nutrition Care Team.

FACTORS AFFECTING NUTRITIONAL CARE

The ventilated child

Mechanical ventilation can remove the need for respiratory muscle exertion, reducing metabolic rate and energy requirements. However, requirements for all other nutrients remain the same. In adults, altering the Respiratory Quotient by increasing the proportion of energy supplied as lipid rather than carbohydrate, reduces carbon dioxide production and can be effective in weaning adults from artificial ventilation (Benotti & Bistrian 1989). A proprietary feed formulated to meet this need in adults has not been tested for suitability in infants and children. If an increased proportion of lipid is utilised then monitoring of tolerance is required. Early detection and avoidance of hyperlipidaemia is essential, since it has been associated with thrombus and emboli formation and impaired pulmonary function (Järnberg et al 1981).

The child requiring cardiac surgery

Cardiac surgery causes major trauma to the chest wall, including a large sternal or thoracic cage incision. This iatrogenic stress increases nutrient requirements, while ventilation, sedation and pharmacological paralysis decrease these. However, many infants requiring cardiac surgery will be malnourished prior to surgery, because of long-term heart failure (Magnay et al 1989, Poskitt 1993). The nutritional requirements of infants with cardiac anomalies are estimated to be 120% to 150% of normal. Cardiac failure and fluid restriction cause difficulties in supplying adequate nutrition within the available volume. Nutritional supplements can be increased prior to surgery, and feeding can be commenced as soon as possible postoperatively. The use of diuretics depletes sodium, potassium, calcium and phosphate levels and it may be difficult to provide sufficient electrolytes to anticipate and replace losses. Intravenous electrolyte supplements may be required to counter these effects.

The child with renal dysfunction

This is very complex, and specialist paediatric renal dietetic advice is essential. Protein requirements depend on the differential diagnosis of renal disease, the type of dialysis used, the serum plasma protein levels and the age of the child. The nature of feed is influenced by fluid restriction and a need to minimise the accumulation of nitrogenous waste products. It is essential that adequate protein is given for growth. To ensure that protein is utilised only for growth, sufficient quantities of fat and carbohydrate must be provided for energy.

Other nutrients that must be provided according to individual requirement are sodium, potassium, phosphate and an energy source. Proprietary feeds are often unsuitable, and a modular feed, calculated by the dietitian, may be indicated.

The child with an infectious disorder

Infections increase metabolic rate and energy requirements because of the presence of pyrexia. For every 1°C of pyrexia an extra 10% of calories is required. Extra fluid, sodium and potassium must also be provided (Micklewright & Todorovic 1989). A competent immune system, to fight infection, has absolute requirements for nutrients, especially vitamins and minerals.

The child with multiple injuries

Head injuries cause an increase in energy requirements similar to those observed in thermal injury: that is, 120% to 140% of normal. Traumatic head injury may not be the only injury. Multiple fractures, wounds and infection may further increase nutrient requirements, to 180% of normal. Fluid restriction to reduce cerebral oedema and possible rises in intracranial pressure make provision of adequate nutrition difficult.

The child with thermal injury

The size and thickness of the burn determine requirements for energy and protein. The greater the size of the burn, the higher the nutritional requirements; 150% to 180% of normal may be needed. The Burn Interest Group of the British Dietetic Association recommends providing twice the Dietary Reference Value of all vitamins and minerals, to avoid possible non-absorption and overdosage. However, high levels of vitamin C supplements may be required for collagen synthesis (Thomas 1994).

The child with gastrointestinal disorders

Each disorder causes unique and specific nutritional requirements, impairing gut digestion and absorption. In these instances, feeds based on hydrolysed proteins, non-milk proteins, peptides or amino acids may be indicated. Alternative carbohydrate and fat sources, such as glucose, sucrose and medium-chain triglycerides may be required to utilise different modes of absorption. Other substances such as the amino acid, glutamine and pectin may be added to an enteral feed to ensure intestinal structure and function is maintained. Malabsorption may be due to a short gut or other malformation, a lack of specific enzymes or a disease such as Crohn's disease. Thorough assessment of the specific problem is essential to plan appropriate nutritional support.

The nutritional care of the critically ill child is complex, the choice and method of feeding are important and should be an integral part of initial care planning.

CHOICE OF ROUTE AND METHOD OF PROVIDING NUTRITIONAL SUPPORT

Nutritional support can be provided using the gastrointestinal tract or the intravenous route. If surgery is anticipated then prior consideration to the mode of nutritional support facilitates the insertion of a feeding tube or intravenous line during the procedure.

Enteral feeding

Enteral feeding includes:

- oral
- nasogastric
- nasoduodenal
- nasojejunal
- gastrostomy
- jejunostomy.

Oral feeding is least likely to be used in PIC. Enteral feeding is widely considered to be the route of choice: *'If the gut works, use it'*. Gastric and colonic stasis may be present, but the small intestine is still capable of digesting and absorbing feed. Absence of bowel sounds should not preclude feeding. Jejunal or duodenal feeding can mean enteral feeding may be started earlier (Anderson & Fearon 1995, Chellis et al 1996). This is desirable, as it:

- prevents gut atrophy

- maintains gut-associated lymphoid tissue
- attenuates the catabolic response to injury
- maintains blood flow to the gut, protecting newly formed anastomoses (Minard & Kudsk 1994).

Early enteral feeding starts within 24 h of surgery, injury, burn or infection. However, it may not be possible to provide all the requirements enterally; therefore, concurrent parenteral and enteral nutrition may be necessary.

Choosing an enteral nutrition catheter

Nasogastric tubes are made of polyvinylchloride or polyurethane plastic. Wide-bore tubes are considered inferior in terms of comfort and erosion of nasal tissue to fine-bore tubes. However, a wider-bore tube may be important for some patients in PIC. Regular aspiration of gastric contents is an easy way to check gastric emptying and reduces the risk of vomiting and aspiration.

Types of enteral feed available

Enteral feeds are divided into two main groups:

- proprietary ready-to-feed
- modular feeds.

They can be further subdivided into whole and modified protein feeds. They may come as 'ready to feed' liquids or powder requiring reconstitution. Any feed used in PIC must be produced in a clean environment, free from microbial contamination. Ready-to-feed and proprietary tube feeds meet these requirements. Any feeds made up in hospital should ideally be prepared in a separate milk kitchen by staff trained to handle feeds. Where possible, all feeds, including expressed breast milk, should be pasteurised before administration. Feeds can be further divided into those suitable for four age groups:

- premature infants under 2 kg
- term infants 2–10 kg (0–12 months)
- children 10–20 kg (1–6 years)
- children above 20 kg (6 years to adult).

Premature infants. Feeds for premature neo-

Table 22.1 Examples of currently available infant formulae

Low-birthweight formulae	Whey-dominant formulae	Casein-dominant formulae	Follow-on formulae
C & G Low-birthweight	C & G Premium	C & G Plus	C & G Step-up
SMA Low-birthweight	SMA Gold	SMA White	SMA Progress
Farley's Premcare	Farley's First	Farley's Second	Farley's Follow on
Milupa Prematil	Milupa Aptamil	Milupa Milumil	

nates are higher in energy, protein, calcium, phosphorus and vitamin D (Table 22.1). Breast milk fortifiers are available; these can be added to expressed breast milk to improve its overall nutrient density. Feeds must be introduced cautiously, as an immature gut may tolerate enteral feed poorly. This can be detected by abdominal bloating, intestinal hurry and increasing gastric aspirate, indicating slow emptying of the stomach.

Infants 2–10 kg. Feeds for term infants are readily available. These are divided into whey-dominant and casein-dominant feeds. There is very little to choose between the various brands, which all meet the Department of Health and Social Security Guidelines (1980) and compare to mature human breast milk. There is no advantage to using the casein-dominant formula, which may be contraindicated as gastric emptying is slowed. Some feeds, for example Aptamil, contain long-chain polyunsaturated fats, which appear to be important in neurological development (Crawford 1993). Follow-on formulae are suitable for infants aged 6 to 12 months, as they are higher in iron and protein.

Breast milk is the optimum choice of feed for babies (Pettit 1992, Watling 1994). For the mother who wishes to breast feed her baby the alternative of expressing breast milk should be discussed and encouraged. PIC nurses must ensure that the mother is able to maintain a regular fluid intake and a nutritious diet. When expressing breast milk a quiet, comfortable setting with facilities for the mother to rest and relax are essential. A nurse/midwife should be available to:

- teach the mother how to use the equipment and to store the expressed milk
- answer questions
- give advice and encouragement.

Table 22.2 Paediatric feeds suitable for children aged 1 to 6 years

Feed	Energy per 100 mL	Protein per 100 mL
Nutrison Paediatric Standard (C & G Nutricia)	100 kcal	2.75 g
Paediasure (Ross)	101 kcal	3.0 g
Nutrison Paediatric Energy Plus (C & G Nutricia)	150 kcal	3.4 g

Children aged 1 to 6 years. Children aged from 1 to 6 years have different protein and energy requirements to very young infants. There are currently three proprietary feeds available for this age group (Table 22.2). Feeds providing 1.5 kcal/mL have an advantage over feeds providing 1 kcal/mL when fluid restrictions minimise the volume available for feed administration.

Children aged 6 to adolescent. The large range of adult proprietary feeds, although not ideal, will meet most of this age group's nutritional requirements. Advice from the NCT should prevent the child receiving too much of any one nutrient, with possible serious metabolic consequences.

Proprietary modified feeds

All the macro nutrients may be modified. These feeds are generally more expensive than whole protein unmodified feeds and they should only be used when clearly indicated. There are many feeds available, designed for different age groups. The advice of the Nutritional Care Team saves time, ensuring the correct feed is used.

Indications for using a proprietary modified feed. These include:

- malabsorption
- intolerance of
  - milk protein
  - lactose or sucrose
  - long-chain fatty acids
- clinical indication: e.g. chylothorax requires a feed low in long-chain triglycerides and high in medium-chain triglycerides
- short-gut syndrome
- gastroschisis
- metabolic problem, for example: phenylketonuria (PKU).

Modification of existing proprietary feeds

A proprietary feed is unlikely to supply sufficient nutrition in the total volume allowance. Modification of the feed is required to maximise nutritional intake. This can be achieved by concentrating the feed or adding energy supplements. All feed modifications should be calculated by a dietitian.

Concentrating the feed. Any feed supplied as a powder can be concentrated, with care, above the level recommended by the manufacture. Infant formulae are commonly a 13% weight/volume solution. Concentrating this to 15% weight/volume increases nutrient density of the feed. Concentration must be increased gradually, allowing the child to become used to the higher osmolarity. It is important to change either concentration or volume, not both at once, to avoid the risk of intolerance due to significant changes in the nature of the feed.

Adding energy supplements to feeds. Energy may be added as glucose polymers, fat emulsion, or a mixture of both (Box 22.4). Fat emulsions are available in long-chain triglycerides (LCT) and medium-chain triglycerides (MCT) fatty acid formulations. Fat alone must not be added to provide more than 50% of the energy, as it encourages the production of ketone bodies causing metabolic instability. Energy should be added gradually. It is usual to add in daily increments of 1% or 2% until the desired concentration is reached. An

infant formula with 5% glucose polymer and 3% of a 50% fat emulsion supplies 100 kcal/100 mL.

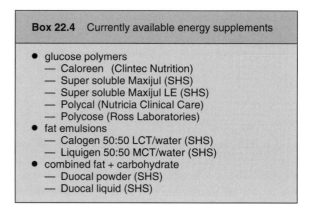

Box 22.4 Currently available energy supplements

- glucose polymers
  - Caloreen (Clintec Nutrition)
  - Super soluble Maxijul (SHS)
  - Super soluble Maxijul LE (SHS)
  - Polycal (Nutricia Clinical Care)
  - Polycose (Ross Laboratories)
- fat emulsions
  - Calogen 50:50 LCT/water (SHS)
  - Liquigen 50:50 MCT/water (SHS)
- combined fat + carbohydrate
  - Duocal powder (SHS)
  - Duocal liquid (SHS)

Modular feeds

These are used when a child has very specific requirements for nutrients that cannot be met by modifying an existing feed. A modular feed consists of:

- nitrogen source — a whole protein powder, comminuted chicken or an amino acid powder
- carbohydrate — glucose, sucrose, fructose, glucose polymer, corn starch
- fat — LCT or MCT emulsion.

Vitamins and minerals, sodium and potassium supplements are added based on daily requirements.

A modular feed is indicated in renal or liver failure, or in malabsorption syndromes and should be calculated by a dietitian experienced in using such feeds.

Feeding regimens

Strength of feeds. Feeds should be introduced at full strength and at a low volume with supplemental IV fluid until enteral feeding is fully established. It may sometimes be necessary to dilute a feed. This should be done in the milk kitchen, allowing the feed to be pasteurised before use, therefore reducing the risk of contamination.

The volume of feed can be increased 4–6 hourly,

depending on how well it is absorbed. Tolerance of the feed can be ascertained by regular (usually 4–6 hourly) aspiration of the stomach contents.

It is difficult to define the volume of gastric aspirate that is normal. The secretion of gastric acid is a normal response to the presence of food in the stomach. It is reasonable to assume that during critical illness this response will not be as sensitive as normal, so relatively more gastric juice may be secreted. It should be remembered that a larger child will produce a greater volume of gastric aspirate. The complete absence of aspirate is not usual, and some aspirate should be expected. Following a period of starvation, gastric emptying can be abnormal for 8 hours after the reintroduction of feeding. It may be necessary to use a drug such as cisapride to stimulate gastric emptying (Goldhill 1997). Parenteral nutrition (PN) is indicated if persistent gastric stasis is present.

Continuous, intermittent or bolus feeds. Continuous regimens minimise potentially adverse reactions on cardiac, respiratory, and renal function.

Bolus feeds are associated with

- an increase in resting metabolic rate of up to 10–15%
- requiring a sudden increase in cardiac output and respiratory rate
- a surge in blood concentration of electrolytes and nitrogen which may not be well tolerated, especially in the child with renal failure.

In the critically ill child these stressors, which can exacerbate organ failure, are not associated with continuous feeding. In addition continuous feeds do not affect dietary induced thermogenesis and are therefore better utilised for repair of damaged tissue. Continuous feeding at a steady rate, for a total of 18–20 h within the 24 h period allows the pH of the gastric contents to fall to below 3.4 during the rest period, thus preventing bacterial growth in the stomach. This may be beneficial since presence of bacteria in gastric contents has been associated with aspiration pneumonia (Lee et al 1990). Continuous feeding for 75–80% of a 24 h period may also prevent

stress ulceration of the gastric mucosa by maintaining a raised gastric pH (greater than pH 4) for much of the day. Bolus feeds should not really be considered in the critically ill child, as the advantages of the continuous regimen are so great. However, bolus feeds do have a role in mimicking the child's usual feeding pattern when the aim is to normalise care.

Monitoring of enteral nutrition

The Paediatric Intensive Care Nurse is responsible for observation and documentation of the amount and nature of gastric aspirate, the volume and type of feed delivered and presence or absence of bowel motions. This also includes monitoring the effectiveness of the feeding regimen (Table 22.3) and anticipation of feeding complications.

Other aspects of nursing care which should be considered are the maintenance of normothermia to reduce oxygen and energy requirements and the planning of the child's care to allow for maximal rest so that the energy provided is directed toward healing and recovery.

Complications of enteral feeding[a]

Nasogastric tube placement. Placement of the nasogastric tube and checking the position are two important aspects of care. When a child is heavily sedated and possibly paralysed, muscle tone and pharyngeal reflexes are reduced or absent and, as a result, inadvertent placement of the nasogastric tube in the bronchi is possible (Miller 1988, Roubenoff & Ravich 1989). Checking the position of the tube prior to commencement of feeding is therefore essential. When the tube is first placed, position may be confirmed with chest radiography but is not appropriate for ongoing management (Metheny 1988).

Aspiration of the feed into the lungs and the development of aspiration pneumonia is a complication that can be avoided by regular monitoring of the tube position, residual contents of the stomach and appropriate positioning of the child.

Problem-solving advice includes the following.

Table 22.3 A guideline for monitoring of enteral and parenteral nutrition

Frequency	Enteral feeding	Parenteral feeding
Daily	• Full blood count • Electrolytes • Blood gases; acid–base balance • Urea and creatinine • Blood glucose • Liver function tests • Urinalysis, for ketone bodies and glucose • Fluid balance, including the type and total volume of feed administered • Weight (ideal)	• Full blood count • Electrolytes • Blood gases; acid–base balance • Urea and creatinine • Blood glucose • Observation for hyperlipidaemia • Serum triglycerides • Liver function tests • Urinalysis, for ketone bodies and glucose • Fluid balance, including the type and total volume of feed administered • Weight (ideal)
Twice weekly	• Weight • Mid-upper arm circumference • Triceps skin fold thickness	• Weight • Mid-upper arm circumference • Triceps skin fold thickness
Once weekly	• Weight (minimum)	• Weight (minimum) • Calcium • Urinary electrolytes
Weekly after third week of nutrition	• Trace elements • Vitamin status	• Trace elements such as magnesium, zinc and selenium • Vitamin status

NB: The frequency of many of these measurements will be determined by severity of illness.

• Check the position of tube regularly by aspiration of stomach contents; the larger the syringe used the less pressure is exerted on the lumen of the tube. Aspirate should be tested for acid with blue litmus paper, at least at the start of each feeding period. A pH range paper should be used for the child receiving antacid therapy or H_2 antagonists such as ranitidine.

• Use a wide-bore tube and 4 hourly aspiration to assess gastric emptying.

• Raise the patient's head, by raising top of the bed.

• Consider medication to facilitate gastric emptying, for example cisapride (Goldhill 1997).

• Consider duodenal or jejunal feeding.

• Consider thickening feed.

• Consider parenteral nutrition.

Diarrhoea. Diarrhoea may be common in enterally fed patients; however, it is not necessarily due to the feed. Use of antibiotics may alter the gut flora sufficiently to cause diarrhoea. A hypertonic feed, or one with added sodium or potassium chloride, may also cause intestinal hurry. The following should be considered before stopping the feed.

Problem solving advice includes the following.

• Ascertain cause of diarrhoea.
• Reduce infusion rate.
• Reduce osmolarity of feed.
• Consider a lactose-free feed.
• Stop broad-spectrum antibiotics.
• Consider a feed containing fibre.

Blocked tube. This is a common complication, and can be avoided in the following ways.

• Flush the tube 4–6 hourly with 2–5 mL of sterile water (even when feed is flowing).

• When administering drugs, stop the feed, check the tube position, administer the drug in liquid form, then flush the tube and restart the feed.

• A blocked tube can be flushed with 2–5 mL of fizzy pop, a pinch of bicarbonate of soda in sterile water or pineapple juice.

• Remove and replace the tube.

Repeated tube removal. This is common when the child is agitated and awake. It is less of a problem if the child is sedated. Anticipation of the problem as sedation is reduced can prevent repeated intubation.

Problem solving advice includes the following.

• Tape the tube securely and comfortably to the face.

• Engage the child in play or distraction therapy.

• Consider mittens or arm splints.

• Consider gastrostomy if enteral feeding is likely to be long term: for example, in some children with severe neurological impairment following head injury.

• If the tube is removed, prompt replacement

is vital to ensure the prescribed amount of feed is delivered.

Infection. The systems and practices used in the delivery of enteral feeds can become a source of infection for the critically ill child (Patchell et al 1994). Therefore it is essential that the PICU has agreed and written standards of practice for infection control during the storage, administration and handling of enteral feeds (Sizer et al 1996).

Metabolic complications. Metabolic complications are rarely due to the feed alone, but regular monitoring will minimise side effects. The frequency of blood sugar measurement depends on several factors, including the age of the child and the nature and severity of illness. Hyperglycaemia (blood glucose >11 mmol/L) must be monitored, documented and reported. In some instances a sliding scale infusion of insulin may be prescribed. Hypoglycaemia (blood glucose <2 mmol/L) should be reported and treated with 0.5–1 g/kg of intravenous 10% dextrose, depending on age. In each instance the feed volume, absorption and tolerance should also be reviewed.

Loss of oral motor skills. A poorly documented, but important complication of enteral feeding is the loss of normal eating behaviour in the child or infant. If enteral feeding is short term and likely to discontinue before the child leaves PIC, then difficulties with re-introduction of oral feeding are unlikely. However, with long-term enteral feeding, early planning of a daily programme designed to retain eating and feeding skills is essential. Involvement of a speech and language therapist may be necessary to devise the best programme for the child.

Problem-solving advice includes the following.

- Encourage the presence of something in the mouth if the child is conscious. For an infant, use of a dummy encourages sucking.
- Play mouth games, kissing and blowing raspberries.
- Stroke the mouth and face with firm strokes, to prevent sensitivity occurring.
- Carry out/encourage regular mouth care and tooth brushing.

Parenteral nutritional support

The provision of nutrients via a route other than the gastrointestinal tract is not a new concept (Ball et al 1993). Parenteral nutrition (PN) is used to administer a 'normal diet' as an intravenous solution when enteral nutrition is either not feasible or not meeting the child's full nutritional requirements. Indications for parenteral nutrition include intestinal failure, multiorgan failure and hypercatabolism (Ball et al 1990).

Parenteral nutrition (PN) consists of protein as amino acids (e.g. vamin), carbohydrate as glucose, and fat, which is administered in droplet form coated in egg phospholipid and dispersed in water (e.g. Intralipid). In addition, water, electrolytes, vitamins and trace elements are added and titrated according to individual patient needs, renal and liver function and electrolyte levels.

Routes of delivery

The preferred mode of access for convenience and reliability in neonates, infants and children requiring PN for a week or more, is central venous catheterisation (Ball et al 1993). In PIC this is most commonly achieved via a dedicated lumen of a triple lumen central line or via a silastic catheter. In neonates the use of a fine central catheter inserted percutaneously via a peripheral vein is a feasible and cheaper alternative to surgical placement (Puntis 1987)

Peripheral intravenous access is not ideal, because of the risks of infection, phlebitis, thrombosed veins and extravasation injury, which may be severe because of the hypertonic nature of the solutions (Ball et al 1990).

Prescribing

The advent of a computer program and software has resulted in a less time-consuming and more accurate process in the prescribing of parenteral nutrition for children (Ball et al 1985, Ball et al 1990). To facilitate this the Nutritional Care Team will require recent anthropometry of the child, information about existing fluid restrictions, the nature of other infusions being administered concurrently and recent serum electrolyte values.

Administration

Standard procedures for the safe administration of any drug should apply to the checking of a PN prescription. The PIC nurse has a primary role in reducing catheter sepsis by ensuring that all staff involved in the insertion and management of the line adhere to unit prevention of infection policies. The use of a line dedicated purely for parenteral nutrition with the minimum number of line connections will reduce the incidence of infection. Filtration of the amino acid/glucose solution through a filter of 0.22 µm pore size should be standard practice, since it reduces the risk of phlebitis (Falchuk et al 1985) and other associated particulate hazards (Puntis et al 1992). Recent developments allow the filtration of all parenteral nutrient mixtures, including lipid emulsions (Latter et al 1996). This is potentially beneficial to the patient, since lipid emulsions support rapid bacterial growth (D'Angio et al 1987).

Monitoring

A systematic approach is required to monitor effectiveness and detect the other potential complications of PN (Box 22.5). A problem-solving approach similar to that described for enteral nutrition will assist in early detection, treatment and correction of problems. Regular screening for infection is essential. If sepsis is suspected then blood and urine cultures should be taken along with blood from the PN line.

CONCLUSION

The evidence for nutritional support in terms of improved outcome, reduced rates of complications and shorter hospital stays has been well documented (Lennard-Jones 1992, are Taylor & Goodinson-McLaren 1992, Silk et al 1994). It is

---

Box 22.5 Potential complications of parenteral nutrition

Intravenous access:
- sepsis (Maki 1980) — Most common complication, with varying rate of incidence (2–29%) thought to be due to the different definitions of catheter sepsis (Taylor & Goodinson-McLaren 1992, ch 18.1)
- thrombus
- embolism
- pneumothorax, hydrothorax
- damage to major veins, arteries, brachial plexus & thoracic duct
- malposition of the catheter
- air embolism

Catheter related:
- blockage
- leakage

Metabolic:
- disturbance of:
  — fluid balance
  — glucose levels
  — electrolytes/trace elements
  — acid–base balance
- cholestasis (Beath et al 1996)
- lipid agglutination
- jaundice

Associated:
- translocation of gut bacteria (Alverdy 1988, Inoue et al 1988, Spaeth et al 1990)

---

essential that each Paediatric Intensive Care Unit utilises a multidisciplinary approach in ensuring the nutritional needs of the critically ill child are met. Each unit should devise its own strategy to guarantee that nutrition is considered as soon as the initial life-threatening phase of the child's illness is stabilised.

ACKNOWLEDGEMENTS

We acknowledge the assistance of Chris Holden, Clinical Nurse Specialist Nutritional Care, Anita MacDonald, Head of Dietetic Service, and Charles Ralston, Director of Intensive Care, The Birmingham Children's Hospital NHS Trust.

REFERENCES

Alexander J W, Saito H, Trocki O et al 1986 The importance of lipid type in the diet following burn injury. Annals of Surgery 204:1–8

Alverdy J C 1988 Total parenteral nutrition promotes bacterial translocation from the gut. Surgery 104:185–190

Anderson I D, Fearon K C H 1995 Paralytic ileus and enteral feeding Part II. British Journal of Intensive Care:117–121

Ball P A, De-Silva D G H, Candy D C A, McNeish A S 1985 The micro-computer: an aid to paediatric parenteral nutrition. International Journal of Monitoring and Computing 1:233–239

Ball P A, Booth I W, Puntis J W L 1990 Paediatric parenteral nutrition. KabiVitrum, Bourne End

Ball P A, Booth I W, Holden C, Puntis J 1993 Paediatric parenteral nutrition. Pharmacia, Milton Keynes

Beath S V, Davies P, Papadopoulou A, Khan A R, Buick R G, Corkery J J, Gornall P, Booth I W 1996 Parenteral nutrition-related cholestasis in postsurgical neonates: multivariate analysis of risk factors. Journal of Pediatric Surgery 31(4):604–606

Benotti P N, Bistrian B 1989 Metabolic and nutritional aspects of weaning from mechanical ventilation. Critical Care Medicine 17(2):181–185

Booth I W 1994 Costing malnutrition: add or multiply? Lancet 342(8897):554–555

Chellis M J, Sanders S V, Webster H, Dean J M, Jackson D 1996 Early enteral feeding in the paediatric intensive care unit. Journal of Parenteral and Enteral Nutrition 20(1):71–73

Crawford M A 1993 The role of essential fatty acids in neurological development: implications for perinatal nutrition. American Journal of Clinical Nutrition 57 (suppl.):703S–710S

D'Angio R, Quercia N K, Treiber J C et al 1987 The growth of microorganisms in total parenteral nutrition admixtures. Journal of Parenteral and Enteral Nutrition 11:394–397

Department of Health and Social Security 1980 Artificial feeds for the young infant. Report on Health and Social Services. HMSO, London

Elia M 1992 Energy expenditure in the whole body. In: Kinney J M, Tucker H N. Energy metabolism: tissue determinants and cellular corollaries. Raven Press, New York

Falchuk K H, Peterson L, McNeil B J 1985 Microparticulate induced phlebitis. New England Journal of Medicine 312:78–82

Francis D 1987 Diets for sick children, 4th edn. Blackwell Scientific, Oxford

Goldhill D R 1997 Cisapride and the ICU patient. Care of the Critically Ill 13(2):61–64

Huddleston K C, Ferraro-McDuffie A, Wolff-Small T 1993 Nutritional support of the critically ill child. Critical Care Nursing Clinics of North America 5(1):65–78

Inoue S, Epstein M, Alexander J W, Trocki O 1988 Prevention of yeast translocation across the gut by a single enteral feed after burn injury. Journal of Parenteral and Enteral Nutrition 12:55

Järnberg P O, Lindholm M, Eklund J 1981 Lipid infusion in critically ill patients: acute effects on haemodynamics and pulmonary gas exchange. Critical Care Medicine 9:27–31

Keithley J K, Eisenberg P 1993 The significance of enteral nutrition in the intensive care unit patient. Critical Care Nursing Clinics of North America 5(1):23–29

Latter M, Ball P R, Hunter A J, et al 1996 Performance of a new endline filter for the filtration of nutrient admixtures and emulsions. Pall Technical Bulletin, Pall Corporation, New York

Lee B, Chang R W S, Jacobs S 1990 Intermittent naso-gastric feeding: a simple and effective method to reduce pnuemonia among ventilated ICU patients. Clinical Intensive Care 1(3):100–102

Lennard-Jones J E 1992 A positive approach to nutrition as a treatment. The King's Fund

Magnay A R, Puntis J W L, Booth I W 1989 Cardiopulmonary bypass surgery in childhood: a nutritional problem for intensive care. Intensive Therapy and Clinical Monitoring April:124–126

Mainous M R, Block E F J, Deitch E A 1994 Nutritional support of the gut: how and why. New Horizons 2(2):193–201

Maki D G 1980 Sepsis associated with infusion therapy. In: Karran S (ed) Controversies in surgical sepsis. Praegar, Eastbourne, pp 207–266

Metheny N 1988 Measures to test placement of nasogastric and nasointestinal feeding tubes: a review: Nursing Research 37(6):324–329

Meyer N A, Muller J M, Hernon D N 1994 Nutrient support of the healing wound. New Horizons 2(2):202–214

Micklewright A, Todorovic V 1989 A pocket guide to clinical nutrition. Parenteral and Enteral Nutrition Group of the British Dietetic Association

Miller T W 1988 Inadvertent tracheobronchial placement of feeding tubes. Radiology 167:875

Minard G, Kudsk K A 1994 Is early feeding beneficial? How early is early? New Horizons 2(2):156–163

Patchell C, Anderton A, MacDonald A, George R H, Booth I W 1994 Bacterial contamination of enteral feeds. Archives of Disease in Childhood 70:327–330

Pettit J 1992 Establishing successful breastfeeding in special care. Paediatric Nursing 4(7):24–25

Poskitt E M 1993 Failure to thrive in congenital heart disease. Archives of Disease in Childhood 68(2):158–160

Puntis J W L 1987 Percutaneous insertion of central feeding catheters — the first choice in paediatric parenteral nutrition. Intensive Therapy and Clinical Monitoring 8:7–10

Puntis J W L, Wilkins K M, Ball P A, Rushton D I, Booth I W 1992 Hazards of parenteral treatment: do particles count? Archives of Diseases in Childhood 67:1475–1477

Roubenoff R, Ravich W J 1989 Pneumothorax due to nasogastric feeding tubes: report of four cases, review of the literature and recommendations for prevention. Archives of Internal Medicine 149:184–188

Schwartz S, Farriol M, Garcia E, Alfonso J J, Rodriguez R 1987 Influence of MCT/LCT ratio in enteral nutrition on liver and jejunal mucosa protein synthesis in post surgical stress. Journal of Clinical Nutrition and Gastroenterology 2:31–37

Sizer T (ed), Russell C A, Wood S, Irwin P, Allison S,

Wheatley C, Whitney S 1996 Standards and guidelines for nutritional support of patients in hospitals. British Association for Parenteral and Enteral Nutrition (BAPEN), Maidenhead

Spaeth G, Specian R D, Berg R D, Deitch E A 1990 Bulk prevents bacterial translocation induced by the oral administration of total parenteral nutrition solution. Journal of Parenteral Enteral Nutrition 14:442–447

Taylor S, Goodinson-McLaren S 1992 Nutritional support: A team approach. Wolfe Publishing, London

Thomas B 1994 The manual of dietetic practice, 2nd edn. Blackwell Scientific, Oxford, ch 5.1, p 605; ch 5.4, pp 627–634

Watling R 1994 Setting off on the right foot. Child Health 2(1):16–18

Wilmore D W, Smith R J, O'Dwyer S T, et al 1988 The gut: a central organ after surgical stress. Surgery 104:917–923

FURTHER READING

Department of Health 1991 Dietary reference values for food energy and nutrients for the United Kingdom (Report 41). HMSO, London

Shaw V, Lawson M (eds) 1995 Clinical paediatric dietetics. Blackwell Scientific, Oxford

Taylor S, Goodinson-McLaren S 1992 Nutritional support: a team approach. Wolfe Publishing, London

Thomas B (ed) 1994 Manual of dietetic practice, 2nd edn. Blackwell Scientific, Oxford

23

Pharmacological support in paediatric intensive care

Rebecca Dallmeyer

INTRODUCTION

The use of drugs in children is fraught with legal and ethical difficulties. Only a small minority of drugs are licensed to be used in children. These drug treatments often fall outside the existing legal framework and have therefore become known as 'therapeutic orphans'. When a drug is used outside the scope of its licence it is the prescriber, not the manufacturer, who must take responsibility for any adverse effects associated with its use. It can be argued that those who dispense and administer the drug also have an ethical responsibility to ensure the child's wellbeing.

Since clinical trials have rarely been conducted in children, paediatric doses must initially be based on adult data. This has obvious limitations since children are not small adults. The physiological development of the child and the effect this has on how the body handles drugs, the rapidly changing body composition of a growing child and the practical difficulties of administering a dose must all be taken into account.

This chapter addresses the safe and appropriate use of drugs in critically ill children by describing:

- the effect a child's physiological development has on drug handling
- routes of drug administration
- the effect of organ failure on drug handling
- drug use in the following therapeutic areas:
  — pain and sedation
  — muscle relaxation
  — antiinfective agents
  — inotropic support

Table 23.1 Classification of childhood by age

Classification	Age
Premature neonates	gestational age < 38 weeks postnatal age < 1 month
Full-term neonates	gestational age > 38 weeks postnatal age < 1 month
Infants	1–12 months
Child	1–10 years
Pubescent or adolescent	10–15 years
Adult	> 15 years

— control of seizures

— maintenance of gastric integrity.

DRUG HANDLING IN NEONATES, INFANTS, CHILDREN AND ADULTS

In order for a drug to produce its clinical effect it must first be absorbed, then distributed to different parts of the body. This is usually followed by metabolism and excretion of the active drug or its metabolites. Some drugs must be metabolised in the body before they exert their effect (e.g. inactive enalapril is metabolised to active enalaprilat) whilst others may be excreted unchanged (e.g. isoflurane). Absorption, distribution, metabolism and excretion can all be influenced by age and are collectively known as pharmacokinetics.

Absorption

Gastrointestinal tract

Drugs are usually absorbed in the gastrointestinal tract. Changes take place in the structure of the gut from birth to adulthood, the most clinically significant of which occur during the first month of life.

Gastric pH. This is high (alkaline) at birth, falling to more acidic values within a few days (Stewart & Hampton 1987). This is attributed to the inability of the neonatal gastric mucosa to secrete hydrochloric acid and to the presence of amniotic fluid in the stomach. As the gastric mucosa develops, gastric acid production rises to adult values at about 3–5 years of age. Alkaline drugs such as ampicillin reach higher plasma concentrations in neonates than in adults. This is

due to the drug remaining as the parent compound and not dissociating, thus being absorbed by passive diffusion in the stomach. However, this theory does not consider other age-related changes which could also result in a higher plasma concentration, such as increased rate of absorption, decreased elimination or decreased volume of distribution. However, significant absorption of most drugs occurs in the duodenum. The duodenum has a much larger surface area than the stomach and undergoes little age-related change. Therefore absorption does not alter significantly with age.

Gastric motility. This is reduced in neonates and reaches adult rates at about 6 months of age. Reduced gastric motility decreases the rate but not the *extent* of absorption of drugs from the gastrointestinal tract. The extent of absorption usually determines the clinical effect of drugs. Preparations which provide a slow release of drug in the gastrointestinal tract are designed for adults and must be used with great caution in infants and children because their absorption is unpredictable.

Gastric microorganisms. These rapidly colonise the gut after birth. The degree of colonisation and variety of gastrointestinal flora does not appear to significantly affect the absorption of most drugs.

Gastrointestinal enzyme activity. This may alter drug absorption. Chloramphenicol palmitate, available as an oral suspension, must be hydrolysed in the gut by α-amylase, a pancreatic enzyme, to chloramphenicol before it is absorbed. The production of α-amylase is greatly reduced in neonates, resulting in ineffective absorption of chloramphenicol. Production of α-amylase reaches adult values at about 4 months of age. Neonates have low lipase concentrations which, in conjunction with low gastric bile acid concentrations, may reduce the absorption of fat-soluble drugs such as phytomenadione and calciferol.

Skin

The structure of the skin changes significantly with age. This limits the use of percutaneous drug administration to produce systemic effects.

The rate of drug absorption through the skin is markedly affected by its degree of hydration and the thickness of the corneal strata. High skin hydration and thin corneal strata facilitates percutaneous absorption in neonates. In addition, their ratio of body surface area to weight is much greater than adults'. This means that plasma concentrations can rapidly reach therapeutic and even toxic levels. The immature percutaneous barrier has been exploited to deliver drugs in neonates. Topical povidone iodine has been applied to the skin of iodine-deficient babies, and fat emulsion has been rubbed into the skin to treat essential fatty acid deficiencies. Unfortunately, absorption of unwanted substances has also been reported. For example, alcohol and hexachlorophene have been extensively absorbed through the skin and caused inadvertent poisoning (Stewart & Hampton 1987). The use of occlusive plastic nappies increases skin hydration, thereby enhancing the absorption of topical creams and ointments. Excessive absorption of steroids from creams has been associated with systemic side effects.

Distribution

Distribution describes the location and concentration of a drug in different parts of the body. Drug concentrations can only be measured in the blood, not at their site of action. When the clinical response is directly related to the plasma concentration of the drug, the relationship of this to the dose is characterised by the apparent volume of distribution, which is expressed as volume per kilogram of body weight (L/kg):

$$\text{apparent volume of distribution} = \frac{\text{dose} \times \text{bioavailability}}{\text{plasma concentration} \times \text{body weight}}$$

The apparent volume of distribution is dependent upon the characteristics of the drug (fat-solubility, protein or tissue binding) and the characteristics of the child (body size and plasma protein concentration). Highly protein-bound drugs which tend to remain in the plasma have a low volume of distribution. Highly fat-soluble drugs, or those that are tissue-bound, have a high volume of distribution.

Percentage body water

Neonates have a much higher water content than adults. At birth, this value is about 75%, which falls to adult values of 60% at about 2 years of age. This is significant, as changes in the ratio of body water to body fat will alter the apparent volume of distribution of drugs. Most drugs have a larger volume of distribution in young children than in adults. Thus relatively higher doses must be given to achieve the same plasma concentrations and therefore a therapeutic effect. For example, the volume of distribution for digoxin is:

- 4–6 L/kg   for pre-term neonates
- 5–7 L/kg   for term neonates
- 8–13 L/kg   for infants
- 11–12 L/kg   for 1–5 years of age
- 7–10 L/kg   for 6–20 years of age

(Hastreiter et al 1985).

Protein binding

During the neonatal period, some drugs show decreased plasma protein binding despite albumin levels being similar to adult values. This can be explained by:

- the presence of fetal albumin, which has a lower binding capacity than adult albumin
- the presence of substances that compete for the protein binding sites, e.g. bilirubin
- lower blood pH
- decreased total plasma protein.

When less drug is bound to plasma proteins, the free level of drug is higher. When this is combined with decreased metabolism and excretion of the drug, free plasma levels will rise, with repeated doses leading to toxicity. For example, the recommended dose of phenytoin (which is highly protein bound) is 2–4 mg/kg twice a day for neonates, compared with 2.5–7.5 mg/kg twice a day in infants and children. The recommended therapeutic range is also decreased to 6–15 mg/L in neonates, compared with 10–20 mg/L in infants and children to decrease the risk of toxicity.

However, bilirubin is often displaced from its

protein-binding sites by drugs, thus increasing free bilirubin levels. Unbound bilirubin is not effectively metabolised by the liver. It readily crosses the immature blood–brain barrier, causing kernicterus and neurological damage. Drugs that are known to displace bilirubin from plasma protein-binding sites include aspirin, sulphonamides and vitamin K analogues. Plasma protein binding usually reaches adult values at about 3 months of age.

Metabolism

Metabolism varies greatly between individuals. During the neonatal period, metabolism is markedly reduced, with some immature liver enzyme systems. These quickly develop and reach adult effectiveness by about 1 month of age. The liver detoxifies drugs using two types of reactions which can be classified as phase 1 and phase 2.

Phase 1 reactions

These modify the drug by oxidation, reduction and hydrolysis and are less affected by age than are Phase 2 reactions. The majority of oxidation reactions occur in microsomes, part of the reticuloendothelial system, utilising the cytochrome P_{450} enzyme system. This enzyme system is important for the metabolism of many drugs.

Phase 2 reactions

This type of reaction combines or conjugates the modified drug with another molecule to make it more water-soluble, thus facilitating excretion. The most important of these reactions are glucoronidation, sulphate conjugation, glycination and N-dealkylation. Phase 2 reactions take longer to mature. During the neonatal period, glucoronidation and N-dealkylation pathways are known to be deficient.

Chloramphenicol is usually conjugated by glucoronidation. Because this pathway is deficient in neonates, chloramphenicol accumulates, leading to cardiovascular shock and 'grey baby syndrome'. Chloramphenicol can be safely used in neonates, but doses must be reduced and plasma concentrations measured to avoid toxic concentrations.

Despite several Phase 2 metabolic pathways being deficient in the immature liver, the neonate or infant adapts to metabolise drugs along other pathways. Paracetamol, for example, is metabolised primarily by glucoronidation in adults; reduced efficiency of this pathway in neonates results in sulphate conjugation becoming its primary route of metabolism.

Theophylline is excreted almost completely unchanged in the urine by neonates. Conversely, children and adults only excrete between 7% and 10% unchanged theophylline in the urine, the rest being metabolised by the liver. The metabolism of caffeine is delayed in neonates and infants. This is explained by the difference in plasma half-life (the time taken for the plasma concentration to fall by half), which is 4 days in neonates and decreases to only 4 h in adults. The long half-life of caffeine in neonates and its wide therapeutic range makes it the drug of choice for neonatal apnoeas.

Many drugs that rely on the liver for metabolism show a decreased rate of metabolism during the neonatal and infant stages of development. Cautious drug regimens, tailored to each child, should be used in these age groups. Drug regimens should be altered according to the clinical response and the measured plasma drug concentration. Older children (3–5 years to puberty) often metabolise drugs at a greater rate than adults. This can be explained by the ratio of liver size to body surface area, which can be twice that of adults in this age group.

Excretion

Drugs and their metabolites are excreted by the kidneys by passive glomerular filtration or active tubular secretion. Once in the renal tubule, some drugs can be reabsorbed into the circulation. The majority of drugs excreted via the kidney rely on passive glomerular filtration to determine their rate of excretion.

A commonly measured indicator of renal function or glomerular filtration rate (GFR) is creatinine clearance, which is usually corrected to an adult body surface area of 1.7 m². The following equation relates creatinine clearance to the child's height and serum creatinine level.

$$\text{creatinine clearance (mL/min)} = \frac{k \times \text{height (cm)}}{\text{serum creatinine (}\mu\text{mol/L)}}$$

where k, a constant = 29 for preterm infants, 40 for full-term infants, 49 for children and adolescent girls, 62 for adolescent boys (Schwarz et al 1987).

This equation is only accurate when the serum creatinine concentration is stable. Creatinine is a breakdown product of muscle, so plasma levels can be increased by muscle damage (e.g. intramuscular injections) or reduced in children who are clinically malnourished. Both the clinical state of the child, together with the calculated glomerular filtration rate, must be used to determine the true renal function. The use of creatinine clearance as a marker of glomerular function is not always accurate, because creatinine is also secreted into renal tubules, which can be blocked by drugs such as cimetidine. Inulin, an inert polysaccharide, is filtered at the glomerulus. It does not interact with other drugs and is excreted unchanged by the kidneys. Measurement of inulin clearance gives a more accurate marker of glomerular filtration.

The kidneys are relatively immature at birth. Neonates have a corrected glomerular filtration rate of about 20 mL/min. Adult values of 100–130 mL/min are not reached until about 6 months of age. The glomerular filtration rate is also directly related to postconceptual age; thus, premature neonates have a lower rate of filtration than full-term neonates.

Renal function must be considered when prescribing drugs, with doses being reduced or intervals increased appropriately — e.g., for digoxin clearance:

- 0.7–1.4 mL/min/kg for preterm neonates
- 1.7–2.2 mL/min/kg for term neonates
- 2.7–3.5 mL/min/kg for infants
- 3.7–4.2 mL/min/kg for 1–5 years of age
- 2.5–3.1 mL/min/kg for 6–20 years of age

(Hastreiter et al 1985). In practice the following dosing regimen is used for digoxin:

- premature neonates: 2–3 µg/kg, twice a day
- neonates to 5 years: 5 µg/kg, twice a day
- 5–10 years: 3 µg/kg, twice a day.

These changes in renal excretion are much greater than the changes in volume of distribution, so it is likely that changes in renal excretion account for changes in digoxin clearance.

Tubular secretion matures slightly later than the glomerular filtration rate, reaching adult values at about 8 months of age. This only becomes significant for drugs which exert their effects within the kidney. If tubular secretion is reduced in neonates and infants, it follows that higher plasma concentrations will be necessary to have the same therapeutic effect. For example, frusemide is actively secreted into the tubule, where it has its diuretic effect. High doses of frusemide must be given in order to achieve a therapeutic effect in neonates and infants.

EFFECT OF SYSTEM FAILURE AND TREATMENT MODALITIES ON DRUG HANDLING

Failure of one or more organs affects the pharmacokinetics of many drugs. This section explores the effects of specific organ failure on drug handling.

Heart failure

Effect on absorption

In heart failure the gastric mucosa can become oedematous and blood flow to the gastrointestinal tract may be reduced as blood is directed to the vital organs. The rate of drug absorption from the gastrointestinal tract may be decreased, but the total amount of drug that is absorbed is not usually affected.

Effect on distribution

Distribution may be altered in cardiac failure as peripheral perfusion is reduced to maintain an adequate blood supply to the vital organs. In theory the plasma levels of some drugs may be elevated, although this does not have significant therapeutic consequences.

Effect on metabolism and excretion

Reduced blood supply to both liver and kidneys may limit the rate of metabolism and excretion of drugs and their active metabolites. The clinical half-life of some drugs may be increased, which can lead to accumulation and toxicity if dosing intervals are not lengthened by a similar ratio.

Poor venous return in heart failure can result in oedema, which may substantially increase body weight. If a drug is fat-soluble, has a narrow therapeutic range, or is bound to protein or tissue, expected body weight should be used initially. Dosing regimens are then altered according to plasma levels or clinical effect.

To establish an oedematous child's expected body weight, the position where the child's height falls on the growth chart must be transposed to the corresponding weight chart (Haycock 1994). Alternatively, recent 'dry' weight can be used. Except for altering the weight on which dosing is based, heart failure has insignificant clinical consequences on drug regimens.

Theoretically, cardiac 'by-pass' can be used to treat a failing heart. However, it is only used during and immediately after cardiac surgery. There are no dosing recommendations for use of drugs during by-pass, other than altering the dose according to clinical response or measured plasma concentrations.

Liver failure

The liver is the major site of drug metabolism. Active drugs are inactivated or made more water-soluble so they can be excreted by the kidneys. The liver is a relatively large organ in children and usually has a vast capacity. However, liver dysfunction can affect the metabolism of drugs in many ways, which makes dosage recommendations difficult.

Effect on absorption

Changes in absorption are usually only associat-

ed with chronic liver disease. Portal hypertension can cause oedema of the small intestine, which reduces absorption from this part of the gastrointestinal tract. In advanced liver disease, complex collateral vessels develop around the gut in response to hypertension in the portal vein. These effectively shunt blood away from the liver and into the systemic circulation. As a result, orally absorbed drugs will directly enter the systemic circulation without undergoing first-pass metabolism in the liver. Drugs which usually undergo extensive first-pass metabolism, such as pethidine, propranolol and chlormethiazole, may reach the systemic circulation in dangerously high concentrations. Oral doses of these drugs must be significantly reduced. Drugs only undergo first-pass metabolism when given orally. When administered by any other route (e.g. percutaneous, intravenous or rectal), first-pass metabolism is avoided.

Effect on distribution

Liver dysfunction can cause changes in protein binding of drugs in the plasma. Albumin, which is manufactured in the liver, usually accounts for about half the total plasma protein. During chronic liver dysfunction, plasma albumin levels fall, decreasing the total number of plasma protein-binding sites available. Thus free (unbound) levels of drugs that are highly protein bound are significantly increased. Bilirubin competes with drugs for protein-binding sites. Liver failure increases plasma bilirubin levels, thus displacing drugs from their binding sites.

Drugs with high extraction ratios (see below) which are highly protein bound will be cleared more quickly because a higher concentration of free drug will be available for metabolism. If the decrease in plasma binding is combined with an increase in hepatic clearance, the total plasma concentration may remain the same, or increase, but the free fraction will be increased. If the drug is highly protein bound, small changes in binding will lead to relatively large increases in the free fraction. An increase in the free fraction of drugs with narrow therapeutic ranges such as theophylline, phenytoin, warfarin and diazepam can lead to unwanted side effects and toxicity.

Effect on metabolism

Intrinsic hepatic clearance describes the amount of drug that is removed from the blood (extraction ratio, E) when it flows at a certain rate through the liver. The metabolism of drugs in the liver is described as flow-limited or capacity-limited.

Flow-limited drugs naturally have a high extraction ratio ($E > 0.7$). The rate at which the liver can metabolise these drugs is limited only by the rate of blood flow through it. The rate of metabolism of morphine is flow-limited and is relatively insensitive to changes in protein binding or hepatic enzyme activity.

Capacity-limited drugs have low extraction ratios and depend upon the plasma concentration of free drug available to interact with hepatic enzymes to determine their rate of metabolism. Capacity-limited drugs can be further divided into those that are highly protein bound and therefore sensitive to changes in protein binding (e.g. phenytoin, warfarin, diazepam) and those that have low protein binding (e.g. paracetamol, theophylline). Drugs whose metabolism is capacity-limited are most likely to accumulate in liver failure.

Effect on excretion

Liver dysfunction has no known clinical effect on excretion of drugs, except those that are required to exert their effect in the bile. Clindamycin does not penetrate the bile in biliary tract obstruction.

Practical implications

In practice it is very difficult to predict the dose that should be used in different types of liver dysfunction. The best indicators of the degree of liver dysfunction are plasma albumin concentrations and prothrombin time, although these are not particularly sensitive and can be altered by other disease states.

In most cases an awareness of the possible con-

sequences of adverse drug reactions, the measurement of plasma levels where appropriate, and adjustment of dosage regimens according to their clinical effect, is the best way to manage a child with liver dysfunction. However, drug use should be kept to a minimum, and alternatives which do not rely on the liver for metabolism should be used wherever possible.

Children with established liver dysfunction are predisposed to hepatic coma. In order to reduce the risk of coma, central and respiratory depressants should be avoided.

No treatment modality is available to compensate for liver dysfunction.

Kidney failure

The kidneys are the major site for excretion of water-soluble drugs or metabolites. In renal failure the kidneys do not excrete these drugs effectively which can lead to accumulation on successive dosing.

Effect on absorption

Renal failure does not affect absorption of drugs from the gastrointestinal tract.

Effect on distribution and metabolism

The inability of failing kidneys to excrete urea effectively causes plasma levels to rise, leading to 'uraemic syndrome'. Acidic drugs, such as warfarin and phenytoin, are displaced from plasma protein-binding sites in uraemic children. Because more free drug is available to be distributed throughout body tissues, the volume of distribution will increase and likewise the amount of drug available for metabolism will be increased.

The binding of alkaline drugs, such as trimethoprim and chloramphenicol, is not affected by uraemia.

Vitamin D (calciferol) is metabolised in the liver to 25-hydroxycholecalciferol and then further hydroxylated to active 1,25-dihydroxycholecalciferol in the kidneys. In renal failure hydroxylation in the kidneys is significantly reduced. Therefore 1-α-hydroxyc-holecalciferol is administered orally for the treatment of renal rickets.

Effect on excretion

Drugs or their metabolites are excreted by the kidneys either by passive glomerular filtration or by active tubular secretion. Once in the renal tubule, some drugs may be reabsorbed back into the circulation. The rate of excretion of drugs cleared by the kidney is determined by the rate of passive glomerular filtration.

The simplest method to quantify the glomerular filtration rate and therefore the degree of renal failure, is to calculate creatinine or inulin clearance (see p. 186). Tubular reabsorption will increase as the glomerular filtration rate falls.

Drug regimens must be altered in renal failure to avoid accumulation on successive dosing whilst maintaining therapeutic plasma levels. Most drug companies are able to recommend dosage adjustments for adults with renal insufficiency which can be safely extrapolated to children with similar corrected glomerular filtration rates. In general, dosing intervals should be increased or doses reduced in renal dysfunction. If the drug can be measured in the plasma and has a narrow therapeutic range, above which unwanted effects may occur, the dosing regimen must be altered according to individual plasma concentrations. Individualisation of drug regimens in altered renal function is recommended for drugs such as vancomycin, gentamicin, aciclovir and digoxin.

Renal replacement therapy

When renal function deteriorates acutely, renal replacement therapy must be initiated. This can be achieved by peritoneal dialysis, haemodialysis or haemofiltration.

Dialysis removes wastes and water-soluble drugs from the body by diffusion across a semi-permeable membrane. The clearance of a drug by dialysis depends on the extent to which it is normally cleared by the kidneys. Thus drugs which are more than 20% protein bound, have a high molecular weight, are highly lipid-soluble, or have a large volume of distribution do not dialyse well.

Peritoneal dialysis. Continuous peritoneal dialysis is approximately equivalent to a glomerular filtration rate of 10 to 20 mL/min (Dade & Ashley 1996).

Haemodialysis. When drugs are removed by haemodialysis (e.g. water-soluble drugs such as vancomycin), dosing should occur after dialysis. Maintenance, or 'top-up', doses may be required between dialysis sessions for drugs that undergo extrarenal clearance. The manufacturer's data sheet or the pharmacy should be contacted for individualisation of dosing regimens in haemodialysis.

Haemofiltration. Haemofiltration removes wastes from the body through convection by ultrafiltration across a membrane. Haemofiltration forces water from the blood into the filtrate and is primarily used to remove water from the body. It is used as an adjunct to haemodialysis to remove a water load without causing an osmotic shift of water into the intracellular space. This reduces the risk of muscle cramps and hypotension.

Haemofiltration is not efficient at removing drug molecules from the plasma. Only a small percentage of water-soluble molecules with low molecular weights will be removed.

Failure of the gastrointestinal tract

The gastrointestinal tract is the site of absorption for orally administered drugs.

Effect on absorption

The gastric emptying rate determines how quickly drugs move from the stomach into the small intestine. This may directly affect the rate, and possibly the extent, to which drugs are absorbed. Gastric emptying rates can be delayed by trauma, pain, intestinal obstruction and raised intracranial pressure. However, changes in gastric emptying rates do not have a significant effect on drug absorption.

Effect on distribution, metabolism and excretion

Failure of the gastrointestinal tract does not affect drug distribution, metabolism or excretion.

Effect of nasogastric and nasojejunal administration of drugs

In paediatric intensive care units, most children are sedated, and often ventilated, which makes oral administration of drugs not only dangerous but impossible. Nasogastric tubes are usually inserted to enable feeding and administration of oral medications. Nasojejunal tubes bypass the stomach altogether.

Thick suspensions or finely crushed tablets can block nasogastric or nasojejunal tubes; therefore they must be flushed with warm water after drugs are administered through them. Drugs can interact with feeds. High electrolyte concentrations 'crack' (destabilisation of the emulsion) feeds. The absorption of phenytoin is severely hindered by the presence of feed in the stomach (Miller & Strom 1988, Pearce 1988). In adults, feeds should be stopped for 2 h before and after a drug is administered. This is obviously not practical for a baby who requires frequent feeds. In these cases enteral feeds should be stopped for at least 30 min before and after drug dosing.

Nasojejunal tubes deliver drugs directly into the jejunum. Erythromycin increases peristalsis and has been used to facilitate the passage of nasojejunal tubes to their correct position. The main problem associated with nasojejunal administration of medicines is diarrhoea. This is often caused by the osmotic load of drugs and feed in the jejunum, which draws water and electrolytes into the small intestine (Adams 1994). Drugs with low osmolality should be used for jejunal administration. Oral syrups with a high osmolality, and liquids containing sorbitol (an osmotic laxative), should be avoided (Heimburger 1990). Dispersible tablets, finely crushed tablets, or injections that are safe and efficacious when given orally are often more useful.

Failure of the lungs

The lungs have a huge surface area which makes them ideal for drug absorption. However, at present, they are only exploited to produce a local action (e.g. ipratropium or salbutamol for bronchodilation) and not for systemic effect.

Extracorporal membrane oxygenation (ECMO) is a technique which oxygenates a child's blood outside his/her body. It is one of a number of techniques used to treat intractable — but reversible — respiratory failure (Donn 1994).

The effect ECMO has on drug disposition is mostly unknown. However, the circuit uses large volumes of transfused blood, which is likely to significantly increase the volume of distribution. Larger doses of water-soluble drugs such as vancomycin may be needed to achieve therapeutic levels. The site of drug administration in the circuit may also affect its distribution (Hoie et al 1993). Drug disposition and therefore dosing in ECMO is largely empirical and based on clinical response and measurement of plasma concentrations where appropriate.

ADMINISTRATION OF DRUGS IN PAEDIATRIC INTENSIVE CARE

The number and variety of drugs that must be administered to critically ill children is often large. Therefore it is important to choose the most appropriate route and ensure that each drug is administered to produce a predictable therapeutic response.

Oral administration

If the critically ill child can absorb medication from the gastrointestinal tract then this route remains the most appropriate for continuing existing drug regimens. When children are sedated, oral medication can be safely administered through a nasogastric or nasojejunal tube.

Rectal administration

Rectal administration can be utilised when the oral and intravenous routes are not available. This route can be used effectively for anti-emetics (prochlorperazine), anticonvulsants (diazepam), pain relief (paracetamol and diclofenac) and for sedation (chloral hydrate). Diarrhoea and constipation obviously limit the effective use of suppositories or rectal solutions.

Percutaneous administration

Percutaneous administration has extremely limited applications despite its theoretical exploitation in neonates. The rate of absorption through the skin varies greatly with age and the degree of skin hydration. Delivery of the required concentration to produce a therapeutic response is therefore unpredictable and not easily reproduced.

Examples of effective percutaneous administration include the following.

• Glyceryl trinitrate (GTN) patches can be applied to the skin to produce a systemic effect. GTN diffuses through the skin and enters the bloodstream, where it causes peripheral vasodilation of veins. This further facilitates its uptake into the systemic circulation.

• Emla® cream is a mixture of lignocaine and prilocaine, which both have a local anaesthetic action when applied to the skin. Absorption is enhanced by covering the cream with an occlusive dressing, thus numbing the area within 1–2 h.

Intramuscular administration

Intramuscular injections should not be used routinely in children except to administer vaccinations. Children have less muscle than adults, which makes intramuscular injections very painful. Distribution of drug from the injection site is often slow and unpredictable. Fat-soluble drugs will diffuse through capillary walls, while water-soluble drugs, with a low molecular weight, can pass through the pores in the capillary membrane. However, lipid-insoluble drugs with high molecular weights are only removed from the injection site by the relatively slow process of lymphatic absorption. When an intramuscular injection is the most appropriate route

of administration, ensuring adequate peripheral circulation, movement and massage can each increase the rate of absorption.

Subcutaneous administration

The subcutaneous route of administration has the same limitations as the intramuscular route, but the injections are less painful. It is not routinely used in paediatric intensive care units.

Intravenous administration

Intravenous administration ensures that all the administered dose enters the bloodstream. Particular care must be taken when drugs are administered by this route to minimise the risk of blood contamination. The advantage of this route is that all the dose reaches the circulation immediately and therefore its clinical effect is quick and predictable. Conversely, the major disadvantage is that any unwanted dose is extremely difficult, if not impossible, to remove from the body.

In paediatric intensive care the child often has several intravenous catheters through which drugs are administered. Central lines, often with two or three lumens, deliver drugs directly into the heart. Central administration will ensure immediate mixing with a large volume of blood, which negates any need for dilution. However, the recommended rate of administration must be followed to minimise the risk of adverse effects on the central nervous or cardiovascular systems. The central route is preferred in the following situations:

• when the drug has either a high or low pH, is hyperosmolar, or is irritant, causing risk of thrombophlebitis
• when the child has a fluid restriction and so dilution of intravenous drugs must be kept to a minimum
• when the drug itself causes peripheral vasoconstriction; it stimulates α_1 adrenoceptors which causes constriction of vascular smooth muscle.

Peripheral access is usually both quicker and

easier to achieve than central access in an emergency. In stable situations, this route is often reserved for the administration of maintenance fluids and for drugs that are less irritant to the vessels. Dextrose solutions of more than 10% should not be administered peripherally, because they are hyperosmolar, leading to thrombophlebitis and possible tissue damage if extravasation occurs. Addition of electrolytes to maintenance fluid must be carefully assessed. The maximum concentration of potassium chloride that can be administered peripherally is 40 mmol/L (British Medical Association 1996). Above this concentration, potassium infusions are extremely irritant and cause vessel damage. Extravasation of the infusion causes burns to the surrounding tissues. Calcium gluconate is preferred to calcium chloride, except in a cardiac emergency, because it is less irritant to veins. When electrolytes are added to dextrose solutions (especially those of 10% or more) their potential to cause thrombophlebitis is compounded.

Reconstitution of intravenous drugs

Many intravenous preparations are available as freeze-dried powders which must be reconstituted before they can be administered intravenously. Most intravenous preparations are formulated for adults, so often only a fraction of the total unit dose is used for children. Therefore it is important to know the exact concentration of the reconstituted injection so that an accurate dose can be given.

The volume of fluid which the freeze-dried drug displaces when reconstituted is known as its displacement value. The displacement value must be subtracted from the final desired volume, and the resulting volume used to reconstitute the injection to ensure an accurate concentration. Once the required dose of drug has been drawn up into a syringe, it often needs to be diluted further before administration, especially when given as an infusion. Acid drugs should usually be diluted in 5% dextrose which has pH 4–5. Alkaline drugs should be diluted with 0.9% sodium chloride (pH 7), as they are incompatible in 5% dextrose.

Rate of administration

Most drugs can be given intermittently as an intravenous bolus over 1–2 min. However, adenosine is an exception which should be given rapidly. Drugs such as metoclopramide which have the potential to cause unpleasant central nervous system or cardiovascular side effects must be administered as a slow bolus over 2–5 min. Drugs which are irritant or cause histamine release should be administered as infusions over 30–60 min, e.g. vancomycin and erythromycin. Drugs that have a short half life and whose plasma level must be maintained within a therapeutic range, e.g. dopamine and dobutamine should be administered as continuous infusions.

Compatibility of intravenous solutions

When intravenous access is limited, or the number of drugs that must be given exceeds the number of lumens available, some drugs will inevitably have to be administered through the same lumen. It is important to know which drugs are physically and chemically compatible or incompatible, as precipitation occurs with incompatible drugs. This may block the lumen, cause thrombophlebitis in a peripheral vein, increase the risk of emboli formation or reduce the amount of drug available to produce a therapeutic response.

In order to assess the risk associated with a combination of infusions the following questions should be asked.

Has it been done before? Because of the number of possible combinations of intravenous solutions and their wide variability in concentration, it is highly unlikely that published compatibilities exactly fit the situation. When there is no published literature, previous experience of the proposed combination, where a therapeutic response with no ill effects was achieved, may exist. Advice can be sought from within the paediatric intensive care unit, from the pharmacist, other specialist paediatric centres, adult intensive care centres or from drug companies.

Are the pH values of the solutions compatible? Alkaline solutions are less likely to be compatible with acid solutions than with other alkalis, and vice versa. The more extreme the pH, the less likely that it will be compatible with other solutions.

What diluent should be used? Some drugs are only physically compatible in 0.9% sodium chloride (e.g. erythromycin and frusemide) while others are only compatible in 5% dextrose (e.g. amiodarone). Obviously, in these cases the different diluents that must be used will not allow them to be mixed. However, many drugs are compatible in both 0.9% sodium chloride and 5% dextrose.

Is the drug known to be unstable? Some diluted solutions are known to be physically unstable and therefore must be given separately. Phenytoin, for example, when diluted with 0.9% sodium chloride, can precipitate, while epoprostenol infusions are only stable for 12 h. Small changes to these solutions may cause them to become unstable and to precipitate.

Through which lumen of the central line should drugs be administered? Central catheters usually have two or three lumens. Each lumen delivers drugs to the body at a different position along the catheter tip. Drugs that enter the bloodstream furthest away from the tip of the catheter (distal position) should be those that have less extreme pH and are most physically stable. The more unstable solutions, which are most likely to be incompatible with others, should enter the bloodstream at the tip of the catheter (proximal position) so that they are immediately mixed in the blood. Thus they will not flow past the relatively high concentrations of potentially incompatible drugs exiting the other lumens.

Having considered these factors, the combination with the lowest risk of incompatibility should be chosen. The most important point to remember is that the drugs must be successfully administered to the child and very often there is no alternative but to 'try it and see'. To minimise the child's risk, he/she must be regularly monitored to ensure the drugs are therapeutically effective. Infusions should be mixed together in the lumen for as long as possible outside the child's body so that any potential precipitation can be seen. If infusions are administered through a filter, as is the practice in some paediatric intensive care units, they will be blocked by the precipitate.

Flushing and purging of intravenous lumens

After each intravenous bolus is administered, the lumen must be flushed with at least its own volume of 0.9% sodium chloride or 5% dextrose. This ensures that all the dose enters the child's bloodstream instead of remaining in the lumen. The solution used to flush the lumen must be physically compatible with the bolus that has just been given. Its compatibility with the next bolus should also be considered and a second compatible flush used if necessary.

The flush or a purge must be administered at the same rate as the previous infusion or bolus so that all the drug is administered at the correct rate. An example, where the lumen volume is 1 mL, is:

- aciclovir 100 mg diluted to 20 mL with 5% dextrose and infused over 1 h
- flush with 1 mL 5% dextrose over 3 min
- flush with 1 mL 0.9% sodium chloride
- frusemide 8 mg diluted to 2 mL with 0.9% sodium chloride given over 4 min
- flush with 1 mL 0.9% sodium chloride over 2 min.

PAIN AND SEDATION

Paediatric intensive care is a stressful place for the child and family. The need for the child to be pain-free whilst adequately sedated is paramount.

Evaluation of pain. Evaluation of pain in paediatric intensive care is hampered by the difficulty children have expressing and quantifying their pain. Usually the child is sedated and unable to respond either verbally or visually to a pain scale. In these cases, the sympathetic nervous system responses — an increase in heart rate, blood pressure or respiratory rate (in the non-ventilated patient) or dilation of the pupils — are the only indicators of pain.

Control of pain. Once pain has been experienced it is more difficult to control with analgesics. Therefore the aim of pain relief is to maintain effective analgesia with regularly timed, or continuous, dosing of one or a combination of analgesics most appropriate for each child's pain.

Sedation. Sedation is an induced state of calmness or sleep without anaesthesia. The level of sedation each child requires will depend upon how they respond to each situation. Sedatives blunt the body's response to stimuli.

Drugs used for pain and sedation. The drugs used to treat pain or cause sedation often have more than one action. They can be divided into the following groups:

- opioids for analgesia and sedation
- benzodiazepines for sedation and amnesia
- non-steroidal antiinflammatory agents for musculoskeletal pain
- paracetamol for analgesia
- chloral hydrate or triclofos for sedation
- ketamine for sedation and analgesia.

Opioids

Opioids act at opioid receptors in the central nervous system and have no antiinflammatory action. At present, four opioid receptors have been described:

- μ/δ receptors: cause miosis, bradycardia, central analgesia, euphoria, dependence and respiratory depression
- κ receptors: cause constriction of pupils, sedation and spinal analgesia
- σ receptors: cause dysphoria, hallucinations, respiratory and vasomotor stimulation.

Opioids also have actions outside the central nervous system. They cause vasodilation, mediated by peripheral histamine release, and constipation by increasing smooth muscle tone throughout the gastrointestinal tract and decreasing peristalsis. This may decrease absorption from nasogastric feeds. A faecal softener such as docusate sodium or lactulose should be prescribed when gastric feeding and regular opioid use are concurrent.

Tolerance occurs when an increase in dose is required to maintain the same analgesic or sedative effect. It can occur within 2 or 3 days of opioid use.

Physical dependence leads to *withdrawal* syndrome when opioids are discontinued abruptly or a reversing agent is used. This is characterised by increased respiratory rate, perspiration, tremors and goosebumps. The severity of the withdrawal syndrome depends upon the individual child, the drug used, the size and frequency of the dose, and the duration of drug use.

Morphine

The most widely used opioid agonist is morphine, which stimulates both μ- and κ-receptors and has a predictable action. Morphine should not be used in children with biliary tract complications, as it causes constriction of the sphincter of Oddi.

The major side effect of morphine is respiratory depression. Infusion rates should be initiated at 10–30 μg/kg/h using the lowest effective dose. The infusion rate in non-ventilated children should not exceed 60 μg/kg/h.

Morphine is metabolised in the liver to active and inactive metabolites. The most active metabolite is morphine-6-glucoronide, which is ten times as potent as morphine. Morphine-6-glucoronide is excreted via the kidneys and accumulates in renal failure and during prolonged use. Care should be taken when administering morphine in renal and liver dysfunction. Neonates are unable to conjugate large doses of morphine, because of an immature liver, prolonging the drug action.

Papaveretum

Papaveretum is a mixture of opium alkaloids; morphine, papaverine and codeine. Noscapine was removed from the formulation in 1993 because of concerns that it may be genotoxic (Committee on the Safety of Medicines 1991). It has been claimed that papaveretum produces less severe side effects than morphine, although this has not been realised in clinical practice.

Pethidine

Pethidine is the analgesic of choice in pancreatitis

associated with biliary tract disease because it does not cause constriction of the sphincter of Oddi. It is metabolised in the liver to both active and inactive metabolites. Norpethidine, an active metabolite, accumulates in renal failure or during prolonged infusions, and has a hallucinogenic and convulsant effect.

Codeine

Codeine is a weak opioid and should only be used for moderate pain. It is the analgesic of choice for head injuries, causing insignificant depression of the central nervous system and thereby not interfering with its assessment. Inadvertent intravenous administration causes a massive release of histamine which results in a fall in cardiac output.

Fentanyl

Fentanyl is between 50 and 100 times more potent than morphine. High doses cause chest wall rigidity which may be so severe that intubation and ventilation requiring heavy sedation and muscle relaxation may be necessary. Fentanyl's high fat-solubility results in a rapid onset of action and a half life of 4–8 h. Initially, fentanyl has a brief duration of action because it redistributes from the brain into fat stores in the body. However, after large or frequent doses the child's lipid stores become saturated and the elimination rate is dependent on its rate of metabolism. Accumulation also occurs in liver and renal dysfunction. Fentanyl skin patches are only suitable for control of chronic pain. Their use for acute analgesia is limited because of the long lag time to achieve therapeutic levels and the current inflexibility of dose. Lower doses of fentanyl are administered percutaneously, compared with the intravenous dose, because first-pass metabolism in the liver is avoided.

Remifentanil

Remifentanil is a recently marketed opioid analgesic which has a rapid onset, and short duration, of action. These properties would allow intermittent assessment of the child (by briefly stopping the infusion) without compromising its care; however, remifentanil has yet to be adopted in adult or paediatric intensive care units.

Buprenorphine

Buprenorphine acts as a partial agonist at μ-receptors. It has a long duration of action and cannot be completely reversed by naloxone.

Opioid reversal

Naloxone. Naxolone is an opioid antagonist which reverses the μ-, δ- and κ-receptor-mediated effects of morphine and other opioid-like substances. It has a short duration of action (1–2 h) compared with most opioids. Thus several doses may need to be given, depending on the child's response. Naloxone reverses both the side effects and analgesic action of opioids.

Benzodiazepines

Benzodiazepines have sedative, anxiolytic and amnesic properties. It is proposed that they act on specific benzodiazepine receptors which enhance the activity of the inhibitory neurotransmitter gamma-amino-butyric acid (GABA) in the brain and spinal cord. GABA has anticonvulsant and muscle-relaxing properties in the motor system and amnesic and anxiolytic actions in the limbic system. Benzodiazepines have no analgesic properties but do reduce the anxiety associated with pain and the memory of pain. When used in conjunction with an opioid they significantly reduce the amount of analgesic required. Benzodiazepines are highly fat-soluble and accumulate in the body's fat stores after prolonged use, which can delay recovery. They are highly protein bound and metabolised by the liver. Long-term use of benzodiazepines can cause physiological dependence.

Diazepam

Diazepam is available as an injection and as a lipid emulsion (Diazemuls®). Diazemuls® must be used for intravenous infusions because this preparation is considerably less irritant to veins than the injection. Diazepam is well absorbed from the rectum, making this the route of choice to control seizures at home. It has a long duration of action (20–40 h) which may delay wakening on stopping an infusion.

Midazolam

Midazolam is more amnesic than diazepam but is also much more expensive. It has a short duration of action (2–3 h) and a rapid onset of action (2–3 min). Once fat stores have become saturated with midazolam, its rate of metabolism determines its effective clinical half-life.

Benzodiazepine reversal

Flumazenil is a benzodiazepine receptor antagonist which rapidly reverses the effects of benzodiazepines. It is used to reverse unwanted central and respiratory depression, which are dangerous in a non-ventilated child. Its use in intensive care is not usually warranted and therefore extremely rare.

Non-steroidal antiinflammatory drugs

Non-steroidal antiinflammatory drugs (NSAIDs) have antipyretic, analgesic and antiinflammatory properties. They are excellent for reducing musculoskeletal pain, and their concurrent use with opioids can reduce opioid requirements. Their major action is to inhibit the enzyme cyclo-oxygenase which is involved in the production of prostaglandin. Reduced levels of circulating prostaglandin decrease inflammation and pain. NSAID side effects, which are a direct result of their antiprostaglandin action, limit their use in paediatric intensive care. These include: gastrointestinal bleeding, inhibition of platelet aggregation and reduced renal function in debilitated children where renal vasodilation and maintenance of renal perfusion are under prostaglandin control. NSAIDs are contraindicated in neonates with cardiac abnormalities where the ductus arteriosus must remain patent. The patency of the ductus arteriosus is dependent on prostaglandin.

Ibuprofen

Ibuprofen is a mild analgesic with a relatively low incidence of side effects.

Diclofenac

Diclofenac is more potent than ibuprofen and has a correspondingly higher incidence of adverse effects. It is available as a tablet, suppository or injection. The injection can be given intramuscularly or by intravenous infusion. The intramuscular route is painful and not recommended. For intravenous administration the injection must be diluted with 0.9% sodium chloride or 5% glucose, both of which must be buffered with sodium bicarbonate.

Paracetamol

Paracetamol is a mild analgesic which has no antiinflammatory action. Its mechanism of action is not fully understood. Paracetamol is a highly effective analgesic when administered regularly and is the analgesic of choice in infants under six months of age. It is available as a suspension or suppositories.

Chloral hydrate and triclofos

Both chloral hydrate and triclofos are rapidly metabolised in the liver to trichloroethanol. Trichloroethanol causes sedation by depressing the central nervous system, whilst having minimal effect on the circulation or respiration.

Chloral hydrate

Chloral hydrate has an unpleasant taste and irritates the gastrointestinal tract. Dilution of the dose with plenty of water reduces gastric irritance and enhances absorption. Doses are given 'as required' when intermittent or light sedation is needed.

Triclofos

Triclofos has less severe gastric side effects than chloral hydrate and is therefore more acceptable to conscious children.

Anaesthetic agents

Ketamine

Ketamine is an intravenous anaesthetic which has sedative, analgesic and amnesic properties. It causes an increase in blood pressure and heart rate whilst having no effect on respiration. Thus it is the sedative of choice in acute asthma. Ketamine's major side effect of unpleasant, vivid, hallucinatory dreams are more common in children over 15 years of age. Concurrent administration of a benzodiazepine reduces the incidence of 'emergence syndrome' as the effect of the ketamine wears off.

Propofol

Propofol is a short-acting intravenous anaesthetic that is available as a lipid emulsion. Propofol should be given by repeated slow intravenous bolus or infusion to maintain light anaesthesia. Plasma lipid levels must be measured during prolonged intravenous infusions to ensure the child is able to eliminate the high fat content of the emulsion from the body. Accumulation of fat has been reported to cause death in children (Committee on the Safety of Medicines 1992a). Propofol is metabolised by the liver, may cause dysrhythmias, convulsions (Committee on the Safety of Medicines 1992b) and rarely alters the colour of urine after prolonged use. Propofol should only be administered using PVC giving sets.

Etomidate

Etomidate causes less hypotension than other intravenous anaesthetics. Its use is limited because long-term administration inhibits the cytochrome P_{450} enzyme system. This enzyme system plays an important role in adrenal steroidogenesis. Inhibition of the cytochrome P_{450} enzyme system reduces steroid production, which may lead to dangerously low cortisol levels.

MUSCLE RELAXANTS ('NEUROMUSCULAR BLOCKERS')

Muscle relaxants are used to produce a state of paralysis for intubation and to stop the child resisting the ventilator when artificial respiration is required. They must be used with sedatives because it is unacceptable, and extremely traumatic, for a child to remain conscious while paralysed.

How do muscle relaxants work? Muscles contract when acetylcholine, which is released at the neuromuscular junction, binds to nicotinic acetylcholine receptors on the muscle and causes depolarisation. Acetylcholine is rapidly inactivated by acetylcholinesterase, an enzyme, and the muscle repolarises and relaxes. Muscle relaxants either produce their action by depolarising the muscle but not allowing repolarisation for further contractions (depolarising muscle relaxants) or by blocking acetylcholine receptors without activating them (non-depolarising muscle relaxants).

Depolarising neuromuscular blockers

Depolarising agents compete with acetylcholine for receptors but cannot be inactivated by acetylcholinesterase. Repolarisation and return of contractility only occurs when the depolarising agent diffuses out of the neuromuscular junction and into the plasma. Here it is inactivated by plasma cholinesterase.

Suxamethonium

Suxamethonium (succinylcholine) is the only depolarising muscle relaxant in clinical use. It acts within a few seconds and has a brief duration of action, usually less than 10 min. These properties make it ideal for rapid intubation in an emergency situation.

Suxamethonium should be administered as a bolus injection. Low doses cause bradycardia, while repeated dosing produces tachycardia because of agonism of muscarinic acetylcholine receptors. If a second dose of suxamethonium is necessary, intravenous atropine should be given just before, to block the muscarinic receptors.

Between 1 in 2500 and 1 in 3000 of the population have a genetically determined atypical plasma cholinesterase which results in poor metabolism of suxamethonium. When suxamethonium is given to children with atypical plasma cholinesterase they will take longer than expected to regain normal muscle tone.

Suxamethonium activates the acetylcholine receptor to cause muscle depolarisation and consequently muscle contractions which can cause muscle ache. Potassium is released during muscle contraction, which raises the plasma concentration by between 0.5 and 1.0 mmol/L (Wheeler 1993). This may precipitate ventricular fibrillation in children who are already hyperkalaemic.

Non-depolarising neuromuscular blockers

The drugs in this therapeutic class vary in their cost, side effects and duration of action. They can either be given as a continuous intravenous infusion, which ensures effective relaxation but may lead to accumulation and overrelaxation, or as intravenous boluses when the child clinically requires them. The latter relies on anticipation of the child's needs by paediatric intensive care staff. The child's level of muscle relaxation can be monitored by close observation or the use of a peripheral nerve stimulator (Wheeler 1993).

Pancuronium

Pancuronium has been in clinical use for a long time, is cheap and has a long duration of action. Pancuronium causes histamine release and has vagolytic effects resulting in tachycardia and hypertension. About 20% is metabolised in the liver to active metabolites while the rest is excreted by the kidneys. Pancuronium should not be used where there is cardiac instability, or renal or liver dysfunction.

Vecuronium

Vecuronium has an intermediate duration of action. It is the drug of choice for children with cardiac instability because it has little effect on the heart. 80% is metabolised by the liver to active and inactive metabolites which are excreted in the bile and by the kidneys. Two active metabolites are excreted by the kidneys and will therefore accumulate in renal failure. Vecuronium is not recommended for use in children with renal or liver dysfunction.

Atracurium

Atracurium has an intermediate duration of action. It is inactivated spontaneously in plasma by Hoffman elimination, a chemical process which requires neither hepatic metabolism nor

Table 23.2   Classification and actions of paralysing agents

Drug	Class	Onset of action	Duration of action	Metabolism/ elimination	Side effects
Pancuronium	Non-depolarising	2–3 min	45 min	Renal>>hepatic	Tachycardia, ↑BP
Atracurium	Non-depolarising	2–3 min	15–40 min	Hoffman elimination	Some histamine release: ↓BP
Vecuronium	Non-depolarising	2–3 min	Infant: 30–40 min Child: 15–20 min	Bile>>renal	No cardiac side effects
Suxamethonium	Depolarising	1 min	3–5 min	Plasma cholinesterases	Bradycardia, ↑BP, ↑K⁺, muscle pain

renal excretion. It is therefore the drug of choice in renal or hepatic dysfunction. However, atracurium has a limited use in children with cardiac instability because it releases histamine which can cause hypotension and flushing of the face and chest.

Cisatracurium

Cisatracurium is a single isomer of atracurium. It is more potent than atracurium and does not cause histamine release, thereby providing greater cardiac stability. Cisatracurium is gaining use in adult units, but experience in children is limited.

Reversal of neuromuscular blockade

There are few clinical situations where reversal of neuromuscular blockade is acceptable or necessary. Neostigmine, pyridostigmine and edrophonium have all been used to reverse muscle relaxation. They are cholinesterase inhibitors which inhibit the breakdown of acetylcholine, increasing transmitter concentrations available to stimulate the receptors. Acetylcholine stimulates nicotinic receptors, reversing neuromuscular blockade. Acetylcholine stimulation of muscarinic receptors causes severe bradycardia and excessive salivation. Glycopyrolate or atropine is administered just before the reversal agent to block these unpleasant and dangerous side effects.

INOTROPES

Inotropes are drugs that increase the force of contraction of the heart. Drugs with α adrenoceptor activity cause vasoconstriction which can lead to gangrene. These drugs should be administered by the central intravenous route to avoid local vasoconstriction and possible extravasation. Phentolamine, a short-acting α-adrenergic blocking agent, can be infused intravenously to minimise the α-adrenergic effects of inotropes. All inotropes have a short half-life and are administered as a continuous infusion. The rate at which the inotrope is infused is altered according to each child's response.

Adrenaline (epinephrine)

Adrenaline is a naturally occurring hormone which is secreted by the adrenal medulla. It stimulates both α and β adrenoceptors. Adrenaline has a much greater affinity for β_1 receptors than for β_2 receptors, but is not selective for either α_1 or α_2 receptors.

Intravenous administration of adrenaline stimulates α receptors to produce a rapid rise in both systolic and diastolic blood pressure and improved venous return. Heart rate, cardiac output and stroke volume all increase because of direct stimulation of β_1 receptors in the heart.

Adrenaline is rapidly metabolised in the mucosa of the gastrointestinal tract and in the liver. Thus it is ineffective when given orally and must be administered parenterally. Following an intravenous injection, adrenaline is rapidly distributed throughout the nervous system and the heart, having a half life of approximately 10 min. Adrenaline is absorbed more rapidly from muscle than from subcutaneous sites because it causes vasoconstriction of subcutaneous blood vessels.

Life-threatening adverse effects of adrenaline include severe hypertension and ventricular arrhythmias. It also causes a decrease in blood flow through the kidneys, as vascular resistance is increased. Other side effects include tremors, restlessness, headache and anxiety.

Interactions and precautions

• Severe hypertension and bradycardia may occur with β adrenoblocker agents, as only α_1 effects can be realised.
• There is an increased risk of arrhythmias with halothane, quinidine and digoxin.
• There may be hypersensitivity to effects of adrenaline if hyperthyroid or hypertensive.
• There is an increased risk of hyperglycaemia, especially in diabetics, because of α_2 suppression of insulin.

Noradrenaline (norepinephrine)

Noradrenaline is the major neurotransmitter of the sympathetic nervous system. It stimulates α and β_1 receptors but has little effect on β_2 receptors. Therefore it increases systolic and diastolic blood pressure as a result of vasoconstriction, increased systemic vascular resistance and increased venous return. Noradrenaline is only used for the treatment of acute hypotension, because it has little effect on cardiac output.

Noradrenaline is metabolised in the liver and excreted in the urine.

As a direct result of its profound vasoconstrictive effect, noradrenaline decreases blood flow to the peripheral circulation, causing tissue necrosis. Phentolamine is administered concurrently to minimise these adverse effects.

Isoprenaline

Isoprenaline is a synthetic catchecholamine which has mainly non-specific β receptor action and little α activity. Isoprenaline has inotropic and chronotropic actions resulting from stimulation of the sinoatrial node. It increases contractility, decreases peripheral resistance and increases renal blood flow.

Isoprenaline is conjugated in the liver, with less than 15% being excreted unchanged in the liver.

Dopamine

Dopamine is a central neurotransmitter which is a precursor of noradrenaline and adrenaline. The pharmacological effects of dopamine vary as the infusion rate is altered.

- At low rates of infusion, such as 0.5–2 mg/kg/min, D_1 and D_2 receptors are stimulated. Activation of D_1 receptors causes vasodilation of renal and coronary vascular smooth muscle. D_2 receptor activation inhibits the release of noradrenaline.
- When infused at a rate of 2–5 mg/kg/min, β_1 receptors are predominately stimulated. This causes an increase in cardiac output and systolic blood pressure.
- When infused at rates exceeding 5 mg/kg/min, α_1 and α_2 adrenoceptors are activated. This increases both systolic and diastolic blood pressure.

Dopamine is metabolised by the liver and excreted by the kidneys. Low-dose dopamine is used with dobutamine to improve renal blood flow.

Dobutamine

Dobutamine is a mixture of two isomers which are mirror images of each other. L-dobutamine has α_1 properties, which causes vasoconstriction and an increase in the force of contraction. D-dobutamine has β_1 and β_2 adrenoceptor activity. This produces an increase in cardiac contractility and vasodilation of skeletal smooth muscle.

Dobutamine is metabolised by the liver and excreted by the kidneys.

CONTROL OF SEIZURES

Seizures occur when acute focal or generalised electrical disturbances are generated within the

Table 23.3 Classification and actions of adrenoceptors

Receptor	Cardiac effect	Extracardiac effect	Main clinical effect
$\alpha_{(1+2)}$		Arterial and venous vasoconstriction	↑ systemic vascular resistance ↑ venous return
β_1	↑ heart rate ↑contractility ↑ AV conduction		↑ cardiac output
β_2	↑ heart rate	Arterial vasodilation Bronchodilation Mast cell stabilisation	↓ systemic vascular resistance ↓ brochospasm ↓ acute allergic response
D_1		Renal and mesenteric vasodilation	↑ renal and mesenteric blood flow

brain. The cause of these abnormal electrical impulses is not known and therefore the mechanisms by which antiepileptic drugs control epilepsy are not completely understood. However, the following mechanisms of action have been suggested for the following antiepileptic drugs which are in common usage.

- Gamma-amino-butyric acid (GABA) is the major inhibitory neurotransmitter in the central nervous system.
- Benzodiazepines increase the effectiveness of GABA, enhancing neuronal inhibition.
- Barbiturates and phenytoin block picrotoxin receptors. Picrotoxin blocks the postsynaptic inhibitory effect of GABA.
- Phenytoin seems to prevent the continuance of epileptic discharges.
- Phenobarbitone depresses all neuronal excitability.
- Clonazepam raises the intra-cerebral levels of 5-hydroxytryptamine, a neurotransmitter which is known to raise the seizure threshold.

Control of status epilepticus

Status epilepticus is a medical emergency which is treated by terminating 'grand mal' seizures.

Diazepam

Diazepam is used for first-line control of seizures, usually in the paediatric accident and emergency department. In these situations, it is most commonly administered rectally. In a paediatric intensive care unit, diazepam is usually administered intravenously in the form of Diazemuls®, an emulsion preparation, as the injection causes thrombophlebitis. See p. 409.

Phenytoin

Phenytoin is given routinely to control status epilepticus. A loading dose must be given to achieve therapeutic plasma concentrations. Subsequent doses are administered twice a day to maintain the desired plasma levels. Phenytoin

metabolism varies greatly between individuals but tends to be faster in infants and children than in adults. Phenytoin has a narrow therapeutic range above which unwanted effects are seen. These include: ataxia, nystagmus, tremor, dysarthria, sedation and paradoxical increased seizures. Phenytoin is metabolised by the liver and is highly (90%) protein bound. In uraemia phenytoin is displaced from its plasma protein-binding sites, increasing the percentage of unbound, active drug and lowering the therapeutic range. For these reasons phenytoin must be used in caution in hepatic and renal failure.

Phenytoin injection is very unstable. It should only be diluted to accurately administer a small dose. When dilution is necessary, 0.9% sodium chloride is used. The diluted injection must be checked for precipitate before it is administered. Administration of the injection can be painful because it is highly alkaline (pH 12) and has the potential to cause thrombophlebitis. It should be administered slowly to avoid cardiac arrhythmias.

Phenytoin induces liver enzymes, which increase the rate of metabolism of drugs (such as warfarin and other antiepileptics) that are inactivated in the liver, significantly reducing their effectiveness unless their doses are increased proportionately.

Clonazepam

Clonazepam is most often used as an infusion. The main side effects of clonazepam are impaired swallowing and respiratory depression. Salivary and bronchial hypersecretion also occur, which increases the need for suction.

Each ampoule of clonazepam must be diluted with at least its accompanying ampoule of diluent before administration. This is necessary because clonazepam injection is not stable. Clonazepam adsorbs onto plastic giving sets, and the infusion should be changed every 12 h.

Chlormethiazole

When a clonazepam infusion does not control the seizures, an intravenous infusion of chlormethiazole is initiated. Chlormethiazole enhances the effects of GABA transmission by blocking the picrotoxin site on the GABA receptor.

Chlormethiazole is available as a ready diluted injection which is unstable at room temperature and so must be stored in the refrigerator. The infusion rate should be titrated according to the child's response. Once the seizures are controlled, the rate should be reduced gradually every 4–6 h.

Chlormethiazole can cause hypotension and respiratory depression which become more pronounced when intravenous therapy is continued for more than 12 h. Intravenous infusions of chlormethiazole cause a tingling sensation in the nose which may be accompanied by sneezing, itchy eyes and bronchorrhoea. The infusion interacts with PVC giving sets increasing the risk of thrombophlebitis and altering the drop size, making administration with a burette inaccurate. The giving set must be checked regularly to ensure no softening of the tubing has occurred. This becomes more significant when the infusion rate is low. The giving set must be changed at least every 24 h.

Thiopentone sodium

Thiopentone sodium is an intravenous anaesthetic which is administered at a rate of 1–8 mg/kg/h after an initial loading dose of 4–8 mg/kg. It is used when other drugs have been unsuccessful at controlling seizures. The injection is alkaline (pH 10.5) and therefore irritant. Thiopentone produces a rapid clinical effect because of its high fat-solubility. Thiopentone distributes to the brain and then into the tissues, which act as a reserve from which redistribution back into the blood can occur.

Thiopentone has serious adverse effects which include hypothermia and cerebral shut-down which are more likely to occur when the infusion rate is above 5 mg/kg/h. Recovery of consciousness may be extremely delayed if the infusion is continued for more than 48 h. Thiopentone is metabolised by the liver to pentobarbitone which is also active. Long-term anaesthesia should be monitored by maintaining a maximum thiopentone plasma concentration of between 60 and 100 mg/L (O'Brien 1990).

ANTIINFECTIVE AGENTS
Encephalitis of unknown origin

When a child presents with decreased cerebral function, such as alteration in consciousness, seizures or changes in personality, it is vital to treat them with anti-infective agents that cover all probable infective pathogens as quickly as possible. Once the causative pathogen is known, treatment is altered according to the reported sensitivities.

Antiviral agents

Aciclovir

Aciclovir inhibits the replication of viral DNA. Doses are calculated using body weight except between the ages of 3 months and 12 years, when dosage is based on body surface area. The use of body surface area stops gross miscalculation for the fat or chubby child. Aciclovir does not penetrate fat. It is excreted renally, and dosing intervals must be adjusted according to the child's corrected glomerular filtration rate (GFR).

Aciclovir injection is extremely irritant, with pH 11. It must be diluted to a concentration of not more than 5 mg/mL with 0.9% sodium chloride or 4% glucose/0.18% sodium chloride before being administered peripherally over at least 1 h. The intravenous course of aciclovir should be continued for 10 days (Whitley et al 1986, Skoldenberg et al 1984) and then reviewed according to the condition of the child.

Antibacterial agents

The bacterium most likely to cause meningitis varies depending upon the age of the child. In neonates *Group B streptococcus*, *Enterobacter* and *Listeria* are common pathogens. However, in infants and older children, *Meningococci*, *H. influenzae* and *S. pneumoniae* are the commonest organisms found.

Cefotaxime

Cefotaxime is a third-generation cephalosporin with activity against both Gram-positive and Gram-negative bacteria. Cephalosporins are bactericidal and act by inhibiting bacteria cell wall synthesis.

Cefotaxime penetrates the meninges and is active against *H. influenzae, N. meningitidis, S. pneumoniae, E. Coli, Klebsiella, Enterobacter* and *Proteus*. Large doses (150–200 mg/kg/day in 2–4 divided doses) must be used initially to ensure effective penetration into the cerebrospinal fluid. These should be continued throughout therapy, as penetration decreases as the meninges become less inflamed and therefore less permeable. Cefotaxime is metabolised by the liver and excreted by the kidneys. Dosage reduction is only required when the GFR falls below 5 mL/min. Cefotaxime does not penetrate the nasal mucosa. Therefore rifampicin is given orally for at least 2 days before hospital discharge to eradicate *H. influenzae* and *N. meningitidis* from the nasal mucosa (Committee on Infectious Diseases et al 1996).

Ceftriaxone

Ceftriaxone has the same spectrum of activity as cefotaxime but has a longer half life. It also eradicates *H. influenzae* and *N. meningitidis* from the nasal mucosa, thereby minimising the risk of passing on the infection. Ceftriaxone is licensed to be given once every 24 h for the treatment of meningitis, although early studies used 12-hourly dosing regimens. This may be of advantage when intravenous access is limited. Ceftriaxone can be reconstituted with lignocaine and administered intramuscularly if intravenous access is not possible.

Erythromycin

Erythromycin is added to cover atypical bacteria such as *Mycoplasma pneumoniae*. Erythromycin is bacteriostatic and acts by inhibiting bacterial protein synthesis.

The injection has a neutral pH of 6.5–7.5, but is extremely irritant. When given peripherally it must be diluted to at least 5 mg/mL with 0.9% sodium chloride and administered over 20–60 min. Erythromycin is incompatible with 5% glucose unless it is buffered with sodium bicarbonate.

Erythromycin can inhibit the metabolism of some drugs in the liver. These include warfarin and theophylline. This reaction can produce a significant clinical effect within 1 or 2 days of initiation of erythromycin therapy (Hansten & Horn 1997).

Ampicillin and amoxycillin

Both ampicillin and amoxycillin are bactericidal and act by inhibiting bacterial cell wall synthesis. They are active against *Listeria* and *Streptococci*. They are excreted in the urine, and the time interval between doses must be increased when renal function is impaired.

DRUGS ACTING ON THE GASTROINTESTINAL TRACT

Protection of the gastrointestinal tract

Children in intensive care are susceptible to stress and infection. This can be manifested in the gastrointestinal tract as stress ulceration or an increase in Gram-negative infections. In healthy children the integrity of the gastric mucosa is maintained by a fine balance between aggressive factors (hydrogen ions, pepsin, bile acids) and protective mechanisms (bicarbonate ions, mucus, cell regeneration, mucosal blood flow). Sucralfate, H_2-antagonists and antacids have all been used in an attempt to protect the gastrointestinal tract in intensive care patients.

Studies in adult patients have shown that, contrary to popular belief, most intensive-care patients produce less gastric acid and pepsin than healthy volunteers. Thus it seems that the body's protective mechanisms are less efficient in a stressful environment, as opposed to there being an increase in aggressive factors.

Sucralfate

Sucralfate is administered to sedated children, via a nasogastric tube, to protect the gastric mucosa from stress ulceration and its associated bleeding. Sucralfate becomes a paste in acid conditions, which binds to the mucosa, protecting it from attack by natural gastrointestinal acid secretions. It also promotes the release of prostaglandin, which increases mucosal blood flow and stimulates mucus and bicarbonate secretion. Sucralfate binds pepsin and bile salts, further protecting the gastric mucosa from aggressive factors.

Sucralfate is an aluminium salt of sucrose octasulphate. It should be used with caution in renal failure because aluminium is excreted renally. The absorption of some drugs from the stomach and duodenum is decreased by sucralfate. They should be administered at least 2 h before or after a dose of sucralfate.

Ranitidine

Ranitidine is an H_2-antagonist which blocks histamine-associated release of acid by parietal cells in the stomach. Ranitidine is used in preference to cimetidine because, at present, it appears to have a better side effect profile. Cimetidine blocks the P_{450} enzyme system, which causes significant drug interactions by reducing the rate of metabolism of drugs such as warfarin, amiodarone, phenytoin and theophylline which rely on this system for inactivation.

Ranitidine is administered as a slow intravenous bolus over at least 2–5 min. Before administration it must be diluted with 0.9% sodium chloride. Ranitidine is excreted by the kidneys; therefore doses must be reduced in renal failure.

Sucralfate or H_2-antagonist?

Sucralfate is as effective as H_2-antagonists at reducing the risk of stress bleeding in adults. H_2-antagonists and antacids both reduce the stomach pH, increasing the risk of bacterial colonisation of the stomach. When the pH of the stomach contents rises above 4, Gram-negative bacteria predominate.

Sucralfate does not alter the stomach pH, and therefore bacterial colonisation is significantly lower compared with the less acid environment created using H_2-antagonists. Colonisation tends to be with oropharyngeal flora rather than Gram-negative bacteria.

The stomach contents of intubated children can be aspirated into their respiratory tract. Therefore the risk of pulmonary infection in ventilated children is directly related to the colonisation of the stomach with bacteria. Sucralfate is recommended for the prophylaxis of stress ulceration bleeding because it reduces the incidence of Gram-negative infection in ventilated children compared with H_2-antagonists (Driks et al 1987).

Gut sterilisation

Some centres advocate sterilising the gut in ventilated children to minimise the risk of bacterial infection originating from the gut. These regimens have included:

- amphotericin for the eradication of fungi
- colistin for the eradication of Gram-negative bacteria, especially *Pseudomonas*
- tobramycin for the eradication of Gram-negative organisms.

REFERENCES

Adams D 1994 Administration of drugs through a jejunostomy tube. British Journal of Intensive Care Jan:10–17

British Medical Association 1999 British national formulary. London: BMA and Royal Pharmaceutical Society of Great Britain, London

Committee on Infectious Diseases, American Academy of Pediatrics, Infectious Diseases and Immunization

Committee, Canadian Paediatric Society 1996 Meningococcal disease prevention and control strategies for practice-based physicians. Pediatrics 97(3):404–411

Committee on the Safety of Medicines 1991 Genotoxicity of papaveretum and noscapine. Current Problems 31

Committee on the Safety of Medicines 1992a Serious adverse effects and fatalities in children associated with the use of propofol for sedation. Current Problems 32

Committee on the Safety of Medicines 1992b Propofol and delayed convulsions. Current Problems 35

Dade J, Ashley C 1996 Renal replacement therapy and the pharmacist. In: Ayers S, Magee P (eds) The beginners' guide to renal pharmacy. UK Renal Pharmacy Group.

Donn S M 1994 Alternatives to ECMO. Archives of Disease in Childhood 70:F81–83

Driks M R, Cranen D E, Gelli B, et al 1987 Nosocomial pneumonia in intubated patients given sucralfate as compared with antacids or histamine type 2 blockers. New England Journal of Medicine 317:1376–1382

Hastreiter A R, van der Horst R L, Voda C, Chow-Tung E 1985 Maintenance digoxin dosage and steady-state plasma concentration in infants and children. Journal of Pediatrics 107:140–146

Hansten P D, Horn J R (eds) 1997 Drug interactions analysis and management. Applied Therapeutics, Vancouver, p 513

Haycock G B 1994 Steroid responsive nephrotic syndrome. In: Postlethwaite R J (ed) Clinical paediatric nephrology, 2nd edn. Butterworth Heinemann, London

Heimburger D 1990 Diarrhoea with enteral feeding; will the real cause please stand up? American Journal of Medicine 88:89–90

Hoie E B, Hall M C, Schaaf L J 1993 Effects of injection site and flow rate on the distribution of injected solutions in an extracorporeal membrane oxygenation circuit. American Journal of Hospital Pharmacy 50:1902–1906

Miller S, Strom J 1988 Stability of phenytoin in three enteral nutrient formulas. American Journal of Hospital Pharmacy 45:2529–2532

O'Brien M D 1990 Management of major status epilepticus in adults. British Medical Journal 301:918

Pearce G 1988 Apparent inhibition of phenytoin absorption by an enteral nutrient formula. Australian Journal of Hospital Pharmacy 18:289–292

Schwarz G J, Brion L P, Spizer A 1987 The use of plasma creatinine concentration for estimating glomerular filtration rate in infants, children and adolescents. Pediatric Clinics of North America 34:571–590

Skoldenberg B, Forsgren M, Alistig K, et al 1984 Acyclovir versus vidarabine in herpes simplex encephalitis. The Lancet ii:707–711

Stewart C F, Hampton E M 1987 Effect of maturation on drug disposition in pediatric patients. Clinical Pharmacy 6:548–562

Wheeler A P 1993 Sedation, analgesia, and paralysis in the intensive care unit. Chest 104(2):566–576

Whitley R J, Alford C A, Hirsch M S, et al 1986 Vidarabine versus acyclovir therapy in herpes simplex encephalitis. New England Journal of Medicine 314:144–149

INDEX